TECHNOLOGY AND MEDICAL SCIENCES – TMS*i* 2010

PROCEEDINGS OF THE 6TH INTERNATIONAL CONFERENCE ON TECHNOLOGY AND MEDICAL SCIENCES – TMS*i* 2010, PORTO, PORTUGAL, 21–23 OCTOBER 2010

Technology and Medical Sciences – TMS*i* 2010

Editors

R.M. Natal Jorge & João Manuel R.S. Tavares
Faculdade de Engenharia da Universidade do Porto, Porto, Portugal

Marcos Pinotti Barbosa
Universidade Federal de Minas Gerais, Brasil

Alan Peter Slade
University of Dundee, Dundee, Scotland

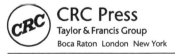
CRC Press
Taylor & Francis Group
Boca Raton London New York

CRC Press is an imprint of the
Taylor & Francis Group, an **informa** business

A BALKEMA BOOK

First issued in paperback 2018

CRC Press/Balkema is an imprint of the Taylor & Francis Group, an informa business

© 2011 Taylor & Francis Group, London, UK

Typeset by Vikatan Publishing Solutions (P) Ltd., Chennai, India

Published by: CRC Press/Balkema
          P.O. Box 447, 2300 AK Leiden, The Netherlands
          e-mail: Pub.NL@taylorandfrancis.com
          www.crcpress.com – www.taylorandfrancis.co.uk – www.balkema.nl

ISBN 13: 978-1-138-11289-6 (pbk)
ISBN 13: 978-0-415-66822-4 (hbk)

Technology and Medical Sciences – Natal Jorge et al. (eds)
© 2011 Taylor & Francis Group, London, ISBN 978-0-415-66822-4

Table of contents

Preface	xi
Acknowledgements	xiii

Full papers

Modelling, designing and simulating living systems with BlenX *P. Lecca*	3
Measurement system of the eye vergence and accommodation with 3D hologram stimulation *J. Dušek, T. Jindra & M. Dostálek*	15
3D modelling for FEM simulation of an obese foot *V.C. Pinto, N.V. Ramos, M.A.P. Vaz & M.A. Marques*	19
A breast modelling application for surgeons *A. Cardoso, H. Costa, V. Sá & G. Smirnov*	23
A framework model for e-Health services *M. Macedo & P. Isaías*	29
A possibility for pos-EVAR surveillance: A novel smart stent-graft *I.C.T. Santos, J.M.R.S. Tavares, L.A. Rocha, S.M. Sampaio & R. Roncon-Albuquerque*	35
Analysis of the contraction of the pelvic floor through the finite element method considering different pathologies *T.H. da Roza, M.P.L. Parente, R.M. Natal Jorge, T. Mascarenhas, J. Loureiro & S. Duarte*	39
Anticipatory postural adjustments in post-stroke subjects during reaching *S. Ferreira, C. Silva, P. Carvalho, A. Silva & R. Santos*	43
Approaches to juxta-pleural nodule detection in CT images *A. Massafra*	51
Blood flow in artificial bypass graft: A numerical study *L.C. Sousa, C.F. Castro, C.C. António & B. Relvas*	57
Calibration of free hand ultrasound probe tracked by optical system *K. Krysztoforski, R. Będziński, E. Świątek-Najwer & P. Krowicki*	63
Contact finite element with surface tension adhesion *R.A.P. Hellmuth & R.G. Lima*	69
Crystalline lens imaging with a slit-scanning system *C. Oliveira, J.B. Almeida & S. Franco*	79
Design of Medical Rehabilitation Devices: A case study *E. Seabra, L.F. Silva, P. Flores & M. Lima*	83
Development of a flexible pressure sensor for measurement of endotension *I.C.T. Santos, J.M.R.S. Tavares, A.T. Sepúlveda, A.J. Pontes, J.C. Viana & L.A. Rocha*	89
Development of an adaptable system for a stationary bike to convert mechanical energy into electric power applied in indoor cyclism training *J.B. Soldati, Jr., L.A. Szmuchrowski, D.N. Rocha, F.L. Corrêa, Jr., T.S.P. Sono, C.B.S. Vimieiro & M. Pinotti*	95

Development of computational model to analyze the influence
of fiber direction in the Tympanic Membrane   101
C. Garbe, F. Gentil, M.P.L. Parente, P. Martins, A.J.M. Ferreira & R.M. Natal Jorge

Electronic device for temperature monitoring during the decompression
surgery of the facial nerve   107
S.S.R.F. Rosa, M.L. Altoé, L.S. Santos, C.P. Silva & M.V.G. Morais

Ethical aspects in the design of medical devices   111
J. Ferreira, F. Soares, J. Machado & M. Curado

Evaluation and implementation of technology in health care   115
R. Santos

Frequency domain validation of a tetrapolar bioimpedance spectroscopy
system with tissue equivalent circuit   119
A.S. Paterno, V.C. Vincence & P. Bertemes-Filho

Highly Focalized Thermotherapy: A minimally invasive technique
for the treatment of solid tumours   123
A. Portela, M. Vasconcelos & J. Cavalheiro

Identification of rib boundaries in chest X-ray images using elliptical models   129
L. Brás, A.M. Jorge, E.F. Gomes & R. Duarte

Improving diagnosis processes through multidimensional analysis in medical institutions   135
O. Belo

In vivo measurement of skeletal muscle impedance from rest to fatigue   143
*O.L. Silva, I.O. Hoffmann, J.C. Aya, S. Rodriguez, E.D.L.B. Camargo,
F.S. Moura, T.H.S. Sousa, R.G. Lima, A.R.C. Martins & D.T. Fantoni*

Influence on the mandible and on a condyle implant of the distribution
of the fixation surgical screws   147
A. Ramos, M. Mesnard, C. Relvas, A. Completo & J.A. Simões

Intensity inhomogeneity corrections in MRI simulated images for segmentation   151
R. Lavrador, L. Caldeira, N.F. Lori & F. Janela

Interactive collaboration for Virtual Reality systems related
to medical education and training   157
B.R.A. Sales, L.S. Machado & R.M. Moraes

Lissajous scanning pattern simulation, for development of a FLO   163
P. Nunes & P. Vieira

Measuring the pressure in a laryngoscope blade   169
A. Silva, J. Teixeira, P. Amorim, J. Gabriel, M. Quintas & R.M. Natal Jorge

Mechanical properties of temporalis muscle: A preliminary study   173
*V.L.A. Trindade, S. Santos, M.P.L. Parente, P. Martins, R.M. Natal Jorge,
A. Santos, L. Santos & J. Fernandes*

Medial-lateral CoP-rearfoot relation during stance   177
T.J.V. Atalaia & J.M.C.S. Abrantes

Multidisciplinary interactions for the development of medical devices   183
R. Simoes

Multi-objective optimization of bypass grafts in arteries   191
C.F. Castro, C.C. António & L.C. Sousa

Multiple Sclerosis subjects plantar pressure—A new tool for postural
instability diagnosis   197
L.F.F. Santos & J.M.C.S. Abrantes

Neurom: A motor treatment system for chronic stroke patients 205
F.L. Corrêa, Jr., R.C. de Araújo, D.N. Rocha, T.S.P. Sono, L.R. dos Santos,
A.M.V.N. Van Petten & M. Pinotti

Non-invasive diagnosis and monitoring of Cystic Fibrosis
by mass spectrometry of the exhaled breath 209
S. Gramacho, M. Piñeiro, A.A.C.C. Pais, A.M.d'A.R. Gonsalves, F. Gambôa & C.R. Cordeiro

Noninvasive assessment of Blood-Retinal Barrier function
by High-Definition Optical Coherence Tomography 215
T. Santos, R. Bernardes, A. Santos & J. Cunha-Vaz

OCT noise despeckling using a 3D nonlinear complex diffusion filter 221
C. Maduro, R. Bernardes, P. Serranho, T. Santos & J. Cunha-Vaz

Possible relations between female pelvic pathologies and soft tissue properties 227
P.A.L.S. Martins, R.M. Natal Jorge, A.L. Silva-Filho, A. Santos, L. Santos,
T. Mascarenhas & A.J.M. Ferreira

Processing and classification of biological images: Application to histology 233
B. Nunes, L.M. Rato, F.C. Silva, A. Rafael & A.S. Cabrita

Reducing and preventing drug interactions–An approach 239
R. Barros & F. Janela

Registration of bone ultrasound images to CT based 3D bone models 245
P.J.S. Gonçalves & P.M.B. Torres

Segmentation and 3D reconstruction of the vocal tract from MR images—A comparative study 251
S.R. Ventura, D.R. Freitas, I.M. Ramos & J.M.R.S. Tavares

Significance of fast and simple determination of catecholamines
and their metabolites in patients with Down syndrome 257
L.I.B. Silva, M.E. Pereira, A.C. Duarte, A.M. Gomes, M.M. Pintado, H. Pinheiro,
D. Moura, A.C. Freitas & T.A.P. Rocha-Santos

Study of pressure sensors placement using an Abdominal Aortic Aneurysm (AAA) model 261
L.A. Rocha, A. Sepulveda, A.J. Pontes, J.C. Viana, I.C.T. Santos & J.M.R.S. Tavares

Termographic assement of internal derangement of the temporomandibular joint 267
M. Clemente, A. Sousa, A. Silva, J. Gabriel & J.C. Pinho

The action of middle ear muscles using the finite element method 271
F. Gentil, C. Garbe, M. Parente, P. Martins & R.M. Natal Jorge

The contribution of the scapular patterns to the amplitude of shoulder external
rotation on thrower athletes 275
A.M. Ribeiro & A.G. Pascoal

Influence of an unstable shoe on compensatory postural adjustments 279
A.S.P. Sousa, R. Macedo, R. Santos & J.M.R.S. Tavares

The use of muscle recruitment algorithms to better assess problems
for children with gait deficiency 285
M. Voinescu, D.P. Soares, M.P. Castro, A.T. Marques & R.M. Natal Jorge

Using an Infra-red sensor to measure the dynamic behaviour
of N_2O gas escaping through different sized holes 289
A.P. Slade, D. Convales, J. Vorstius & G. Thomson

Visual tracking of surgical instruments, application to laparoscopy 293
P.J.S. Gonçalves & A.M.D. Gonçalves

Wavelet analysis of the pupil's autonomic flow 297
G. Leal, P. Vieira & C. Neves

White matter segmentation in simulated MRI images using the Channeler Ant Model   301
E. Fiorina

Abstracts

In-silico models as a tool for the design of medical device technologies   307
J.M. García-Aznar, M.A. Pérez, M.J. Gómez-Benito, J.A. Sanz-Herrera & E. Reina-Romo

3D biomechanical model of the human hand using FEM   309
D.N. Rocha, R.M. Natal Jorge & M. Pinotti

Using radiobiology simulators for evaluation of ^{99m}Tc Auger electrons
for targeted tumor radiotherapy   311
A.A.S. Tavares & J.M.R.S. Tavares

Therapeutic contact lenses obtained by SCF-assisted imprinting processes:
Improved drug loading/release capacity   313
*M.E.M. Braga, M.H. Gil, H.C. de Sousa, F. Yañez, C. Alvarez-Lorenzo,
A. Concheiro & C.M.M. Duarte*

Supercritical solvent impregnation of natural bioactive compounds in *N*-carboxybutyl chitosan
membranes for the development of topical wound healing applications   315
A.M.A. Dias, I.J. Seabra, M.E.M. Braga, M.H. Gil & H.C. de Sousa

Potential and suitability of Ion Mobility Spectrometry (IMS) for breath analysis   317
V. Vassilenko, A.M. Bragança, V. Ruzsanyi & S. Sielemann

Phosphonium-based ionic liquids as new *Greener* plasticizers
for poly(vinyl chloride) biomedical applications   319
*S. Marceneiro, A.M.A. Dias, J.F.J. Coelho, A.G.M. Ferreira, P.N. Simões, M.E.M. Braga,
H.C. de Sousa, C.M.M. Duarte, I.M. Marrucho, J.M.S.S. Esperança & L.P.N. Rebelo*

New approach to bone surface reconstruction from 2.5D sonographic dataset   321
P. Krowicki, K. Krysztoforski, E. Świątek-Najwer & R. Będziński

Metal-Organic Framework as potential drug carriers against inflammation   325
I.B.V. Santos, T.G. da Silva & S. Alves, Jr.

Knowledge based system for medical applications   327
C.S. Moura, P.J. Bártolo & H.A. Almeida

In vitro method for test and measure the accuracy of implant impression   329
F.J. Caramelo, P. Brito, J. Santos, A. Carvalho, G. Veiga, B. Vasconcelos, J.N. Pires & M.F. Botelho

Improving the resolution of scintigraphic images with super-resolution:
Development of a dedicated device   333
R. Oliveira, F.J. Caramelo & N.C. Ferreira

Hyperbolic surfaces for scaffold design   337
H.A. Almeida & P.J. Bártolo

Finite element analysis of a three layered cartilage   339
D.M. Freitas, P.J. Bártolo & H.A. Almeida

External breast radiotherapy treatment planning verification
using advanced anthropomorphic phantoms   341
J.A.M. Santos, J. Lencart, A.G. Dias, L.T. Cunha, C. Relvas, A. Ramos & V.F. Neto

Blood Volume Pulse peak detector with a double adaptive threshold   345
J. Medeiros, R. Martins, S. Palma, H. Gamboa & M. Reis

Bilateral study on arterial stiffness assessment by a non-invasive optical
technique of Photoplethysmography   349
V. Vassilenko, A.C. Silva, A.M. Martin & J.G. O'Neill

A biomimetic strategy to prepare silica- and silica/biopolymer-based
composites for biomedical applications   351
R.B. Chim, M.E.M. Braga, M.M. Figueiredo, H.C. de Sousa, C.R. Ziegler & J.J. Watkins

Non-invasive biomonitoring of human health: Technical developments in breath analysis   353
V. Vassilenko

Author index   355

Technology and Medical Sciences – Natal Jorge et al. (eds)
© 2011 Taylor & Francis Group, London, ISBN 978-0-415-66822-4

Preface

The International Conference on Technology and Medical Sciences – TMS*i* is a roving meeting, organized every two years since 2000 alternating between cities in Brazil and Europe, devoted to be an open and multidisciplinary discussion forum on novel concepts, new developments and innovations relating to Technology and Medical Sciences in order to solidify knowledge in these fields and define their key stakeholders.

This book contains keynote lectures and full papers presented at TMS*i* 2010, the 6th International Conference on Technology and Medical Sciences, which was held in Faculdade de Engenharia da Universidade do Porto (FEUP), Portugal, during the period 21–23 October 2010.

TMS*i* 2010 had 4 invited lectures, 57 oral presentations in ten sessions and 13 posters, representing contributions from 12 countries: Brazil, Cuba, Czech Republic, France, Italy, Japan, Lithuania, Poland, Portugal, Romania, United Kingdom and the United States of America. The received contributions addressed many different topics, including Analysis and diagnosis, Applications in medicine, Bioengineering, Biomedical devices, Computational methods, Computer aided diagnosis, Computer assisted surgery, Imaging, Minimally invasive devices and techniques, Prosthesis and orthosis, Rehabilitation, Technical aids, Telemedicine and Virtual reality.

TMS*i* 2010 brought together researchers representing several scientific domains, including Biomechanics, Computational Vision, Computational Mechanics, Computer Graphics, Mathematics, Medicine, Robotics, Simulation and Statistics, that spanned a broad range of techniques and technologies.

The organizers of TMS*i* 2010 would like to take this opportunity to thank all the sponsors, members of the Scientific Committee, Invited Lecturers and the Authors for submitting and sharing their work.

R.M. Natal Jorge
João Manuel R.S. Tavares
Marcos Pinotti Barbosa
Alan Peter Slade

Acknowledgements

The organizers of the 6th International Conference on Technology and Medical Sciences – TMS*i* 2010 acknowledge the support towards the publication of this book and the organization of **TMS***i* 2010 by the following organizations:

- Faculdade de Engenharia da Universidade do Porto
- Fundação para a Ciência e a Tecnologia (FCT)
- Instituto de Engenharia Mecânica—Pólo FEUP (IDMEC-Polo FEUP)
- Instituto de Engenharia Mecânica e Gestão Industrial (INEGI)
- Associação Brasileira de Engenharia e Ciências Mecânicas (ABCM)
- Grupo Publindústria

Full papers

Technology and Medical Sciences – Natal Jorge et al. (eds)
© 2011 Taylor & Francis Group, London, ISBN 978-0-415-66822-4

Modelling, designing and simulating living systems with BlenX

P. Lecca
The Microsoft Research—University of Trento, Trento, Italy
Centre for Computational and Systems Biology, Povo, Trento, Italy

ABSTRACT: In the past, many scientists and philosophers have been inspired by the parallel between nature and human design, in mathematics and engineering. Today, the huge increase in biological knowledge, together with the developments in computer simulation modelling, and in design engineering systems, have made more comprehensive system-level studies of nature possible. The modern biological, medical, and pharmaceutical research approaches computing not only under the need of data mining and processing, but also under the need of using new languages for describing, designing and simulating biological entities and interactions. Although the techniques of the infinitesimal calculus have been recognized to provide valuable computational tools in simulating dynamic systems, they often do not offer the possibility to nimbly capture the intrinsic concurrency, causality, compositionality and probabilistic nature of biological interactions. This talk will present the BlenX language, that has been recently developed at CoSBi. BlenX is a programming language implementing the Beta-binders calculus. This calculus is a process algebra developed to model the time evolution of biological systems at any scale (from molecular to ecological systems). Namely, its syntactical and semantic structures have been specifically built to represent a biological entities and the network of its interactions with the other entities and components of a system. The richness and the level of abstraction of its syntax enable the modeler to describe through this calculus either the biochemical interactions between atom, molecules, functional complexes, cells, tissues at the micro- and meso-scale or the interactions and the relationships among the individuals of an ecological system. Some examples of application of BlenX to model living systems are given.

1 INTRODUCTION

In these years the experimental and the computational research approaches in the life sciences are abandoning the reductionist vision to adopt a system-level point of view. Unlike the reductionist approach, the framework of the systems theory proposes an integrative planning out to model complex biological phenomena. The integrative modelling is the main aspect of the systems biology. This emerging discipline describes the activity of biological entities, such as biochemical networks, cells, tissues, organs, and organisms, as the result of the properties and the mutual interactions of the single components of these systems. In particular, systems biology integrates the knowledge about structure and functions of the components of a systems obtained by the past reductionist investigation methodologies with the current knowledge about the dynamical processes concerning those components.

Systems of living entities are composed of several interacting elements. This implies that mathematical models can be designed at various observation and representation scales. The microscopic scale corresponds to model, by integro-differential equations the time evolution of the state of each single variable of the system. If the system is composed by a large number of elements it is possible to obtain suitable local in space averages of their state in an elementary space volume ideally tending to zero (Bellomo 2008). In this case the modelling can be developed at the macroscopic scale, which describes the time behavior of locally averaged quantities called *macroscopic variables*. Moreover, generally the modelling is deterministic. i.e., it follows deterministic causality principles: unless some external noise is added, once a cause is given, the effect is determined. The macroscopic modelling scale can still be applied when the number of system components is sufficiently large and a sufficiently small volume still contains enough elements to allow the averaging process mentioned above.

It is generally believed that understanding the properties and the time evolution of a system follow from a detailed knowledge of the state of each of its elements. Consider as an illustrative example a system composed by a certain number of particles (proteins, molecules, ions, functional complex, etc). At microscopic molecular level the states of the particles evolve according to the laws of classical mechanics that describes with a system of first order differential equations the time behavior of the position and velocity of each particle of the system. If the initial values position and velocity are known, the system of differential equations can be solved. and the macroscopic properties of the physical system can be obtained as averages involving the microscopic information contained in such a solution. However, it is very hard to implement such a program. Even in principle, it is impossible to predict the exact molecular population levels at some future time unless we know the exact positions and velocities of all the particles of the systems. D. Gillespie in (Gillespie 1977) points out that a reacting system of classical molecules is a deterministic process in the position-momentum phase space, but it is not a deterministic process in the multidimensional subspace of the species population numbers.

An alternative to the deterministic approach is the stochastic representation, where the state of the whole system is described by a suitable probability distribution function over the macroscopic state of the interacting system. In this article, we will focus on the discrete-space continuous-time stochastic modelling, because the living systems either at the molecular scale or at the ecological scale are composed by a discrete number of particles and individuals, respectively. At the molecular scale the adoption of stochastic representation is recommended when the number of molecules is small, whereas at the large scale typical of ecological systems it is recommended when the network of interactions among species is inherently affected by factors of random noise.

The deterministic and the stochastic essence of a natural process depends on the properties of the components of the system and on the physics of the characteristic interactions among them. For example, chemical reactions are due to random colisions between interacting particles. Another example: random motion of genetic particles imbues the cellular environment with intrinsic noise that frequently causes cell to cell variability and even significant phenotypic differences within a clonal cell population. Extending our glance to ecosystems, if population sizes are small, then models should be stochastic: the effects of fluctuations due of population size must be explicitly analyzed. Nowadays, stochastic models in ecology have begun to be systematically studied because of their relevance to biological conservation.

The difference between the deterministic and the stochastic nature of a biological or physical process requires also different modelling languages. In life science differential equations are appropriate for continuous time, continuous space modelling of systems composed by a large number of elements. The stochasticity manifests itself when the number of the system components is small and it is exalted when the system includes parallel and/or concurrent interactions. Biological processes often are stochastic, parallel and concurrent. Therefore, living systems require a descriptive approach substantially different from differential equations. It has to be able to represent parallelism and concurrency of the interactions, that at the microscopic scale derive from the multiple functionalities of the proteins and molecular functional complexes, whereas at the ecological scale are the engine of Darwinian selection.

In this article we first describe the BlenX language and then we present two time-continuous discrete stochastic models specified in BlenX language (Dematté et al. 2008b) and simulated with Beta WB simulator (Dematté et al. 2008a): (i) a model of ubiquitin-proteasome system, and (ii) a simple predatory-prey model. BlenX implements a stochastic process calculus explicitly developed to represent biochemical entities and their interactions at the micro- and meso-scale. BlenX is part of the software platform *CoS-BiLab*, on which our group is currently working and that implements a new conceptual modeling, analysis and simulation approach—primarily inspired by *algorithmic systems biology* (Priami 2009)—to biological processes. Algorithmic systems biology grounds on the belief that algorithms and computer-science formalisms—like processes calculi—can help not only in modelling well established knowledge but also in coherently extracting the key biological principles that underlie the experimental observations (Priami 2009).

The BlenX language offers to the modeler the possibility to address parallelism and concurrency of interactions, to express causality of the interactions, to represent multifunctionality of living entities. Moreover, BlenX formalisms is quantitative, interaction-driven, composable, scalable and modular, and thus able to represent not only the main static features of modularity and compositionality of a living system, but also the principal characteristic of its quantitative time evolution.

2 THE BLENX LANGUAGE

BlenX is a programming language implementing the Beta-binders calculus. here we provide a descriptive user-point-of-view introduction to the fundamental units, operators, and "actions" of this language. We refer the reader to (Dematté et al. 2008a, Dematté et al. 2008b, cos) for a detailed technical description of the language.

In computer science, the process calculi (or process algebras) are a diverse family of related approaches to formally modelling concurrent systems. Beta-binders in particular is an extension of the stochastic π-calculus (Priami 1995). Beta-binders calculus, as the other members of the family of process algebras, is based on the notion of *communication* described through a set of temporally ordered *actions*. The fundamental units of the calculus are the interlocutors of this communication, represented by *computational processes*. Just as in a conversation, the main actions that a computational process can take are sending and receiving messages. To denote a chain of events, the action prefix operator is used, which is written as an infix dot. For instance, a! . b? . P denotes a process that may offer action on a, then offers an action on b, and finally behaves as process P. a and b are the *channels* through which the communication take place. The behaviour of the process a!.b?.P consists of sending a signal over the channel a (a!) and waiting for a message over a channel b (b?). The processes can be composed in parallel. Parallel composition (denoted by the infix operator |, for instance P|Q) allows the description of processes which may run independently in parallel and also synchronize on *complementary actions* (by complementary action we mean a *send* and a *receive* over the same channel). Communication between processes is always binary and synchronous. The rep operator replicates copies of the process passed as argument. Only guarded replication is used, i.e. the process argument of this operator must be prefixed by an action that forbids any other action of the process untile the first action has been executed. In addiction to the parallel composition processes can be also composed through a *non deterministic choice,* indicated with the summation operator "+". The sum of processes P and Q, P + Q behaves either as P or as Q and selection of an alternative discards the other forever. To represent a deadlock situation, where the process is unable to perform any sort of action or co-action, the nil operator is used.

Beta-binders calculus adds to these simple syntactical elements *boxes*, also called *bio-processes*, that can be intuitively pictured as shapes encapsulating processes. Formally, the boxes are defined by unique identifiers that express the interaction capabilities of the processes encapsulated. These identifiers, called *binders* can be pictured as interaction sites put in charge of allowing the inter-boxes communication. Consider Fig. 1. A binder is a pair (x, A), written as x, A, where x is the name used by the internal process P to perform send/receive actions, while the binder identifier A, called *type*, expresses the interaction capabilities at the site x. The usefulness of the type of binder can be understood if we consider the interaction between boxes. The type A is a syntactical structure through which it is possible to quantitatively express the affinity

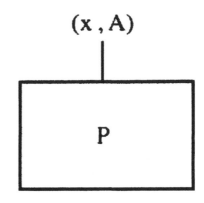

Figure 1. A pictorial view of a box. The sites of interaction are represented as binders on the box surface. In this figure, the box has only one binder identified by its name x and its type A, and an internal process P.

of the interaction between boxes. Two boxes are likely to interact if their interface contains binders whose types are affine, i.e. binders whose affinity if non null.

The BlenX language adds to the actions defined in the original Beta-binders calculus new actions that extend the possibilities to define and control the way in which a box evolves. The evolution of the interfaces of a box is driven by suitable actions that are defined by the processes inside the box. Such actions are named hide, unhide, ch (i.e. "change") and expose. These actions corresponds to the following transformation of the status of a binder: hide disables any communication through the binder, by hiding it from the tentatives of communication with binders of other boxes; unhide takes the opposit action: it enable communication through the binder, by undisclosing it to the view of other boxes; change changes the type of the binder; and expose adds a new binder to the box interface. The evolution of the processes inside a box that do not directly affects the interface can be defined by the following actions: send/receive action between processes (called *intra-communication*; and delay action that imposes a delay of a certain amount of time before the execution of subsequent actions.

The execution of the actions can be controlled with if-then statements, used to express conditions that need to be satisfied before executing the actions defined in the statement. Finally, a box can be eliminated from the system by executing the action die.

Boxes can interact in different ways: the can join (join is the action verb), they can form complexes, they can send/receive information each to other through dedicated binders (*inter-communication*, and a box can split in tow boxes (split is the

5

verb of this event). New boxes can be created (new is the corresponding action verb), boxes can be eliminated (delete is the action verb). join, split, new, delete are verbs of *events*. An event is the composition of a condition and an action verb. namely, events are used to express actions that are enabled by global conditions.

Boxes can be interpreted as biological entities, i.e. components that interact in a model to accomplish some biological function: proteins, enzymes, organic or inorganic compounds as well as cells or tissues. Binders of boxes are models of molecules interaction sites, protein sensing and effecting domains. The biochemical interactions between the biological entities are abstracted as communications between boxes and join events, whereas conformational changes, allosteric reactions, and zero-th order degradation or production are established respectively by the processes inside the box, by split actions, by delete and new actions. Regard to conformational change and allosteric reaction, for instance, the internal structure of a box can codify for the mechanism that transforms an input signal into a protein conformational change, which can result in the activation or deactivation of another domain.

In order to obtain quantitative simulations of a BlenX model, a specific speed (or rate constant) is associated to each action. This attribute is a generalization of the rate constant of a biochemical interaction. The affinity between two binder types is a number that can quantify chemical affinity in a reaction, but also the degree of structural complementarity in key-lock reaction mechanisms. The magnitude The dynamics of a BlenX model is governed by the values of these rate constants and is stochastically defined an efficient adaptation of the Gillespie algorithm (Gillespie 1977). The physical basis of the algorithm is the collision of molecules within a reaction vessel. It is assumed that collisions are frequent, but collisions with the proper orientation and energy are infrequent. Therefore, all reactions within the Gillespie framework must involve at most two molecules. Reactions involving three molecules are assumed to be extremely rare and are modeled as a sequence of binary reactions. It is also assumed that the reaction environment is well mixed. The algorithm executes four main steps: 1. initialization of the number of molecules in the system, reactions constants, and random number generators; 2. (Monte Carlo step) generation of random numbers to sample from an uniform and an exponential probability density respectively the next reaction to occur as well as the time interval. The probability of a given reaction to be chosen is proportional to the number of substrate molecules. 3. Update: the time step is increased by the randomly generated time in step 2., and the molecule count is updated on the basis of the reaction that occurred. 4. Iteration: the algorithm execute all the steps from Step 1 unless the number of reactants is zero or the simulation time has been exceeded.

In order to enable the reader to catch the potentialities and teh essence of BlenX, we show in Fig. 2 the result of the execution of an inter-communication, that will be largely used in our models. The process inside the first box can receive a message on channel x, that is bound to an active binder of the box ((x:1, A)). The process inside the second box sends a message through the active binder ((x:1, A)) through the action y!(). The empty brackets in these actions mean that, in this model, there is no need to specify the object of communication. The exchange of information between the two box is permitted only if the binders involved in the communication are compatible, i.e., if their affinity is non null. Once the communication has occurred, their change of state if reflected by the modification of the internal processes: the execution of the inter-communication results in the "disappearance" of the channels x and y and with the exposure of the subsequent action, that in this example is simply the deadlock process.

In Fig. 3 a small model of the interaction between a nascent protein and a chaperone, and between mis-folded protein and proteasome.

A Nascent Protein (NP) is a box. Its interface is defined by two binders (y:1, P) and (prot:1, PTSP). The number 1 after the name of the binder indicate the value of th especific speed of the activity involving the binder. The internal structure is specified by the process in (1). This process expresses a non deterministic choice ("+") between the process y?(). ch(100,y,DR).hide(1,ubi).nil and

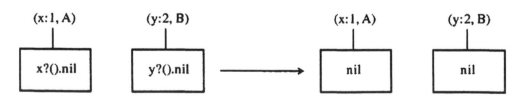

Figure 2.   Graphical representation of an inter-communcation.

6

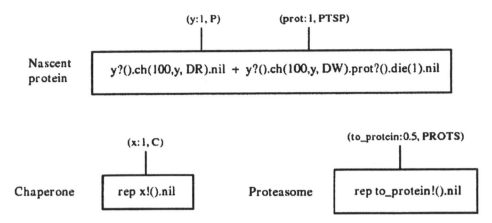

Figure 3. Pictorial scheme of a model of chaperone-protein interaction. The system includes a nascent protein, a molecular chaperone, and a proteasome. After the interaction with chaperone through the binders x and y, the protein can result correctly folded or misfolded. The type P of the protein binder changes to DR if the protein assumes the healthy 3D shape, whereas it changes to DW if it assumes the faulty shape. In the second case it is ready to undergo an interaction with the proteasome through the binders prot and to_protein. More details in the text.

process y?().ch(100,y,DW).prot?(). die(1).nil, Let call NP₁ the first process and NP₂ the second process. NP₁ can receive a message on channel y (y?()), then it can change—at a specific speed set to 100—the type of binder (y:1,P) into (y:1,DR) (ch(100,y,DR)), and finally it ends with a deadlock (nil), i.e. a process that can do nothing. NP₂ can receive a message on channel y (y?()), then it can change—at a specific speed set to 100—the type of binder (y:1,P) into (y:1,DW) (ch(100,y,DR)), then it can receive on channel prot (prot?()) and finally it can perform a die action that eliminate the box with a specific speed equal to 1 (die(1)).

y?().ch(100,y,DR).nil

+y?().ch(100,y,DW).prot?()
.die(1).nil   (1)

The chaperone is represented by a box with one binder, (x:1,C) and an internal process that replicates the sending action of channel x. Similarly, the proteasome is represented by a box with one binder, to_protein:0.5,PROT, and an internal process replicating the sending action on channel to_protein.

Since a nascent protein has to be sequestered by the chaperone to be folded, an interaction between box Nascent protein and Chaperone has to be enabled. The way to enable a possible interaction is to define a non null affinity between the binders (y:1,P) and (x:1,C). Given a non null affinities between the binder, an inter-communication thorough these binders on the complementary channels y and x is enabled.

In stochastic regime, according to the Gillespie algorithm (Gillespie 1977), the eventuality that the inter-communication involves process NP₁ or process NP₂ is quantitatively determined by the number of available chaperones, nascent proteins and the rates of interaction associated to channels x and y.

The non deterministic choice NP₁ + NP₂ reflect the possibility that the interaction between chaperone and misfolded protein through the binders (y:1,P) and (x:1,C) can result in a healthy protein or a faulty protein. In fact, after the inter-intercommunication is fired, a change action is enabled to change the type of (y:1,P) into (y:1,DR) to denote a right-folded protein *or* into (y:1,DW) to denoted a "wrong" protein. If the process NP₁ is stochastically selected for the inter-communication the interaction between chaperone and nascent protein ends in a healthy protein that does not undergo any further interaction with the other components of the system (the process terminates in a deadlock nil). If the process NP₂ is stochastically selected for the intercommunication the interaction between chaperone and nascent protein produces a faulty protein that is going to interact with the proteasome though the binders (prot:1,PTSP) and (to_protein:0.5, PROT) on the channels prot and to_protein, provided that in the model the affinity between (prot:1,PTSP) and (to_protein:0.5, PROT) has been defined non null. After this interaction has occurred the misfolded proteins is eliminated from the system with the execution pf a die action.

The internal behaviors of the chaperone and proteasome is defined by a replicated process,

Table 1. The BlenX model coding for the interaction between nascent protein and chaperone and between misfolded protein and proteasome. The system is defined as the parallel composition (||) of three boxes: `protein` (line 4), `chaperone` (line 8), and `proteasome` (line 11). The absolute simulation time is set to 100 (line 3), and the initial amounts of the model components is set to 1000 (lines 14–15–16).

```
1  // File: example.prog
2
3  [time = 100]
4  let protein: bproc =
6  #(y:1, P), #(prot:1, PTSP)
6  [y?().ch(100,y, DR).nil
7  + y?().ch(100,y, DW).prot?().die(1).
   nil];
8
8  let chaperone: bproc =
9  #(x:1, C) [rep x!().nil];
10
11 let proteasome: bproc =
11 #(to_protein:0.5, PROTS)
12 [rep to_protein!().nil];
13
14 run 1000 protein
15    || 1000 chaperone
16    || 1000 proteasome
```

Table 2. The binder definition file stores all the binders identifiers and the affinities between binders associated with a particular identifier.

```
1  // example.types
2
3  {P, PTSP, C, PROTS, DW, DR}
4  %%
5  {
6  (P,C,1),
7  (DW,C,1),
8  (PTSP, PROTS,10)
8  }
```

to express the fact that after the interaction with nascent protein and misfolded protein, respectively, they remain unaltered.

The BlenX code for this example is reported in Tables 1 and 2, that shows the program file and the files for the definition of binder types and affinities, respectively. The code in Table 2 says that couple of binders having non null affinities are (P,C), (DW,C), (PTSP,PROTS), and the value of their affinities are 1, 1, and 10, respectively.

A possible trajectory of the time evolution of the protein-chaperone-proteaseome system is sketched in Figs. 4 and 5. After the interaction with the chaper one, the nascent protein is still not correctly folded (the box represent the protein has changed (y,P) into (y,DW)) and undergoes an interaction with proteasome at the end of which the protein is degraded and is eliminated from the system (in the the BlenX code, its corresponding box dies and becomes the deadlock box).

3 THE UBIQUITIN-PROTEASOME SYSTEM

The ubiquitin-proteasome system is the major pathway that mediates the degradation of unwanted intracellular soluble proteins (i.e., mutant, misfolded, denatured, misplaced, or damaged) in the cytoplasm, nucleus, and endoplasmic reticulum of eukaryocytic cells. The process whereby the ubiquitin-proteasome system clears these unwanted proteins mainly involves two steps: (i) labeling of unwanted/damaged proteins with chains of activated ubiquitin molecules transported by parkin proteins; (ii) transport of ubiquitinated proteins to the proteasome by chaperone molecules (e.g., heat shock proteins).

Multiple molecules of ubiquitin, a small highly-conserved polypeptide, attached to the target protein, constitute the signal for proteasome attack. Mutant variants of α-synuclein protein can interfere with normal ubiquitin-proteasome system function, by inhibiting the signal transmitted by the ubiquitinated mis-foeld protein to protesome (Lang and Lozano 1998, Olanow and McNaught 2006, Vila and Przedborski 2004). The switch off of the signal sent by aberrant ubiquitinate proteins to the regulatory complex of proteasome causes proteolytic stress, protein accumulation and aggregation, and finally cell death.

Our BlenX model of the ubiquitin-protesome system consists of the parallel composition of seven boxes representing the nascent protein, the chaperone, that parkin and the ubiquitine (Fig. 6); the stress factor, the α-synuclein protein and the proteasome (Fig. 7).

The box of the nascent protein has three binders (y:1, P), (ubi:10, U), and (prot:1, PTSP) through which the communication with chaperone, ubiquitin and proteasome are respectively enabled. The process inside the nascent protein box is given by

```
y?().ch(100,y, DR).hide(1,ubi).nil
```

$$+y?().ch(100,y, DW).ubi?().prot?().die(1).nil \qquad (2)$$

where a non deterministic choice models the eventuality of a correctly folded protein or a faulty protein as a result of the interaction between chaperone and nascent protein. In the case in which the nascent protein is correctly shaped (i.e., the first term of the summation is selected the action `y!()` and `ch(100,y,DR)` are executed), the internal process first disables with a `hide` action any further communication through the binder (ubi:10,U), that is dedicated to the ubiquitylation's activities, and then terminates in a deadlock, meaning that

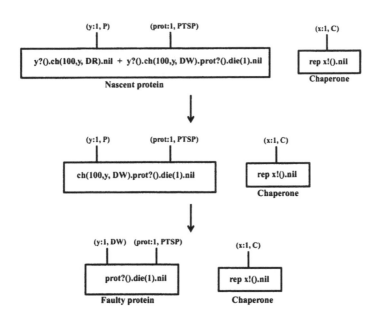

Figure 4. Inter-communication between nascent protein and chaperone represents the biochemical interaction between these two entities. In this figure a porssible trajectory of the system is shown: the intereaction results in a faulty protein.

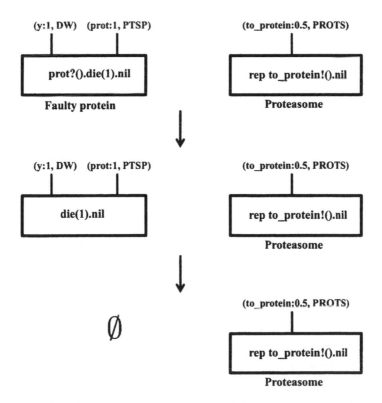

Figure 5. The faulty protein undergoes an inter-communcation with the proteasome and then it becomes the deadlock process, i.e., it degrades.

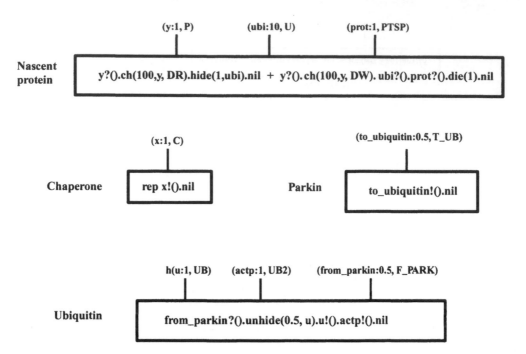

Figure 6. Sketch of the boxes representing nascent protein, molecular chaperone, parkin and ubiquitin molecules (see in the text the detailed description).

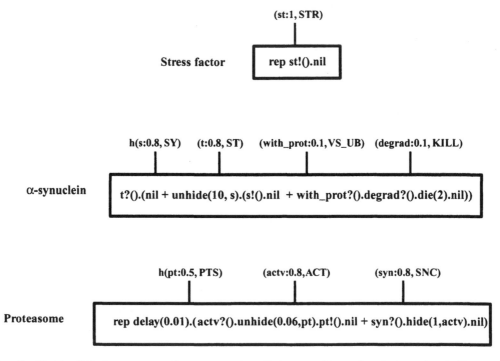

Figure 7. Sketch of the boxes representing enzymes stress factor, synuclein, and proteasome (see in the text the detailed description).

the correctly faulty protein does not perform any another reaction with the other component for the system. On the contrary, in the case in which the nascent protein did not assume the healthy shape, it is going to be ubiquitinated (i.e., it is willing to receive through channel ubi bound to the bidner (ubi:10,U)) and than degraded by the proteasome (i.e., if first communicates with the proteasome box thorugh prot?() and then "dies" (due to the execution of die(1).nil).

The parkin is represented as a box having a binder devoted to communicate with ubiquitin:(to_ubiquitin:0.5,T_UB). The internal process is a send action on the channel to_ubiquitin. The ubiquitin molecule is a box having three binders:(from_parkin:0.5, F_PARK),h(u:1,UB),and (actp:1,UB2) allowing communications with parkin, misfolded protein and proteasome, respectively. At the beginning the binder(u:1,UB) is hidden (an "h" prefixes the definition of the binder), and thus it is invisible to any another system's boxes.

The box representing the stress factor contains a replicated send action through the binder(st:1,STR). The α-synuclein box has four binders: h(s:0.8,SY), (t:0.8,ST), (with_prot:0.1,VS_UB), (degrad:0.1, KILL) for the communications with the proteasome, the stress factor, the ubiquitin, respectively.

As shown in Fig. 7, the protein α-synuclein first interacts with the stress factor through the binders (t:0.8,ST) and (st:1,STR), respectively. Then, since we assume also the possibility that this interaction does not change the protein, the internal process of the α-synuclein box can evolve also into a deadloack process. If the stress factor changes the structure of the α-synclein, the Fig. 7 discloses the binder h(s:0.8,SY) by performing an unhide action. Now, a second non deterministic choice is enabled. The first term of the sum describes the effective interaction of the mutant α-synclein and the proteasome through the binders (s:0.8,SY) and (syn:0.8,SNC), that results in the inactivation of the proteasome. Formally, this inactivation is described by the masking of binder (actv:0.8,SNC) performed by the execution of the action hide(1,actv). On the contrary, the second term of the sum describes first the activation of the proteasome by the mutant ubiquitinated α-synuclein (i.e., the communication through the binders (with_prot:0.1,VS_UB) and(actv:0.8,ACT), and its subsequent degradation realized by the executions of the inter-communication between binders degrad:0.1,KILL) and (pt:0.5,PTS) of α-synuclein and proteasome, respectively. At the end of this inter-communication, the action die in the internal process of α-synuclein is finally

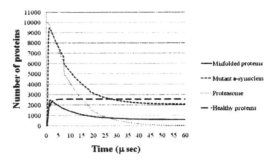

Model with mutant α-synuclein

Figure 8. Simulated time-behavior of the number of misfolded proteins, mutant α-synuclein, proteasomes and healthy proteins. Each curve is the average of 100 simulation runs.

enabled and determine the deletion of the box of mutant α-synuclein.

The Fig. 8 shows the time behavior of the number of misfolded proteins, healthy proteins, mutant variant of α-synuclein, and proteasomes. The values of the rate constants, and of the affinities of interaction producing these behavior are reported in the "pictorial" codes in Figs. 6–7. All the rates are expressed in units of μ sec ^{1}, that is the typical scale of α-synuclein folding (Ferreon et al. 2009). Their values are fictitious, but their orders of magnitude respect the typical temporal scale of the processes involved in ubiquitin-proteasome system functioning. The initial values for the numbers of molecules of the species have been chosen as follows: 5×10^3 nascent proteins, 10^4 molecules of parkin and ubiquitin, 10^4 proteasomes. They are fictitious values chosen used with the only purposes of experimenting *in silico* possible kinetics and dynamics of the systems. The number of bio-processes representing the stress factor has been varied over the range from 10 to 10^5 without obtaining significant changes in the dynamics. This number is an indicator of the intensity of the perturbation with which the stress factor causes the formation of aberrant molecules of α-synuclein. In Fig. 8 we can see that the number of mutant α-synuclein proteins has a fast linear growth within the first 5 μ sec, then it decreases and reach a stable value at 55 μ sec. Simultaneously, the number of available proteasomes decreases proportionally to the number of mutant α-synucleins and it vanishes as soon as the number of mutant α-synuclein becomes constant. The decrement of the number of α-synuclein proteins is due to the action of the protesomes that attack and degrade them. In particular, within the first 9 μ sec the curve of the number of proteasome and the one of mutant α-synuclein are superimposed, i.e. the decrement of these two species occur at the same rate. We see also that the number of faulty proteins experiences a rapid linear growth within the first 5 μ sec, then it slowly decreases and stabilizes as soon as the number of available proteasome is approximately zero (around 45 μ sec). This behavior correctly reflect the obvious impossibility of degrading faulty proteins if the systems does not have a sufficient number of available proteasomes. Finally, the simulations of our model show that the number of healthy proteins also linearly grows during the first 5 μ sec. Then, since these proteins are not involved in any other processes, their number remain constant for the rest of the time.

This model also includes a mechanism of production of free molecules of ubiquitin and parkin to guarantee the reactions of ubiquitination of the new formed nascent proteins, if the number of free ubiquitin and parkin molecules drops below a critical threshold, that does not allow the sustenance of the ubiquitation process. Free molecules of ubiquitin are returned to the systems as a consequence of possible unbinding reactions that break the complexes ubiquitin-parkin. The production of parkin and ubiquitin molecules is modeled in BlenX with events:

```
when(ubiquitin:|ubiquitin| = 0:inf)
          new(10000);
when(parkin:|parkin|=0:inf)
          new(10000);
```

and the eventuality that the complex ubiquitin-parkin breaks to free new molecules of ubiquitin and parkin is modeled by assigning a non-null value to the rate constant of unbinding reaction in the affinity definition for the complex ubiquitin-parkin (0.34 is the value of the rate constant of the unbinding reaction), as follows

```
(F_PARK,T_UB,0.7,0.34,1.2).
```

4 A PREDATOR-PREY MODEL

Here, the main parts of a simple predator/prey developed in collaboration with our student is presented (Livi 2009). The code is listed in Table 3. Teh reader is referred to (Livi 2009) for the complete model and the simulation results.

Table 3. Part of the BlenX predator-prey model.
```
1 // file: predator_prey.prog
2
3 let Transorca: bproc =
4  #(eat,transorca_hunts),#(dupl:0,A)
5 [ rep proc<<y,ptransorca>> ];
6
7 let ptransorca: pproc =
8   eat! ().y! ().nil
```

```
9   + eat!().ch(0.00005,dupl,
      duplication).nil
10 + die(inf).nil;
11
12 let Pinniped: bproc =
13  #(eat,hunts_pinni),#(food,pinni_
    lifes),
14     #(dupl:0,A)
15 [ repproc<<x,ppinni >> ];
16
17 let ppinni: pproc =
18   food! ().x! ().nil
19 + food!().ch(0.0043,dupl,
      duplication).nil
20 + eat?().die(inf)
21 + die(inf).nil;
22 ...
```

Consider a top-predator, for instance the transient orca. The predator is defined as a box with the communication channel eat and the additional duplication channel dupl.

Orca's eat channel is affine to the eat channel of the prey species to enable an inter-communication between prey and predator. The internal process ptransorca is composed of the three subprocesses linked by the non-deterministic choice operator + (see lines 8–9–10 in Table 3).

The process eat!() creates an inter-communication over the eat channel with the corresponding *eat* channel of the prey species when the predator "hunts" and "eats" the prey. Then, one instance of the prey pinniped disappears from the system. The eat-process has two possibilities to be executed, with two different successive behaviours: (i) eat!().ch(0.00005,dupl,duplication).nil. In this case the sequence of the processes is "eat" and then "reproduce". The change command ch changes the binder type A into the binder type dupl (with a propensity rate of 0.00005) which causes a split action. (ii) eat!().y!().nil. This second possibility is the sequence of the processes "eat" and then "go back to life". With the command rep the ptransorca process replicates a copy of itself and starts from the beginning, without changes in the interface or in the internal behaviour.

Finally, the death of the predator is modeled as at line 14 of Table 3. The third process and internal evolution is the abstraction for the death of the transient orca box, implemented as *die(inf).nil*.

Now, consider the prey species or intermediate species pinniped. Similarly to the predator, the prey is defined as a box with the communication channels eat, food and the additional duplication channel dupl. The food channel creates an inter-communication with the corresponding eat channel of another prey species (e.g. the salmon), or creates an inter-communication with the corresponding *food* channel of the food species (e.g. macroalges). After this communication, one instance of the hunted species disappears from the system. The addition of the specific replication rate, which is unique for every species is implemented identically as in the predator. The food-process has two possibilities to be executed, with two different results: the duplication of the box or "going on with life" without changes neither in interface nor in the internal processes. The death without being hunted is also implemented in the prey as in the predator. The *delay* command retards the execution of the *die* command, which causes the deletion of the box from the system.

5 CONCLUSIONS

As all the other sciences, computational systems biology makes progress in three different fields: (i) solution of new problems, (ii) elaboration of new methods, and (iii) development of new symbolisms. This article focused particularly on this last aspect and presents a language developed by the CoSBi team for modelling and simulating complex living systems. The language is born from the convergence of computer science and biology. Namely, the language spoken by biologists to describe the mechanisms of the dynamics of a biological pathway is similar to the formal languages spoken by computer scientists to describe the functioning of mobile communicating systems. Living systems and computational and communication systems of devices share many features, principally the parallelism and concurrency of the interactions driving the time evolution of these systems. We believe that taking this convergence far biology can benefit from the use of formal languages for the purposes of modeling, simulations and ultimately, understanding of living system dynamics. At the same time, computer science can be inspired by the way in which nature build complex systems and interaction networks.

ACKNOWLEDGEMENTS

The author would like to thank Corrado Priami and Ferenc Jordan of CoSBi for the inspiring discussions and useful suggestions, and Carmen M. Livi of University of Trento for having worked on the BlenX predator-prey model.

REFERENCES

Bellomo, N. (2008). *Modelling complex living systems. A kinetic theory and stochastic game approach.* Birkhaeuser.

Dematté, L., Priami, C. & Romanel, A. (2008a). The beta workbench: a computational tool to study the dynamics of biological systems. *Briefings in Bioinformatics* 9(5), 437–448.

Dematté, L., Priami, C. & Romanel, A. (2008b). The blenx language: A tutorial. *SFM 2008 LNCS 5016,* 313–365.

Ferreon, F.C.M., Gambin, Y., Lemke, E.A. & Deniz, A.A. (2009, April). Interplay of α-synuclein binding and confromational switching probed by single-molecule fluorescence. *PNAS 106,* 5645–5650.

Gillespie, D.T. (1977). Exact stochastic simulation of coupled chemical reactions. *The Journal of Physical Chemistry 81(25),* 2340–2361.

http://www.cosbi.eu/index.php/research/prototypes/overview

Lang, A.E. & Lozano, A.M. (1998). Parkinson's disease—first of two parts. *The New England Journal of Medicine 339(15),* 1044–1053.

Livi, C.M. (2009). Modelling and simulating ecological networks with blenx. the food web of prince william sound: a case study. Master's thesis, Alma Mater Studiorum—University of Bologna, Italy.

Olanow, C.W. & McNaught, K.S.P. (2006). Ubiquitin-proteasome system and parkinson's disease. *Movement Disorders 21(11),* 1806–1823.

Priami, C. (1995). Stochastic π-calculus. *The Computer Journal 38(6),* 578–589.

Priami, C. (2009). Algorithmic systems biology. *Communications of the ACM 52,* 80–88.

Vila, M. & Przedborski, S. (2004, July). Genetic clues to the pathogenesis of parkinson's disease. *Nature Medicine,* 58–62.

Technology and Medical Sciences – Natal Jorge et al. (eds)
© *2011 Taylor & Francis Group, London, ISBN 978-0-415-66822-4*

Measurement system of the eye vergence and accommodation with 3D hologram stimulation

J. Dušek & T. Jindra
Institute of Biophysics and Informatics, First Faculty of Medicine, Charles University, Prague, Czech Republic

M. Dostálek
Centre for Functional Disorders of Vision, Litomysl's Hospital, Litomysl, Czech Republic

ABSTRACT: We deal with strabismus measurements. Our system is designed for noninvasive simultaneous measurement of eye vergence and accommodation dynamics in infants. Co-ordination of these two phenomenons is fundamental for the motoric component of single binocular vision. Disturbances of the convergence-accommodation synkinesis are related to strabismus. As it is important to start diagnostics and consequent treatment early because the rise of treatment success, it is considerable to design the system convenient to youngest children as well as easy and fast for personnel.

Keywords: Hirschberg principle, excentric photorefraction, simultaneous recording, accommodation, vergence, image analysis, applied holography

1 INTRODUCTION

Binocular function's disturbances are the most frequent eye disorder in childhood. Standard binocular function's investigation assess sensoric (Landolt, Pfluger, Snellen optotypes, Bagolini test, Wort test, synoptophore etc.) and motoric parametres (Hess screen, Weiss screen, Cover test, NPC, etc.) in isolation and statically. Simultaneous and dynamic measurements are not commonly available in clinical practice. There is not any quick and easy proved routine clinical methodology for dynamic measurement synkinesis between vergence and accommodation.

2 METHODS

Our measuring system is designed especially for infants. The near reaction is used as a standardized stimulus for accommodation-vergence reaction. The two fixation pictures (farand near) are generated by two holograms in one holographic plane. These holograms are stimulated by divergent laser beam. Holograms have interesting feature in their characteristic geometric layout of stimuling sources. To one reconstructed picture correspondsone position of one laser. It enables to display different pictures only by switching between laser sources in different position. Next interesting feature of holograms is registration of real distance between scanned object and holographic plate during recording hologram. During reconstruction displayed picture is in the same virtual distance as it was during the recording of hologram. The implementation of hologram allows us to decrease the size of the whole system. For the stimulation of eyes is far fixation pointin the distance 2–3 m and near fixation point is in 0.25 m. Application of this system with real optical distances in clinical practice would be spacious and is not suitable for common use. Using virtual space pictures recorded on one holographic plate can be whole system built in a small box that is suitable for clinical practice. On the Fig. 1 and Fig. 2 are displayed reconstruceted far and near fixation pictures recorded in 2 m and 0.25 m.

Patient is placed behind holographic plate and is forced to change vergence and accommodation by consequent switching on this two 3D fixation images. For dynamic refraction measurement is used near infrared eccentric video-refraction [3]. Source of near infrared (NIR) beam (Fig. 3) is designed as array (25 × 5 mm) of four NIR light emitting diodes (λ = 850 nm, 80 m W/30°) placed near optical axis of camera's lens (with respecting of the eccentric photo-refraction conditions).

Measuring infrared light beam passes through optical system of eye to retina. 2% of light is reflected and passes back. Eccentric shield placed

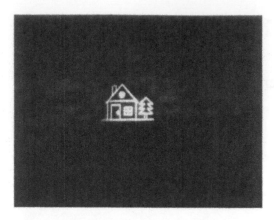

Figure 1. Far fixation picture 2 m.

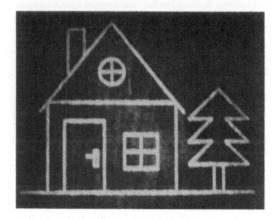

Figure 2. Near fixation picture 0,25 m.

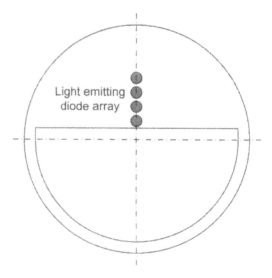

Figure 3. Eccentric shield with array light source.

behind objective remove part of modified beam and adjust resulting image. The steepness of the luminance profile in pupil (recorded by camera) is equivalent to refractive state of eye (accommodation). For determination of vergence the Hirschberg's principle is implemented. This method detects relative distance between the 1st Purkinje image and the center of pupil that is equivalent to vergence position. The near infrared light source is used as the measuring light due to its invisibility for humanvision system and do not evoke physiological miosis. Dynamic reactions of both eyes during the standardized near reaction stimulation are recorded by high-speed (372 fps) NIR camera in 640 × 240 pixel resolution. Light power reflected by eye's layer is about 2% of power emitted by NIR light source. Therefore high sensitivity of camera and right eliminating of visible light is important for capturing high—quality image. Obtained image sequences will be used for future image analysis. The above described methodology of image analysis [1] is used for simultaneous measurement of accommodation (vertical average luminance profile of retinal reflex) and vergence (distance between 1st Purkinje image and pupil's centre measured in average horizontal luminance profile).

3 RESULTS

The scheme of designed optical measurement system is presented in Fig. 4.

Whole system is placed in dark box inlaid with light absorbing tissue towards eliminating danger parasite reflections of laser beam. Divergent laser beam reconstruct image corresponding with source position. Fixation image reflected by dichroic mirror is displayed to patient. The mirror has character of cold mirror. Visible beam is reflected and infrared beam passes through. Mirror also eliminates undesired visible light coming from outer space of the box around patient's head. In front of the camera's lens, the there is bi-prims. It is located in the optical trajectory of backward modified measuring beam. It removesunwanted image area (nose—that is between eyes). This is not diagnostic important and enable to increase resolution of recorded regions of interest. Experimental image captured by this system is presented in Fig. 5.

The 1st Purkinje image important for relative vergence establishment is conspicuous point close to center of eye pupil. High contrast in comparison with surroundings is suitable for automatical software processing. Vertical slope luminance profile of retinal reflex is important to determination of relative eye accommodation.

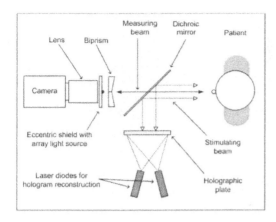

Figure 4. Optical scheme of measuring system.

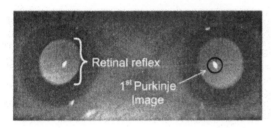

Figure 5. Image recorded by the measurement system.

The clinical applicability was confirmed in small clinical study with children of various ages and diagnoses.

4 CONCLUSION

We have designed optical measuring system for fast, reliable, non-invasive measurement of simultaneous dynamics of vergence and accommodation (Fig. 4).This system is suitable for common clinical practice especially for strabismology and ophthalmology.

ACKNOWLEDGEMENT

This work was supported by grant GAUK 0880/2010.

REFERENCES

[1] Dostalek, M. & Dusek, J. 2004. E.M.A.N. (Eye Movement and Accommodation Analyzer) device for vergence accommodation synkinesis recording and analysis. Transactions, 28th European Strabismological Association Meeting. J.-T. de Faber. London, New York, Taylor & Francis: 357–361.
[2] Jindra, T. 2009. Infrared measurement of accommodation and eye movements - Hardware design. Bachelor work, Prague, Charles University in Prague, p. 43.
[3] Schaeffel, F., Farkas, L. & Holand, H.C. 1987. Infrared photoretinoscope, Appl. Opt 26, 1987, pp. 1505–1509.

Technology and Medical Sciences – Natal Jorge et al. (eds)
© 2011 Taylor & Francis Group, London, ISBN 978-0-415-66822-4

3D modelling for FEM simulation of an obese foot

V.C. Pinto, N.V. Ramos & M.A.P. Vaz
INEGI—Instituto de Engenharia Mecânica e Gestão Industrial, Porto, Portugal

M.A. Marques
ISEP—Instituto Superior de Engenharia do Porto, Porto, Portugal

ABSTRACT: The objective of this paper is to validate a procedure to build a 3D model of the foot and to simulate three different instances during the gait cycle and also for the balanced standing posture, to obtain pressure and tensions distributions in the foot. From CT images, one obtains mesh clouds of the 3D objects using Mimics® software. The different solid parts are obtained using Solidworks® software, and the FEM analysis was done using Ansys® software. This methodoly was applied to the study of an obese foot in situations that can cause pain and discomfort, in order to define the best orthosis solution.

1   INTRODUCTION

Several problems are associated to obesity, and this study is looking for a way to minimize some of these problems in the foot. If the anatomical structure of the foot is geometrically well defined it's possible to simulate all types of situations that can affect gait and stability of an obese patient.

In the attempt to find a new, reliable and efficient method to build 3D anatomical structures for FEM simulation this study validates a process that includes software correlation, starting in medical imaging files, through CAD software, to FEM simulation is possible to obtain a 3D foot model of an obese patient.

The objective of this study is to find the deformations in the foot and the stress tensions in the bone structure, related to patient's weight and plantar pressure distribution to determine best orthoses solutions for obesity, by minimizing plantar pressure in the more affected areas of the foot, helping gait and balanced standing.

Beyond this simulation, done with software Ansys®, the goal is to identify the tensions inside the foot during the three stages that characterizes gait cycle.

2   METHODOLOGY

2.1   3D modeling of the foot

From Computed Tomography (CT) medical images (DICOM files) of obese patient feet whose body mass is 121 kg, a single file with the corresponding mesh clouds was obtained, using Mimics® v9.1,

according to tissue density. The use of different masks provided by the software, one could obtain bones with cartilage and soft tissues with muscles, fat tissue and skin, according to tissue density, by using different masks, that are provided by the software. These mesh clouds were divided into two groups: bone structure (that includes bones and cartilage) and soft tissue (Fig. 1).

Then, the mesh cloud files were exported as STL files, to a CAD software, Solidworks® 2009, where they were edited and improved. Finally, a solid part for each 3D object was generated (Fig. 2).

However, bone structure is a complex object and it is difficult for the software to generate surfaces along all the structure. Therefore the bone structure was anatomically divided into five pieces: tibia and fibula; calcaneous and talus; cuboid, cuneiforms and navicular; all the metatarsals and all the phalanges; then solid parts for all the objects were generated.

Finally they were combined, resulting in an unified bone structure, which was assembled with the soft tissue (Fig. 2). A rigid support was added to the full assembled foot to simulate the ground.

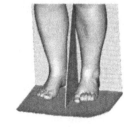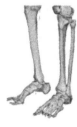

Figure 1.   Bone structure and soft tissues from CT by Mimics®.

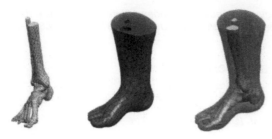

Figure 2. Solid parts of bone structure and soft tissues in Solidworks® and final assembly.

2.2 *FEM simulation*

In the several simulations, done with Ansys® v.11 software, it was defined that the bone structure and the soft tissues were bonded in the corresponding contact surfaces and edges. It was also added five springs to the bone structure simulating the tendons in the plantar fascia during balanced standing and during gait cycle.

In the simulation of balanced standing position a mesh was generated for all anatomic structures with 173399 nodes and 97759 elements, with 3D tetrahedral elements due to its complexity; for the ground support quadrilaterals elements were used. For the first stage gait simulation, the mesh was generated with 169879 nodes and 95594 elements, with the same type of elements, and for the third stage gait simulation, the mesh had 169533 nodes and 95517 elements.

Bone structure, soft tissue and tendons were considered linearly elastic, isotropic and homogeneous (Cheung et al. 2004). Mechanical properties, such as Young's modulus and Poisson's ratio were found in the literature and used in previous work (Marques et al. 2008). For bone, Young's modulus and Poisson's ratio, were calculated by taking into account the relative weight of cortical and trabecular bone, resulting in a value of 7300 MPa and 0.3, respectively; for soft tissue used were 0.15 MPa and 0.45, respectively, and for the plantar fascia the Young's modulus is 350 MPa.

For the first simulation, related to balanced standing posture, a vertical force on the ground of 605N was applied, in order to get the foot and stress distributions, due to the patient's weight.

In the second simulation, related to the three stages of gait cycle, it was applied, separately, vertical forces with different values corresponding to these three stages, described in Table 1.

Due to different contact areas in each stage, there was the need to apply different initial conditions related to contact between soft tissue and the ground. For both simulations, the ground was

vertically recessed, with no longitudinal expansion and rigid. Also in both situations tibia and fibula were fixed.

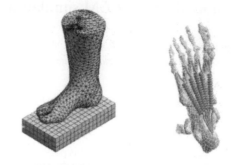

Figure 3. Mesh of the assembly: Bone structure, soft tissues and ground, in Ansys® (left). Springs that simulates tendons on the plantar fascia (right).

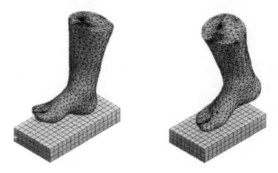

Figure 4. Mesh of the assembly for first and third stage of gait.

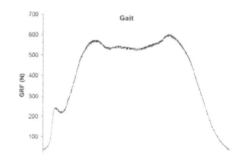

Figure 5. Ground reaction force during gait.

Table 1. Ground reaction forces during the stages of the gait.

Stages	GRFx	GRFy	GRFz
1st	5.02966	−48.2619	384.964
3rd	5.83626	50.7321	307.299

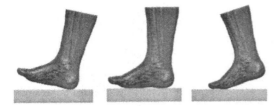

Figure 6. 3D foot model for three stages of the gait.

3 RESULTS AND DISCUSSION

3.1 Balanced standing

As expected, deformation of bone structure is more significant in the toes, being the maximum displacement of 10.593 mm. The stress tension distribution was also the expected one, having a maximum of 475.46 MPa, with the highest values near anatomical joints of the ankle.

Analyzing the results, it is possible to assume that patient's foot isn't isometric align when he stands in a balanced position, showing some signs of supinated foot. This makes the ankle rolls away from the center, making the little toe down, meaning that the foot rolls to outside (lateral) and describing an high plantar arch.

One of this signs is that contact between tibia and fibula has the maximum displacement as Figure 8 shows.

The maximum plantar pressure value is 0.50958 MPa for the balanced standing posture and it is located in the calcaneous.

The second phase of the gait, it was assumed the foot was completely in the ground, so it's similar to the balanced standing (first simulation).

3.2 Gait

For the first stage of the gait and right after initial contact the calcaneous has a more important role in the stress distribution (maximum), leaving the metatarsal without significant stress, since there is no contact with the ground. The maximum displacement is 30,613 mm, the maximum stress peak is 73,498 MPa and it is in the between tibia and fibula.

For the propulsive stage (third simulation), the first metatarsal was still in contact with the ground so the tension distribution shows the highest values of stress under the metatarsal heads and insignificant under the calcaneous. The maximum displacement is 28.049 mm, the maximum stress peak is 477.76 MPa and it is in the first metatarsal.

For gait's first stage plantar pressure maximum value is 0.19594 MPa and for third is 0.868 MPa.

Soft tissue experiments traction and compression by the ground and the bone structure, so negative

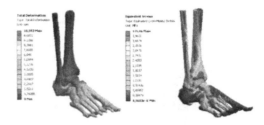

Figure 7. Displacement and equivalent stress (von Mises) in the bone structure in balanced standing posture.

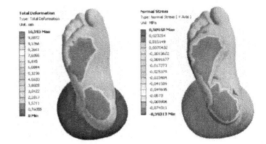

Figure 8. Displacement and pressure distribution during balanced standing posture.

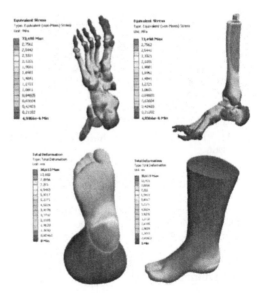

Figure 9. Displacement and equivalent stress during gait's first stage.

values of the pressure could be explained by that. If values scale is translated for positive values, the maximum pressure value is 0.90271 MPa for the balanced standing posture, 0.90971 MPa for gait's first stage and 3.6946 MPa for gait's third stage.

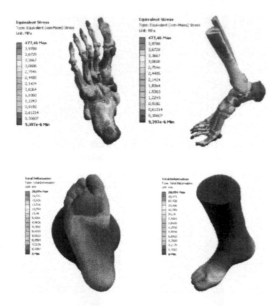

Figure 10. Displacement and equivalent stress during gait's third stage.

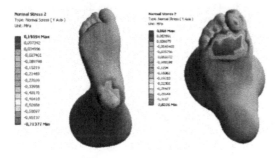

Figure 11. Pressure distribution during first and third stage of gait.

4 CONCLUSION AND FUTURE WORK

To get displacement of the foot in balanced standing position it was difficult to align foot and ground in the model, due to foot position in the CT. So this method is extremely useful if the position of the foot can be controlled in CT and is correctly vertically align during it.

Speaking in results, it's possible to see that displacement and pressure are distributed more in lateral area, in metatarsal and in calcaneous in balanced standing posture, more in calcaneous during first stage of gait and more in metatarsal during third stage of gait. So the foot of this obese patient has a deviation from the center to the lateral (outside) comparing to a normal foot.

In the balanced standing position it is possible to see the patient's plantar stress distribution showing regions representative of hyper pressures, enabling the search for the best orthosis for this obese patient, since these pressures were very well localized in the plantar surface of the foot, especially near the area of the calcaneous and the metatarsal heads.

Since it was an obese patient, values of displacement, equivalent stress and pressure were higher than if it was a normal weigh individual.

It is a future goal to validate these results in experiments with pressure mapping sensors and compare them to an normal weigh individual.

Having these validated, CAD construction of an orthosis for minimizing the plantar pressure to incorporate in a simulation using this method is another goal.

Future work will take into account hyperelastic behavior for soft tissue and viscoelastic behavior for bone.

REFERENCES

Antunes, P.J., Dias G.R., Coelho, A.T., Rebelo, F. & Pereira T. 2007. Non-Linear Finite Element Modelling of Anatomically Detailed 3D Foot Model. MIA 2207.

Birtane, M. & Tuna, H. 2004. The evaluation of plantar pressure distribution in obese and non-obese adults. Clinical Biomechanics, 19 (2004): 1055–1059.

Cheung, J.T., Luximon, A. & Zhang, M., Parametrical Design of foot orthoses for plantar pressure relieve based on computational modelling.

Cheung, J.T., Zhang, M. & An, K. 2004. Effects of plantar fascia stiffness on the biomechanical responses of the ankle-foot complex. Clinical Biomechanics, 19 (2004): 839–846.

Cheung, J.T., Zhang, M., Leung., A.K. & Fan, Y. 2004. Three-dimensional finite element analysis of the foot during standing—a material sensitivity study. Journal of Biomechanics, 38 (2005): 1045–1054.

Gefen, A. 2002. Stress analysis of the standing foot following surgical plantar fascia release. Journal of Biomechanics, 35 (2002): 629–637.

Gefen A. 2003, Plantar soft tissue loading under the m edial metatarsals in the standing diabetic foot. Medical Engineering & Physics 25 (2003): 491–499.

Lemmon, D., Shiang, T.Y., Hashmi, A., Ulbrecht, J.S. & Cavanagh, P.R. 1997. The effect of insoles in therapeutic footwear—A finite element approach. Journal of Biomechancis, 30, 6(1997): 615–620.

Marques, M.A., Nabais, C., Ramos, N.V., Ribeiro, R. & Vaz, M.A.P. 2008. Modelação do pé para o estudo de tensões internas localizadas. 7º Congresso de Mecânica Experimental 2008.

Simkin, A. 1982. Structural Analysis of the Human Foot in Standing posture 1982. Phd tesis, Tel Aviv University, 1982.

Technology and Medical Sciences – Natal Jorge et al. (eds)
© *2011 Taylor & Francis Group, London, ISBN 978-0-415-66822-4*

A breast modelling application for surgeons

Augusta Cardoso & Horácio Costa
Centro Hospitalar de Vila Nova de Gaia/Espinho EPE, Portugal

Vera Sá
Departamento da Matemática, Faculdade de Ciências, Universidade do Porto, Portugal

Georgi Smirnov
Centro de Matemática da Universidade do Porto
Departamento de Matemática e Aplicações, Universidade do Minho, Portugal

ABSTRACT: Although the number of works on breast soft tissue modelling significantly increased during the last few years, the development of an adequate breast model still continues to be a challenging problem. The main areas of application of breast modelling are: aesthetic surgery and medical imaging analysis. One of the main goals is to provide surgeons with a reliable forecast of the breast's final geometry. In this work we present the prototype of a program that allows one to represent the pre and post-operatory breast geometries. This program aims to be an easy instrument to use and may reveal itself specially helpful to inexperienced surgeons. With this tools they can test, for example, if a small variation in the incision angle could influence the final geometry of the patient's breast, or not. The program allows the surgeons, considering their pacient's opinion, to choose the final form of the breast. The breast tissue is modelled using 3D finite elements, the skin is modelled using 2D finite elements, and the Chassaignac space is modelled as a system of springs.

Keywords: Surgery planning, Breast modelling, Finite element method, Breast reduction surgery

1 INTRODUCTION

Plastic surgery of the breast and particularly breast reduction, is considered a difficult and distinct area. Breast reduction is one of the most common procedures in breast surgery and has been gaining increasing importance, especially in women over 40 years of age. Surgical techniques are very personalized and there are innumerable variations described in the literature. Mastering the techniques is a long path, and it can become a challenge for a less experienced surgeon to understand exactly what to do when facing a particular type of breast. The aim of this work is to develop a prototype of a program that allows one to represent the pre and post-operatory breast geometries, according to the incision marking parameters. This program aims to be an easy instrument to use and may reveal itself specially helpful to inexperienced surgeons. The program allows the surgeons, considering their pacient's opinion, to choose the final form of the breast.

Although the number of works on the breast soft tissue modelling significantly increased during the last few years (Delingette 1998, del Palomar,

Calvo, Herrero, López & Doblar 2008, Whiteley & Gavaghan 2007), the development of an adequate breast model still continues to be an unsolved problem. The main areas of the breast modelling application are: aesthetic surgery (Ayache & (Eds.) 2003, Balaniuk, Costa & Melo 2006, Cardoso, Smirnov, Costa & Sá 2009, Rajagopal, Nielsen & Nash 2004, Smirnov & Sá 2007, Smirnov & Sá 2009) and medical imaging analysis (Azar, Metaxas & Schnall 2002).

The breast reduction surgery simulator described in this paper is based on numerical solution of what we call a general problem of plastic surgery. From the mathematical point of view this is a problem of calculus of variations with unusual boundary conditions, known as knitting conditions. The breast tissue is considered as a hyperelastic material, i.e. a material satisfying the standard thermodynamic axiom of non-negative work in closed processes (Gurtin 1981). Although most of soft tissues are incompressible (Fung. 1993), we consider the breast as a compressible Neo-Hookean material (Zienkiewicz & R.L.Taylor 2005). The complex structure of the breast involves several tissues whose elastic properties cannot be readily deduced from the elastic properties of the tissues forming it.

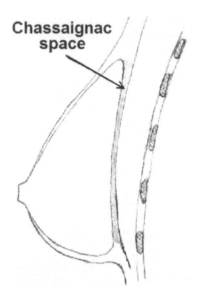

Chassaignac space

Figure 1. Transversal section of the breast showing the Chassaignac space.

The compressibility of the breast is an experimental fact. Indeed, the breast reduction surgery where only a part of the skin is removed from the breast (breast lift), diminishes the breast volume without removing any part of its internal tissue. The skin has elastic properties very different from those of the breast gland and fat tissue, and therefore, must be modelled differently (Retel, Vescovo, Jacquet, Trivaudey, Varchon & Burtheret 2001). The breast tissue is modelled using three-dimensional finite elements, the skin is modelled using two-dimensional finite elements (Zienkiewicz & R.L. Taylor 2005, Whiteley & Gavaghan 2007), and the Chassaignac space (Bono 2008) as a spring system (Mollemans, Schutyser, Cleynenbreugel & Suetens 2004). The Chassaignac space plays a special role in the breast mobility and is responsible for the connection between the breast and the chest (Fig. 1).

There are many papers, dedicated to the problem of the elastic parameters determination (Akamatsu 1993, Fehrenbach, Masmoudi, Souchon & Trompette 2006). In this work, the determination of the elastic parameters is carried out from the breast geometry observation. This methodology is new and is based on the fact that when the patient changes her position (upright, prone, on the back, etc.), the breast geometry also changes and these transformations depend on the elastic properties of the breast.

2 MATHEMATICAL FORMULATION OF THE PROBLEM

In this section we include a short description of the mathematical model used in our simulations.

Let f be the deformation of the elastic body $\mathcal{B}$ and let W be the strain-energy density (Gurtin 1981). The boundary Γ of $\mathcal{B}$ is represented as $\Gamma = \Gamma 1 \cup \Gamma_2 \cup \Gamma_3 \cup \Gamma_4$, where $\Gamma_3 = \Gamma_+ \cup F_-$. This means that we consider the boundary of the elastic body as being formed by a fixed part $\Gamma 1$, a free part Γ_2, a part Γ_3 where two of the incised tissues are sutured to each other, and another part where the incised tissues are sutured to a fixed surface Γ_4 (see Fig. 2).

Consider the following variational problem

$$I(f) = \int_{\mathcal{B}} W(\nabla f(p))\, dp \rightarrow \inf \qquad (1)$$

with the boundary conditions:

$$f(p) = 0,\, p \in \Gamma_1, \qquad (2)$$

$$f(g(p)) = f(p),\, p \in \Gamma_+, \qquad (3)$$

$$h(f(p)) = 0,\, p \in \Gamma_4, \qquad (4)$$

where $g: \Gamma_+ \rightarrow \Gamma_-$ is a map. It can be fixed or variable and describes the suturing. We call problem (1)–(4) a general plastic surgery problem. To model the Chassaignac space we consider a system of springs situated at the breast base. From the mathematical point of view this means that we add the functional

$$\int_{\Gamma_{ch}} c(p)\,\| f(p) - p \|^2\, dp$$

to functional (1). Here $c(p)$ is a given function (springs' stiffness). When we introduce the Chassaignac space to the model we add a movable part to the boundary that we have called $\Gamma_{ch} \subset \Gamma_4$.

As we mentioned above, we consider a neo-Hookean compressible (Zienkiewicz & R.L. Taylor 2005) material. This means that the strain energy density function is given by

$$W(F) = \frac{\mu}{2}\left(tr\left(FF^{T} \right) - 3 - 2\ln \det(F) \right) + \frac{\lambda}{2}\left(\det(F) - 1 \right)^{2}, \qquad (5)$$

where $F = \nabla f$ is the Jacobi matrix of f. The parameters λ and μ are different for the skin and the interior tissue.

This problem has already been studied in (Cardoso, Smirnov, Costa & Sá 2009, Smirnov &

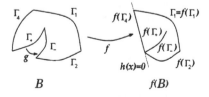

Figure 2. Scheme of the elastic body boundary parts before and after the surgery.

Sá 2007, Smirnov & Sá 2009). In those works the finite element method equations are deduced for this problem and it is placed among other elasticity theory problems. The introduction of the Chassaignac space in the model was presented in (Cardoso, Smirnov, Costa & Sá2010).

3 COMPUTATIONAL ASPECTS

We use the finite element method (Zienkiewicz, R.L. Taylor & Zhu 2005) to obtain a reliable computational model of the breast. The breast tissue is modelled using three-dimensional finite elements and the skin is modelled using two-dimensional finite elements. The Chassaignac space is modelled by a spring system.

We assume that there exists a "neutral state" of the breast (Smirnov & Sá 2009), i.e. a state of the breast in which all forces (elastic and mass) are zero. Although the existence of this state is a very strong and unrealistic hypothesis, it is absolutely necessary for the modelling.

The breast reduction surgery modelling contains the following main steps:

1. determination of the elastic parameters λ and μ in (5), and of the original breast neutral state,
2. incision of the tissue to be removed,
3. tissues suturing,
4. determination of the final breast neutral state.

3.1 Breast reduction surgery modelling first step

To fulfil the first step we use a methodology based on the study of the breast deformation as a function of the patient position. The corresponding mathematical problem consists of the minimization of the discrepancy between what is observed and what is modelled (Smirnov & Sá 2009). Using this methodology we determine the parameters λ and μ in (5) and obtain the pre-operative breast model (see Figure 3).

It took several measurements with patients in different positions, in order to choose the parameters of the model and to determine the elastic coefficients of the breast and of the skin according to this methodology.

3.2 Breast reduction surgery modelling second step

The second step is a simple geometric construction applied to the breast in the neutral state. In the former works (Smirnov & Sá 2009, Cardoso, Smirnov, Costa & Sá 2009), based on the incised surgery marking (see Figure 4) we considered the breast as a symmetric body. The symmetry plane is ortogonal to the chest and passes through the nipple dividing

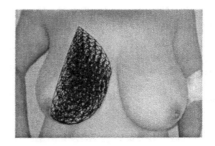

Figure 3. Pre-operative breast model.

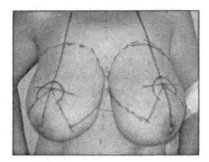

Figure 4. Cutting lines.

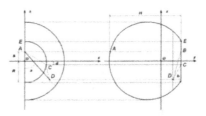

Figure 5. Neutral state of the breast and tissues incision scheme depending on the parameters a, s, h, and d.

the breast in almost two equal parts. It is assumed that in the neutral state the breast is a spherical cap with the base radius R and the height H (see Figure 5). In our experiments we did not take into account the type of nipple pedicle. The scheme of the surgery is shown in Figure 5. Half of the breast is incised by the planes ABD and BCD and the other half of the breast by planes symmetrics to this ones. The point A represents a new position of the nipple. The point C belongs to the breast base and D is a point on the breast surface.

To describe the cutting planes ABD and BCD we use the angle a between the planes ABD and $0yz$ (see Figures 5), the distance s between the point A and the plane $0xy$, the distance d between the point C and the plane $0xy$, and the distance h between the point D and the base of the breast.

Considering now the breast as an ellipsoid, and performing the incision along planes different from the symmetric ones, one obtains two non symmetric surfaces (see Figure 6).

3.3 Breast reduction surgery modelling third step

If we consider the incision on the breast to draw a symmetric body, to perform the suture, we must match all vertices with their symmetrics, relative to the symmetry plane *Oyz*. Otherwise, if the incision does not produce symmetry, we need to improve the matching method, enabling it to handle two non symmetric surface meshes.

Both curvilinear triangles *BCD* and *BC'D'* are sutured to the "chest", meaning the plane *0xz*. Here, the points labeled with primes, represent the vertices of the other half of the breast. The curvilinear triangle *ABD* will be sutured to the curvilinear triangle *ABD'*. To suture this two curvilinear triangles to each other we need to match, vertex by vertex, the two correspondent surface meshes. In our model we represent the breast as a set of tetrahedron, and after the incision we obtain two surfaces with different mesh configurations. We want the same configuration in both meshes, therefore we create the following procedure, based on what was already described in (Smirnov & Sá 2007). Consider the meshes shown in Figure 7. To automatically reconfigure the meshes shown in Figure 7 one executes the following steps:

1. Create two arrays: one with surface S_1 boundary vertices, the other with surface S_2 boundary vertices;
2. Identify the vertices that are common to both surface meshes (these are boundary vertices). In case of Figure 7 these vertices are: A, P_1 and B;
3. Arrange the boundary vertices array beginning by the common vertices;
4. If the identified boundary vertices number is not the same in both surface meshes, then:

   (a) Calculate the quantity of vertices that one needs to insert. In the case of Figure 7 we need to insert one vertex in S_1 surface mesh boundary (see Figure 8);
   (b) Measure the segments lengths between all the vertices that form the surface mesh boundary, except the ones that are common with the other surface mesh boundary;

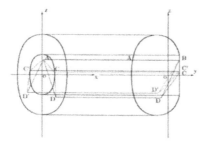

Figure 6.   Eliptical breast cutting scheme.

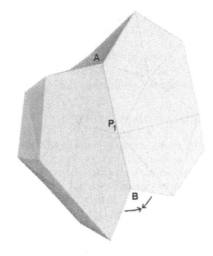

Figure 7.   Surface meshes—S_1 at left and S_2 on right.

   (c) Find the biggest segment and create a vertex in the middle of the segment, effectively splitting the segment in two parts. In the example case the biggest segment is [*PQ*], and P_{new} is the middle point of the segment;
   (d) Find all the tetrahedron that include the split segment and divide them as well (see: dashed line in Figure 8).

Repeat steps (b) to (d) until all the needed vertices have been inserted. Figure 8 shows the result after the fourth step, where P_{new} is the added vertex.

5. Couple the vertices of the two arrays and save these couples in a new array, labeled *suture array*;
6. For both surface meshes create a convex polygon made by their boundary vertices;
7. Compute the centroid of each convex polygon and connect all its vertices to its centroid. The result is the first triangulation of each convex polygon and consequently of both surface meshes (see Figure 9).
8. Couple the centroids and add them to the *suture array*;
9. If the requested precision does not demand for a thinner mesh proceed to step ten, otherwise do:

   (a) Refine the before mentioned triangle mesh by bisecting each triangle edge in two equal parts. While refining the mesh, one ends up creating new surface mesh boundary vertices, therefore one must divide their correspondent tetrahedron as well;
   (b) Couple all new vertices and add them to the *suture array;*
   (c) Repeat this process till the surface meshes respect the required precision.

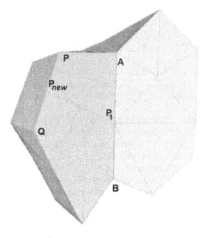

Figure 8. Surface meshes with same number of boundary vertices.

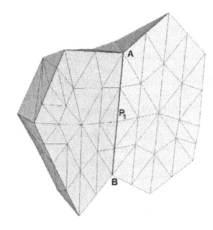

Figure 10. The reconfigured surface meshes.

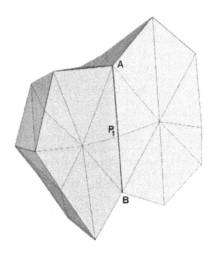

Figure 9. Surface meshes with the first triangulation.

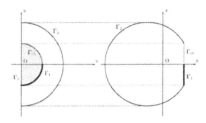

Figure 11. Breast scheme showing the consider boundary parts.

10. Destroy all tetrahedron that are now invalid. Call the Delaunay triangulation method to remesh both surfaces. This, creates new tetrahedron which respect the new mesh vextex configuration;

The end result is an array with the suture information, vertex by vertex. Figure 10 shows the result of our example case after only one step of mesh refining. Now we may proceed to determine the final breast geometry.

3.4 Breast reduction surgery modelling fourth step

To fulfil this step we numerically solve variational problem (1)–(4). To get the final breast neutral state

we set all stresses equal to zero. This last step can be considered as the breast recovering modelling.

To obtain the surgery forecast in states different from the neutral one, for example when the patient is standing up, we have to apply mass forces to the previously obtained neutral state and to solve problem (1).

When we simulate the surgery, if we consider the breast as symmetric the knitting problem reduces to a problem with constraints (2) and (4), (Smirnov & Sá 2009, Cardoso, Smirnov, Costa & Sá 2009). In Figure 11 we schematically represent on the left a front view and on the right a side view of the breast. We represent Γ_{ch} in grey, Γ_1 with a thick line on the left and as a segment on the right; Γ_2 is the surface of the sphere.

4 THE CHASSAIGNAC'S SPACE INFLUENCE

As we mentioned in the introduction to this paper, the breast has a complex structure, involving several tissues. We came to the conclusion, in (Cardoso, Smirnov, Coelho, Zenha, Costa & Sá 2010), that no realistic breast model is possible without the Chassaignac space, which plays special role in breast mobility and is responsible for the connection between the breast and the chest. The mobility of the breast base is an experimental fact. For example, we drew in the patients skin, the breast base. Then we measured the length of this line when the patients were standing up, and when the patients were lying supine. The difference between two measurements was about 20–30%. However, the breast cannot arbitrarily move along the body because it is fixed in its lower part, known as inframammary fold. All these tissues should be included in a realistic breast model.

5 CONCLUSIONS

Breast reduction is a complex surgical area and a non-experienced surgeon faces serious difficulties in the process of estimation and analysis of the surgery results. The application of computer models based on biomechanical engineering provides a possibility to simulate breast reduction with reliable end-results. In this paper presents the prototype of a program that allows us to represent the pre and post-operatory breast geometries. This program aims to be an easy instrument to use and may reveal itself specially helpful to inexperienced surgeons. The method allows them to estimate the form of the breast after surgery knowing its form before the intervention and considering the parameters of incision they are going to apply at the time of surgery. With this the surgeons, considering their pacient's opinion, can choose the final form of the breast.

Nevertheless, the work is not already complet because tissues like fascia have not been considered yet. In our future work we plan to consider more involved breast models including the fascia.

ACKNOWLEDGEMENT

To Fundação para a Ciência e a Tecnologia (SFRH/BD/40119/2007), for the financial support.

REFERENCES

Akamatsu, M. (1993). Identification of Lam coefficients from tangencial boundary observations. *J. Fac. Sci. Univ. Tokyo 6*, 623–634.
Ayache, N. & H.D. (Eds.) (2003). Surgery Simulation and Soft Tissue Modeling. In *Lecture Notes in Computing Science*, p. 2673. Berlin: Springer.
Azar, F., Metaxas, D. & Schnall, M. (2002). Methods for modelling and predicting mechanical deformations of the breast under external perturbations. *Medical Image Analysis 6*, 1–27.

Balaniuk, R., Costa, I. & Melo, J. (2006). Cosmetic Breast Surgery Simulation. *Anais do VIII Symposium on Virtual Reality.*
Bono, J. (2008). Ligamental mammaplasty. *Rev. Bras. Cir. Plást. 23(3)*, 192–199.
Cardoso, A., Smirnov, G., Coelho, G., Zenha, H., Costa, H. & Sá, V. (2010). Computer Simulation of Breast Reduction Surgery. *European Journal of Plastic Surgery.*
Cardoso, A., Smirnov, G., Costa, H. & Sá, V. (2009). Métodos variacionais de engenharia biomecânica em cirurgia plástica de tecidos moles. In *Conferência de Engenharia 2009.* Covilhã.
Cardoso, A., Smirnov, G., Costa, H. & Sá, V. (2010). On the importance of Chassaignac's space in breast modelling. In *IV European Conference on Computational Mechanics.* Paris.
del Palomar, A.P., Calvo, B., Herrero, J., López, J. & Doblar, M. (2008). A finite element model to accurately predict real deformations of the breast. *Medical Engeneering & Phisics 30*, 1089–1097.
Delingette, H. (1998). Towards Realistic Soft Tissue Modeling in Medical Simulation. *IEEE: Special Issue on Surgery Simulation*, 512–523.
Fehrenbach, J., Masmoudi, M., Souchon, R. & Trompette, P. (2006). Relative Young's modulus identification using elas-tography. *Revue Europenne de Mcanique Numrique 15*, 167–174.
Fung, Y. (1993). *Biomechanics—Mechanical Properties of Living Tissues* (2nd ed.). Springer-Verlag.
Gurtin, M. (1981). *An Introduction to Continuum Mechanics.* New York: Acad. Press.
Mollemans, W., Schutyser, F., Cleynenbreugel, J.V. & Suetens, P. (2004). Fast Soft Tissue Deformation with Tetrahedral Mass Spring Model for Maxillofacial Surgery Planning Systems. *Springer Berlin /Heidelberg 3217/2004*, 371–379.
Rajagopal, V., Nielsen, P. & Nash, M. (2004). *Development of a Three-Dimensional Finite Element Model of Breast Mechanics.* IEEE-EMBS 26th Ann. Intl. Conf.
Retel, V., Vescovo, P., Jacquet, E. Trivaudey, F., Varchon, D. & Burtheret, A. (2001). Nonlineal model of skin mechanical behaviour analysis with finite element method. *Skin Research and Technology 7*, 152–158.
Smirnov, G. & Sá, V. (2007). Simulação Numérica da Cirurgia Plástica da Mama. In *CMNE/CILAMCE, Porto, 13–15 de Junho, 2007.* Porto: FEUP, APMTAC.
Smirnov, G. & Sá, V. (2009). Métodos de determinação dos parâmetros que influenciam os resultados da cirurgia plástica de redução mamária. In *Congreso de Métodos Numéricos en Ingeniería 2009, Barcelona, 29 de Junho a 2 de Julho, 2009.* Barcelona: SEMNI.
Whiteley, J.P. & Gavaghan, D.J. (2007). Non-linear modelling of breast tissue. *Mathematical Medicine and Biology 24*, 327–345.
Zienkiewicz, O. & Taylor, R.L. (2005). *The Finite Element Method for Solid and Structural Mechanics* (6th ed.). Amsterdam: Elsevier.
Zienkiewicz, O., Taylor, R.L. & Zhu, J. (2005). *The Finite Element Method: Its Basis and Fundamentals* (6th ed.). Amsterdam: Elsevier.

Technology and Medical Sciences – Natal Jorge et al. (eds)
© 2011 Taylor & Francis Group, London, ISBN 978-0-415-66822-4

A framework model for e-Health services

Mario Macedo
Instituto Politécnico de Tomar

Pedro Isaías
Universidade Alberta

ABSTRACT: The normalization and integration of clinical data is a main issue to promote the evidence based medicine, the medical research and hospitals' administration.
Some barriers already exist due to some reasons:

1. Inadequate information systems' architectures;
2. Proprietary databases;
3. Lack of terminology and of medical ontologies alignment.

This paper aims to show firstly that there are norms and regulations sufficient and suitable to develop a normalized information system. Secondly this paper suggests a framework to develop a normalized platform.
The expected deliveries of normalized clinical repositories are an improvement in data accessibility, ubiquity and medical knowledge construction.

Keywords: Healthcare, EHR, Archetype, ISO 18308, ISO 21090, ISO 13606, TC215, RIM, SNOMED

1 INTRODUCTION

The ontologies are very useful in the medical sciences because they describe the knowledge related to pathologies, micro organisms, drugs, medical acts, medical devices, anatomic structures and other concepts related with healthcare.

Due to a huge diversity of guidelines, cultures, science progress, variables and terminologies, it can happen that the clinical records of each a person only can be understood by its own author.

This fact is a real barrier to the development of scientific knowledge of each person, sharing of data, development of collaborative treatment plans and sharing of research information. The lack of aligned terminologies is also a barrier to the drop of clinical risk.

It is possible to conclude that aligned ontologies are crucial to the rise of quality in healthcare services.

The development of models to improve the sharing of clinical data increases the longevity and quality and at same time to make the data independent of the used technology is a main goal nowadays.

The concept of EHR (Electronic Health Record) has different definitions. According to a report published by a working group of ISO organization, TC215-WG1, [1], the EHR definition had some equivalences such as EHCR (Electronic Health Care Record), CPR (Computarized Patient Record) and EPR (Electronic Patient Record). All these terms had the same meaning with different origins.

The Centre for Health Informatics and Multiprofessional Education of the University College London defined the requirements of an EHR [2]. The main objectives of these requirements for an EHR are completeness, to be communicable, pervasive, coherent and suitable for interoperability between different systems, countries and cultures. At the same time the EHR should be compliant with the law of different regions and ethical practices.

In 2004 the ISO published a norm named 18308 to establish the requirements for a normalized clinical information system.

Different working groups have developed recommendations about this subject. The TC215 working group has proposed some of the ISO norms.

2 THE NORMALIZED METADATA

One of the goals of metadata normalization is to create databases which could be shared by different systems. These systems can use standardized messages' structures. The logic of these messages and correspondent workflows guarantees the data alignment.

There are a set of ISO rules for normalization and standardization of variables related to demographic data and quantitative metrics.

The ISO 11404 [3] specifies a set of data types available to model data structures. These atomic data types are the boolean, the integer, the real, the nominal and the class among others.

The main goal of this rule is to define a set of data types and their aggregation to guarantee the software code portability among different programming languages, different versions of each language and promote new technologies like for example JBI (Java for Business Integration), data representation in XML using namespaces and XLST.

The usage of this rule allows software sharing among different entities. This improves the development of the Open Source industry.

The ISO 21090 rule [4] defines a set of metadata structures related to healthcare services.

The model is developed with UML 2 terminology and uses classes with attributes whose data types are defined by ISO 11404.

The ISO 21090 has an enormous improvement for clinical text. This particularity is named *Nullfavor*. This new type allows specifying situations that the clinical variable is unknown because of many reasons like for instance disability of the person, lack of knowledge, impossible to know, ethical reasons, privacy and confidentiality.

The Openehr organization [5] has developed the *Nullfavor* data type and created some normalized values to this type of situations.

The ISO 18308 [6] defined the requirements of an electronic health record. These rules specify the structure, data architecture and terminologies to provide a reliable platform to manage the processes and their orchestration, security and privacy.

In the field of communications, ISO published a rule named 13606, [7]. This rule described the data and structures of messages for the system interoperability.

The rules referred so far and others in this domain were developed by TC215 [8] which is formed by 8 working groups.

The clinical data has multidimensional characteristics from other domains and specific metrics.

It is also possible that data from other software applications like, for instance, geographic coordinates can be included in health record.

It is possible to replicate identical structures, so the isomorphism propriety is confirmed like hereditary.

It is also possible to use the data aggregation to build more complex structures.

These properties motivate the usage of the concept of business objects for clinical data like it is defined by OMG.

The definition of clinical objects can be achieved with the usage of OML (Object Modeling Language). In addition, the development of patterns of business objects will make viable different data repositories with normalized structures.

Some attributes of these objects can be complex variables structured by different rules.

There are some rules for data acquisition. The ECGs, the EEGs, the laboratory systems, and so on use different data types and protocols to communicate. The data from these systems can be included in other clinical objects.

At the end it is possible to have complex objects that encapsulate atomic objects and so on.

According to [9], *Semantic interoperability and secondary use of data are important informatics challenges in modern healthcare.* The author argues that the implementations of Archetypes model accomplishes with ISO 18308.

The HL7 version 3 (Health Level 7) is an implementation of communication and data repository rules. The metadata definition is made with a language named CDA (Clinical Document Architecture). This language can define not only the data structures but also the messages and the constraints of the objects.

The communication of clinical data in this norm is made by XML documents.

The HL7 has a RIM (Reference Information Model) [10]. This RIM has an archive of metadata structures and links to a terminology database.

According to [11] *HL7 Templates and EN/ISO 13606 Archetypes are essential components for a semantically interoperable exchange of Electronic Health Record (EHR) data.*

The main object definitions available are the following:

- Entities
- Roles
- Structured documents
- Acts
- Communications

A very important issue in clinical data records is the information about relatives.

The genealogic tree establishes the relationships between persons and it is a very important tool to know the probability of genetic diseases.

This information should be kept in a clinical record. So, HL7 can provide objects to archive genetic data.

There are situations in which the patient is not able to describe the relationship with a relative.

The HL7 has proposed a set of codes for special situations like this one, [12].

The OpenEHR organization presented an architecture based on archetypes. An archetype is an object class that can be described with XML language.

The model of OpenEHR [13] is based in three components:

- RM (Reference Model);
- AM (Archetype Model);
- SM (Service Model).

The Reference Model is composed by all the metadata definitions and terminologies. The Archetype Model defines all the semantic contents using a language called ADL (Archetype Definition Language).

To query the data records was developed an HER query language. This language is not yet standardized. According to [14], *EQL is neutral to EHR systems, programming languages and system environments and depends only on the openEHR archetype model and semantics.*

3 CLINICAL ONTOLOGIES

According to MEdline a clinical ontology is defined as a set of linked concepts. An ontology is intended to describe evidences to preserve the knowledge. There are several ontologies in information systems context. The OASIS organization normalized a language to share knowledge in the Web, the OWL.

The ontologies in the medical sciences are named terminologies.

There are some different terminologies in healthcare domain.

The selection of one terminology is related to the semantic objectives.

Some organizations like IHTSDO promoted the SNOMED-CT terminology, but other like ICD, LOINC and ICPC are also well known.

The discussion and analysis of the different terminologies is out of the scope of this paper.

The SNOMED-CT is widely used in medical services. This terminology has the possibility to add synonymous and cross tables to others codifications. It has also the possibility to be multilingual.

4 PROPOSED FRAMEWORK

This Framework is based on a RIM. The proposal of the RIM is in accordance with the ISO 21090. The model is based on archetypes to archive clinical data and to communicate between different systems.

The development goal is to use the classes defined in ISO 21090 and to model a system in which the archetypes are a specialization of this rule.

The classes defined by ISO 21090 are of different types. With these classes and the related basic data types it is possible to specify all the necessary variables associated with terminologies, persons' identification, locations, binary files from medical equipments and so on.

A new approach of enterprise modeling shows the benefit of business archetype pattern and Model Driven Architectures [15]. The model is formed by classes of objects with some mandatory implementations and others optional.

With the classes defined by this ISO 21090 it is possible to define a clinical data model using MDA (Model Drives Architectures), [15] and develop data patterns.

The terminology repository can be included in the RIM and modeled with MDA techniques. Using this methodology it is possible to have one or more sets of a terminology inside the RIM or even more than one terminology.

The services available on the platform can be modeled with MDA techniques. Once again it is possible to implement some or all the services in each platform. This benefit guarantees the portability and interoperability of the platform.

The platform developed with this framework will accomplish all the requirements defined by the ISO 18308.

The proposed model has a Service Model component to access the terminologies, archetype model, ISO rules repository and Data repository.

The available methods are:

- Creation of objects and their instancing;
- Query of data objects;
- Update of data objects;
- Maintenance of MDA model;
- Browsing of terminologies;
- Maintenance of terminology.

The objects are defined by the MDA model of classes.

There are some archetypes editors available to edit the metadata structures. One of these editors is LinkEHR-Ed [16].

The Service Model consults the class model and instances the object with defined attributes and methods.

The type of each object and the ID that identifies the terminology concept are verified by the Service Model.

If an object is related with another already created object, the service model will establish the necessary links.

The queries and updates of data objects are made by the semantic contents, relationships and values of the attributes.

The MDA model can be created and updated with an MDA pattern. This pattern has all

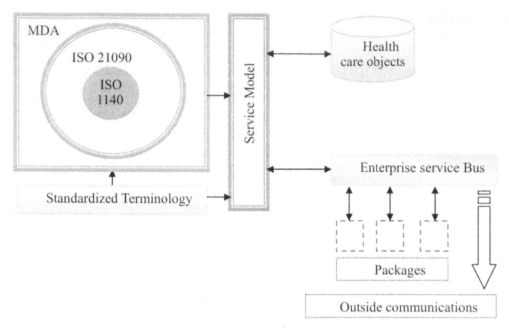

Figure 1. Framework model for e-Health services (authors' proposal).

mandatory classes, attributes and methods. The optional elements are marked and can be excluded from the model.

The Enterprise Service Bus is the component that establishes the communications with internal software applications and external services.

The Enterprise Service Bus has an engine of the business rules that is responsible for the integrity of transactions and its completeness.

There are a set of webservices which are available to integrate the internal software applications.

The communication with external software applications is also available by webservices.

This platform uses the ISO 13606 rule in order to normalize the communication of data with external applications.

This rule is available in the framework and normalizes the XML messages used to communicate clinical data.

The XML documents are available by webservices functions. These components are a part of a complete SOA (Service Oriented Architectute).

The SOA architecture to share clinical information as services has been cited by many authors, like Bridges [17].

The SOA architecture can include BPMS (Business Process Management System) to negotiate de services with ESB and to automate the workflows with the users and other external software applications. This approach was argued by Papakonstantinou [18].

To guarantee the semantic alignment, each message has an ID that identifies the used terminology and its version.

The data integrity and semantic alignment are by this way guaranteed.

5 CONCLUSIONS

The usage of ISO 13606, ISO 21090 and other related rules to model clinical information systems is undoubtedly the most suitable way to develop interoperability.

According to [19], *CEN EN13606 is one of the most promising approaches. It covers the technical needs for semantic interoperability and, at the same time, it incorporates a mechanism (archetype model) that enables clinical domain experts to participate in building an EHR system.*

The proposed framework has some benefits that makes possible a total integration of data and services.

This framework can be adapted to the needs and sizes of the different hospitals.

It is also possible to upgrade the models without losing their integrity.

The usage of an Enterprise Service Bus allows the integration with all the software applications that use this technology.

The usage of an engine of business rules makes the model very flexible and robust.

The usage of ISO 13606 to communicate with other platforms makes this model suitable with any other normalized platform.

Finally, the framework is independent of the programming languages, database management systems and other technologies selected.

REFERENCES

[1] TC215, I. *Requirements for an Electronic Health Record Reference Architecture.* 2000; Available from: http://secure.cihi.ca/cihiweb/en/downloads/info-stand_ihisd_isowg1_TSV0.5_e.pdf

[2] Lloyd, D. and D. Kalra. *EHR Requirements.* n.d.; Available from: http://eprints.ucl.ac.uk/1583/1/A5.pdf

[3] ISO 11404, *Information technology—General Purpose Datatypes (GPD),* 2007.

[4] ISO 21090, *Health Informatics—Harmonized data types for information interchange.*

[5] Beale, T. *Null Flavours and Boolean data in openEHR* 2007; Available from: http://www.openehr.org/wiki/display/spec/Null+Flavours+and+Boolean+data+in+openEHR

[6] ISO 18308, in *Meetings ISO/TC 215/WG1* 2002.

[7] ISO 13606, *Health informatics—Electronic health record communication.*

[8] ISO TC215. *TC215 Working Group.* Available from: http://www.tc215wg3.nhs.uk/documents/docs09

[9] Bernstein, K., et al., *Can openEHR archetypes be used in a national context? The Danish archetype proof-of-concept project.* Stud Health Technol Inform, 2009. 150: pp. 147–51.

[10] HL7, *HL7 Reference Information Model* 2003.

[11] Bointner, K. and Duftschmid, G. *HL7 template model and EN/ISO 13606 archetype object model— a comparison.* Stud Health Technol Inform, 2009. 150: p. 249.

[12] Wendy Huang. *Proposal: New PersonalRelationship-RoleType codes.* 2009; Available from: http://wiki.hl7.org/index.php?title = Proposal:_New_Personal-RelationshipRoleType_codes

[13] OpenEhr. *openEHR Architecture.* 2007.

[14] Ma, C. et al., *EHR query language (EQL)—a query language for archetype-based health records.* Stud Health Technol Inform, 2007. 129 (Pt 1): pp. 397–401.

[15] Arlow, J. and Neustadt, I. *Enterprise Patterns and MDA,* ed. Szyperski, C. 2004: Addison Wesley.

[16] Maldonado, J.A. et al., *LinkEHR-Ed: a multi-reference model archetype editor based on formal semantics.* Int J Med Inform, 2009. 78(8): pp. 559–70.

[17] Bridges, M.W., *SOA in healthcare, Sharing system resources while enhancing interoperability within and between healthcare organizations with service-oriented architecture.* Health Manag Technol, 2007. 28(6): p. 6, 8, 10.

[18] Papakonstantinou, D., Malamateniou, F. and Vassilacopoulos, G. *Using ESB and BPEL for evolving healthcare systems towards SOA.* Stud Health Technol Inform, 2008. 136: pp. 747–52.

[19] Brass, A. et al., *Standardized and Flexible Health Data Management with an Archetype Driven EHR System (EHRflex).* Stud Health Technol Inform, 2010. 155: pp. 212–8.

Technology and Medical Sciences – Natal Jorge et al. (eds)
© 2011 Taylor & Francis Group, London, ISBN 978-0-415-66822-4

A possibility for pos-EVAR surveillance: A novel smart stent-graft

Isa C.T. Santos & João Manuel R.S. Tavares
Instituto de Engenharia Mecânica e Gestão Industrial / Faculdade de Engenharia, Universidade do Porto, Portugal

L.A. Rocha
Institute for Polymers and Composites/I3 N, University of Minho, Portugal

S.M. Sampaio & R. Roncon-Albuquerque
Vascular Surgery Hospital S. João, Faculdade de Medicina, Universidade do Porto, Portugal

ABSTRACT: Aortic aneurysms can be deadly if not treated. Their modern treatment commenced in the early 1950's, but it was during the 1990's that was revolutionized by the introduction of EndoVascular Aneurysm Repair (EVAR). This minimally invasive procedure is frequently associated with advantages such as shortened hospital stays and the possibility to treat patients unfit for surgery. However, it requires long-term surveillance, which has important implications in the total cost. The development of a smart stent-graft, i.e., a stent-graft with some in-device mechanism to perform a given function and can communicate with an external element, could help mitigate this problem. This paper identifies the main users of a smart stent-graft and presentsitskey characteristics.

1 INTRODUCTION

An aneurysm is a localized, blood-filled dilation of an artery that, if not treated, may lead to death. It can appear anywhere but it occurs most commonly in the aorta, as well as in arteries located at the base of the brain and in the legs.

Abdominal Aortic Aneurysms (AAA), Figure 1, are the most frequent arterial aneurysm and, in spite of being relatively indolent, they are one of the causes of sudden death. In fact, in Europe, they represent the 12th cause of death and, in the U.S., the 13th (Wilt et al. 2006), affecting around 12 to 15 per 100 000 persons-year (Ricotta II et al. 2009).

Among the AAA's risk factors age is an important one andmales over 65 years oldare predominantly affected by this disease (McPhee et al. 2009). Taking into consideration that, currently, approximately 16% of the European population is aged 65 or over and projections estimate that this value will boom to more than 28% in the year 2050, the disease's incidence is expected to increase.

Since the early 1950's, aneurysms' standard treatment has consisted in an open surgery (done under general anesthesia) and the replacement of the diseased segment of the aorta by a synthetic prosthetic graft (Myers et al. 2001), Figure 2. In spite of its invasiveness and the fact of being limited to fit patients, this treatment is still a current practice and less invasive techniques are being studied to minimize its disadvantages.

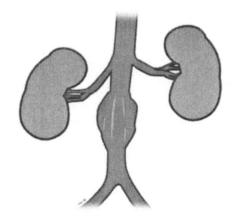

Figure 1. Abdominal Aortic Aneurysm (AAA).

In the beginning of the 1990's, the treatment was revolutionized when Parodi et al. demonstrated that endovascular aneurysm repair (EVAR) was a safe and feasible practice (Parodi et al. 1991).

EVAR is a minimally invasive procedure done percutaneously, Figure 3. Typically, a small incision is made in each groin to expose the femoral arteries. Then, with the aid of catheters and guidewires, a stent-graft is guidedto the affected artery segment allowing blood to pass without exerting pressure in the aneurysm sac and, thus, preventing wall rupture.

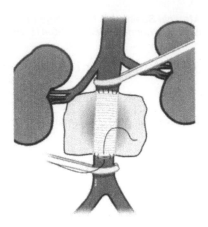

Figure 2. Conventional treatment of AAA's, open surgery.

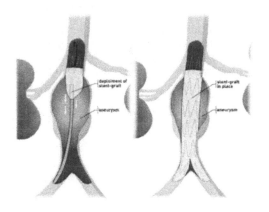

Figure 3. EndoVascular Aneurysm Repair (EVAR), stent-graft deployment sequence.

This surgical procedure is commonly associated with less physiological derangement, lower morbidity and mortality, and early return to full activity. Nonetheless, late complications, such as stent-graft migration, endoleaks or module disconnection, still occur (Katzen et al. 2006), compelling long-term surveillance that is responsible for increased costs and, thus, compromises the cost-benefit relation.

This paper describes the early stages of the development of a smart stent-graft, i.e., a stent-graft with monitoring capabilities. Such device would help to attenuate surveillance costs and improve the patient's quality of life, since it could regularly send information regarding the patient's health and the prosthesis performance to the doctor avoiding the dependence of expensive and potentially harmful imaging exams.

This paper is organized as follows. After a brief introduction to the disease and its treatment options, a review of the results of some EVAR cost-benefit analysis will be presented to clarify the need of a new medical device. Following, the potential users of the novel device will be identified and the device's key characteristics will be indicated. Finally, the conclusions and perspectives of future work will be pointed out.

2 EVAR COST BENEFIT

Comparing EVAR with conventional surgery, the first is preferable due to the fact of being less stressful and reducing significantly systemic complications (Rutherford et al. 2004), as well as having lower costs of inpatient stay and less or no need for intensive care facilities during recovery (Myers et al. 2001; Hayter et al. 2005). While a number of early studies appeared to support this claim, nowadays, data shows otherwise (Rutherford et al. 2004). Shorter stays at both intensive care units and the hospital, reduced use of blood, fewer laboratory studies and fewer resources lead to cost savings, but later,additional cost exist due to surveillance procedures. Currently, EVAR's surveillance protocol involves imaging at 1, 6, and 12 months after the procedure, and thereafter, on an annual basis (Milner et al. 2006).

The durability of open surgery, established with long-term follow-up studies, is excellent (Rutherford et al. 2004), so good that there is little or no requirement for long-term surveillance.

Hayter (Hayter et al. 2005) compared both hospital and follow-up costs of patients who had undergone EVAR or open surgery and concluded that EVAR costs were higher. One of the justifications presented was the endograft's high price.

Primary studies describe EVAR as being more economical because the price of the first stent-grafts was lower and excluded surveillance costs. Nowadays, EVAR can be considered cost-effective only for very elderly patients or those with a reduced life expectancy and doubtful for young patients, those who would benefit more from the short hospital stay and early return to full activity.

Considering the longer life expectancies and the rising public expectations for quality of life, EVAR is an attractive treatment. However, its cost-benefit relation can be jeopardized by the requirement of long-term surveillance. In order to reduce and even eliminate these exams, new surveillance technologies are being investigated and the most promising technique identified thus far is remote pressure sensing (Milner et al. 2006).

The authors believe that including sensing capabilities in a stent-graft will benefit EVAR's future. Yet, that may not be enough. Preliminary results of a recent survey regarding the ideal features of a stent-graft show that attention should be given to the devices adaptability and delivery profile. Another issue that should be considered is the price of the devices: a less expensive stent-graft is desirable.

3 STENT-GRAFT'S USERS

It has been proven that involving users in the medical device development process leads to sundry benefits for manufacturers. Not only they favor product innovation, as they give ideas for new products as well. Knowing the user's actual requirements and expectations it is possible to reduce development costs by identifying potential problems in an early stage. Another benefit is the possibility to improve the device's design, usability and safety (Shah et al. 2007).

Doctors, nurses and patients can be quoted as only few within the myriad of medical devices' possible users. Besides the variety, each group has a distinctive perspective given the fact the device is used differently and with dissimilar expectations by each of them. Nonetheless, all perspectives are important for the medical device's success, even if they are competing.

In Shah (Shah et al. 2008) a definition and a classification for medical device's users are proposed. The authors distinguish *medical device user* from *end-user*. The first refers to 'a person who uses a medical device for the treatment and/or care of him-/her-self or someone else', while the second refers to 'a person who is the ultimate beneficiary of the usage of a medical device and who can also be the user of a medical device if using the medical device for him-/her-self'.

In the case of stent-grafts, the *medical device user* is different from the *end-user*. While the first are the doctors involved in the treatment and the follow-up of the aortic diseases, the later are the patients that suffer from them.

With stent-graft's current design, patients only benefit from the protection against the blood pressure. However, if sensing capabilities are added, patients could also gain from less invasive follow-up protocols since imaging exams, and the consequent use of radiation and nephrotoxic contrast agents, would only be performed to confirm an alarm issued by the device. Reduction of costs is also expectable since patients would perform fewer imaging exams and reduce the number of doctor's appointments to verify the state of the stent-graft. A decrease in the number of visits to the doctor, would eliminate the inherent cost of the appointment, and would also contribute to the reduction of work hours lost by the patient and the person that eventually accompanies him. Ultimately, such device could lead to an improvement of the

quality of life since patients would be constantly monitored and a health professional would be warned if a problem occurred.

Stent-grafts are prostheses that are used inside the human body. As most patients are laymen concerning diseases of the aorta, they trust their surgeon to decide which device is best. A stent-graft with sensing capabilities will do more than just protect the artery, it will also transmit data which may make patients feel uncomfortable and ask doctors not to use such a device. Even if a smart stent-graft is cheaper, more efficient and pleases doctor's, it will only be successful if patients are willing to use it.

Doctors use stent-grafts to treat aortic diseases and, after the endovascular procedure, they have to perform imaging exams to verify both the health of the patient and the performance of the device. If sensing capabilities are added, doctors can learn about the aneurysm behavior after the introduction of a stent-graft. The information gathered could also alert doctors to problems that currently are difficult or impossible to detect, namely graft wear.

Doctors' involvement is essential for the development of a (smart) stent-graft because they not only know the disease, as well as they can identify potential complications and difficulties with current state-of-the-art treatment solutions.

4 SMART STENT-GRAFT CHARACTERISTICS

A smart stent-graft can be defined as a stent-graft with some in-device mechanism to perform a given function and can communicate with an external element.

Although there is still no commercial device available, it could be decomposed in three elements: a stent-graft, a sensing element and a display, Figure 4. The stent-graft, besides protecting the aneurysm from the blood pressure, has built-in sensing elements that are able to gather information concerning the patient's health and/or the prosthesis performance. The information gathered is then sent to an external element—a display—and can be used in the patient's diagnose or in the comprehension of the aneurysm's sac behavior after the implementation of the stent-graft.

Like a conventional stent-graft, the novel device will be classified as a class III medical device and,

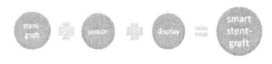

Figure 4. Decomposition of a smart stent-graft.

as such, will have to be biocompatible, biostable, non-toxic, non-allergic and non- carcinogenic. Furthermore, it will have to be tolerated by the human body not causing a foreign body reaction or an inflammatory reaction.

Regarding the mechanical requisites, the device should be durable, flexible, tough and yet ductile. Its components should also present resistance to both wear and tear, as well as excellent corrosion resistance.

For a successful protection of the blood vessel, the device should have a design as less invasive as possible in order to minimize flow resistance and pressure drops. Radial force is another relevant feature, not only for stents to stay open without being crushed with muscular activity, but also to provide a good seal and to ensure fixation.

The deployment of the device is a critical step for the procedure's success, thus, the stent-graft should have a low profile to facilitate the deployment and minimize lesions in the access arteries. At this stage, radiopacity is also crucial to ensure the correct positioning of the prosthesis.

From the commercial point of view, the device must be capable of being adequately sterilized and stored as an "off-the-shelf" product. A broad range of sizes is desirable since it allows the treatment of a wider array of anatomies.

One of the key questions in the design of a smart stent-graft regards the instrumentation capabilities required. Ideally, the device should be able to monitor its material degradation, detect migration and leakages.

Regarding the transmission of the measured data, the device must be able to transmit the data without any internal power. Moreover, the data cannot interfere with other implants nor be influenced by other electronic signals.

To assure patient's comfort and even reduce costs, the measurement protocol should be done duringthe doctor's appointmentor at home and the results transmitted to the doctor's office. Regardless where measurements are taken, the procedure should be quick, the least invasive as possible and avoid any kind of pain or even discomfort.

5 CONCLUSIONS AND FUTURE WORK

A stent-graft with sensing capabilities could help to alleviate the costs associated to EVAR follow-up protocols. Even so, it will not be surprising if, initially, the procedure costs increase since the introduction of new functions usually results in more expensive devices.

The success of the new endoprosthesis will depend on the ability to develop a stent-graft with an excellent performance and a lower price than the existent devices. Another factor that will surely influence the device's success is its adoption by the medical community. Thus, to effectively address the doctor's needs, the device must be developed jointly with them.

ACKNOWLEDGMENTS

The first author wishes to thank FCT—Fundação para a Ciência e Tecnologia, in Portugal, for the financial support provided by the grant SFRH/BD/42967/2008.

This work is partially supported by FCT under the project MIT-Pt/EDAM-EMD/0007/2008.

The authors also wish to thanks Miguel Marafuz (http://illustration-mfz.wordpress.com) for the illustrations.

REFERENCES

Hayter, C.L., Bradshaw, S.R. et al. 2005. Follow-up costs increase the cost disparity between endovascular and open abdominal aortic aneurysm repair. *Journal of Vascular Surgery* 42(5): 912–918.

Katzen, B.T. & MacLean, A.A. 2006. Complications of endovascular repair of abdominal aortic aneurysms: A review. *Cardio Vascular and Interventional Radiology* 29(6): 935–946.

McPhee, S.J. & Papadakis, M.A. 2009. Current medical diagnosis & treatment 2009. New York, Lange Medical Books/McGraw-Hill, Medical Publishing Division.

Milner, R., Kasirajan, K. et al. 2006. Future of endograft surveillance. *Seminars in Vascular Surgery* 19(2): 75–82.

Myers, K., Devine, T. et al. 2001. Endoluminal Versus Open repair for abdominal aortic aneurysms. *2nd Virtual Congress of Cardiology*.

Parodi, J.C., Palmaz, J.C. et al. 1991. Transfemoral intraluminal graft implantation for abdominal aortic aneurysms. *Annals of Vascular Surgery* 5(6): 491–499.

Ricotta II, J.J., Malgor, R.D. et al. 2009. Endovascular abdominal aortic aneurysm repair: Part I. *Annals of Vascular Surgery* 23(6): 799–812.

Rutherford, R.B. & Krupski, W.C. 2004. Current status of open versus endovascular stent-graft repair of abdominal aortic aneurysm. *Journal of Vascular Surgery* 39(5): 1129–1139.

Shah, S.G.S. & Robinson, I. 2007. Benefits of and barriers to involving users in medical device technology development and evaluation. *International Journal of Technology Assessment in Health Care* 23(01): 131–137.

Shah, S.G.S. & Robinson, I. 2008. Medical device technologies: who is the user? *International Journal of Healthcare Technology and Management* 9(2): 181–197.

Wilt, T., Lederle, F. et al. 2006. Comparison of endovascular and open surgical repairs for abdominal aortic aneurysm. Evidence report/technology assessment (144): 210.

Technology and Medical Sciences – Natal Jorge et al. (eds)
© 2011 Taylor & Francis Group, London, ISBN 978-0-415-66822-4

Analysis of the contraction of the pelvic floor through the finite element method considering different pathologies

T.H. da Roza, M.P.L. Parente & R.M. Natal Jorge
IDMEC—Faculty of Engineering, University of Porto, Porto, Portugal

T. Mascarenhas, J. Loureiro & S. Duarte
Faculty of Medicine, University of Porto, São João Hospital, Porto, Portugal

ABSTRACT: Pelvic floor disorders are high prevalent diseases that affect different aged women. Two of the most common conditions are urinary incontinence and Pelvic Organ Prolapse (POP) which is a major health care problem, with of 11% of women undergoing surgery for POP and/or urinary incontinence during life time. Statistical studies show that 30% of those women will be subject to a repeated surgery. Dynamic magnetic resonance (MRI) imaging is an important diagnostic tool used to stage or evaluate POP. The acquisition speed during imaging makes these dynamic assessments possible. MRI allows to generate 3D solids of pelvic floor muscles through manual segmentation. These 3D solids are discretized to apply the Finite Element Method (FEM) to study the biomechanical behavior of pelvic floor muscles contributing to analyze this complex musculature structure. The aim of this study is to build the pelvic floor muscle and simulate, through the finite element method the contraction into two distinct disorders: urinary incontinence and prolapsed. It was found that women with incontinence can keep the force of contraction in higher values than with prolapsed. The present work shows a methodology that can be applied in the pelvic floor biomechanics.

1 INTRODUCTION

Pelvic Floor Muscles (PFM) play an essential role in the support and functioning of the pelvic organs. 'Levator ani' is the collective term used to describe the deep PFM. The levator ani consists primarily of the striated muscles pubococcygeus (PC), puborectalis (PR) and iliococcygeus (IC) (Wall, 1993). In healthy women at rest, the levator ani muscles are in contraction, thereby keeping the rectum, vagina, and urethra elevated and closed by pressing them anteriorly toward the pubic symphysis (DeLancey, 1993).

Pelvic floor disorders include a group of conditions that affect adult women including pelvic organ prolapse, urinary incontinence, fecal incontinence, and other sensory and emptying abnormalities of the lower urinary and gastrointestinal tracts. It is estimated that one or more of these conditions affect up to one-third of adult women (Olsen et al. 1997).

Pelvic Organ Prolapsed (POP) is a major health care problem, with 11% of women undergoing surgery for POP and/or urinary incontinence during life time. Statistical studies show that 30% of those women will be subject to a repeated surgery (Olsen et al. 1997).

Pelvic floor prolapsed is a common female condition characterized by symptomatic descent of the bladder (cystocele), uterus or vagina (uterine or vaginal vault prolapse), small bowel (enterocele), or rectum (rectocele) (Fielding, 2002).

Urinary Incontinence (UI) is a manifestation of several different types of injury and disease processes of the lower urinary tract or the part of the nervous system that regulates it. According to the International Continence Society (ICS) (Abrams et al. 2002), UI is defined as any involuntary leakage of urine. The pathophysiology of UI involves an overactive detrusor or an incompetent urethral sphincter. Therefore, the three most common types of UI are Stress Urinary Incontinence (SUI), Urge Urinary Incontinence (UUI) or a combination of stress and urge known as Mixed Urinary Incontinence (MUI).

Magnetic Resonance Imaging (MRI) is increasingly used to assess pelvic anatomy in women with pelvic floor disorders, where his image produces detailed pictures of the soft tissues of the pelvic floor (Klutke et al. 1995). This technique holds great promise because of its potential for identifying injuries to the muscles and fascia of the pelvic floor.

MR images allows to generate three-dimensional (3D) solids of pelvic floor muscles through manual segmentation. To study the biomechanical behavior of pelvic floor muscles contributing to analyze this complex musculature structure (Janda et al. 2003), these 3D solids are descritezed to apply the Finite Element Method (FEM) (Parente et al. 2008).

The purpose of this study is to simulatethe contraction of pubovisceral muscle (composed of the pubococcygeal and puborectal muscles,) using the finite element method on computational meshes based on MR images.

2 MATERIALS AND METHODS

Were selected two women with the same age (64 years) but with different dysfunctions, one of them had mixed urinary incontinenceand the other had prolapse in the anterior and posterior compartment.

The MR images were acquired from the subject supine position, using a 3.0 T system. Field view of the exam was 25×25 cm, 2 mm thick with no gap. The subjects were asked not to contract the pelvic floor during imaging. This study used twenty consecutive images obtained in the axial plane for each of the women.

2.1 Building procedure

Each model was built, from a set of MR images obtained in DICOM -Digital Imaging and Communications in Medicine- format and subsequently converted to jpeg format, with all dimensions of the initial image. After the preparation of images to use, one can start the construction of the model, using CAD software. Thus it is created a set of parallel plans, separated according to the value at which the MR images were obtained.

The images were inserted in the plans and the outline of the pubovisceral muscle is drawn, then, all the images are linked and finally, the 3D geometrical model is generated, this process can be seen in Figure 1.

2.2 Finite element method

After the construction of the 3D solid, the model is saved in format STEP—Standard for the Exchange of product model data- and exported to the softher of numerical simulation "ABAQUS" to create the numerical model.

The finite element mesh (Figure 2) was generated using ABAQUS finite element tool. The meshconsisted of tetrahedron solid elements type C3D4, and the analyses were made through

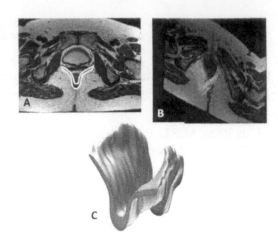

Figure 1. We can see the contour spline around the structure (A) then, all the images are linked (B) and the 3D model (C).

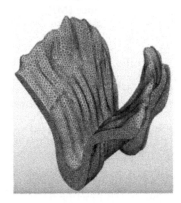

Figure 2. Pubovisceral muscle of the prolapsed woman under finite element method.

the same software. The methodologies presented by D'Aulignac (2005) and Parente (2008) were followed.

This new numerical model is now ready to be used in Finite Element Method simulations. For the simulation of the PF contraction the ABAQUS software was used based on a UMAT subroutine containing such formulation of the active muscle (Parente et al. 2009). This mathematical model is based in the following strain energy density function:

$$U = U_I\left(\bar{I}_1^C\right) + U_J\left(J\right) + U_f\left(\bar{\lambda}_f, \alpha\right) \tag{1}$$

where the first term is related to the embedding matrix, the second one is associated with volume change and third one is the fiber term.

In order to simulate the intra-abdominal pressure a distributed load of 1×10^{-1} MPa was applied—in

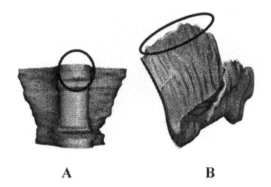

A   **B**

Figure 3. Boundary conditions in coccix (A) and the tops of laterals (B).

ventral surface. After that and while that pressure was maintained, the muscle activation ranged between 10%, 50% and 100% of maximum contraction puboviceral muscle is then applied.

2.3 Boundary Conditions (BC)

Two boundary conditions were applied:

- One in the region in which the levator ani makes contact with the coccyx (in the posterior part);
- Another one in the top of the sides, where the pelvic floor muscles is linked with the obturator fascia (right and left) and tendinous arch of levator ani muscle.

Displacements were restricted in the directions X, Y and Z, for the two boundaries.

Pathological anatomy refers that women with prolapse present some lack of connection between the puboviceral with the fascia and/or with the tendinous arch. Thus we can consider that this part was "lost", without boundary conditions (see in Figure 3).

3   RESULTS AND DISCUSSION

In order to compute the final deformation of the puboviceral muscle, three levels of forces were applied: 10%, 50% and 100% from maximal contraction. Displacements were recorded in cranium-caudal direction (Graphics 1 and 2).

These graphs show different behaviors between women with prolapse and with incontinence. The curves from women with prolapse present very small movements (on the left of the graph) when compared with the other graph. The women with prolapse can not reach the movement of women with incontinence even with maximum contraction (100%).

Another finding (see graphics 1 and 2) is that women with incontinence can keep the force of

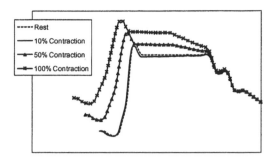

Graph 1.   Simulation of contraction pelvic floor in woman with prolapse.

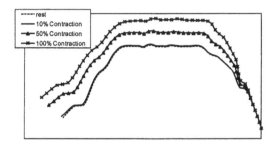

Graph 2.   Simulation of contraction pelvic floor in woman with incontinence.

Table 1.   Displacements' average found in cranium-caudal direction in both women.

	Displacement (mm)	
	Prolapse woman	Incontinence woman
10% Contraction	0.22	0.12
50% Contraction	1.87	1.84
100% Contraction	3.62	3.39

contraction in higher values than with prolapse in the 2 compartment.

In women with prolapsed can be noted, manly, in the posterior compartment she cannot perform the contraction. This region is one where we did not perform the boundary conditions, because in MRI we can see that there was no connection with the fascia or the arch.

4   CONCLUSIONS

The present work shows a methodology that can be applied in the pelvic floor biomechanics. The constitutive law and parameters used here to compose biomechanics finite element analyses were adequate to simulate contraction in a pelvic floor in 3D model.

It is important to highlight that awareness of the correct contraction of the pelvic floor is difficult to learn. However, this methodology is a technique, to obtain 3D models of anatomical structures based on MR images. It may bepossible to analyze the different behaviors of the contraction of pelvic floor in distinct pathologies. Should be evaluated with the useof more 3D models including different types of pathology and compare them with the medical findings on MRI.

ACKNOWLEDGEMENTS

The authors truly acknowledge the funding provided by Ministério da Ciência, Tecnologia e Ensino Superior—Fundação para a Ciência e a Tecnologia (Portugal) and by FEDER, under grant PTDC/SAU-BEB/71459/2006.

REFERENCES

Abrams, P. Cardoso, L. Griffiths, D. Rosier, P. Uvan Kerrebroeck, P. Victor, A. & Wein, A. 2002. Standardisation Sub-committee of the International Continence Society. The standardization of terminology of lower urinary tract function: report from the standardization sub-committee of the international Continence society. Neurourol Urodyn. 21:167–178.

Aulignac, D. Martins, J. Pires, E. Mascarenhas, T. & Natal Jorge, R. 2005. A shell finite element model of the pelvic floor muscles. Comp Met Biomech and Biom Eng. 8: 339–347.

DeLancey J.O.L. 1993. Anatomy and biomechanics of genital prolapse. Clin Obstet Gynecol. 36: 897–909.

Fielding, J.R. 2002. Practical MR Imaging of Female Pelvic Floor Weakness. RadioGraphics. 22: 295–304.

Janda, S. Van der Helm, F.C.T. & Blok, S.B. 2003. Mensuring morphological parameters of the pelvic floor for finite elements modeling purpose. J Biomech. 36: 749–757.

Klutke, C.G. & Siegel, C.L. 1995. Functional female pelvic anatomy. Urol Clin North Am. 22: 487–98.

Olsen, A.L. Smith, V.J. Bergstrom, J.O. et al. 1997. Epidemiology of surgically managed pelvic organ prolapse and urinary incontinence. Obstet Gynecol. 89: 501–506.

Parente, M.P.L. Natal Jorge, R.M. Mascarenhas, T. Fernandes, A.A. & Martins, J.A.C. 2008. Deformation of the pelvi floor muscles during a vaginal delivery. International Urogynecology J. 19: 65–71.

Parente, M.P.L. Natal Jorge, R.M. Mascarenhas, T. Fernandes, A.A. & Martins, J.A.C. 2009. The influence of the material properties on the biomechanical behavior of the pelvic floor during a vaginal delivery. Journal of Biomechanics. 42: 1301–1306.

Wall, N. 1993. The muscles of the pelvic floor. Clin Obstet Gynaecol. 36: 911–923.

Technology and Medical Sciences – Natal Jorge et al. (eds)
© *2011 Taylor & Francis Group, London, ISBN 978-0-415-66822-4*

Anticipatory postural adjustments in post-stroke subjects during reaching

S. Ferreira, C. Silva, P. Carvalho, A. Silva & R. Santos
Centro de Estudos do Movimento e Actividade Humana (CEMAH-ESTSP), Oporto, Portugal

ABSTRACT: The Anticipatory Postural Adjustments (APAs) study in post-stroke subjects during reaching, aimed to explore the existence of impairments at the activation timings of the serratus anterior, superior, middle and inferior trapezius fibers, in relation to the contralateral upper limb and healthy subjects. Methods: Electromyographic and kinematic analysis was performed during reaching of a glass placed ipsilaterally to the upper limb in study, in the seated postural set; both upper limbs were assessed separately. Results: At the inferior fibers of the left trapezius and the serratus anterior bilaterally, were found differences in the activation timings between the studied groups. No differences were found in the activation timings between the two sides of the subjects; no relation was established between the first and the velocity or handedness. Through these data, the neuronal activation patterns were inferred in cortical and subcortical lesions.
Conclusion: APAs were found in some muscles in post-stroke subjects.

Keywords: Anticipatory postural adjustments; Stroke; Electromyography; Scapular stabilizers; Reaching

1 INTRODUCTION

In order to preserve the equilibrium during voluntary movement, the Central Nervous System (CNS) uses internal models to anticipate and adapt to the forces exerted. One of the mechanisms of the postural control is the Anticipatory Postural Adjustments (APAs) that, based on the movement experience and using somatossensorial information, consist of the muscular activation previously to the perturbation inducted by the movement, occurring between the 100 ms preceding and lasting till 50 ms following a prime mover's instant of activation (Shumway-Cook & Woollacott 2007; Matias et al. 2006; Aruin 2002; Ghez & Krakauer 2000, Massion 1992).

They can be separated in preparatory APAs (pAPAs) and accompanying APAs (aAPAs). The first, precede the movement often for more than 100 ms, contributing to its initiation as they maintain the stability, whereas the last occur in order to stabilize the body or body segment during the movement; a APAs are also anticipatory as they occur before any possibility of feedback (Schepens & Drew 2004).

The APAsare influenced by the postural task, action associated with the perturbation, magnitude and direction of the perturbation (Aruin 2002). Besides, there is controversy over the relation between the APAs and the movement velocity (Shiratori & Aruin 2007; Aruin 2002).

In individuals post-stroke the APAs are abolished or have a higher latencyin relation to healthy subjects (Aruin 2002, Cirstea & Levin 2000). For this reason, the study of the muscular activation patterns in these subjects is essential as a way to infer the neuronal activation patterns, as well as, the differences existing in cortical and subcortical lesions as in the last. Consequently, the aim of this study was to explore the existence of impairments in the muscular activation timings at the scapular stabilizers, mainly at the serratus anterior, superior, middle and inferior trapezius fibers, during reaching, in post-stroke subjects, comparing them between the two sides of each subject and establishing their relation to the handedness and velocity. Besides, it meant to compare the activation timings between the healthy subjects and post-stroke subjects, as well as, between cortical and subcortical lesions.

2 METHODS

2.1 Participants

A pilot study was developed in order to correct the questionnaire and the study protocol. A reliability study was also performed.

The sample consisted of 17 volunteers, selected by a questionnaire. These subjects were divided into 2 groups: Group 1and Group 2 with n = 10 and n = 7, respectively.

In Group 1 were selected healthy subjects without pain at least for 3 months and/or pathology in the shoulder or the neck (Matias et al. 2006); minimum of 45 years-old; absence of any neurological pathology. This group consisted of 10 subjects in which mean ± standard deviation were 52.40 ± 5.28 and 26.70 ± 2.91 for the age (in years) and the Body Mass Index (BMI), respectively.

The inclusion criteria for Group 2, i.e. post-stroke subjects, were: first cortical or subcortical isquemic stroke occurring in the middle cerebral artery, confirmed with Computerized Axial Tomography, with a minimum of 3 months of recovery (Fridman et al. 2004); absence of neglect as noted by a score of 52 ± 54 on the Star Cancellation Test (Zachowski et al. 2004); active range of motion on the predominantly affected side of at least 15° in the shoulder and elbow (Zachowski et al. 2004); absence of biomechanical impairments in soft tissue confirmed by two expert Physiotherapists with more than 10 years of experience in the neurological field; ability to remain in the sitting postural set without support for at least 5 minutes; Mini-mental State Examination with a minimum score of 23 (Canadian Stroke Network 2010a). As exclusion criteria were selected: elevation of the upper limb restricted to the coronal plane (Takahashi & Reinkensmeyer 2003); pain or subluxation of the shoulder (Cirstea & Levin 2000). Therefore, Group 2 consisted of 7 post-stroke subjects in which mean ± standard deviation were 56.57 ± 7.39 and 32.86 ± 4.91 for the age and the BMI, respectively. Their characteristics are exposed in Table 1, including the score of the "Arm Section" of the Rivermead Motor Assessment Scale (RMA).

Every post-stroke subject, with the exception of subject 6, presented subcortical lesions in the internal capsule, involving the diencephalon. The referred subject had a lesion affecting the corona radiata. Due to this fact, we compared the results of this group with the existing evidence relative

Table 1. Characteristics of the post-stroke subjects composing Group 2.

| Subject | Hemisphere | Time since stroke | |
		Months	RMA*
1	Right	7	5
2	Left	6	12
3	Right	92	1
4	Left	20	3
5	Right	87	4
6	Right	37	11
7	Left	11	2

RMA*: indicates Rivermead Motor Assessment.

to the neuronal activation patterns post-cortical stroke.

Every participant presented right upper limb dominance.

2.2 Instruments

The Star Cancellation Test has an excellent test-retest reliability (Intraclass Correlation Coefficient, ICC = 0.89) and a predictive validity of 0.55 (Bailey et al. 2004). On the other hand, the Mini-mental State Examination presents moderate sensitivity (62%) and good specificity (88%) (Canadian Stroke Network 2010b). Finally, the RMA has an excellent test-retest reliability (r = 0.88) (Canadian Stroke Network 2010c).

The electromyographic activity (EMG) of the anterior deltoid (considered the prime mover), serratus anterior, superior, middle and inferiortrapezius fiberswas registeredwith MP100 WSW Data Acquisition System and Acqknowledge 3.9.0 Data Acquisition and Analysis Software version(sampling frequency: 1000 Hz) (BIOPAC Systems, Inc., Goleta, USA), using TSD150B active electrodes (BIOPAC Systems, Inc., Goleta, USA).

Kinematics were recordedusing one camera Sony Handycam DCR-HC53 (sampling frequency: 50 Hz) (Sony Portugal, Lisbon, Portugal) and subsequently analyzed with 12.1.0.10 APAS Software version (Ariel Performance Analysis System, Ariel Dynamics Inc., Canyon, USA). In the reliability study was determined an intra-rater reliability (ICC) of 0.991 and a Standard Error of Measurement (SEM) of 2.447 (cm).

2.3 Procedure

In order to determine their dominant upper limb, the subjects were asked about which upper limb they used to perform several daily tasks (Coelho 2006).

The assessment was performed in the seated postural set (without trunk support) and the feet in full contact with the ground or a stable foot stool (Levin et al. 2002, Tyler & Hasan 1995). The experimental seat height was normalized by placing it at a height equivalent to each subject's lower leg length, that was measured from the lateral knee joint line to the ground, with the subject standing barefoot. Besides, 75% of the thigh length, measured from the lateral knee joint line to the greater trochanter, was supported on the marquise (Levin et al. 2002).

The subjects reached a glass placed ipsilaterally to the upper limb in study, with both upper limbs separately, at 30° from the frontal plane (Faria et al. 2008). The glass was placed according to the subject's stretched upper limb length, measured from the medial axilla to the distal wrist crease (i.e. within the anatomical reaching distance for the hand) (Levin et al. 2002; Michaelsen et al. 2001), on the top of a table with 73 cm of height, which limit was coincident with the distal border of the subject's thigh.

After the skin preparation, the active electrodes were placed over the surface of the Anterior Deltoid (AD), Serratus Anterior (SA), Superior (ST), Middle (MT) and Inferior (IT) Trapezius fibers (interelectrode distance 20 mm) according to the SENIAM Project (n.d.) and Faria et al. (2008) references. The reference electrode was placed over the contralateral olecranon and the signal's quality was verified as stated by Faria et al. (2008) and Matias et al. (2006).

Reflective markers were placed at the dominant upper limb in Group 1 and at the predominantly affected upper limb in Group 2 on the following landmarks: dorsal surface of the head of the second metacarpal, lateral epicondyle of the humerus, mid-sternum, acromion process, tragus, greater trochanter and spinous process of the seventh cervical vertebrae (Levin et al. 2002; Fits et al. 1998).

The subjects maintained the upper limb in study resting in the ipsilateral thigh, with the shoulder at 0° of flexion / extension, or abduction / adduction, with the elbow close to the side of the body (Michaelsen et al. 2001).

The subjects were asked to reach the glass as fast as possible (Barthélémy and Boulinguez 2002) after an auditory signal; no instructions relatively to the trunk behavior were transmitted (Tyler and Hasan 1995). Three trials were performed separately by one minute in order to avoid fatigue (Wolf et al. 1998).

2.4 Data analysis

A temporal analysis of the EMG data was performed off-line with the Acqknowledge 3.9.0. (BIOPAC Systems, Inc., Goleta, USA). The signal was filtered with a high-pass filter of 50 Hz (www. biopac.com) and a band-pass filter of 20 and 450 Hz (Matias et al. 2006). The onset of EMG activity was determined by the time at which the EMG activity exceeded the mean level of 500 ms of baseline activity by 2 standard deviations, for a minimum of 30 ms (Dickstein et al. 2004). It was considered that an APA preceded the movement by 100 ms and lasted till 50 ms after the onset of the EMG activity of the anterior deltoid muscle (Shumway-Cook & Woollacott 2007, Matias et al. 2006; Latash et al. 1995). The axioscapular muscles' latency was estimated through the mean value obtained by the subtraction of their activationtimings to the value determined for the

anterior deltoid in the trials performed (Matias et al. 2006).

In order to establish the relation between the activation timings and the velocity, the movement duration was defined as the time elapsed between the moment at which the hand started to move, till the moment at which it reached the glass. The movement distance (i.e. upper limb length) was divided by the movement duration to determine the velocity.

The trunk displacement was estimated through the kinematic analysis of the x and y coordinates of the acromion using the 12.1.0.10 APAS software (Ariel Dynamics Inc., Canyon, USA).

2.5 Ethics

All subjects gave their informed consent according to the Declaration of Helsinki (1964).

2.6 Statistics

SPSS Statistics 17.0 (IBM SPSS Statistics, Chicago, USA) was used for the statistical analysis. Because of the small sample size and non-normal distribution of the data, non-parametric statistical tests were used.

The descriptive statistics was used to describe the activation timings of Groups 1 and 2 subjects. Besides, the Wilcoxon test was used to compare the activation timings between the two sides of each subject and the trunk displacement (in Group 2), allowing, in the first case, the inference of their relation to the handedness. On the other hand, the Mann-Whitney test was performed to compare the activation timings, as well as, the velocity and the trunk displacement, between Group 1 and Group 2 subjects. Finally, the correlation between the activation timings and the movement velocity, in addition to the correlation between the activation timings and the trunk displacement, was established through the Spearman's correlation coefficient.

Differences with a P value < 0.05 were considered to be statistically significant.

3 RESULTS

The medians / means and respective interquartile deviations / standard deviations of the EMG signals were estimated and are displayed in Tables 2 and 3.

The median was selected as the comparison measure of the results, as it represents a real value of the sample (Matias et al. 2006).

Due to the anthropometric characteristics of subjects 3 and 6 of Group 2, it wasn't possible to record EMG signals from both the serratus anterior

Table 2. Medians / means, respective interquartile deviations / standard deviations of the activation timings of the muscles in study in Group 1, in milliseconds (ms), relatively to the anterior deltoid, and P values of the Wilcoxon test.

Muscle	Left median (ms)	Left mean (ms)	Right median (ms)	Right mean (ms)	P value
ST*	52.8 (35.2)	61.5 (69.4)	59.3 (26.4)	118.8 (244.3)	0.867
MT**	17.3 (35.3)	14.1 (54.4)	8.8 (29.8)	18.8 (41.2)	0.846
IT***	3.0 (36.4)	15.7 (55.8)	−3.0 (25.9)	19.7 (38.4)	0.322
SA****	24.5 (40.9)	40.9 (64.9)	34.8 (51.5)	50.8 (69.2)	0.770

ST*, MT**, IT***: indicates superior, middle and inferior trapezius fibers, respectively; SA****: serratus anterior.

Table 3. Medians / means and respective interquartile deviations / standard deviations of the activation timings of the muscles in study in Group 2, in milliseconds (ms), relatively to the anterior deltoid, and P values of the Wilcoxon test.

Muscle	Left median (ms)	Left mean (ms)	Right median (ms)	Right mean (ms)	P value
ST*	14.0 (93.5)	−40.1 (110.9)	23.5 (127.8)	120.3 (239.8)	0.469
MT**	−5.5 (33.5)	−1.7 (88.3)	−23.0 (44.0)	−25.6 (152.0)	0.688
IT***	126.5 (49.3)	97.6 (72.6)	31.0 (160.5)	54.1 (182.2)	0.578
SA****	216.5 (144.2)	194.1 (148.2)	153.5 (237.9)	292.6 (334.5)	0.625

ST*, MT**, IT***: indicates superior, middle and inferior trapezius fibers, respectively; SA****: serratus anterior.

muscles; so, these results were considered missing values. In these Tables are also referred the P values of the Wilcoxon test for the activation timings of the muscles in study. Therefore, there weren't significant differences in the distribution of the activation timings of the muscles in study between both sides of each subject of Groups 1 and 2, i.e. it can't be affirmed that the distribution of the activation timings was statistically different according to the dominant upper limb.

There were statistical evidences to conclude that the distributions of the variables activation timings of the inferior fibers of the left trapezius ($P = 0.043$), right and left serratus anterior ($P = 0.028$), were significantly different in Groups

1 and 2, which was not verified in the rest of the muscles (P (left ST) = 0.055, P (left MT) = 0.740, P (right ST) = 0.459, P (right MT) = 0.270, P (right IT) = 0.887).

Besides, there were statistical evidences that the distribution of the variable velocity was significantly different in the right and left movements of both Groups ($P = 0.000$ and $P = 0.009$, respectively). However, there weren't sufficient statistical evidences that this variable was significantly correlated with the activation timings of the muscles in study (Group 1: P (left TS) = 0.726, P (left TM) = 0.446, P (left TI) = 0.556, P (left SA) = 0.385, P (right TS) = 0.894, P (right TM) = 0.521, P (right TI) = 0.220, P (right SA) = 0.498 / Group 2: P (left TS) = 0.432, P (left TM) = 0.535, P (left TI) = 0.645, P (left SA) = 0.188, P (right TS) = 0.337, P (right TM) = 0.432, P (right TI) = 0.939, P (right SA) = 0.624).

There weren't sufficient statistical evidences that the variable trunk displacement was significantly different in both sides of Groups 2 subjects ($P = 0.688$), as well as, between Groups 1 and 2 ($P = 0.669$ and $P = 0.813$, respectively). On the other hand, this variable wasn't significantly correlated with the activation timings of the muscles in study, with the exception of the left superior trapezius fibersin Group 2 (Group 1: P (left TS) = 0.489, P (left TM) = 0.829, P (left TI) = 0.803, P (left SA) = 0.934, P (right TS) = 0.089, P (right TM) = 0.108, P (right TI) = 0.556, P (right SA) = 0.048 / Group 2: P (left TS) = 0.036, P (left TM) = 0.645, P (left TI) = 0.294, P (left SA) = 0.624, P (right TS) = 0.939, P (right TM) = 0.383, P (right TI) = 0.294, P (right SA) = 0.285).

4 DISCUSSION

In the present study were verified significant differences in the activation timings of the serratus anterior bilaterally and the inferior left trapezius fibers between Groups 1 and 2. No differences were found in the other muscles in study, which may be related to impairments in the scapular alignment, particularly observed in Group 2 subjects; on the other hand, these differences might, as well, be associated with the typical shifting of the body weight towards the less affected side observed in post-stroke subjects (Slijper et al. 2002).

On the other hand, no statistically significant differences were found in the activation timings of the serratus anterior, superior, middle and inferior trapezius fibers in both sides of each subject in Groups 1 and 2. Teyssèdre et al. (2000) found a similar muscular pattern of APAs in the dominant and non-dominant upper limb in healthy subjects as well, in the pointing movement, but with an inferior latency at the external oblique in the dominant upper limb. This may be relatedto the task's constraintsand aims, that are distinct from the reaching movement (Shumway-Cook & Woollacott 2007).

These results might reflect the existence of homolog neuronal activation patterns between both sides of each subject, as verified by Luft et al. (2004) in subcortical lesions, i.e. in the population in study the handedness might not have a significant influence in the referred patterns.

The neuronal activation patterns are the outcome of the cortical reorganization that occurs after stroke and presenta high variability, probably related with the location, extension and duration of the respective lesion (Fridman et al. 2004, Byrnes et al. 2001, Cao et al. 1998). Therefore, several studies report an increase in the cortical activation of secondary motor areas such as the premotor cortex, supplementary motor area and cingulate motor area, with variation in the activation magnitude between subjects (Ward et al. 2006, Cao et al. 1998).

According to Fridman et al. (2004), in subcortical lesions, the ipsilesional premotor cortex presents corticomotoneuronal connections, at least as strong as those that remain intact in the ipsilesional primary motor cortex. Besides, the first connects with the rubrospinal and reticulospinal systems; the last, on the other hand, has connections with the vestibulospinal system through the vestibulocerebellum (Brodal 2004; Shelton & Reding 2001). Hence, the premotor cortex and other medial cortical areas as the supplementary motor area and the cingulate motor area, present corticospinal neurons that form a bilateral corticoreticulospinal route (Brodal 2004; Seitz et al. 1998). The activation of contralesional precentral areas in subjects with lesions at the internal capsule and corona radiata (Luft et al. 2004), as well as, the activation of the corticoreticulospinal route (also performed by ipsilesional areas) (Mazevet et al. 2003) might, in part, explain the presence of APAs in Group 2 subjects, in some of the muscles in study.

It also would be important to perform statistical tests to verify the distribution of the variables activation timing, velocity and trunk displacement in subjects post-stroke divided by the affected hemisphere. However, the reduced number of subjects present in each sub-group, restricted the referred tests.

No significant correlation was found between the activation timings and the velocity; thus, these results point up the absence of a significant relation between the activation timings and the velocity during reaching in this population. Similar results were found by Teyssèdre et al. (2000), in the pointing movement; Shiratori & Aruin (2007)

reported that in voluntary movements, the velocity didn't modulate the APAs in lower limb and trunk muscles.

Furthermore, no significant differences in trunk displacement were found between the two sides of each Group 2 subject, in addition to between Groups 1 and 2 subjects; no significant correlation was found between the activation timings and the trunk displacement in both groups, with the exception of the left superior trapezius fibers, which can be due to the cited alignment impairments and weight shifting, or the SEM of 2,447 cm in the kinematic analysis that could impede the detection of more significant differences. Consequently, it can be concluded that the trunk displacement probably wasn't used as a compensatory strategy in Group 2 subjects, which might be related to the presence of APAs in part of the studied muscles (depending on the side considered).

According to Shelton & Reding (2001) and Seitz et al. (1999), after cortical strokes, occurs the activation of cortical areas as the premotor cortex; in more extensive lesions, occurs the activation of the ipsilesional premotor cortex and supplementary motor area, as well as, the contralesional premotor cortex and primary motor cortex. Therefore, there isn't a complete interruption of the cortical output to the rubrospinal, reticulospinal and vestibulospinal systems (Shelton & Reding 2001). These facts indicate that subjects with cortical lesions may present APAs.

In subjects with excellent recovery post-stroke, in either cortical or subcortical lesions, occurs a bilateral enhanced activation or overactivation of non-affected sensory and primary / secondary motor areas. However, in cortical lesions there's a strong activation of peri-lesioned areas, in addition to the ipsilesional premotor cortex (Calautti & Baron 2003).

The ipsilesional activation of other areas may be the result of the recruitment of neuronal projections normally inhibited, composing the anterolateral corticospinal tract, that is involved in the upper limb proximal activity, presenting projections from secondary motor areas (Caramia et al. 2000).

Slijper et al. (2002) reported the preservation of the APAs in post-stroke subjects, as well as, the increased latency particularly in the predominantly affected limb, or their absence in the performance of movements at the subject's maximal velocity, which demonstrates the variability of muscular activation patterns probably resultant of the variability of neuronal activation patterns (Ward et al. 2006, Fridman et al. 2004, Byrnes et al. 2001).

This study presents as limitations the reduced sample size and external validity, as well as, the absence of participants and observers blindness.

5 CONCLUSION

This study points up the absence of a relation between the activation timings and the handedness in healthy and post-subcortical subjects, as well as, between the first and the movement velocity. In addition, were found significant differences in the activation timings of the serratus anterior bilaterally and the inferior fibers of the left trapezius between the referred groups of subjects.

A vast variability of muscular patterns was found, which emphasizes the necessity for an adequate individual assessment and consequent individualized Physical Therapy intervention. These are probably related with the variability of neuronal activation patterns dependent of the location, extension and duration of the lesion.

REFERENCES

Aruin, A. 2002. The organization of anticipatory postural adjustments. *Journal of Automatic Control* 12: 31–37.

Barthélémy, S. & Boulinguez, P. 2002. Manual asymmetries in the directional coding of reaching: Further evidence for hemispatial effects and right hemisphere dominance for movement planning. *Exp Brain Res* 147: 305–312.

BIOPAC Systems, Inc. n.d. *ECG Artifact in EMG Signal*. http://www.biopac.com/FAQ-Details.asp?ID=233. (accessed March 5, 2010).

Brodal, P. 2004. *Central Nervous System: The Structure and Function*. 3rd ed. New York: Oxford University Press.

Byrnes, M., Thickbroom, G., Phillips, B. & Mastaglia, F. 2001. Long-term changes in motor cortical organization after recovery from subcortical stroke. *Brain Res* 889: 278–287.

Calautti, C. & Baron, J. 2003. Functional neuroimaging studies of motor recovery after stroke in adults: A review. *Stroke* 34: 1553–1566.

Canadian Stroke Network. 2010a. *In Depth Review of Star Cancellation Test*. http://www.medicine.mcgill.ca/strokengine-assess/module_sct_indepth-en.html. (accessed March 6, 2010).

Canadian Stroke Network. 2010b. *Psychometric Properties*. http://www.medicine.mcgill.ca/sess/module_mmse_psycho-en.html#section6. (accessed March 6, 2010).

Canadian Stroke Network. 2010c. *Psychometric Properties*. http://www.medicine.mcgill.ca/strokengine-assess/module_rma_psycho-en.html#section6. (accessed March 6, 2010).

Cao, Y., D'Olhaberriague, L., Vikinstag, E., Levine, S. & Welch, K. 1998. Pilot study of functional MRI to assess cerebral activation of motor function after poststroke hemiparesis. *Stroke* 29: 112–122.

Caramia, M., Palmieri, M., Giacomini, P., Iani, C., Dally, L. & Silvestrini, M. 2000. Ipsilateral activation of the unaffected motor cortex in patients with hemiparetic stroke. *Clinical Neurophysiology* 111: 1990–1996.

Cirstea, M. & Levin, M. 2000. Compensatory strategies for reaching in stroke. *Brain* 123: 940–953.

Coelho, P. 2006. *Assimetria Manual na Antecipação – Coincidência: Efeitos da Idade e da Complexidade da Tarefa*. Tese de Mestrado. Porto: Faculdade de Desporto da Universidade do Porto.

Dickstein, R., Shefi, S., Marcovitz, E. & Villa, Y. 2004. Anticipatory postural adjustments in selected trunk muscles in poststroke hemiparetic patients. *Arch Phys Med Rehabil* 85: 261–267.

Faria, C., Teixeira-Salmela, L., Goulart, F. & Gomes, P. 2008. Comparisons of electromyographic activity of scapular muscles between elevation and lowering of the arms. *Physiotherapy Theory and Practice* 24 (5): 360–371.

Fridman, E., Hanakawa, T., Chung, M, Hummel, F., Leiguarda, R. & Cohen, L. 2004. Reorganization of the human ipsilesional premotor cortex after stroke. *Brain* 127: 747–758.

Ghez, C. & Krakauer, J. 2000. The Organization of Movement. In E. Kandel, J. Schwartz & T. Jessell (eds), *Principles of Neural Science*, 4th ed: 655–674. Nova Iorque: McGraw-Hill.

Latash, M., Aruin, A., Neyman, I. & Nicholas, J. 1995. Anticipatory postural adjustments during self inflicted and predictable perturbations in Parkinson's disease. *J Neurol Neurosurg Psychiatry* 58: 326–334.

Levin, M., Michaelsen, S., Cirstea, C. & Roby-Brami, A. 2002. Use of the trunk for reaching targets placed within and beyond the reach in adult hemiparesis. *Exp Brain Res* 143: 171–180.

Luft, A., Waller, S., Forrester, L., Smith, G., Whitall, J., Macko, R., Schulz, J. & Hanley, D. 2004. Lesion location alters brain activation in chronically impaired stroke survivors. *NeuroImage* 21: 924–935.

Marsh, N. & Kersel, D. 1993. Screening tests for visual neglect following stroke. *Neuropsychological Rehabilitation* 3: 245–257.

Massion, J. 1992. Movement, posture and equilibrium: Interaction and coordination. *Prog Neurobio* 38: 35–56.

Matias, R., Batata, D., Morais, D., Miguel, J. & Estiveira, R. 2006. Estudo do comportamento motor dos músculos deltóide, trapézio, e grande dentado durante a elevação do braço em sujeitos assintomáticos. *EssFisiOnline* 2 (4): 3–23.

Mazevet, D., Meunier, S., Pradat-Diehl, P., Marchand-Pauvert, V. & Pierrot-Deseilligny, E. 2003. Changes in propriospinally mediated excitation of upper limb motoneurons in stroke patients. *Brain* 126: 988–1000.

Michaelsen, S., Luta, A., Roby-Brami, A. & Levin, M. 2001. Effect of trunk restraint on the recovery of reaching movements in hemiparetic patients. *Stroke* 32: 1875–1883.

Mieschke, P. & Elliott, D. 2001. Manual asymmetries in the preparation and control of goal-directed movements. *Brain Cogn* 45, 129–140.

Schepens, B. & Drew, T. 2004. Independent and convergent signals from the pontomedullary reticular formation contribute to the control of posture and movement during reaching in the cat. *J Neurophysiol* 92: 2217–2238.

Seitz R., Höflich, P., Binkofski, F., Tellmann, L., Herzog, H. & Freund, H. 1998. Role of the premotor cortex in recovery from middle cerebral cortex artery infarction. *Arch Neurol* 55: 1081–1088.

Seitz, R., Azari, N., Knorr, U., Binkofski, F., Herzog, H. & Freund, H. 1999. The role of diaschisis in stroke recovery. *Stroke* 30: 1844–1850.

SENIAM. n.d. *Recommendations for Sensor Locations in Shoulder or Neck Muscles.* http://www.seniam.org/ (accessed March 6, 2010).

Shelton, F. & Reding, M. 2001. Effect of lesion location on upper limb motor recovery after stroke. *Stroke* 32: 107–112.

Shiratori, T. & Aruin, A. 2007. Modulation of anticipatory postural adjustments associated with unloading perturbation: Effects of characteristics of a motor action. *Exp Brain Res* 178: 206–215.

Shumway-Cook, A. & Woollacott, M. 2007. *Motor Control: Translating Research into Clinical Practice.* 3rd ed. Maryland: Lippincott Williams & Wilkins.

Slijper, H., Latash, M., Rao, N. & Aruin, A. 2002. Task-specific modulation of anticipatory postural adjustments in individuals with hemiparesis. *Clinical Neurophysiology* 113: 642–655.

Takahashi, C. & Reinkensmeyer, D. 2003. Hemiparetic stroke impairs anticipatory control of arm movement. *Exp Brain Res* 149: 131–140.

Teyssèdre, C., Lino, F., Zattara, M. & Bouisset, S. 2000. Anticipatory EMG patterns associated with preferred and non-preferred arm pointing movements. *Exp Brain Res* 134: 435–440.

Tyler, A. & Hasan, Z. 1995. Qualitative discrepancies between trunk muscle activity and dynamic postural requirements at the initiation of reaching movements performed while sitting. *Exp Brain Res* 107: 87–95.

Ward N., Newton, J., Swayne, O., Lee, L., Thompson, A., Greenwood, R., Rothwell, J. & Frackowiak, R. 2006. Motor system activation after subcortical stroke depends on corticospinal system integrity. *Brain* 129: 809–819.

Wolf, S., Slijper, H. & Latash, M. 1998. Anticipatory postural adjustments during self-paced and reaction-time movements. *Exp Brain Res* 121: 7–19.

Zachowski, K., Dromerick, A., Sahrmann, S., Thach, W. & Bastian, A. 2004. How do strenght, sensation, spasticity and joint individuation relate to the reaching deficits of people with chronic hemiparesis. *Brain* 127: 1035–1046.

Technology and Medical Sciences – Natal Jorge et al. (eds)
© *2011 Taylor & Francis Group, London, ISBN 978-0-415-66822-4*

Approaches to juxta-pleural nodule detection in CT images

A. Massafra*

Physics Department & Istituto Nazionale di Fisica Nucleare (INFN), University of Salento, Lecce, Italy

ABSTRACT: This work is part of the MAGIC-5 (Medical Applications on a Grid Infrastructure Connection) experiment of the Italian INFN (Istituto Nazionale di Fisica Nucleare). A simple CAD (Computer-Assisted Detection) system for juxta-pleural lung nodules in CT images is presented, with the purpose of comparing different 2D concavity-patching techniques and assessing the respective efficiency in locating nodules. After a short introduction on the motivation, and a review of some CAD systems for lung nodules already published by the MAGIC-5 Collaboration, the paper describes the main lines of this particular approach, giving preliminary results and comments. In our procedure, candidate nodules are identified by patching lung border concavities in a hierarchical multi-scale framework. Once located, they are fed to an artificial neural network for false positive reduction. The system has a modular structure that easily allows the insertion of arbitrary border-smoothing functions for concavity detection and nodule searching. In this paper the α-hull and morphological closing are compared, proving the higher sensitivity of the former, which also appears computationally less heavy.

Keywords: juxta-pleural lung-nodule detection; Computer Assisted Detection; medical image processing

1 INTRODUCTION

1.1 *The lung cancer*

Lung cancer is one of the main causes [1, 2] of death among both men and women. The 5-year survival rate is strictly related to the stage in which the disease is diagnosed: [3] early detection and subsequent resection can significantly improve the prognosis. The development of 'Computer-Assisted Detection' (CAD) techniques to automatically locate nodules can enhance diagnosis accuracy in the usual clinical practice. [4] Computed Tomography (CT) is considered the best imaging modality for the detection of lung nodules, see e.g. [5–7].

1.2 *Project description*

This work is part of the development of a composite CAD system for the detection of pulmonary nodules in CT scans, carried out in the framework of the "Medical Applications in a Grid Infrastructure Connection" (MAGIC-5) Collaboration, an experiment of the Italian INFN ("Istituto Nazionale di Fisica Nucleare"). Different kinds of tumor nodules may be found in the lung parenchyma: shape, size, position vary considerably, so that no unique detection approach exists. Dense nodules may be in

contact with the pleura ("juxta-pleural" nodules), because either they grew near, or originated from, the pleural sheet. Segmentation algorithms often fail in returning correct lung borders with all the juxta-pleural nodules included, due to their high density: in this case, nodules appear in the segmentation masks as small border concavities. In this work we focus on the problem of efficiently locating juxta-pleural nodules, comparing the success of two concavity-patching methods in discriminating them from other structures.

The MAGIC-5 lung CAD system already allows the detection of lung nodules, both internal and juxta-pleural, with various approaches and good accuracy, e.g. [8–12] In particular, concerning juxta-pleural nodules, in [10] the directional-gradient concentration method is applied to the pleural surface (identified as a triangulated isosurface) and combined with a morphological-opening based procedure to generate a list of pleural nodule candidates. Each candidate is characterized by 12 geometrical and textural features, which are analyzed by a rule-based filter and a neural classifier. The latter generates a list of CAD findings. Care is devoted to the reduction of False Positives (FPs) by the application of a Self Organizing Map (SOM) which helps in identifying a representative subset of the FP population, for efficient network training. In the approach described in [11] the lung parenchymal volume is segmented by

---

*on behalf of MAGIC-5 collaboration

means of a Region Growing (RG) algorithm, and pleural nodules are included through an original ACM technique. Then, RG is iteratively applied to the previously segmented volume in order to detect candidate nodules. A double-threshold cut and a supervised feed-forward neural network are applied for FP reduction. The leave-one-out cross validation is used to exploit the highest possible number of True Positives (TP) during the training phase. Finally, in [12] ant colonies are able to segment artificially-generated and natural objects of different shape, intensity, background. The CT analysis makes use of a Channeler Ant Model (CAM) to segment the bronchial and vascular tree and remove it from the CT before searching for nodular structures in the image with a dedicated filter. The moving rules depend on the pheromone content at destination. The ant colony behaviour is related to the original image features via their influence on the pheromone release rules.

The interest in developing complementary methods comes from the possibility of integrating the results given by diverse procedures with the purpose of obtaining a "composite" CAD system more accurate than each component. [13] Therefore we decided to plan a further system devoted to juxta-pleural nodules: it is based on the α-hull [14,15], a concavity-patching method far less known than its well-spread counterpart, i.e. morphological closing. This explorative paper is our first attempt at the development of an α-hull CAD tool and, while it succeeds in building a working system, it anyway does not try yet to optimize it in terms of classification accuracy, focusing instead on a comparison with morphological closing, with the purpose of selecting the more performing concavity-patching technique. Moreover, the idea of performing nodule search in a hierarchical framework [15] is pursued.

The nodule-inclusion procedure starts from the segmented pulmonary volume, where dense juxta-pleural nodules remain outside the lung mask, and appear as small concavities of the lung border. Following and generalizing [15], morphological closing and α-hull were implemented in a hierarchical framework, depending on a suitable parameter (the curvature of the circular SE and the α value, respectively): this approach allows a multiscale analysis, by which a tree of nested concavities can be built.

2 MATERIALS AND METHODS

2.1 Materials

The procedure described in this paper was tested on a database composed of 57 high-resolution, low-dose (140 kV, 20 mA · s) CT scans with internal

and juxta-pleural nodules, or belonging to patients without nodules. Slices are 512 × 512 pixel, 12-bit grey level matrices; pixel size ranges from 0.53 mm to 0.74 mm in the xy axial plane, while z size is 1 mm. The images were annotated by experienced radiologists, giving a list of found nodules with position and size. The database contains 78 diagnosed juxta-pleural nodules, of which 28 at direct contact with the pleura, and the others connected to it by peduncles.

2.2 Methods

Our comparison procedure follows the classical scheme of a CAD system: a) segmentation of the volume of interest (i.e. the lungs), b) juxta-pleural candidate nodule detection, c) feature choice and calculation, d) classification. In this work, we stress on stage (b), where candidate nodules are identified by a concavity-patching method, which can be the alpha hull, morphological closing, ACMs, or some other technique to be tested. The features we calculated in step (c) are not necessarily the best: in this preliminary work we chose some reasonable ones (some borrowed from [15], some already used in the lung CAD systems developed by the MAGIC-5 Collaboration, e.g. [11]), with the only purpose of setting up a procedure to discriminate between concavity-patching techniques.

2.2.1 Segmentation

The segmentation algorithm can be found in [17]. The result is a pair of binary masks for the two lungs. Dense nodules (and vessels) are not contained in the segmented volume. Therefore, regions containing nodules and vessels now show cavities and concavities. The concavities originated by juxta-pleural nodules (and larger vessels) are dealt with in the next phase by concavity-patching procedures that allow concavity (i.e. candidate nodule) detection.

2.2.2 Detection of juxta-pleural candidate nodules

By using a concavity-patching method, which allows the reconstruction of a smoothed lung border (where concavities are 'closed'), and by applying a difference operation between the old and the new border, we can detect concavities where the two borders differ. Moreover, if the procedure relies on a spatial parameter (related to a concavity scale), we obtain a multiscale procedure [15] which also retains information about nesting: this can be useful to better understand the relation between concavities (e.g., a nodule being contained in the hilus concavity). In this paper 2D morphological closing and alpha hull are implemented, and the respective efficiencies compared.

Morphological closing is defined as a dilation operation followed by erosion, both using the same Structural Element (SE). Here a disk with varying radius r is used. The α-hull [14,15] is a convex hull generalization, able to detect concavities, whose shape depends on a curvature parameter α. A definition of α-hull is the following: given a set S of points in the plane, and a positive number α, the global α-hull of S is the intersection of the closed complements of all the circles of radius $r = 1/\alpha$ such that the intersection of these circles with S is empty. By definition, the α-hull when α = 0 is the convex hull. The effect of calculating the α-hull of a closed and dense spatial distribution of points (such as the segmentation mask of a lung slice), is the gradual closing of concavities, depending on the value of α.

Following and generalizing [15], morphological closing and α-hull were tested in a hierarchical framework, respectively depending on the inverse of the radius of the SE (the disk), hereafter also called α, and on the α value: this approach allowed a hierarchical, multiscale analysis of concavities, leading to juxta-pleural nodule detection. The programming environment was Matlab R2008a for Linux, with the Image Processing Toolbox. Morphological closing was implemented by the standard toolbox function, while the C code for the α-hull is available on the Web. [16].

As pointed out, concavities are found, slice by slice, by calculating the difference between the borders of the original lung slice B, and the smoothed one B_α: $D = B-B_\alpha$. D is a list of pixels belonging to the original border but not to the smoothed one, therefore it consists of groups of pixels identifying the concavities at the α value of the scale parameter. Concavities are spotted by finding groups of contiguous pixels separated by gaps. Figure 1 shows the result of the described operation on a lung slice at an arbitrary α value, for the α-hull. By repeating, for a suitable set of α values, the difference operation in and the search for concavities, a hierarchy for each slice is determined. The choice of a useful set A of α values involved much experimenting, because of competing requests: a richer A set means a finer description of concavities, but also longer calculation times and, even, a larger number of False Positives (FPs). Too small α's (large radii) are useless because they reveal noise and are not able to detect nested concavities. Too large α's (small radii) are useless, too, because they give negligible border difference (no detection). Because of the geometrical meaning of the α parameter (a curvature, i.e. the inverse of a radius) we populated A according to the range of nodule sizes (2 to 12 mm) (Figure 2). In our preliminary tests we arbitrarily used five α values: {0.083, 0.100, 0.125, 0.154, 0.182} mm [1], corresponding to radii equal to about {12 mm, 10 mm, 8 mm, 6.5 mm, 5.5 mm}, because this A set was able

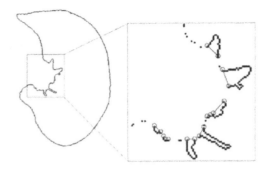

Figure 1. Concavity detection. A lung slice after concavity detection at an arbitrary α value; the concavity-patching technique used for border smoothing (followed by border difference and concavity spotting) was the α-hull.

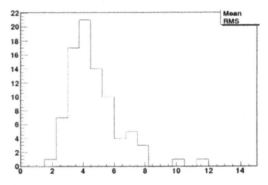

Figure 2. The histogram of nodule radii (mm) in the database of 57 CT scans on which the CAD system was developed and tested.

to detect most of the nodules. Nevertheless, we realized that small radii would alter feature values: thus we decided to reduce the A set cardinality to three, preserving {0.083, 0.100, 0.125} mm [1]. We verified that this set optimized both nodule-searching sensitivity in the detection phase, and classification performance.

2.2.3 Features

After maximizing sensitivity in the detection step, the next goal is the reduction of FPs, i.e. how to identify and reject the concavities that are not juxta-pleural nodules. This task can be obtained by suitable characterizing features calculated on the nodule candidates, which discriminate between nodules and FP. In our simple approach, FP reduction will be performed by straightforward linear filters (thresholds on the feature values), followed by the use of an Artificial Neural Network (ANN). We decided to employ, as a preliminary test, geometrical features (some from [15]), and first-order grey-value features (like in [11]). Thus, our set of features was:

$F = G \cup T \cup \{\alpha\}$, where α is the scale value at which the concavity was detected, and:

$G = \{span, depth, borderLength, area, depthOverSpan, radius, circularity\}$

$T = \{grayMean, grayStd, graySkew, grayKurt, grayEntrpy\}$

The *span* of a concavity is the length of the segment that joins its extremal points; *depth* is the length of the longest perpendicular segment between the concavity pixels and the segment defining the *span*; *borderLength* is the number of boundary points composing the concavity profile; the *area* is the number of pixels between the span segment and the concavity boundary; *depthOverSpan* is *depth/span*; the *radius* is the mean distance of the boundary pixels from the concavity centroid; *circularity* is the ratio of its area A and that of the circle having the same perimeter p (i.e. *borderLength*): $c = 4\,\alpha\,A/p^2$. First order textural features are gray mean, standard deviation, skewness, kurtosis, and entropy, calculated for the pixels within the concavity. Feature distributions were examined and gross intervals of values for a preliminary filtering were identified.

2.2.4 *Classification*

A supervised two-layer, 13-input, 20-hidden-neuron, 1-output feed-forward neural network, trained with gradient descent learning rule with momentum, was chosen as the classifier system. To calculate classification efficiency for each of the concavity-patching methods, we define as True Positives (TPs) the candidate nodules that meet the radiologists' diagnosis according to the following condition: the Euclidean distance between the centroid of the concavity, and the centroid of a diagnosed nodule, is lower than $1.5 \cdot r_R$, where r_R is the nodule radius according to the radiologists. All the other candidates are considered as false positives. The 1.5 factor takes into account radius measurement uncertainty. K-fold cross validation [18] (with $K = 10$) was used. The ANN output, calculated on the concavity list, is distributed in the range [0,1]. By varying a decision threshold, and assigning target $t = 1$ to candidates above threshold (probably positive), $t = 0$ to candidates below threshold (probably negative), sensitivity and specificity referred to the known diagnosis can be calculated. By plotting (for each threshold value) sensitivity vs [1-specificity], and smoothly joining points, the Receiver Operating Characteristic (ROC) curve can be drawn.

3 RESULTS

3.1 *Execution time of the detection step*

A CT scan of about 300 slices takes about 3 minutes per α value for the α-hull, quite more (about 10 minute) for morphological closing, on a modern Dell Precision T5500 (two quad-core Intel Xeon E5540@2.53GHz, 12 GB RAM).

3.2 *Sensitivity of the concavity-detection systems*

The number of juxta-pleural nodules contained in the set of concavities detected by the α-hull is 72 out of 78, while only 66 are collected by morphological closing (sensitivity: 92.3% and 84.6%). All the neglected nodules are not in direct contact with the pleura, but are connected to it by subtle peduncles, with small concavities in the lung border. This fact justifies the failures. All the nodules lost by the α-hull are also lost by the morphological closing. As to the influence of the multiscale approach on detection accuracy, we tried A sets with one element: the result was an increased loss of nodules. On the contrary, increasing A cardinality did not help us recovering already lost lesions.

3.3 *ROC curves*

ROC curve calculation allows quantification of the classifier performance on the collected data, strongly related to the detection method fitness and to the feature choice.

In our tests, the ROC curves (Figure 3) for both methods look similar. The Area Under the Curve (AUC), and sensitivity and specificity, in the point where they have the same value, are (0.80, 72%) and (0.84, 75%) respectively. It is remarkable that ROC curves obtained when only one α value is inserted in the A set show AUC values just a little lower (e.g. 0.76), but the curve shape is far less regular.

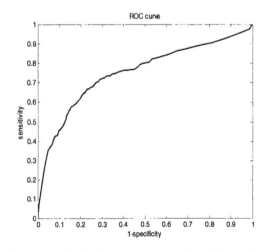

Figure 3. The ROC curve assessing the ability of the neural network in classifying the result of concavity detection by the α-hull.

Moreover, using an A set with more than three elements does not give any accuracy enhancement, because the number of FPs is increased too.

4 CONCLUSIONS AND PROSPECTS

A CAD system for juxta-pleural nodule detection in thorax CT images was developed, with the purpose of being a test framework for different concavity-patching algorithms used for multiscale nodule localization.

Nodule-candidate search is followed by an ANN for FP reduction. In particular, two concavity-patching techniques were compared: the α-hull and morphological closing.

At detection level, the former had better sensitivity (92.3% vs 84.6%), marking as positive some nodules connected to the pleura by subtle peduncles, that morphological closing did not see.

At classification level, the two methods proved roughly equivalent, with sensitivity and specificity around 72–75% and AUC around 0.80–0.84. On the other hand, the two approaches really differed in the computational cost: calculation time for morphological closing (at least in the MATLAB implementation) largely exceeds the α-hull. The preceding considerations lead to prefer the latter approach. In conclusion, the α-hull appears as a powerful method for the detection of concavities.

In the next future the system will be applied to a larger number of images, by also diversifying the source (the LIDC database will be used). The Active Contour Model already implemented in the MAGIC-5 framework and described in [11] will also be tested as an alternative concavity-patching method. Finally, the code will be parallelized to increase efficiency.

ACKNOWLEDGMENTS

This work was carried out in the framework of the MAGIC-5 Collaboration, supported by the Italian "Istituto Nazionale di Fisica Nucleare" (INFN, CSN 5) and by the Italian "Ministero dell'Istruzione, dell'Università e della Ricerca (MIUR)". We also acknowledge: F. Falaschi, C. Spinelli, L. Battolla and A. De Liperi of "U.O. Radiodiagnostica 2", Azienda Ospedaliera Universitaria Pisana; D. Caramella, T. Tarantino, and M. Barattini of the "Divisione di Radiologia Diagnostica e Interventistica", Dipartimento di "Oncologia, Trapianti e Nuove Tecnologie in Medicina" dell'Università di Pisa"; Anna Margiotta, Marinella Foti, Luigi Pignatelli of the "Unità Operativa di Radiologia", Azienda Ospedaliera Vito Fazzi, Lecce, for providing the dataset of CT scans.

REFERENCES

[1] The Lancet, vol. 365, May 14, 2005.

[2] Alberg, A.J. and Samet, J.M. "Epidemiology of Lung Cancer", Chest 123, 2003.

[3] Picozzi, G. et al., "Screening of lung cancer with low dose spiral CT: results of a three year pilot study and design of the randomised controlled trial 'Italung-CT'", Radiol. Med. (Torino) 109 (1–2): 17–26, 2005. See also: http://www.cspo.it/

[4] Sahiner, B. et al., "Effect of CAD on Radiologists' Detection of Lung Nodules on Thoracic CT Scans: Analysis of an Observer Performance Study by Nodule Size", Academic Radiology, Volume 16, Issue 12, December 2009, pp. 1518–1530.

[5] Heitzman, E.R. "The role of computed tomography in the diagnosis and management of lung cancer: an overview," Chest 1986, 89 (suppl 4), pp. 237S–241S.

[6] Howe, M.A. and Gross, B.H. "CT evaluation of the equivocal pulmonary nodule," Computer Radiology 1987, vol. 11, pp. 61–67.

[7] Remy-Jardin, M. et al., "Pulmonary nodules: detection with thick-section spiral CT versus conventional CT" Radiology 1993; 187:513–520.

[8] Gori, I. et al., "Multi-scale analysis of lung computed tomography images", 2007 JINST 2 P09007;

[9] Retico, A. et al., "Lung nodule detection in low-dose and thin-slice computed tomography", Comput Biol Med. 2008 Apr;38(4):525–34.

[10] Retico A. et al., "Pleural nodule identification in low-dose and thin-slice lung computed tomography", Computers in Biology and Medicine 39(2009) 1137–1144.

[11] Bellotti, R. et al., "A CAD system for nodule detection in low-dose lung CTs based on region growing and a new active contour model", Med. Phys. 34 (12), December 2007, pp. 4901–4910.

[12] Cerello, P. et al., "3-D Object Segmentation using Ant Colonies", Pattern Recognition (2009), doi:10.1016/j.patcog.2009.10.007.

[13] van Ginneken, B. et al., "Comparing and combining algorithms for computer-aided detection of pulmonary nodules in computed tomography scans: The ANODE09 study", Medical Image Analysis Volume 14, Issue 6, pp. 707–722 (2010).

[14] Edelsbrunner, H. et al., '"On the Shape of a Set of Points in the Plane", IEEE TRANSACTIONS ON INFORMATION THEORY, VOL. IT-29, No. 4, July 1983 pp. 551–559.

[15] Sensakovic, W.F. et al., "A General Method for the Identification and Repair of Concavities in Segmented Medical Images", Medical Image Conference 2008, Dresden.

[16] www.netlib.org/voronoi/hull.html (see also: weblog.bocoup.com/compiling-clarksons-hull-in-os-x).

[17] De Nunzio, G. et al., "Automatic Lung Segmentation in CT Images with Accurate Handling of the Hilar Region", Journal of Digital Imaging ISSN0897–1889 (Print) 1618–727X (Online) DOI:10.1007/s10278–009–9229–11 (2009), pp. 10–20.

[18] Stone, M. "Cross-validatory choice and assessment of statistical predictions", J.R. Stat. Soc. Ser. B Methodol. 36, pp. 111–147, 1974.

Technology and Medical Sciences – Natal Jorge et al. (eds)
© 2011 Taylor & Francis Group, London, ISBN 978-0-415-66822-4

Blood flow in artificial bypass graft: A numerical study

L.C. Sousa, C.F. Castro & C.C. António
IDMEC—FEUP, University of Porto, Porto, Portugal

B. Relvas
IDMEC—Pólo FEUP, Porto, Portugal

ABSTRACT: The purpose of this study is to obtain a first insight of blood physics behaviour through a bypass graft. The paper describes a numerical analysis by the finite element method of steady blood flow through an idealized bypass graft around a stenosed artery. In this study the biochemical and mechanical interactions between blood and vascular tissue are neglected and no-slip boundary conditions including the graft are considered. Results are visualized for a better understanding of the flow characteristics such as distributions of the flow pattern, stagnation flow and recirculation zones. The outcomes will contribute to characterize the physiology of bypass grafts in the human circulatory system.

1 MOTIVATION

Arterial diseases such as wall conditions may cause blood flow disturbances leading to clinical complications in areas of complex flow like in coronary and carotid bifurcations or stenosed arteries. It is well established that once a mild stenosis is formed in the artery, biomechanical parameters resulting from the blood flow and stress distribution in the arterial wall contribute to further progression of the disease (Deplano & Siouffi 1999). Although blood flow is normally laminar, the periodic unsteadiness or pulsatile nature of the flow makes possible the transition to turbulence when the artery diameter decreases and velocities increase.

A detailed understanding of local hemodynamicenvironment, influence of wall modifications on flow patternsand long-term adaptations of the vascular wall can have useful clinical applications, especially in view of reconstruction and revascularization operations helping doctors or surgeons to make a diagnosis or to plan a surgery.

Nowadays, the use of computational techniques in fluid dynamics in the study of physiological flows involving blood is an area of intensive research (Taylor et al. 1998; Quarteroni et al. 2003). Flow visualization techniques and non-invasive medical imaging data acquisition such as computed tomography, angiography or magnetic resonance imaging, make feasible to construct three dimensional models of blood vessels. Measuring techniques such as Doppler ultrasound have improved to provide accurate information on the flow fields.

In medical practice bypass grafts are commonly used as an alternative route around strongly stenosed or occluded arteries. For inflow operations artificial grafts are considered (Abraham et al. 2004; Huang et al. 1995; Su et al. 2005). They perform well when the arterial flow is high and it has been shown over the years that they provide durable results. The main goal of this work is to obtain a first insight into the simulation flow through an idealized bypass graft using a developed computer program based on the finite element method. Modelling the fluid flow in idealized geometries will help to investigate the issues related to bypass anastomosisas knowing the blood flow, the velocity and stress fields it is possible to find a geometry that leads to small gradient hemodynamic flow and recirculation zones.

2 COMPUTATIONAL STRATEGY

In this current study, due to the complexity of the cardiovascular system, a preliminary analysis aiming suitable simplifying assumptions for the mathematical modelling process is needed.

The numerical analysis of the blood flow phenomena uses the finite element method approach and a geometrical model of the artery and artificial bypass graft. Blood flow is described by the incompressible Navier-Stokes equations and the simulation is carried out under steady flow conditions. Although blood flow in arteries is substantially influenced by unsteady flow phenomena steady state results allow to gain an in-depth understanding of the fluid physics.

In diseased vessels which are often the subject of interest, the arteries are even less compliant and wall motion is further reduced and the assumption of zero wall motion is utilized in most approximations. In the present work, blood flow in an idealized bypass graft is studied considering boundary conditions similar to physiological circumstances. Biochemical and mechanical interactions between blood and vascular tissue are neglected.

2.1 Mathematical model

The fluid flow is governed by the equation of Navier-Stokes. This equation results from the application of the principle of mass conservation. A non-Newtonian viscosity model for simulating pulsatile flow in artery is adopted in this study. Considering blood flow an incompressible non-Newtonian flow and neglecting body forces, the equation of continuity and the Navier-Stokes equations become:

$$\nabla \cdot \mathbf{v} = 0$$
$$\frac{\partial \mathbf{v}}{\partial t} + \mathbf{v} \cdot \nabla \mathbf{v} = -\frac{1}{\rho} \nabla p + \mu \nabla^2 \mathbf{v} \qquad (1)$$

where $\mathbf{v}$ is the velocity field, μ the dynamic viscosity, ρ the blood density and p the pressure. Considering the pseudo-constitutive relation for the incompressibility constraint the continuity equation is replaced by (Babuska 1973; Babuska et al. 1980):

$$p = -\frac{1}{\varepsilon} \nabla \cdot \mathbf{v} \qquad (2)$$

where ε is the penalty parameter generally assigned to 10^{-8} or 10^{-9}. The first set of Equation (1) is eliminated and the Navier-Stokes equations become:

$$\rho \left(\frac{\partial \mathbf{v}}{\partial t} + \mathbf{v} \cdot \nabla \mathbf{v} \right) = +\frac{1}{\varepsilon} \nabla (\nabla \cdot \mathbf{v}) + \mu \nabla^2 \mathbf{v} \qquad (3)$$

Under such conditions the pressure is eliminated as a field variable since it can be recovered by the approximation of Equation (2). If the standard Galerkin formulation is applied it is necessary to use compatible spaces for the velocity and the pressure in order to satisfy the Babuska-Brezzi stability (Babuska 1973; Babuska et al. 1980; Sousa et al. 2002). Unfortunately, not every combination of interpolation functions for pressure and velocity works, as they are required to satisfy the Babuska-Brezzi conditions or pass the mixed patch test in the incompressible limit. In this work reduced integration is used for the terms related with pressure in order to avoid locking effects and to obtain a stabilized finite element solution. A smoothing technique is applied to get continuous fields for pressure and deviatoric stresses.

In blood flow high Reynolds numbers appear and loss of unicity of solution, hydro dynamical instabilities and turbulence are caused by the convective term in Equation (3). If Navier-Stokes equation is solved numerically by the Galerkin method, an unstable and oscillating solution is observed at higher speeds. A severely refined mesh can be used to avoid this phenomenon, but computation time might then become unacceptable.

The numerical scheme requires a stabilization technique in order to avoid oscillations in the numerical solution. In this study the streamline upwind Petrov-Galerkinmethod is applied in order to avoid the loss of accuracy (Brooks & Hughes 1982). This method is applied using modified velocity shape functions, W_i:

$$W_i = N_i + K_{SUPG} \frac{\mathbf{v} \nabla N_i}{\|\mathbf{v}\|} \qquad (4)$$

where N_i are the Galerkin shape functions and K_{SUPG} denotes the upwind parameter that controls the factor of upwind weighting. The resulting system of nonlinear equations is characterized by a non-symmetric matrix, and a special solver is adopted in order to reduce the bandwidth and the storage of the sparse system matrix; the skyline method is used in addition to some improvement of the Gauss elimination.

In this work a steady blood flow is considered and the first term of Equation (3) disappears becoming:

$$\rho \mathbf{v} \cdot \nabla \mathbf{v} = \frac{1}{\varepsilon} \nabla (\nabla \cdot \mathbf{v}) + \mu \nabla^2 \mathbf{v} \qquad (5)$$

Non-Newtonian property of blood is important in the hemodynamic effect and plays a significant role in vascular biology and pathology. In this study two non-Newtonian viscosity modelsare adopted. In the first, the viscosity is empirically obtained using Casson law for the shear stress relation (Perktold et al. 1991). Considering D_{II} the second invariant of the strain rate and c the red cell concentration, the shear stress τ given by the generalized Casson relation is:

$$\sqrt{\tau} = k_0 + k_1(c)\sqrt{2\sqrt{D_{II}}} \qquad (6)$$

and the apparent dynamic viscosity $\mu = \mu(c, D_{II})$, a function of the red cell concentration,

$$\mu = \frac{1}{2\sqrt{D_{II}}} \left(k_0 + k_1(c)\sqrt{2\sqrt{D_{II}}} \right)^2 \qquad (7)$$

where parameters $\mu_0 = 0.124$ Ns, $k_0 = 0.6125$ and $k_1 = 0.174$ were obtained fitting experimental data and considering $c = 45\%$. For the second approach the Carreau-Yasuda constitutive model is adopted and dynamic viscosity is given by (Abraham et al. 2004):

$$\mu(\dot{\gamma}) = \mu_\infty + \frac{\mu_0 - \mu_\infty}{\left(1 + (\lambda\dot{\gamma})^b\right)^a} \tag{8}$$

where $\mu_0 = 0.116$ Ns, $\mu_\infty = 0.0035$ Ns, $a = 1.23$, $b = 0.64$ and $\lambda = 8.2$ s. The shear rate, $\dot{\gamma}$, is related to the second invariant of the strain rate tensor and can be directly obtained from the flow field as:

$$\dot{\gamma} = \sqrt{2\dot{\varepsilon}(\mathbf{v}) : \dot{\varepsilon}(\mathbf{v})} \tag{9}$$

where $\dot{\varepsilon}$ is the strain rate tensor.

3 NUMERICAL RESULTS

3.1 *Finite element approach*

A graft is attached around an occlusion in the coronary artery, as an alternative route for blood flow. The first results presented here consider a 3D simulation. The boundary conditions for the flow field are parabolic inlet velocity, no-slip boundary conditions including graft and artery and a parallel flow condition at the outlet. Considering a 3D analysis the results are presented for Reynolds number equal to 50, defining the Reynolds number as $Re = \rho v_{max} D/\mu$, where v_{max} is the maximum velocity at the inlet and D the artery diameter. Figure 1 shows the geometry and finite element mesh for the arterial bypass system analysed where the artery diameter is $D = 10$ mm and the graft diameter $d = 7$ mm. Due to symmetry only half of the bypass geometry is considered for the numerical simulation. The mesh consists of 11607 nodes and 9272 elements. Considering Casson constitutive model the velocity field is shown in Figure 2.

Figures 3 and 4 show the longitudinal velocity and pressure contours on the plane of symmetry. It is observed that there are no recirculation zones as Reynolds number is not high; pressure increases as the flow exits the graft and the fluid pressure along the centerline is a constant function of axial

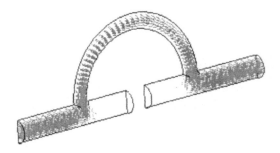

Figure 2. Velocity field using Casson model, $Re = 50$, $d = 7$ mm.

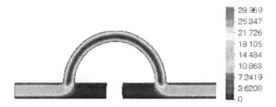

Figure 3. Plane of simmetry of 3D simulation. Velocity field (mm/s) using Casson model, $Re = 50$, $d = 7$ mm.

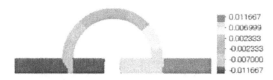

Figure 4. Plane of simmetry of 3D simulation. Pressure distribution (10^4 Pa) using Casson model, $Re = 50$, $d = 7$ mm.

distances. The 3D simulation is compared with a 2D one for the same geometry; simulated 2D velocity and pressure distributions presented in Figures 5 and 6 are similar to those obtained in the 3D simulation.

Since 3D and 2D simulations present similar results the following discussion considering Reynolds number equal to 300 and comparing two viscosity models is based on 2D simulations. In Figures 7 and 8 the results are obtained using Casson's law while Figures 9 and 10 correspond to the Carreau-Yasuda viscosity model. For these analyses two recirculation zones are observed one near the proximal entrance of the bypass graft and another near the toe of the distal anastomosis; it can also be deduced from Figures 7 and 9 that the size of these two regions is more extended when Carreau-Yasuda model is adopted.

3.2 *Aspect ratio variation*

Defining aspect ratio as the ratio of the graft diameter d to artery diameter D, simulations for

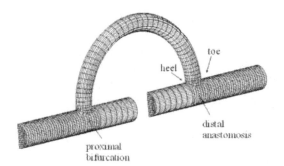

Figure 1. Geometry and finite element mesh for the arterial bypass system analysed.

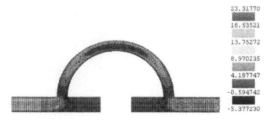

Figure 5. 2D simulation. Velocity field (mm/s) using Casson model, Re = 50, d = 7 mm.

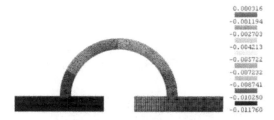

Figure 6. 2D simulation. Pressure distribution (10⁴ Pa) using Casson model, Re = 50, d = 7 mm.

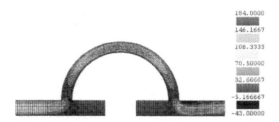

Figure 7. Longitudinal velocity profile (mm/s) using Casson model, Re = 300, d = 7 mm.

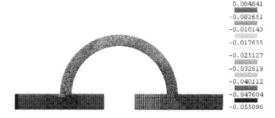

Figure 8. Pressure distribution (10⁴ Pa) using Casson model, Re = 300, d = 7 mm.

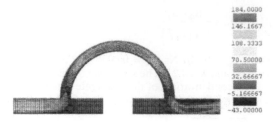

Figure 9. Longitudinal velocity profile (mm/s) using Carreau-Yasuda constitutive model, Re = 300, d = 7 mm.

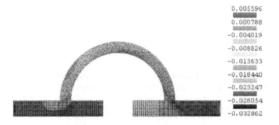

Figure 10. Pressure distribution (10⁴ Pa) using Carreau-Yasuda constitutive model, Re = 300, d = 7 mm.

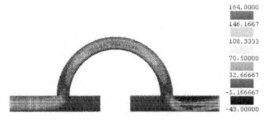

Figure 11. Longitudinal velocity profile (mm/s) using Carreau-Yasuda constitutive model, Re = 300, d/D = 0.8.

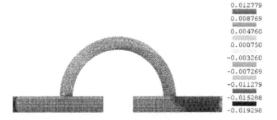

Figure 12. Pressure distribution (10⁴ Pa) using Carreau-Yasuda constitutive model, Re = 300, d/D = 0.8.

different aspect ratios are analysed in this work. Considering Carreau-Yasuda constitutive model the previous results given in Figures 9 and 10 corresponding to d/D = 0.7 are compared with new simulations for higher aspect ratio values. Velocity and pressure distributions for an aspect ratio of 0.8 are presented in Figures 11 and 12 respectively. Figures 13 and 14 present the results corresponding to an aspect ratio of 1.0. The maximum

velocity is observed after distal anastomosis zone corresponding to 184 mm/s, 169 mm/s and 147 mm/s for the diameter aspect ratios equal to 0.7, 0.8 and 1.0 respectively. It can be seen that stagnation zones are larger for the bypass geometry corresponding to an aspect ratio of 0.7.

From the simulations it can be concluded that as the diameter aspect ratio increases the velocities decreases as well the pressures. A graft with a larger

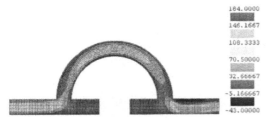

Figure 13. Longitudinal velocity profile (mm/s) using Carreau-Yasuda constitutive model, Re = 300, d/D = 1.

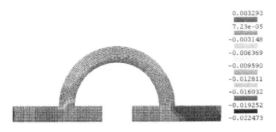

Figure 14. Pressure distribution (10^4 Pa) using Carreau-Yasuda constitutive model, Re = 300, d/D = 1.

diameter produces smaller longitudinal velocity and smaller pressure in the host artery having positive effects for improving the hemodynamics of bypassing surgery.

4 CONCLUSIONS

Results from numerical modelling of blood flow through a bypass artery system using a developed finite element method are validated here by presenting velocity and pressure values obtained for different Reynolds numbers, using two viscosity laws and variable graft artery aspect ratio. By varying the aspect ratios from 1 to 0.7 this study indicates that pressures and velocities decrease by about 20%.

The outcomes will contribute to characterize the physiology of bypass grafts in circulatory system, and detect stagnation flow in recirculation zones. The objective of this preliminary study is also to test the capabilities of the developed mathematical model in order to build robust software for the optimization of bypass grafts shape aiming small gradient hemodynamic flow and minimizing recirculation zones.

Further studies could build more complicated computational models as considering unsteady flow and vessels deformation leading to even more realistic values for flow velocity and pressure profiles.

ACKNOWLEDGEMENTS

The authors thank the financial support by FCT, Portugal, project PTDC/SAU-BEB/102547/2008.

REFERENCES

Abraham, F., Behr, M. & Heinkensgchloss, M. 2004. Shape optimization in stationary blood flow: a numerical study of non-Newtonian effets. *Comp. Meth. In Biomechanics. and Biomedical Eng.* 8: 127–137.

Babuska, I. 1973. The finite element method with Lagrangian multipliers. *Numer Math.* 20: 179–192.

Babuska, I., Osborn, J. & Pitkaranta, J. 1980. Analysis of mixed methods using, mesh dependent norms. *Math. Comp* 35: 1039–1062.

Brooks, N. & Hughes, J.R. 1982. Streamline Upwind/Petrov-Galerkin Formulations for convection dominated flows with particular emphasis on the incompressible Navier-Stokes equations. *Comp. Met. in Appl. Mec. and Eng.* 32: 199–259.

Deplano, V. & Siouffi, M. 1999. Experimental and numerical study of pulsatile flows through stenosis: wall shear stress analysis. *Journal of Biomechanics* 32: 1081–1090.

Huang, H., Modi, V.J. & Seymour, B.R. 1995. Fluid mechanics of stenosed arteries. *Int. J. Engng. Sci.* 33: 815–828.

Quarteroni, A., Tuveri, M. & Veneziani, A. 2003. Computational Vascular Fluid dynamics: problems, models and methods. *Computer and Visualization in Science* 2: 163–197.

Sousa, L.C., Castro, C.F., António, C.A.C. & Santos A.D. 2002. Inverse methods in design of industrial forging processes. *Journal of Materials Processing Technology* 128(1–3): 266–273.

Su, C.M., Lee, D., Tran-Son-Tay, R. & Shyy, W. 2005. Fluid flow structure in arterial bypass anastomosis. *Journal of Biomechanical Eng.* 127: 611–618.

Taylor, C.A., Hughes, T.J.R. & Zarins, C.K. 1998. Finite element modeling of blood flow in arteries. *Comput. Methods Appl. Mech. Eng.* 158: 155–196.

Perktold, K., Peter, R.O., Resch, M. & Langs, G. 1991. Pulsatile non-Newtonian flow in three-dimensional carotid bifurcation models: A numerical Study of flow phenomena under different bifurcation angles, *Journal of Biomedical Eng.* 13: 507–515.

Technology and Medical Sciences – Natal Jorge et al. (eds)
© 2011 Taylor & Francis Group, London, ISBN 978-0-415-66822-4

Calibration of free hand ultrasound probe tracked by optical system

K. Krysztoforski, R. Będziński, E. Świątek-Najwer & P. Krowicki
Division of Biomedical Engineering and Experimental Mechanics, Institute of Machine Design and Operation, Wroclaw University of Technology, Wroclaw, Poland

ABSTRACT: The main aim of study was to develop a method of calibration for ultrasound probe to provide high accuracy of 3D ultrasonic imaging. A system combining an ultrasound linear probe (EchoBlaster128, Telemed) equipped in optical sensor and infrared camera (Polaris Spectra, NDI) was developed. Procedure of calibration is necessary to determine the transformation between the coordinate system combined with on-probe sensor and coordinate system of ultrasound image. The paper describes two algorithms of ultrasound probe calibration. Input dataset for calibration is ultrasound image of five level double N-structures wire phantom and registered 6 DOF position of on-probe sensor related to the coordinate system of on-phantom sensor. Minimal distance between proper and calculated coordinates of fiducial registered on image equaled 0.15 mm. The navigated ultrasound probe is applied in 3D measurements of soft and bone tissue geometry including landmarks and shape identification. Validated on the 3D Calibration phantom (CIRS) accuracy of length measurement was as high as 1.5 mm.

1 INTRODUCTION

1.1 Aim of study

The aim of study was to develop a method of ultrasound probe calibration to apply in 3D measurement of bone and soft tissues to provide high resolution and accuracy.

1.2 State of the art in ultrasound imaging

Ultrasound imaging is a noninvasive technique of tissues examination. Imaging applies the reflection of sound waves from imaged structures, in particular the boundaries between objects with different acoustic impedances. The phenomenon of ultrasounds reflection depends on the angle of the sound beam and the acoustic impedance of materials. Today's development of ultrasound imaging technique brings the possibility of harmonic imaging with a resolution close to the quality of magnetic resonance imaging. Developed contrast media injected to the patient significantly improve the quality of images. Recent trends in the development of ultrasound imaging concern the spatial imaging techniques, integration and monitoring of diagnostic and therapeutic methods, such as control of targeted ultrasound drug delivery (P.A. Lewin, 2004).

1.3 State of the art in 3D ultrasound imaging

The most common method of ultrasound spatial imaging is to record three-dimensional ultrasound dataset registered while changing the position of the ultrasonic beam. This method allows to reconstruct the shape of objects of limited size. Control of the ultrasonic beam is automated and achieved through precise electronic controls and mechanical engines. Automatic scanning movement is provided by phase array and controlled selection of acting transmitters.

To reconstruct objects of unlimited size one needs to apply a specially designed ultrasound probe controlling the direction of sound beam and a localizer tracking the position of the probe in space. Applied sensors are magnetic, optical or mechanical arms. Proposed by Prager (Prager R.W. et al., 2002) Stradx system for three-dimensional reconstruction of ultrasound images allows precise measurement of the tissues. Developed by Prager method of data acquisition was to record scans in arbitrary positions and reconstruct the geometry of the fetus using the nearest neighbor voxel algorithm.

1.4 State of the art in 3D ultrasound system calibration

Calibration of ultrasound head is the procedure allowing a full description of the scanning image plane position in relation to the reference sensor mounted on the probe housing. Measurement of head geometry and location of the sensor mounted on it, is not sufficient to calculate the calibration matrix, since the tilt of scanning plane is not considered.

One method of calibration is to scan a phantom of known geometry. The literature describes the concepts of phantoms consisting of the network of markers (R.W. Prager et al., 1998), (F. Lindseth et al., 2003), (C.D. Barry et al., 1997), (R. Detmer et al., 1994), (M. Blackall et al., 2000), phantoms for visualization of the plane—(R.W. Prager et al., 1998), the phantoms of single markers—(Lindseth F. et al., 2003), phantoms structures "N" or "Z"—(L. Mercier et al., 2005), (Lindseth F. et al., 2003) and Cambridge phantom (imaging of steel lines)—(A. Ali et al., 2007), (L. Mercier et al., 2005). Comparing the results of the ultrasound head calibration phantom with network of markers, three wire markers, and the Cambridgephantom, Prager has shown that the best method of calibration, taking into account the spatial location of the ultrasound head is a phantom with network of markers or Cambridge phantom (Prager R.W. et al., 1998).

According to Prager precision of calibration depends on the angle of viewing of the markers, position of markers on the image, quality of imaging (resolution and artifacts) and methods of navigation (which influence on precision of ultrasound probe location). A substantial error is introduced by manual marking of the fiducials on the ultrasound image. The automatic identification of fiducials would allow significant improvement in the precise calculation of the calibration matrix. It is also recommended to limit the impact of speed changes on the ultrasound measurement through the systems stabilizing the temperature of the liquid, in which phantom is immersed.

According to Mercier ultrasound imaging spatial error obtained as result of calibration using different phantom constructions range from 0.15 mm to 1.04 mm (L. Mercier et al., 2005). This error is expressed as the distance between the calculated fiducial position and the position measured applying more accurate techniques.

In conclusion, the analysis of methods to calibrate ultrasound head showed that the most efficient is application of phantom with network of markers. Improved results of analysis can be achieved through careful registration of optimal image, that is, when the scanning plane is perpendicular to the imaged markers. When the ultrasound image is stored it is recommended to select focal areas of ultrasound beams, depending on the marker location to get the best contrast of the echo.

2 MATERIAL AND METHODS

2.1 *Hardware*

A system combining ultrasound machine EchoBlaster128 (Telemed, Lithuania) with linear probe of width equaling 60 mm and Transducer Central Frequency equaling 9 MHz, and Optical Tracking System Polaris Spectra, (NDI, Canada) providing localization with 0.25 mm RMS error (see Figure 1). The devices are connected to a PC via USB interface.

The Polaris Spectra system is an infrared camera providing up to six degrees of freedom, high resolution and functionality in a wide field of view.

Wireless sensors are frames with unique geometry and four spheres coated with retroreflexive surface, reflecting IR. Each sensor constitutes a rigid body, object with constant geometry.

Passive rigid bodies were calibrated using NDI 6D Architect software, to describe the relative position of markers (infrared reflective spheres) and save the calibration data in the file.

2.2 *Transformation matrix*

To describe the position of ultrasound image in the reference coordinate system (reference frame mounted on patient body) it is necessary to calculate the relative position of probe basing on transformations given by the tracking system for reference frame (B) and sensor on ultrasound probe (A).

To determine the position of each US image pixel in the reference coordinate system (expressed by matrix X), two matrices are required: one describing the position of probe in the patient reference coordinate system (Y) and second—the sought calibration matrix (C). The notation is presented on the Figure 2.

2.3 *Calibration phantom*

To calibrate ultrasound probe a wire phantom creating five levels of double "N" was designed (see Figures 3, 5). The levels of double N structures are alternately identical (similar levels are odd—down on the Figure 3 and even—upper on the Figure 3). The "N" structures differ in geometry. The wire creating "N" structures characterizes 0.5 mm diameter.

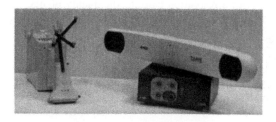

Figure 1.   3D ultrasound measuring system consisting of ultrasound machine and optical localizer.

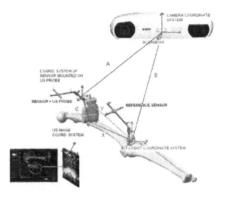

Figure 2. Scheme of matrix transformations for the navigation of ultrasound probe.

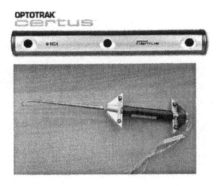

Figure 4. System Optotrak of higher precision and specially designed pointer to measure the position of holes in calibration phantom.

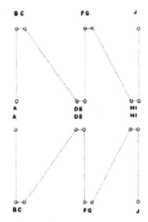

Figure 3. Configuration of double N levels.

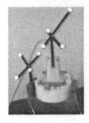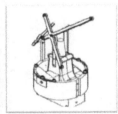

Figure 5. Calibration phantom and navigated ultrasound probe.

2.4 Method of measurement

Measurement of holes in the calibration phantom was carried out using OptotrakCertus system, NDI (see Figure 4). To measure the phantom, a special pointer with curled tip was designed (see Figure 4). The measured positions of holes were related to the reference coordinate system associated with the sensor mounted on a phantom.

Coordinates of holes of particular levels were marked as points A, B, C, D, E, F, G, H, I, J (see Figure 3).

2.5 Methods of calibration

The second phase of calibration was to scan the phantom wires when it is immersed in the tank with dimensions of 45 cm × 30 cm × 15 cm, filled with water. Stabilization of water temperature is provided by a heater controlled by temperature controller BTC9100 measuring the temperature using Pt100. The controller starts the heater through the transmitter SSR, when the fluid temperature is lower than expected. Measurements were carried out at a temperature of 37.0 degrees. In a circular overlay phantom ultrasound head had a determined position (see Figure 6).

On the ultrasound image the locations of 25 echoes from the wires were identified manually (see Figure 7).

The distances between the echoes at each level were determined. Coordinates in pixels were scaled to the values in millimeters, based on width of the head and the selected depth of the scan.

Using assertion about the similarity of triangles for each level of double "N" structures, the spatial coordinates of the fiducials echoes M, K, L, N, O in phantom reference coordinate system were determined. The idea is presented in the work of Kozak for a phantom containing three levels of single "N" structures (Kozak, J. 2009).

Using the formula:

$$\frac{|MK|}{|MN|} = \frac{|KX|}{|YX|}$$

where X is the intersection of lines AB and CD, and Y means the intersection point of lines CD and EF and basing on the dependence:

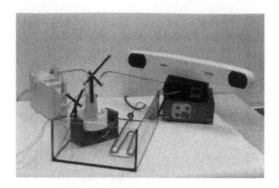

Figure 6. Set for calibration of linear ultrasonic probe.

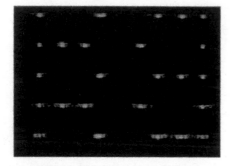

Figure 7. Ultrasound image of wire fiducials.

$$\frac{|NL|}{|NO|} = \frac{|LU|}{|WU|}$$

where U is the intersection point of lines EF and GH, and W represents the intersection of the lines GH and IJ. The coordinates of the points K and L which are intersection of wires with scanning plane, were calculated according to dependences:

$$\vec{K} = X + \frac{|MK|}{|MN|}(Y - X)$$

$$\vec{L} = U + \frac{|NL|}{|NO|}(W - U)$$

The coordinates of the remaining echoes were calculated basing on the assumptions:

- point M lies on lines AB and KL
- point N lies on lines EF and KL
- point O lies on lines IJ and KL

The navigation system tracks the position of the sensor mounted on ultrasound head which is placed in the construction of the phantom and phantom reference sensor. Transformation matrix between the image coordinate system and the phantom coordinate system is the product of the transformation matrix from the phantom to the on-probe sensor coordinate system and unknown calibration matrix.

The mathematical issue is to calculate the calibration matrix. First approach to calculate the matrix was to optimize the sum of distances (formula 2) between proper echoes positions in phantom reference frame and the positions of ultrasound echoes transformed by sought calibration matrix (formula 1).

$$T_{phantom-probe} * M_{calibration} * \begin{bmatrix} xUS_i \\ yUS_i \\ 0 \\ 1 \end{bmatrix} = \begin{bmatrix} xF_i \\ yF_i \\ zF_i \\ 1 \end{bmatrix} \tag{1}$$

$$Min\left(\sum_{i=1}^{15} \sqrt{(xF_i - xP_i)^2 + (yF_i - yP_i)^2 + (zF_i - zP_i)^2} \right) \tag{2}$$

Second approach to calculation of calibration matrix was first to approximate the plane to the positions of echoes using Singular Value Decomposition. Least square orthogonal plane contains centroid (x_0, y_0, z_0) of the echoes dataset and the normal vector of the plane is the column of eigenvector of matrix M (formula 3) corresponding to the lowest eigenvalue of this matrix.

$$M = \begin{bmatrix} x_1 - x_0 & y_1 - y_0 & z_1 - z_0 \\ | & | & | \\ | & | & | \\ x_N - x_0 & y_N - y_0 & z_N - z_0 \end{bmatrix} \tag{3}$$

$$A = M^T M \tag{4}$$

The function f (v) is minimized by the vector A corresponding to the smallest eigenvalue. Decomposition of the matrix M can be expressed according to the formula:

$$M = USV^T \tag{5}$$

where:

- S is a—diagonal matrix containing the singular values of M,
- columns of V matrix—are its singular vectors
- U is orthogonal—matrix

$$A = M^T M = (USV^T)^T (USV^T) \\ = (VS^T U^T)^T (USV^T) = VS^2 V^T \tag{6}$$

It means that the eigenvalues of a matrix A are square of singular values of matrix M and eigenvectors of the matrix A are eigenvectors of the matrix M.

Finally, orthogonal least-squares plane passes through the centroid and its normal vector is a vector of singular matrix M corresponding to the smallest singular value.

The transformation between coordinate system of ultrasound image and phantom coordinate system was defined according to formula (7) where the vx, vy and vz are the direction vector of ultrasound image coordinate system, and t is translation vector from phantom coordinate system origin to the designed origin of the ultrasound image coordinate system.

$$M_{phantom-image} = \begin{bmatrix} vx1 & vx2 & vx3 & -(t \circ vx) \\ vy1 & vy2 & vy3 & -(t \circ vy) \\ vz1 & vz2 & vz3 & -(t \circ vz) \\ 0 & 0 & 0 & 1 \end{bmatrix} \quad (7)$$

In the end the calibration matrix is calculated according to formula (8):

$$M_{calibration} = M_{probe-phantom}^{-1} * M_{phantom-image}^{-1} \quad (8)$$

3 RESULTS

Obtained calibration matrices equaled: using optimization technique:

$$M_{calibration} = \begin{pmatrix} -0.926974 & 0.0131002 & -0.35332 & -54.7083 \\ -0.381023 & -0.965834 & 0.349794 & -194.651 \\ -0.248496 & 0.365218 & 0.868169 & -102.03 \\ 0 & 0 & 0 & 1 \end{pmatrix}$$

and using SVD plane approximation:

$$M_{calibration} = \begin{pmatrix} -0.89249 & 0.23607 & -0.99905 & -60.83392 \\ -0.14107 & -0.85360 & 0.46785 & -195.44594 \\ -0.32010 & 0.41828 & -1 & -104.40520 \\ 0 & 0 & 0 & 1 \end{pmatrix}$$

Sum of distances between proper and calculated using the first matrix, calculated using optimization technique described in section 2.5, equaled about 3 mm. For the single echo the minimal distance equaled 0.15 mm and the maximum distance equaled 2.4 mm

For the second method of calibration (SVD plane approximation) the value of summarized error is higher than 4 mm. The result of the second method of calibration is worse than in first case, since it is strongly affected by imprecise determination of directional vectors vx, vy, vz defining the rotation matrix between phantom and image coordinate system.

4 DISCUSSION

4.1 *Conclusions*

The main achievement of this work is efficient calibration of ultrasound probe using a phantom of unique construction (5 levels of double "N" structures). The novelty in the proposed phantom is increased number of fiducials and differences in double "N" structures geometry.

Obtained accuracy of calibration using optimization technique is comparable to the best values described by Prager 1998 and Mercier 2005.

The stabilization of temperature is realized with accuracy of 0.1 degrees so the influence of temperature on the results of measurement can be excluded.

The important factor influencing on the calibration results is the assumption in ultrasonic imaging, saying that the velocity of ultrasounds in all tissues equals 1540 m/s which is not true in general.

The second element which could influence the results of calibration is manual marking of fiducials echoes, however the results are enough accurate in medical applications.

4.2 *Application*

The developed system found an application (see Figures 8, 9) in measurements and reconstruction of soft and bone tissues geometry (Keppler P. et al., 2007). The validation tests and tests on probands (see Figure 9) revealed good repeatability and accuracy of measurements (Swiatek-Najwer E. et al., 2008).

On the Figures 10 and 11 the results of segmentation and reconstruction procedures for bone tissue imaging are presented. The designed software enables also the virtual planning of osteotomy—correction of limb deformities with online presentation of changing geometrical parameters (see Figure 12).

Performed tests of system accuracy revealed high precision of length measurements on phantom from CIRS company, made of Zerdine water-based polymer. The deviation equaled maximally 1.5 mm (Swiatek-Najwer E. et al., 2008).

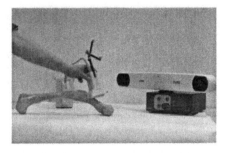

Figure 8. System for bone geometry measurement.

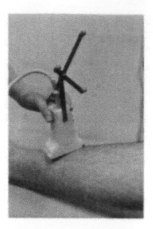

Figure 9. Measuremen: of human limb geometry.

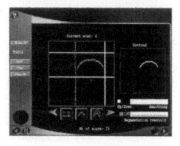

Figure 10. Segmentation of bone tissue applying 3D sonography.

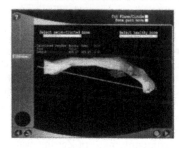

Figure 11. Reconstruction of bone tissue applying 3D sonography.

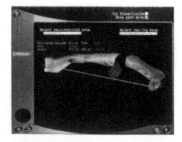

Figure 12. Virtual planning of bone correction basing on 3D sonography da:aset.

The system is now applied in clinical conditions for analysis of mechanical axes of lower limbs for patients with deformities.

ACKNOWLEDGMENTS

The research work is funded by the National Centre for Research and Development, project number NR 13 00 12 04.

REFERENCES

Ali A., Logeswaran R., 2007: A visual probe localization and calibration system for cost-efective computer-aided 3D ultrasound. Computers in Biology and Medicine, 37:1141–1147.

Barry C.D., Allott C.P., John N.W., Mellor P.M., Arundel P.A., Thomson D.S., Waterton J.C. 1997: Three-dimensional freehand ultrasound: image reconstruction and volume analysis. Ultrasound in Medicine & Biology, 23(8):1209–1224.

Blackall M., Rueckert D., Maurer Jr. C.R., Penney Hill D.L.G., Hawkes G.P., Hawkes D.J. 2000: An image registration approach to automated calibration for freehand 3D ultrasound. Proceedings of the 3rd International Conference on Medical Image Computing and Computer-Assisted Intervention, Lecture Notes in Computer Science, Springer, 1935:462–471.

Detmer R., Bashein G., Hodges T., Beach K.W., Filer E.P., Burns D.H., Stradness Jr. D.E. 1994: 3D ultrasonic image feature localization based on magnetic scan head tracking: in vitro calibration and validation. Ultrasound in Medicine & Biology, 20(9):923–936.

Keppler P., Krysztoforski K., Swiatek-Najwer E., Krowicki P., Kozak J., Gebhard F., Pinzuti J.B. 2007: A new experimental measurement and planning tool for sonographic-assisted navigation. Orthopedics (Thorofare, N.J.), Vol. 30, nr 10, suppl., s. 144–147.

Kozak J. 2009: Nawigacja w chirurgii wspomaganej komputerowo: porownanie nawigacji stosujacej obrazy ultrasonograficzne z innymi technikami nawigacji medycznej. Works of Institute of Biocibernetics and Biomedical Engineering, No. 73.

Kremer H., Dobrinski W. 1996: Diagnostykaultrasonograficzna. Elsevier Urban & Partner, Wroclaw.

Lewin P.A. 2004: Quo vadis medical ultrasound? Ultrasonics, 42(1–9):1–7.

Lindseth F., Tangen G.A., Lango T., Bang J. 2003: Probe calibration for freehand 3-D ultrasound. Ultrasound in Medicine & Biology; 29(11):1607–1623.

Mercier L, Lango T, Lindseth F, Collins D.L. 2005: A review of calibration techniques for freehand 3D ultrasound systems. Ultrasound Med Biol 31(4): 449–471.

Prager R.W., Rohling R.N., Gee A.H., Berman L. 1998: Rapid calibration for 3-D freehand ultrasound, Ultrasound in medicine and biology 24 (6): 855–869.

Swiatek-Najwer E., Bedzinski R., Krowicki P., Krysztoforski K., Keppler P., Kozak J. 2008: Improving surgical precision—application of navigation system in orthopedic surgery, Acta of Bioengineering and Biomechanics, Vol. 10, no. 4.

Technology and Medical Sciences – Natal Jorge et al. (eds)
© 2011 Taylor & Francis Group, London, ISBN 978-0-415-66822-4

Contact finite element with surface tension adhesion

R.A.P. Hellmuth & R.G. Lima
Mechanical Engineering Department, Polytechnic School at University of São Paulo, São Paulo, Brazil

ABSTRACT: This work is a contribution on the development of a computational model of lung parenchyma capable to simulate mechanical ventilation manoeuvres. This computational model should be able to represent adhesion caused by surface tension and be able suffer collapse and alveolar recruitment. Therefore, a contact finite element was developed and then simulated in a structure with structural properties of the same order of magnitude of a real alveolus. The simulation was performed with the nonlinear finite element method. The implementation of the arc-length method was also necessary in order to prevent divergence at limit points. The numerical results of the simulation of a single alveolus, including the surface tension and adhesion, are qualitatively similar to experimental data obtained from whole excised lungs. Both present hysteretic behaviour with transmural pressures of the same order of magnitude.

1 INTRODUCTION

Many patients in Intensive Care Units (ICU) are unable to breathe spontaneously and therefore they can only survive by means of mechanical ventilation. In many clinical cases the patient's condition is so weak that the physician must choose between a ventilation manoeuvre or other procedures that would perhaps help in the recovery of the patient. However, he hasn't got complete information about the lung's current condition and doesn't know for sure the efficacy of such therapeutic procedure. So, any improvement in knowledge about the physical and biological phenomena involved in lung dynamics would be very useful both for critical decisions at the bedside as for the development of new pulmonary therapy manoeuvres.

In order to exchange gases the lung depends on a harmonious relationship between ventilation and perfusion. The air and blood are guided by a complex branching system (Moore & Dalley, 2001), where they are exposed to variations of transmural and transpulmonary pressures (Fung, 975b). Thus, the ability of this organ to perform its essential function is intimately related to its mechanical behaviour (expansion and contraction) and geometry, what relates to a strong dependence of function and structure (Fung, 975a). A major challenge for the next generations of physiologists is to integrate the large amount of biological information (in rapid growth) in consistent quantitative models (Bassingthwaighte, 2000). The models summarize briefly the information, and interacting with experiments, show properties and remove contradictions, which are not evident by simple description of its parts.

1.1 Mechanical properties of lung parenchyma

The lung parenchyma is the tissue where the exchange of gases occurs. This soft tissue is composed of alveoli and alveolar ducts. The extracellular matrix of soft tissue is rich in collagen and elastin fibers. The concentration and spatial organization of collagen and elastin fibers are the main factors which defines the mechanical properties of each type of soft tissue (Fung, 1993). At small deformations elastin provides stiffness and stores most of the strain energy. The collagen fibers are comparatively inextensible and usually wavy at rest. With increasing deformation the collagen bundles are gradually stretched at the direction of deformation, what strongly increases the tissue's stiffness. This composite behaviour is analogous to the fibrous tissue of a nylon stocking, where elastin does the role of the rubber band and collagen the nylon's.

1.2 Idealized geometry of the pulmonary alveolus

Recent descriptions based on histological analysis have shown that the alveolar walls are shared between neighbour alveoli and form a structure similar to a honeycomb (Hansen, Ampaya, Bryant & Navin, 1975, Hansen & Ampaya, 1975). Therefore, the airways in the lung parenchyma are series of branching corridors with polygonal walls and their dead ends are called alveoli. There are no "inner" and "outer" parts of the alveoli, instead there are septa which divide either an alveolus from another or an alveolus from an alveolar duct.

Dale, Matthews & Schroter (1980) proposed a geometric model in which the parenchyma takes the form of a tessellation of second order regular polyhedra with 14 faces, see Figure 1. This kind of polyhedra is also know as tetrakaidecahedra, truncated octahedron or simply 14-hedron. It has the advantages of being regular, being convex, fills the space when tessellated and has the smallest ratio of surface to volume among the space filling polyhedra (Fung, 1988). The airways are formed by removing some walls from the tessellated 14-hedra. The estimated difference for the surface-volume ratio between the parenchyma modelled and actual values found in literature is 2.7% (Tawhai & Burrowes, 2003).

1.3 Surface tension in alveoli

Because the lungs are very efficient mass exchangers with very thin wall between air and blood, some water diffuses from the blood vessels to alveolar cavity. The surface tension of the water film on the septa affects significantly the alveolar mechanics. To reduce surface tension of the air-water interface, some epithelial cells produce a very efficient surfactant mixture. Surfactant molecules have a water affinity polar side and an air affinity apolar side.

1.4 Structural effect and hysteresis

The surface tension magnitude depends on the concentration of the surfactant molecules at the air-liquid interface. During the respiratory cycle changes in the total area of the lung alter the air-liquid interface area. Consequently the surfactant concentration at the interface vary together with the surface tension magnitude. That is, surface tension increases during inspiration and decreases during expiration. During inspiration, an excess surfactant molecules are recruited to the interface when the concentration there drops below the saturation level, and at expiration the decrease in interface area causes the expulsion of surplus molecules. The dynamics of interface area, concentration of surfactant at the interface and surface tension causes part of the lung hysteresis, see Figure 2 (Levitzky, 2003).

The surface tension also has structural function in the lung parenchyma, because it increases the stiffness of the lung and supports part of the load. Fortunately, this increased stiffness is much higher in lung volumes near total lung capacity, since the increased surface area of parenchyma reduces the concentration of surfactant at the interface (Schurch, Bachofen, Goerke & Possmayer, 2001).

1.5 Atelectasis

A telectasis is a lung condition in which part of the lung collapses preventing air flow there. A telectasis can be acute or chronic and can affect the entire lung or part of it. From the physical point of view atelectasis occurs when moist membranes of the parenchyma touch themselves, leading to the fusion of the liquid layers, what consequently reduces the surface energy. The collapsed region can only be recruited if subjected to a higher contrary pressure to the adhesion pressure. The surfactant is very important to detach the adhered membranes because it makes easier to increase the area of the interface liquid-air with lower surface tension.

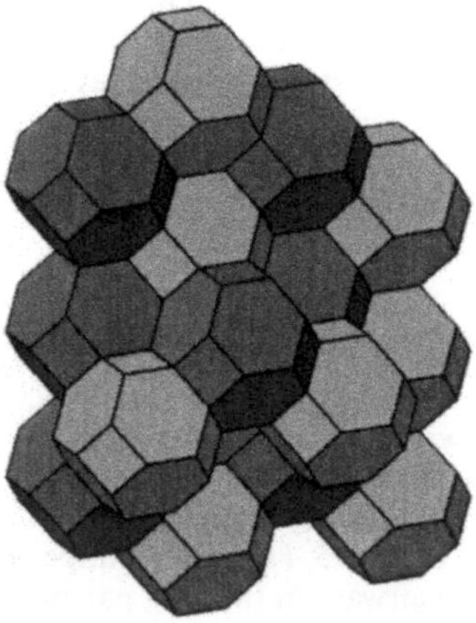

Figure 1.   14-hedra tessellation filling the space.

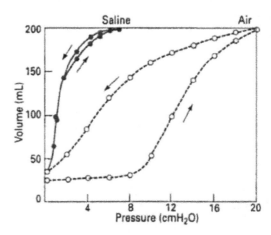

Figure 2.   Pressure-volume graphs of cat excised lungs. Lungs inflated with saline (solid line) and air (dashed line).

Despite the biomedical literature addressing the surface tension as the cause of atelectasis, no tribological studies of the septa surfaces were found. The mechanism of adhesion of the septa and the forces involved in it are still not well understood.

2 OBJECTIVE

A fundamental building block for developing a structural model capable of simulating pulmonary alveolar recruitment manoeuvres is an element of contact with adhesion caused by surface tension. A constitutive equation for this element is proposed and evaluated numerically in a simple structure using the nonlinear finite element method.

3 METHODOLOGY

A constitutive equation for the contact with adhesion finite element will be now presented. In order to validate this model a contact simulation of a simplified membrane structure will be shown. This simulation is done with the Finite Element Method (FEM). As problems involving large deformations, rotations, and particularly contact are not linear, an algorithm for finding equilibrium configurations of non-linear systems had to be used. Since the contact element's constitutive equation introduce critical points to the system, the arc-length method was implemented to avoid numerical instabilities.

3.1 *Adhesion contact function*

The adhesive contact model developed here is simplified, it considers the surface tension constant and ignores the geometry of the meniscus. Its formulation is based on a number of assumptions announced below and illustrated in the Figure 3.

1. The liquid film is continuous on both membrane surfaces. At height h from the surface, molecular attraction forces start to be significant (see Figure (3g)). At greater distances, $d > 2h$, the attraction forces are negligible.
2. At a distance $d \approx 2h = d_2$ the liquid films begin to attract each other (see Figure (3b)) and a meniscus is formed between both surfaces (see Figure (3c)).
3. In the meniscus (or contact) region there is an adhesion pressure as stated by the Young-Laplace Law (Butt & Kappl, 2010),

$$p = \gamma \left(\frac{1}{r_1} + \frac{1}{r_2} \right). \tag{1}$$

4. The surface of the meniscus has two curvature radii, but only the one proportional to

distance is considered $r = r_1 = d/2$ (see Fig. (3d)). The second radius is neglected in equation 1, because it is much higher than the first ($r_2 \gg r_1$). The adhesion pressure becomes

$$\tilde{p}_{ad}(d) = -\frac{2\gamma}{d}. \tag{2}$$

5. At a distance d_1 when the roughness of the surfaces touch each other a contact reaction force arises (see Figure (3d)). At this distance the pressure of adhesion is maximal, i.e. max $(p_{ad}(d)) = p_{ad}(d_1)$. The contact reaction force increases with greater intensity than that of adhesion, when the distance approaches zero.
6. The adhesion work is reversible. That is, the work to detach the surfaces is equal to the work to join them.

3.2 *Formulation*

The Equation 2 has some practical problems. It is always a negative hyperbole, since $d \in \mathbb{R}_+$. In order to include the hypotheses h1 and h5 the adhesion shall act only within the range of $d_1 < d < d_2$. It is also needed to include the contact condition that prevents the interpenetration of the surfaces. To satisfy all hypotheses a pressure equation $p_\gamma(d)$ should be formulated with the following characteristics: $p_\gamma(0) > 0$, $p_\gamma(d) \approx \tilde{p}_{ad}(d) < 0$ within $d_1 < d < d_2$, $p_\gamma(d) \approx 0$ for $d > d_2$ and smooth $p'_\gamma(d)$.

There are some possibilities for $p_\gamma(d)$ function, which can be split in a portion of contact reaction $p_c(d)$ and another of adhesion $p_{ad}(d)$,

$$p_\gamma(d) = p_c(d) + p_{ad}(d), \tag{3}$$

whose derivative is

$$p'_\gamma(d) = p'_c(d) + p'_{ab}(d). \tag{4}$$

The contact reaction was defined as

$$p_c(d) = p_{c_0} e^{-\alpha d}, \tag{5}$$

where $p_{c_0} = p_c(0)$. It is defined such that at the distance d_1 the contact pressure is one percent of that at $d = 0$, therefore α is a constant obtained by

$$p_c(d_1) = 0,01 p_c(0) \quad \Leftrightarrow \quad \alpha = \ln \frac{100}{d_1}. \tag{6}$$

The derivative of the contact pressure is

$$p_c^1(d) = -\alpha p_{c_0} e^{-\alpha d}. \tag{7}$$

The class of sigmoid functions have interesting properties to approximate equation 2 in $d_1 < d < d_2$. They form a smooth step function

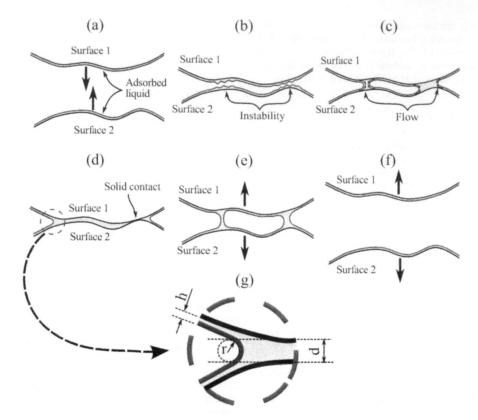

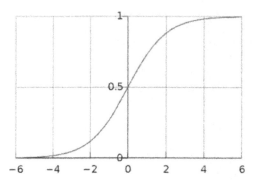

Figure 3. Outline of the adhesive contact between two surfaces. (a) Approaching. (b) The force of molecular attraction draws the liquid into the region where the surfaces are closer. (c) When liquid films fuse and the meniscus is formed, more liquid is attracted to the region. (d) The approach ends when the roughness of the surfaces touch themselves. (e) Withdrawing. (f) Detached surfaces. (g) Detail of the contact showing the geometric variables.

("S" shaped curve in Figure 4) inside the range and are asymptotically constant outside it. Some examples of sigmoid functions are the logistic function, arctangent, hyperbolic tangent and erf error function. For convenience, the logistic function will be used:

$$p_{lg}(t) = \frac{1}{1+e^{-t}}, \tag{8}$$

whose derivative is

$$p'_{lg}(t) = \frac{e^{-t}}{\left(1+e^{-t}\right)^2} = p_{lg}\left(1-p_{lg}\right), \tag{9}$$

whose graphic can be seen in Figure 4.

For 8 to approximate 2 some adjustments must be made. Transforming the range d: $[d_1, d_2]$ to t: $[-5, 5]$ of 8 leads to

$$t(d) = \frac{10}{d_2-d_1}\left[d - \left(\frac{d_1+d_2}{2}\right)\right] \tag{10}$$

Figure 4. Graph of the logistic function, equation 8.

and

$$t'(d) = \frac{10}{d_2-d_1}. \tag{11}$$

To $p_{ad}(d_1) \approx \tilde{p}_{ad}(d_1)$ and $p_{ad}(d_2) \approx 0$, equations 8 and 9 are transformed into

$$p_{ad}\left(d\right)\frac{2\gamma}{d_1}\left[1-p_{lg}\left(t(d)\right)\right] \tag{12}$$

and

$$p_{ad}\left(d\right)=\frac{2\gamma}{d_1}t'\left(d\right)p'_{lg}\left(t(d)\right). \tag{13}$$

Finally a value for p_{c_0} of 5 is chosen, such that $p_\gamma(0)=\tilde{p}_{c_0}$, with a defined value of $\tilde{p}_{c_0}$ With 5 and 12 inside (3) and $d=0$,

$$p_\gamma(0)=p_{c_0}-\frac{2\gamma}{d_1}=\tilde{p}_{c_0}\Leftrightarrow p_{c_0}=\tilde{p}_{c_0}+\frac{2\gamma}{d_1} \tag{14}$$

and 3 e (4) are complete. They can be visualized respectively in Figures 5 and 6. 4 is the derivative of 3, which is necessary for the solution of the Newton-Raphson method.

3.3 Viability test

A simple geometry was used to approximate an alveolus. The human alveoli have an average diameter of $D \approx 0, 3$ mm (McArdle, Katch & Katch, 2006). Simplifying to 2D, a central section of a sphere with this diameter is a circle with perimeter $P = nD \approx 0, 9$ mm. A rectangle with the same perimeter can then be taken $P = 2(l_1 + l_2) \approx 2(0, 30 + 0, 15)$ mm, as shows Figure 7. This is a fairly reasonable approximation since some portions of the lung tend to deform in a non-uniform way.

The membrane of the inter-alveolar septum is simulated with non-linear first-order isoparametric truss elements (Felippa, 2001), with the Kirchhoff

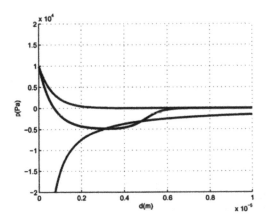

Figure 5. Graphs showing the pressure of Young-La-place's Law in blue (p_{ad} of 2), dry contact in red (p_c of 5) and the constitutive equation of surface tension adhesive contact in black (p_γ of 3). The equations parameters are: $\gamma = 7.5 \cdot 10^{-3}$ N/m, $d_1 = 3 \cdot 10^{-6}$m, $d_2 = 7 \cdot 10^{-6}$m $p_{c_0} = 2 \cdot 10^4 Pa$.

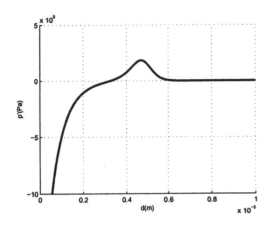

Figure 6. Graphs of the constitutive equation of surface tension adhesive contact derivative (p'_γ of 4). Same parameters of Figure 5.

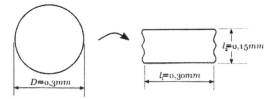

Figure 7. Geometric approximation of a circle to a rectangle with the same perimeter.

material model (Reddy, 2008) as constitutive equation. The value of Young's modulus for collagen, $E = 10^9 Pa$ (Fung, 1993), was chosen as material constant. Despite the Young's modulus and Kirchhoff material's constant relate different strain measures, they differ very little when only small uniaxial strains are accounted. That is, at small strains the first Piola-Kirchhoff stress tensor is approximately equal to the second Piola-Kirchhoff: $P_{11} \approx S_{11}$, and the engineering strain is approximately equal to the Green-Lagrange's: $\epsilon_{11} \approx E_{11}$). As the collagen maximum strain is low, $\epsilon_{max} = 2\%$ (Fung, 1993) (Maksym & Bates, 1997), the approximation error of E to C^{SE} to this strain level is 1%, which makes this approach acceptable. Using the collagen Young's module is reasonable since this is the fibre that resists large soft tissues' deformations.

The thickness of the collagen structural section is difficult to estimate, since at this scale the collagen is viewed as fibre bundles and not as continuum. However the collagen bundles usually have an average diameter between 0.2 and 12 μm (Fung, 1993). Considering the section of the membrane geometry as seen in Figure 7, which by one side has the length of the alveolus (l_1) and by the other the height (h) equivalent to the fibre thickness, a reasonable area for the bar section could be $A_{bar} = l_1 \cdot h = 3 \cdot 10^{-4} \cdot 1, 3 \cdot 10^{-6} \approx 4 \cdot 10^{-10}$ mm.

The height of the liquid film was arbitrarily defined as 3, 5 µm, which means by the hypothesis h2 that the adhesion starts at a distance between membranes $d_2 = 7 \cdot 10^{-6}$ m. The distance of the roughness interference (hypothesis h5) was also chosen arbitrarily as $d_1 = 3 \cdot 10^{-6}$ m. The value of surface tension was chosen as 7, 5 $\cdot 10^{-3}$ N/m, which is a physiological value (Schurch, Lee & Gehr, 1992).

3.4 Numerical stability

The algorithm used to search the nonlinear solution was the Newton-Raphson method (Wriggers, 2008). Because the system has limit points, it was necessary to employ a continuation method to prevent divergence close to these points. The continuation method here applied was the Crisfield (1981) arc-length method linearised by Schweizerhof & Wriggers, (1986).

4 RESULTS

Figures 8 to 16 show a sequence of configurations related to different transmural pressures p_{tm}. The thick red lines represent the truss elements current settings, the dash red lines their the initial position and the black circles the nodes. The fixed black thin line indicate the opposed surface and the dash-dot blue line the position where the adhesion starts and ends.

It is interesting to observe the free nodes vertical trajectory. In Figure 17 the trajectory of half-symmetric structure is seen. Figure 17 shows the adhesion of the central nodes in detail.

Figure 19 is a graph of pressure to cross-sectional area of the alveolus (analogous to the volume in excised lungs), which clearly shows the hysteresis caused by the adhesion. The magnitude of the cross-sectional area

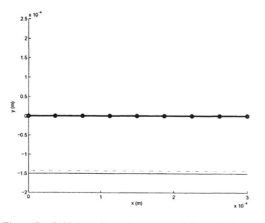

Figure 8.   Initial configuration at $p_{tm} = 0.0$ cm H_2O.

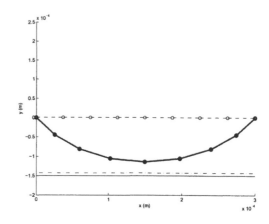

Figure 9.   Configuration at $p_{tm} = -4.0$ cm H_2O.

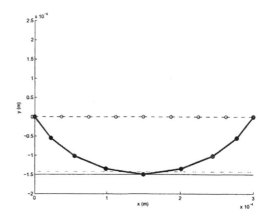

Figure 10.   Initial configuration at $p_{tm} = -8.0$ cm H_2O.

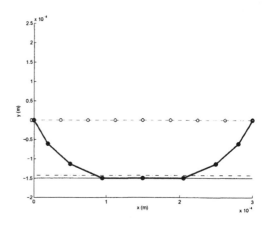

Figure 11.   Configuration at $p_{tm} = -12.0$ cm H_2O.

was calculated by the trapezoid integration method. Each point in evidence in Figure 19 is a configuration of a pre-set transmural pressure. Most of these configurations are shown in Figures 8 to 16.

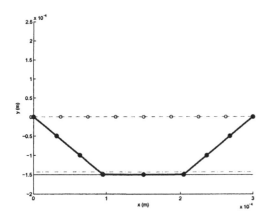

Figure 12. Initial configuration at $p_{tm} = 0.0$ cm H_2O.

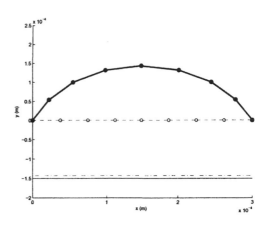

Figure 15. Configuration at $p_{tm} = 8.0$ cm H_2O.

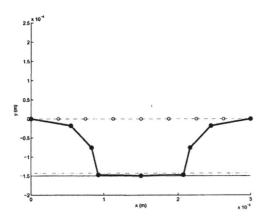

Figure 13. Configuration at $p_{tm} = 30.0$ cm H_2O.

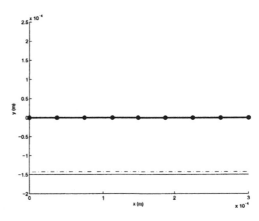

Figure 16. End configuration at $p_{tm} = 0.0$ cm H_2O.

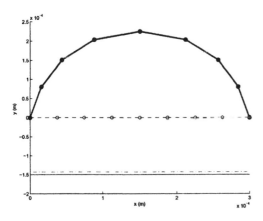

Figure 14. Initial configuration at $p_{tm} = 30.5$ cm H_2O.

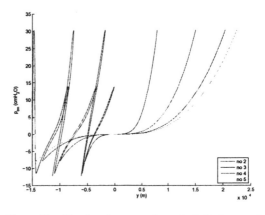

Figure 17. Graphs of pressure to vertical displacement of the nodes of the membrane half-symmetric part.

75

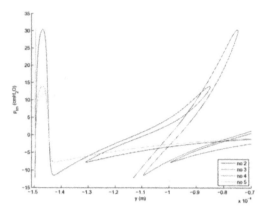

Figure 18. The same curves of Figure 17, highlighting the central nodes 4 and 5.

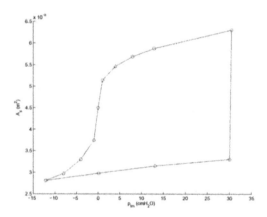

Figure 19. Graph of pressure vs. cross-sectional area of the alveolus, showing hysteresis.

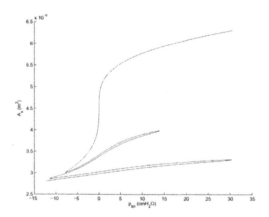

Figure 20. Graph of pressure vs. cross-sectional area of the alveolus, showing the equilibrium path.

Figure 20 shows the equilibrium trajectory got by the arc-length method.

5 DISCUSSION

The sequel from Figure 8 to 16 rebuilds the intuitively expected mechanics. The curve in Figure 19 has the same hysterectical morphology observed experimentally for whole lung in Figure 2. The difference in inclination between the recruitment paths of Figures 19 and 2 comes from the fact that in the whole lung there are many collapsed alveoli being recruited with different pressure levels. The variation of surfactant interface concentration also affects the curve loop in Figure 19, but is neglected in Figure 2.

Figure 17 shows the element nodes vertical trajectory as a function of transmural pressure. Two peaks of pressure can be seen, which correspond to attachment and detachment of the central node (node 5) and the nodes next to it (node 4 and its symmetric pair, node 6). The lowest transmural pressure level ($p_{tm} \approx 14$ cm H_2O) corresponds to the adhesion pressure of the central node and the highest ($p_{tm} \approx 30$ cm H_2O) to the nodes next to the central one. Figure 18 highlights the movement of the central nodes, the ones which undergo adhesion. It is important to remember hypothesis h6, which means that the work needed either to attach or detach are conservative.

From the standpoint of structural stability, there are limit points at the adhesion zone border, and therefore it was necessary to apply the arc-length method. Without the arc-length method each node entering or quitting the adhesion configuration shows snap-through, which leads to numerical instabilities. The degrees of freedom near limit points present almost horizontal derivatives at stiffness softening configuration. Then big displacements are inevitably produced by the Newton-Raphson method, which may unduly drag other degrees of freedom to either inside or outside the adhesion zones. Besides the wrong results, abrupt variations of derivative magnitudes usually lead to numerical instability.

The controlled solution makes it possible to find intermediate results to snap-throughs and snapbacks. These equilibrium positions require a controled loading that does not exist in reality, thus very difficult to be observed experimentally. To reconcile the numerical results with ones experimentally observed, Figure 19 shows only some stable equilibrium configurations found for desired transmural pressure levels (points in evidence) and disregards the equilibrium path that could show unstable configurations. If the whole arc-length trajectories were regarded, path morphology would be like in Figure 20. It would not be a closed curve and the energy barriers of the adhesive contact would be visible.

The open curve in Figure 20 indicates that the adhesion work with continuous surface tension is conservative, which is consistent with the hypothesis of h6. Hysteresis is a characteristic of non-conservative systems and it just appears in the results when snap-throughs are considered. The snap-throughs occur when the equilibrium of the whole system is not quasi-statically controlled. Since it is impracticable to completely control a continuum medium, a theoretical conservative system end up becoming non-conservative. Both the attached and detached conditions are conditions of minimum potential energy, with an energy barrier between them. In Figure 20 it is possible to see the nodes 4 and 5 getting up and down not through an energy barrier but through a transmural pressure barrier, with peaks near $y = -1,43 \cdot 10^{-4}$ m.

6 CONCLUSIONS

The adhesive contact element proposed here can reproduce the hysteresis loop observed in the collapse and recruitment of a group of alveoli, in agreement with the order of magnitude of the involved physical measures. Recruitment is triggered at higher pressures than the collapse, which is the same asymmetry observed experimentally. However it does not reproduce the viscous dissipative aspects of lung dynamics, such as liquid flow, variation of surfactant concentration and tissue viscoelasticity.

This finite element simulations can be applied to large populations of alveoli, which would allow a structural analysis more realistic. Another big advantage of this element is that its parameters can be adjusted with experimental measurements. However the adhesion magnitude on the surface of the alveoli still has to be measured by tribological experiments. The relationship between the surfactant, the liquid film and the surface of the epithelial cell membrane also needs to be better understood.

Even without reliable parameters for a more accurate assessment for the estimation of the intensity of the adhesion forces, this contact element can already simulate aspects not found in the literature.

ACKNOWLEDGEMENTS

This work was supported by the National Counsel of Technological and Scientific Development ("Con-selho Nacional de Desenvolvimento Cientfico e Tecnolgico"—CNPq) 135262/2007-0.

REFERENCES

Bassingthwaighte, J.B. (2000). Strategies for the physiome project. *Annals of Biomedical Engineering* 28, 1043–1058.

Butt, H.-J. & Kappl, M. (2010). *Surface and Interfacial Forces.* Weinheim, Alemanha: Wiley-VCH Verlag GmbH & Co. KGaA.

Crisfield, M.A. (1981). A fast incremental/iterative solution procedure that handles "snap-through". *Computer & Structures* 13, 55–62.

Dale, P.J., Matthews, F.L. & Schroter, R.C. (1980). Finite element analysis of lung alveolus. *Journal of Biomechanics* 13, 865–873.

Felippa, C. (2001). *Nonlinear Finite Element Method.* Boulder, Colorado, USA: Department of Aerospace Engineering Sciences and Center for Space Structures and Controls: University of Colorado.

Fung, Y.-C. (1975a, October). Stress, deformation, and atelectasis of the lung. *Circulation Research* 37, 481–96.

Fung, Y.-C. (1975b, October). Does the surface tension make the lung inherenthly unstable? *Circulation Research* 37, 497–502.

Fung, Y.-C. (1988). A model of the lung structure and its validation. *Journal of Applied Physiology* 64, 2132–2141.

Fung, Y.-C. (1993). *Biomechanics: Mechanical Properties of Living Tissues* (2 ed.). New York, EUA: Springer-Verlag.

Hansen, J.E. & Ampaya, E.P. (1975). Human air space shapes, sizes, areas, and volumes. *Journal of Applied Physiology* 38(6), 990–995.

Hansen, J.E., Ampaya, E.P. Bryant, G.H. & Navin, J.J. (1975). The branching pattern of airways and air spaces of a single human terminal bronchiole. *Journal of Applied Physiology* 38(6), 983–989.

Levitzky, M.G. (2003). *Pulmonary Physiology* (6 ed.). New York, USA: Mc-Hill.

Maksym, G.N. & Bates, J.H.T. (1997). A distributed nonlinear model of lung tissue elasticity. *Journal of Applied Physiology* 82(1), 32–41.

McArdle, W.D., Katch, F.I. & Katch, V.L. (2006). *Exercise Physiology: Energy, Nutrition, and Human Performance* (6 ed.). Baltimore, EUA: Lippincott Williams & Wilkins.

Moore, K.L. & Dalley, A.F. (2001). *Anatomia orientada para a clnica* (4 ed.). Rio de Janeiro: Guanabara Koogan.

Reddy, J.N. (2008). *An Introduction to Continuum Mechanics.* Cambridge, Reino Unido: Cambridge University Press.

Schurch, S., Bachofen, H., Goerke, J. & Possmayer, F. (2001, February). Surface activity in situ, in vivo, and in the captive bubble surfactometer. *Comparative Biochemistry and Physiology Part A* 129, 195–207.

Schurch, S., Lee, M. & Gehr, P. (1992, November). Pulmonary surfactant: Surface properties and function of alveolar and airway surfactant. *Pure and Applied Chemistry* 64, 1745–1750.

Schweizerhof, K.H. & Wriggers, P. (1986). Consistent linearization for path following methods in nonlinear FE analysis. *Computer Methods in Applied Mechanics and Engineering* 59, 261–279.

Tawhai, M.H. & Burrowes, K.S. (2003). Developing integrative computational models of pulmonary structure. *The Anatomical Record Part B: The New Anatomist* 275B, 207–218.

Wriggers, P. (2008). *Nonlinear Finite Element Methods.* Berlin, Alemanha: Springer-Verlag.

Technology and Medical Sciences – Natal Jorge et al. (eds)
© 2011 Taylor & Francis Group, London, ISBN 978-0-415-66822-4

Crystalline lens imaging with a slit-scanning system

C. Oliveira, J.B. Almeida & S. Franco
Centre of Physics, University of Minho, Braga, Portugal

ABSTRACT: Accurate geometric measurements of the human crystalline lens are crucial for a better understanding of the accommodation mechanism and the origin of the presbyopia. Determining the lens shape and curvature can provide key information on the growth and aging of the lens. We present a slit-scanning optical system that is suitable for imaging the human crystalline lens and has the ability to measure its surface shape and curvature.

Keywords: Crystalline Lens, Slit-scanning, Image processing

1 INTRODUCTION

The human crystalline lens plays a fundamental role on the retinal image quality. The ability of the lens to change its shape and, consequently, the total refractive power of the eye, during accommodation, enables one to focus objects at a wide range of distances.

Knowledge regarding the crystalline lens' geometric properties provides insights into the focusing mechanism of the visual system. Namely, the study of changes in surface shape and curvatures of the lens during accommodation is essential for a better understanding of the accommodation mechanism itself (Chien, Huang, and Schachar 2006), (Dubbelman, Van Der Heijde, and Weeber 2005). Age-related changes in these geometric properties of the lens are often invoked to explain the etiology and progression of presbyopia (Koretz, Cook, and Kaufman 1997), (Weeber and van Der Heijde 2007).

Crystalline lens' optical properties, such as focal length and spherical aberrations, are closely related to its geometric properties (Goncharov and Dainty 2007). By measuring the surface's shape and curvature, along with parameters such as the refractive gradient index and thickness, we can determine the optical power of the lens. Studying the changes in optical properties of the lens during accommodation and aging improves the investigation on the relative contribution of lens geometry and refractive index distribution of the lens (Dubbelman and Van Der Heijde 2001).

We are currently developing a slit-scanning tomography system that's capable of imaging the anterior chamber of the eye. This system has already been successfully used to perform complete three-dimensional analyses of the cornea, including shape, curvature, thickness (Franco, Almeida and Parafita 2002) and aberrations; in this document we overview the applicability of our device to the crystalline lens.

2 SYSTEM DESCRIPTION

2.1 *System configuration and image acquisition*

Currently our system (Figure 1) integrates two Charge Coupled Device (CCD) cameras with a compact illumination system. Both CCD cameras

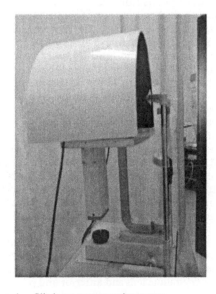

Figure 1. Slit-lamp tomography system.

are mounted to a fixed stand and inclined at 60° from the optical axis of the device. The illumination system is composed by a monochromatic blue Light-Emitting Diode (LED), a collimator, a cylindrical lens, a convex lens and an apodizing aperture slit. After the beam is collimated, the cylindrical lens expands it into a fan. This cylindrical lens, which is rod-shaped, has a diameter of 5 mm and is attached to a rotational motion system controlled by the customized software. The fan is focused on the cornea surface by the convex lens and the light diffused from the cornea produces an optical section. The orientation of the optical sections coincides with the cylinder lens orientation.

The fan automatically rotates along the optical axis, performing scans from 0° to 180° so that the cameras are able to obtain several slit images (the number of captures is user-definable). In each rotation the cameras acquire the images of the optical sections of the cornea.

We opted for this two-camera solution because it affords us a higher capture speed than would be possible with a single camera rotating concomitantly with the fan.

2.2 Image processing

After the captures are performed, a gray-level adaptive thresholding algorithm is applied to each image in order to obtain the edges of the anterior segment structures, including anterior and posterior corneal surfaces and anterior and posterior lens surfaces. The algorithm analyzes the gray-level along a scan line crossing the corneal section image and compares it to a predefined threshold level. This process is repeated for each meridian and provides a set of points from each surface.

Due to the inclined position of the CCD cameras in relation to the eye surface, the captured images suffer a constant geometric distortion. To counter this we used a calibration grid (in other words, of known dimensions) to compute a geometric transformation that we apply to the images in order to eliminate the distortion. This computation is also leveraged to map the set of points from each optical section image into a Cartesian plane.

Furthermore, due to the differences in refractive indices and the several radius of curvature of the refractive surfaces, the posterior corneal surface and both the surfaces of the crystalline lens are also affected by the optical distortion. The anterior surface of the cornea only suffers from geometrical distortion; the posterior cornea is seen refracted from the anterior cornea surface, anterior crystalline lens is seen refracted by both posterior and anterior cornea surfaces, and the posterior crystalline lens is seen refracted by anterior crystalline lens and anterior and posterior

cornea. With all the geometric and/or optical corrections accomplished, the real coordinates of both surfaces of the cornea and crystalline are known. A polynomial is then fitted to the data points of each surface.

3 RESULTS

Figure 2 shows an optical section acquired with our slit-scanning system and the detection of the edges of both surfaces of the lens. The developed algorithm, based on gray-scale analyses, provided an effective detection of the anterior and posterior surfaces of the crystalline lens.

In order to reconstruct the 3 dimensional structure of the crystalline lens, we acquired six slit images of the eye with our optical slit-scanning system. From the complete analysis of the images, we are capable of modeling both cornea and crystalline lens structures (Figure 3).

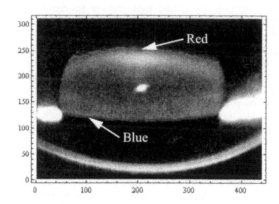

Figure 2. Image of an optical section after the detection of anterior and posterior surfaces of the crystalline lens (blue and red points, respectively).

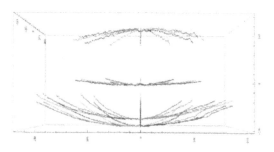

Figure 3. Profile of anterior and posterior surfaces of the cornea and of the crystalline lens (from bottom to top).

4 CONCLUSION

The main focus of this paper is the description of a slit-scanning technique capable of imaging the crystalline lens. Digital image processing and polynomial fitting are used for processing the human crystalline lens images and finally the 3 dimensional reconstruction of the crystalline lens is achieved.

REFERENCES

Chien, Chang-Hai, M., Tseng Huang, and Ronald, A. Schachar. 2006. Analysis of human crystalline lens accommodation. *Journal of biomechanics* 39, no. 4: 672–80.

Dubbelman, M., and Van Der Heijde, G.L. 2001. The shape of the aging human lens: curvature, equivalent refractive index and the lens paradox. *Vision research* 41, no. 14: 1867–77.

Dubbelman, M., Van Der Heijde, G.L. and Weeber, HA 2005. Change in shape of the aging human crystalline lens with accommodation. *Vision research* 45, no. 1: 117–32.

Franco, S., Almeida, J.B., and Parafita, M. 2002. Measuring corneal thickness with a rotary scanning system. *J Refract Surg*, 18, S630–S633.

Goncharov, Alexander, V, and Chris Dainty. 2007. Wide-field schematic eye models with gradient-index lens. *Journal of the Optical Society of America. A, Optics, image science, and vision* 24, no. 8: 2157–74.

Koretz, J.F., Cook, C.A. and Kaufman, P.L. 1997. Accommodation and presbyopia in the human eye. Changes in the anterior segment and crystalline lens with focus. *Investigative ophthalmology & visual science* 38, no. 3: 569–78.

Weeber, Henk, A. and van Der Heijde Rob, G.L. 2007. On the relationship between lens stiffness and accommodative amplitude. *Experimental eye research* 85, no. 5: 602–7.

Technology and Medical Sciences – Natal Jorge et al. (eds)
© 2011 Taylor & Francis Group, London, ISBN 978-0-415-66822-4

Design of Medical Rehabilitation Devices: A case study

E. Seabra, L.F. Silva, P. Flores & M. Lima
Mechanical Engineering Department, Enginnering School, University of Minho, Guimarães, Portugal

ABSTRACT: The paper explains how some fundamental concepts associated with Competence-Based Education are applied in Biomechanical project teaching at the Mechanical Engineering Department of the University of Minho. In the sequel of this process, the most relevant projects carried out in the scope of the Curricular Unit "Design of Medical and Rehabilitation Devices" of the Integrated Master course in Biomedical Engineering, specialization area of Biomaterials, Rehabilitation, and Biomechanics, are presented and discussed. Finally, it will be analyzed in detail a case study related to the conceptual design of a feeding device to assist motor or mental handicapped people.

1 INTRODUCTION

It is known that, to reduce the potential health care costs arising from a rapidly aging industrial world population, the problem of sustaining independent living for the elderly and persons with low to high levels of disabilities must be addressed.

There are many examples of assistive devices for people with manipulative and locomotive disabilities. These devices enable disabled people to perform many activities of daily living thus improving their quality of life. Disabled people are increasingly able to lead an independent life and play a more productive role in society (Butler, 1986).

This paper focus on the development of assistive devices that replace or enhance function, which is the scope of the Curricular Unit "Design of Medical and Rehabilitation Devices" of the Integrated Master course in Biomedical Engineering, specialization area of Biomaterials, Rehabilitation, and Biomechanics. The concepts associated with Competence-Based Education are applied in this Curricular Unit using the methodology of problem-based learning/teaching strategies. The students are active participants rather than passive observers in the Biomechanical project learning process, because the knowledge is learned and applied in a realistic problem solving where the student must make decisions, solve problems and analyze the achieved results. A summary of the research and parallel teaching activities related to the design of medical and rehabilitation devices, and, with more detail, a case study related with the conceptual design of a feeding device to assist motor or mental handicapped people will be presented in this paper.

2 OUTLINE OF THE MEDICAL AND REHABILITATION DEVICES

There are many examples of assistive devices for people with manipulative and locomotive disabilities.

Listed below are the titles of the main projects that were offered within the Curricular Unit mentioned, regarding the design of assistive devices for people with manipulative and locomotive disabilities:

- Active and passive system for shoulder rehabilitation;
- Standing frame for rehabilitation of children with mental deficiency;
- System to help dress and undress activities of disabled individuals in wheel chairs;
- Feeding device to assist motor or mental handicapped people.

2.1 Shoulder rehabilitation device project

The aim of this project was to develop a new device for the rehabilitation of the shoulder. To accomplish this objective a survey of the physiological characteristics of the shoulder was performed, regarding the different types of movements provided by this articulation and its most common pathologies.

The idea behind this project came from the internet analysis of an existing equipment, the Rotater (Rotater, 2010). A device was then developed that fulfills all the characteristic features needed for rehabilitation mechanisms, regarding safety and comfort, as well as being capable to provide an adaptive rehabilitation which is quite useful during all stages of recovery. To accomplish this latter issue, one of the important aspects on this design was the fact that it must be able to rehabilitate the patient in an active and passive scheme, i.e. the device must rehabilitate the shoulder when the patient is unable to exercise it, also enabling the operator or supervisor (usually a physiotherapist, a medical doctor or any other health or rehabilitation professional) to control the rehabilitation procedure to permit the patient to perform some force to improve and/or accelerate the recovery (commanding and controlling the torque developed by the motor that moves the rehabilitation shoulder device).

Therefore, a new system was proposed that adapts an existing arrangement (where the patient exerted his strength by using the other arm), to which a motor was attached to act the mechanism to exercise the shoulder of the patient, without exerting any force during the rehabilitation procedure. Figure 1 shows the 3D modeling of the device designed for passive and active rehabilitation of the shoulder.

2.2 Standing frame project

A standing frame is a mechanical or mechatronic equipment that aims to correct the inability of individuals to assume the vertical position. The available standing frames do not enable an easy positioning and placement of the individual on the device, do not permit full mobility (inside and outside buildings), are not versatile, modular and do not allow children to have occupational activities during treatments. The standing frame developed here and to be used in the treatment of children mental handicapped, takes into account the drawbacks mentioned above and it is perfectly adapted to this specific targeted individuals. The main features of the developed equipment is the modularity, being easily operated and used, especially when the handicapped, and family, need to travel and need to carry with them the standing frame. Figure 2 illustrates the 3D models developed for the standing frame in two different perspectives, where the most important mechanical components can be observed.

2.3 Dress and undress aid device project

The main objectives of this project were to design and develop a device to help individuals with paraplegia

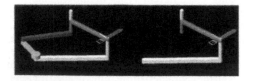

Figure 1. Configuration of the shoulder rehabilitation device: (left) active device and (right) passive device.

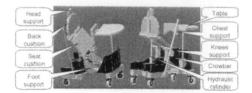

Figure 2. Overall 3D views of the developed standing frame.

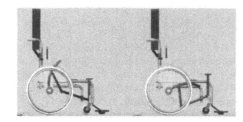

Figure 3. Schematic representation of the lifting solution for the handicapped legs (using pulleys): (left) minimum point and (right) maximum point.

to dress and/or undress. The whole design was based on the procedure for dressing or undressing pants and for individuals with a maximum weight of 120 kg. The proposed solution is a system to be adapted to a common wheelchair, which will have a ramp or a hydraulic pump that be driven by the handicapped individual. Therefore, the individual can elevate her/his legs through a crank or pump, and using a vest and a simple device (attached to the back of the wheelchair) may also elevate the pelvis to pull up or down the pants. The designed alternative to enable the lifting or lowering of the handicapped legs provides a more extensive use of the device, since the use of the pump can cover other handicapped individual groups, as is the case of amputees. Figure 3 displays the 3D modeling of the designed helping device, where the major components are also depicted.

2.4 Feeding aid device project

Eating process is one of the most important activities in everyday life. Eating activity influences many aspects of our overall medical, physical, and social well being. Gustafsson (1995) evaluated the psychological effects of self-feeding and found that disabled individuals who attained their goals of self-nourishment had a heightened sense of control, security, and hope for the future. The inability to feed oneself has been linked to shame for human incompetence, decreased self-esteem, and feelings of panic or fear. This information supports attempts to study feeding devices that assist individuals unable to feed themselves. With this motivation, in the present work it will be presented in more detail the design and development of a new feeding aid device.

3 THE DEVELOPMENT OF A FEEDING AID DEVICE

3.1 Establishing functions

Figure 4 shows the overall flowchart of the sub-functions considered in the conceptual design (Cross, N. 1994) of the feeding aid device.

To begin the process, the patient has to press a button to activate the feeding device. The first device operation will take the spoon to the container for the patient to select the food that he intends to ingest. After the food selection, the system will perform the food capture and drag operation; afterwards it will carry out the elevation of the spoon to deliver the food to the patient's mouth.

3.2 Setting requirements

Usually, the set of requirements considered in the design process of equipment goods are related to the following specifications: Safety, Durability, and Comfort. Based on these specifications, a list of requirements was drawn, in which it is crucial to distinguish the ones that are wishes (W) or demands (D) (Cross, N. 1994).

Therefore, a list of requirements based was obtained (Table 1) to guarantee a good performance of the feeding aid device.

3.3 Development of the adopted solution

In order to be possible to develop the mechanical system of an aid device, it is of paramount importance to know the natural feeding trajectory.

For that reason, an experimental analysis of the feeding movement was performed. It was concluded that the feeding trajectory is not linear; it approaches to a parabola or even of a Sigmoid function (see Figure 5).

This path is the most appropriate for the use in a mechanism with just a motor, since it transmits a continuous and progressive movement. However, it is essential to find a suitable mechanism to replicate this trajectory with one driven motor only. Besides this, it is important to stop the mechanism in a specific point to allow the patients' feeding. It is also desirable that the described trajectory is cyclical and that it should incorporate the individual's mouth in one of the trajectory points.

For that purpose it was necessary to select the most appropriate mechanism to accomplish these requirements.

It was first considered the Watt mechanism (see Figure 6a). This four bars linkage returns a trajectory in form of "eight", which could satisfy the initially imposed conditions. However, the

Table 1. Specification for a feeding aid device.

D or W	Requirements
	A. Structure
D	1. Maximum volume of 0,060 m³
D	2. Maximum height of 0,4 m
D	3. Maximum base area of 0,25 m²
D	4. Maximum weight of 5,5 kg
W	5. Conical geometry of the food container
	B. Operation parameters
D	6. Active system
D	7. Arm angular velocity: 60 and 100 degrees/s
	C. Functionality and operationality
D	8. Easy operation
W	9. Multi-driven system
W	10. Components easy wash and cleaning
	D. Adaptability and comfort
W	11. Possibility of container replacement
W	12. Possibility of cutlery/silverware replacement
D	13. Modular construction
W	14. Support base for different surfaces
W	15. Head and arms supports.
D	16. Adjustment of the supports position
	E. Security
D	17. High accuracy of movements
D	18. High precision of movements
D	19. "Round" ends edges
	F. Durability
D	20. Materials with mechanical, thermal and corrosion resistance
W	21. Life cycle higher than 15 years
	G. Cost
W	22. Price less than 2400 €
	H. Ecology
W	23. Material biodegradable and/or recyclable

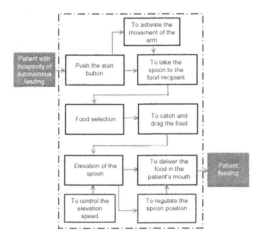

Figure 4. Flowchart of the sub-functions adopted.

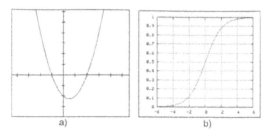

a)   b)

Figure 5.   a) Quadratic function; b) Sigmoid function.

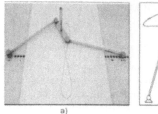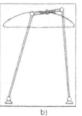

a)   b)

Figure 6.   Mechanisms, a) Watt; b) Chebyshev.

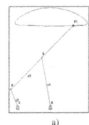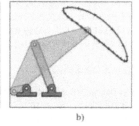

a)   b)

Figure 7.   Mechanisms, a) Hoekens; b) Burmester.

Watt mechanism presents two problems: first, the point that describes the intended trajectory it is the medium point of the central bar (coupler link), which represents a physical obstruction for placing the spoon; second, this mechanism is driven by a bar with alternate motion (input link), which requires the change of the rotation of the motor; this aspect does not satisfy the needed requirements. Despite these problems, the difficulty of maintaining to maintain the horizontal position the spoon during the whole trajectory still exists.

Furthermore, it was studied the possibility to use of the Chebyshev mechanism (see Figure 6b). This returns a "half moon" trajectory that is much easier to maintain the horizontality required for the spoon during the trajectory. However, this mechanism presents the same problems as the previous one, because the point that describes the trajectory is the medium point of the central bar (coupler link), also requiring an alternate driven motor.

In this project, the Hoekens mechanism (see Figure 7a, a variation of the Chebyshev mechanism), was also analyzed with the advantage of having the trajectory defined by the end of one bar (point P1 of Figure 7a). With this mechanism it is possible to fulfill the two main system requirements: to perform the trajectory with the intended end point, while the mechanism is driven in only one rotation direction, since the driven bar carries out a motion of 360°.

Finally, the four bar linkage selected was the Burmester mechanism (see Figure 7b) which is similar to the Hoekens mechanism. The orientation of the fixed body in this mechanism relatively to the obtained trajectory is different and, due to this reason, it was considered more appropriate to the aid feeding system to be developed. The following section presents the mathematical formulation of the equations of motion of this multibody system.

3.4 Equations of motion for a constrained multibody system

When a configuration of the multibody system is described by n Cartesian coordinates $\mathbf{q}$, then a set of m algebraic kinematic independent holonomic constraints $\mathbf{\Phi}$ can be written in a compact form as (Nikravesh, 1988):

$$\mathbf{\Phi}(\mathbf{q}, t) = 0 \qquad (1)$$

Differentiating equation (1), with respect to time, yields the velocity constraint equation. Behind a second differentiation, with respect to time, the acceleration constraint equation is obtained:

$$\mathbf{\Phi}_\mathbf{q}\dot{\mathbf{q}} = \upsilon \qquad (2)$$

$$\mathbf{\Phi}_\mathbf{q}\ddot{\mathbf{q}} = \gamma \qquad (3)$$

where $\mathbf{\Phi q}$ is the Jacobian matrix of the constraint equations, υ is the right hand side of velocity equations and γ is the right hand side of acceleration equations, which contains the terms that are exclusively function of velocity, position and time.

The equations of motion for a constrained multibody system of rigid bodies are written as (Nikravesh, 1988):

$$\mathbf{M}\ddot{\mathbf{q}} = \mathbf{g} + \mathbf{g}^{(c)} \qquad (4)$$

in which $\mathbf{M}$ is the system mass matrix, $\ddot{\mathbf{q}}$ is the vector that contains the state accelerations, $\mathbf{g}$ is the generalized force vector, which contains all external forces and moments, and $\mathbf{g}^{(c)}$ is the vector of constraint reaction equations.

The joint reaction forces can be expressed in terms of the Jacobian matrix of the constraint equations and the vector of Lagrange multipliers as (Garcia de Jalon & Bayo, 1994):

$$\mathbf{g}^{(c)} = -\mathbf{\Phi}_\mathbf{q}^T \lambda \qquad (5)$$

where λ is the vector that contains m unknown Lagrange multipliers associated with m holonomic constraints. Replacing equation (5) in equation (4) yields:

$$\mathbf{M\ddot{q}} + \mathbf{\Phi}_q^T \mathbf{\lambda} = \mathbf{g} \qquad (6)$$

In dynamic analysis, a unique solution is obtained when the constraint equations are considered simultaneously with the differential equations of motion with proper set of initial conditions (Nikravesh, 1988). Therefore, equation (3) is appended to equation (6), yielding a system of ordinary algebraic equations that are solved for $\mathbf{\ddot{q}}$ and $\mathbf{\lambda}$. This system is given by:

$$\begin{bmatrix} \mathbf{M} & \mathbf{\Phi}_q^T \\ \mathbf{\Phi}_q & \mathbf{0} \end{bmatrix} \begin{Bmatrix} \mathbf{\ddot{q}} \\ \mathbf{\lambda} \end{Bmatrix} = \begin{Bmatrix} \mathbf{g} \\ \mathbf{\gamma} \end{Bmatrix} \qquad (7)$$

In each integration time step, the accelerations vector, $\mathbf{\ddot{q}}$, together with velocities vector, $\mathbf{\dot{q}}$, are integrated in order to obtain the system velocities and positions at the next time step. This procedure is repeated until the final time step is reached.

The set of ordinary algebraic equations of motion (7) does not use explicitly the position and velocity equations associated with the kinematic constraints, equations (1) and (2), respectively.

Consequently, for moderate or long time simulations, the original constraint equations are rapidly violated due to the integration process. Thus, in order to stabilize or keep under control the constraints violation, equation (7) is solved by using the Baumgarte stabilization method and the integration process is performed using a predictor corrector algorithm with variable step and order (Baumgarte, 1972 & Flores *et al.*, 2007).

The use of numerical algorithms with automated adjust of step size is particularly important in contact problems whose dynamic response is quite complex due to the suddenly change in kinematic configuration. In such events, the use of a constant time step is computationally inefficient and the system could be overlooked due to insufficient time resolution. Thus, automated time step size adaptability is therefore a crucial part of the dynamic solution procedure. Moreover, the abrupt configuration changes caused by rapidly variation of contact forces are source of stiffness, since the natural frequency of the system is widely spread. Thus, the time step size must be adjusted in order to capture the fast and low components of the system response.

3.5 *Feeding device modeling and simulation*

After the selection of the mechanism that best fits the intended trajectory, a 3D CAD model was built to permit its analysis, as shown in Figure 8. It was necessary to consider the maximum height of the movement that allowed the correct feeding of the individual, as well as the minimum height to make possible the filling of the spoon.

Using the AutoCAD* software, from Autodesk, it was possible to find the appropriate relation between the lengths of the bars that can describe the required trajectory using the Burmester mechanism. It was obtained a length ratio of 2:1 between the fixed bar (B1) and the driven bar (B2) and of 1:2 between the fixed bar (B1) and the remaining bars (B3, B4 and B5). For the bars linkage was used rotation joints (four in the main mechanism and one in the rotation system of the food container).

It must be emphasized, that having been used five bars, the Burmester mechanism is a mechanism with only four bars; the bar of different geometry was replaced by two bars (B4 and B5) linked together.

Finally, in order to evaluate and validate the proposed feeding aid device, the motion of the mechanism was also analyzed using a commercial software specially dedicated to these type of mechanical systems. The computational program Working Model 4D (by MSC Software) was used to carry out the kinematic analysis of the displacement of the spoon, to determine the performance of the feeding system.

After positioning all components (bars, spoon, food container and other components), the mechanism is completed with all its characteristics, that is, the kinematic pairs, the generator of the movement, the friction and restitution coefficients, etc. Once defined the characteristics of the four bar linkage mechanism, it was possible to carry out the kinematic analysis where, for the present simulation, the output variables are the position, velocity and spoon acceleration. The obtained results are presented in the Figure 9, according to the displacement movement of the spoon mechanism.

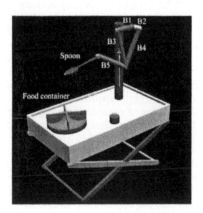

Figure 8. 3D Model of the developed feeding aid device.

87

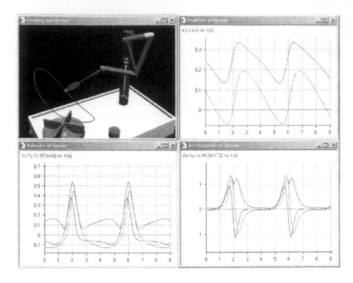

Figure 9. Kinematic analysis of the developed feeding aid device.

Based on the obtained simulation results, it can be concluded that the developed mechanical system is appropriate as a feeding aid device, because it enables to obtain the required spoon trajectory in a continuous motion.

4 CONCLUDING REMARKS

The integration of knowledge, skills and performance relating to Competency-Based Education (Biemans, 2003 & Blank, 1982) in the teaching of engineering design methods for the design and development of medical and rehabilitation devices (at the Department, of Mechanical Engineering University of Minho) was implemented based on case studies. Some of these case studies have been presented and discussed in this paper, with a special focus on the design of a feeding device to assist motor or mental handicapped individuals.

The results of the implementation of these learning methodologies were very positive, since good results have been obtained, for all students, in all assessment stages throughout the semester. The students were motivated and happy to the syllabus of the course and the skills acquired by these students were the knowledge of engineering design methods, mechanical engineering design and mechanisms analysis, the use of AutoCAD (from Autodesk) and specific motion simulation software (Working Model 4D, from MSC.Software), as well as some of the automation knowledge on the development stages. Group work, the ability to collect relevant information and the opportunity to extend the students work to R&D activities in the field of science and technology was also encouraged in this course.

REFERENCES

Baumgarte, J. 1972. Stabilization of Constraints and Integrals of Motion in Dynamical Systems, *Computer Methods in Applied Mechanics and Engineering*, 1: 1–16.

Biemans, H.J.A., Poell, R., Nieuwenhuis, A.F.M. & Mulder, M. 2003. *Investigating competence-based education in The Netherlands: backgrounds, pitfalls and implications.* Conference Paper ECER 2003, Education and Competence Studies. Wageningen, Netherlands.

Blank, W.E. 1982. *Handbook for developing competency-based training programs*, New Jersey: Prentice-Hall, Inc., Englewood Cliffs.

Butler, C. 1986. Effect of powered mobility on self-initiated behaviours of very young children with locomotor disability, *Developmental Medicine and Child Neurology*, 28: 325–332.

Cross, N. 1994. *Engineering Design Methods: Strategies for Product Design*, John Wiley & Sons, 2ª ed.

Flores, P., Ambrósio, J., Claro, J.C.P. & Lankarani, H.M. 2007. Dynamic behaviour of planar rigid multibody systems including revolute joints with clearance, Proceedings of the Institution of Mechanical Engineers, *Part-K Journal of Multi-body Dynamics*, 221(2): 161–174.

Garcia de Jalon, & Bayo, J.E. 1994. *Kinematic and Dynamic Simulations of Multibody Systems*, Springer.

Gustafsson, B. 1995. The experiential meaning of eating, handicap, adaptedness, and confirmation in liming with esophageal dysphagia, *Dysphagia*, 10: 68–85.

Nikravesh, P. 1988. *Computer-aided analysis of mechanical systems*, Prentice-Hall.

Rotater, 2010. *Rotater*. Available in http://therotater.com/wp/ (consulted in March 5th, 2010).

Technology and Medical Sciences – Natal Jorge et al. (eds)
© 2011 Taylor & Francis Group, London, ISBN 978-0-415-66822-4

Development of a flexible pressure sensor for measurement of endotension

Isa C.T. Santos & João Manuel R.S. Tavares
*Instituto de Engenharia Mecânica e Gestão Industrial/Faculdade de Engenharia,
Universidade do Porto, Porto, Portugal*

A.T. Sepúlveda, A.J. Pontes, J.C. Viana & L.A. Rocha
Institute for Polymers and Composites, University of Minho, Guimarães, Portugal

ABSTRACT: An aneurysm is a bulge in a weakened portion of a blood vessel wall much like the bulge that results from over-inflating an inner tube. If left untreated, it may burst or rupture causing shock and/or death due to massive blood loss. EndoVascular Aneurysm Repair (EVAR) is one of the treatments available for aortic aneurysms but, in spite of major advances in the operating techniques, complications still occur and lifelong surveillance is recommended. Current surveillance protocols are based on medical imaging exams that besides being expensive are time consuming. After a brief introduction to EVAR and its complications, this paper reviews post-EVAR surveillance protocols and the current devices to measure endotension. Finally, are introduced two new concepts for a flexible pressure sensor with passive telemetry.

1 INTRODUCTION

An aneurysm is a bulge in a weakened portion of a blood vessel wall, Figure 1. It can be defined as a permanent and irreversible localized dilatation of an artery, having at least a 50% increase in diameter compared with the common one (Johnston et al. 1991).

An aortic aneurysm, Figure 2, if left untreated may burst or rupture causing shock, and even death, due to massive blood loss. EndoVascular Aneurysm Repair (EVAR) is one of the treatments available for this serious disease. It is a minimally invasive procedure in which a stent-graft, Figure 3, is guided from the femoral artery to the affected artery segment to prevent aneurysm rupture by exclusion of the aneurysm sac from systemic pressure. Since it was proposed by Parodi (Parodi et al. 1991), in the early 1990's, has become widely accepted due to advantages such as decreased blood loss, early morbidity and mortality, shorter hospitalization (Ricotta II et al. 2009), reduced patient discomforts and potentially lower costs.

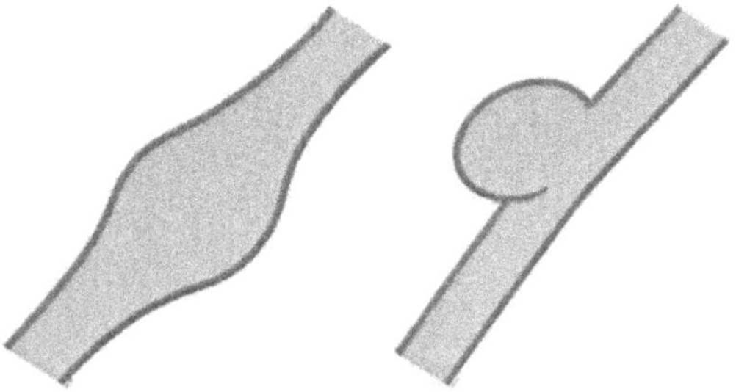

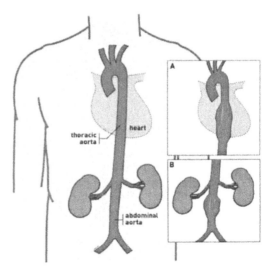

Figure 2.   Representation of a normal aorta, (A) a Thoracic Aortic Aneurysm (TAA), and (B) an Abdominal Aortic Aneurysm (AAA).

Figure 1.   Representation of a fusiform aneurysm (on the left) and a saccular aneurysm (on the right).

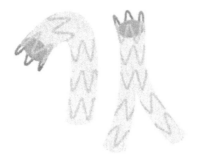

Figure 3. Representation of a thoracic stent-graft (on the left) and an abdominal stent-graft (on the right).

Albeit major advances in EVAR techniques, complications still occur and lifelong surveillance is recommended (Baril et al. 2007).

Presently, follow-up protocols are based in imaging exams that aim to evaluate the size of the aneurysm sac, detect endoleaks, endograft migration, module disconnection, or component fatigue and failure (stent fracture, graft tears). The medical imaging exams provide great information about aneurysm exclusion and sac morphology but do not provide any direct measurement of pressure within the aneurysm sac (Baril et al. 2007).

This paper presents the development of a novel pressure sensor for the measurement of endotension. Its distinctive feature is flexibility, which will allow the conformability of the sensor to the stent-graft and thus the aorta. Such device, in comparison with others, can be attached to the stent-graft and delivered in a single procedure. Furthermore, it enables the placement of more than one sensor, a sensor cluster, contributing to a better pos-endovascular aneurysm study that so far has not been possible.

After an introduction to the topic, EVAR complications will be identified as well as current surveillance protocols. Next, a review on the existing devices and methods for the measurement of the aneurysm sac pressure will be presented. Finally, the development of the new sensor will be considered.

2 EVAR COMPLICATIONS

EVAR has a unique set of possible complications, which occur at a pertinent rate (Ricotta II et al. 2009). However, as surgeons have gained experience with the procedure, the frequency of complications has decreased. Furthermore, it must be taken into account that all devices are subjected to these possible complications, i.e., they are not exclusive of a specific device.

EVAR complications can be described as early, if they occur less than 30 days after the procedure, or as late, otherwise. They can be further categorized as being related to the delivery, the deployment, the devices, systemic problems, and operator errors (Katzen et al. 2006). Table 1 summarizes the complications concerning the deployment and the device.

Stent-graft migration refers to an inappropriate movement of the device. It can be explained by the failure of the attachment with an unchanged aorta or as a failure related to changes in aneurysm morphology. This complication can be prevented oversizing the endoprosthesis to promote friction and/or barb or hook penetration. Other factors that may contribute to fixation of the device include suprarenal attachment, column strength, and arterial ingrowth (Li et al. 2006).

Endoleak is a term that describes persistent aneurysm sac perfusion and pressurization (Katzen et al. 2006). It is the most common complication after stent-graft implantation (Mita et al. 2000) and occur mainly due to incompleteseal of the endovascular graft. Endoleaks have been categorized as follows in Table 2 and are treated by a variety of means, including conversion to surgical repair, or insertion of a new stent or graft.

Endotension is defined as increased pressure within the sac without the presence of an endoleak. This condition may result from the accumulation of fluid within the aneurysm sac or due to the

Table 1. Complications specific to endovascular grafts (adapted from (Katzen et al. 2006)).

Early	Late
Graft kink	Graft migration
Endoleaks	Neck dilatation
Stent-graft structural failure	Sac enlargement
Graft infection	Endoleaks
	Endotension
	Graft tear or failure
	Material fatigue
	Stent breakage
	Component separation

Table 2. Classification of endoleaks (adapted from (Katzen et al. 2006)).

Type	Description
I	Attachment site leaks
II	Branch leaks (without attachment site connection)
III	Graft defect
IV	Graft wall (fabric) porosity

transmission through the wall of the endograft, around its ends at the attachment zones (White 2001). Its consequences are unknown so far.

3 SURVEILLANCE PROTOCOLS AFTER EVAR

Nowadays, imaging exams, such as Computed Tomography (CT) scan, and Magnetic Resonance Angiography (MRA), are the first choice examination to identify inadequate aneurysm exclusion, device migration, and secondary markers of sac pressurization, namely aneurysm expansion and endoleaks.

The standard surveillance protocol involves exams at 1, 6, and 12 months after the EVAR procedure, and thereafter, on an annual basis (Milner et al. 2006).

Device migration and stent fractures or other indication of device fatigue are clear in plain abdominal radiography. Ultrasonography allows the measurement of the aneurysm sac and is effective in the detection of endoleaks but, even with enhanced sensitivity obtained with the use of contrast agents, requires a skilled technician to interpret the exams. CTA (Computed Tomography Angiography), MRI (Magnetic Resonance Imaging) and MRA are sensitive tools to detect endoleaks but cannot be repeated often due to radiation and/or the use of nephrotoxic contrast agents. Furthermore, these exams can be considered time consuming and expensive.

4 MEASUREMENT OF ANEURYSM SAC PRESSURE

Published data describe the use of catheters to measure pressure in the residual aneurysm sac (Carnero et al. 2007). However, although these methods provide precise measurements (Baril et al. 2007), they are invasive and bear multiple risks.

An alternative method for the measurement of the aneurysm sac's pressure is the implant of remote pressure transducers during EVAR. This solution is advantageous since measurements can be done as needed (hourly, weekly, etc.) in the patient's home or office instead of a hospital once or twice a year. Another important feature is the fact of, without risks for the patients, being possible to measure both the mean pressure and the pulsatile pressure. Currently, three telemetric pressure sensors are available: the Impressure AAA Sac Pressure Transducer or Remon AAA (Remon Medical, Tel Aviv, Israel), the EndoSure Wireless Pressure Sensor (CardioMEMS, Inc, Atlanta, USA) and, the TPS Telemetric Pressure Sensor developed by the

Helmholtz-Institute for Biomedical Engineering, RWTH Aachen in cooperation with the Institute of Materials in Electrical Engineering, RWTH Aachen (Springer et al. 2007a).

The Remon Impressure AAA Sac Pressure Transducer measures 3 mm × 9 mm × 1.5 mm and is sewn to the outside of the stent-graft, which is then repackaged in the delivery sheath. It consists of a piezoelectric membrane that when actuated by ultrasound waves from a hand-held probe charges a capacitor. Once charged, the transducer measures ambient pressure, then generates an ultrasound signal, which is relayed to the probe. The data can be downloaded and exported as an Excel data file consisting of pressure measurements and the corresponding times at which the measurements were taken (Ellozy et al. 2004).

The EndoSure Wireless Pressure Sensor measures approximately 30 mm × 5 mm × 1.5 mm and is delivered into the aneurysm sac through its own sheath (completely separate from the aortic endograft). It is made by laminating together several layers to form a capacitor. Metal spirals in the first and last layer form the inductor components of an electrical circuit. Current induction in the sensor results in energy oscillation that varies with frequency. Changes in the circuit's resonant frequency are directly proportional to the force applied to the sensor's surface (in this case, the pressure within the aneurysm sac). The inductor allows electromagnetic coupling between the sensor and the electronic system. The latter consists of an antenna held against the patient's side or back in the area where the sensor is located; it measures the resonant frequency, which is then displayed on a computer screen (Silveira et al. 2008).

The TPS Telemetric Pressure Sensor consists of an implantable sensor capsule and an external readout station. The capsule comprises a capacitive absolute pressure sensor and an in-capsule signal-processing microchip including an inductive telemetry unit. Like the other devices previously described, does not require an internal power source.

The TPS measures 26 mm in length and 3.3 mm in diameter. It has fixation holes at both ends allowing to either suture to the outer wall of the endovascular prosthesis before the EVAR procedure and deployed as a complete system or introduced separately through a regular 11 French catheter system and stabilized within the aneurysm sac, using e.g. self-inflating wires (Springer et al. 2007b).

5 DEVELOPMENT OF A NOVEL SENSOR

A new flexible pressure sensor with passive telemetry to be integrated in a stent graft is currently under development by the authors. The focus is on the use of a flexible substrate enabling the conformability of the sensor to the stent-graft and thus the aorta.

Given the characteristics of the application (the sensor will be attached to the stent-graft) the capacitive sensor must be foldable, extremely flexible and characterized by a very small profile. In addition, the technology should be simple and biocompatible. Silicon based microtechnologies are widely used in implantable medical devices (Receveur et al. 2007), but due to the application specifications, a new fabrication process is being developed.

The pressure monitoring system uses a passive telemetry system, based on an implantable LC resonant network, for the external readout of the pressure sensor signal. The use of passive telemetry in implantable medical devices is common (Mokwa 2007) and enables the realization of active implants with no power constraints.

The fabrication of the implantable pressure monitoring system (capacitive sensor and inductor) is being pursued using two different approaches, both based on a thin flexible substrate made of polydimethylsiloxane (PDMS) and constructed through the use of acrylic molds. While the first approach uses nano-engineered Aligned Carbon Nano-Tubes (ACNT) for the implementation of the passive electronic components, the second uses inkjet printed conductive inks. Figures 4 and 5 show the process flow for each of these approaches.

Both processes start with the production of acrylic molds, using CNC milling, for posterior fabrication of the PDMS membranes. This technique has low costs and fast production times, but it is associated with poor dimensional control.

In the case of the CNT based approach, Chemical Vapor Deposition (CVD) is used to growth forests or "carpets" of vertically-aligned CNTs (Bello et al. 2008). A silicon substrate with patterned Fe/Al_2O_3 catalyst is placed on a horizontal quartz tube furnace at atmospheric pressure at 750°C for the CNTs growth. This method has the advantage of allowing the growth of high purity, high yield and vertically aligned CNTs.

Afterward, the CNTs are embedded into the polymer matrix (PDMS). This step is schematically represented in Figure 4c. The substrate with the CNTs is placed against the moulds, and the PDMS is introduced in the cavities through a hole, followed by the curing of the elastomer. A similar process is used in the case of the second approach, to produce the PDMS membranes for posterior inkjet printing of the conductive inks. The main

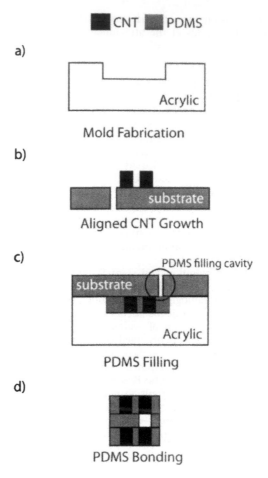

Figure 4. Fabrication process flow for the development of a flexible pressure sensor using CNTs.

concern here is the adhesion between the inks and the PDMS, which may require surface treatment of the PDMS membranes.

Finally, and since the flexible pressure sensor is composed of three thin layers, with the top and bottom layers defining the inductor and the electrodes, and the middle one defining the dielectric (air), a bonding step is performed. The PDMS membranes are bonded using uncured PDMS adhesive techniques.

Both methodologies present several challenges. The use of ACNT technology requires improvements in the growth control of the carbon nanotubes and enhancement of the electric conductivity of ACNT embedded polymeric matrixes. Printing the components requires developments on conductive inks, in order to achieve enough conductivity and adherence to PDMS.

a)

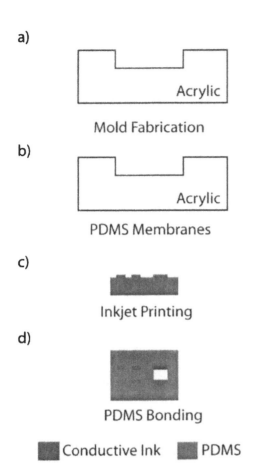

Mold Fabrication

b)

Acrylic

PDMS Membranes

c)

Inkjet Printing

d)

PDMS Bonding

■ Conductive Ink   ■ PDMS

Figure 5.   Fabrication process flow for the development of a flexible pressure sensor using conductive inks.

In both cases, the mechanical and electric behaviors of the flexible film need further studies.

6   CONCLUSION

Although medical imaging exams provide ample information regarding the aneurysm exclusion and the sac morphology, they are time consuming and expensive. As an alternative method, implantable remote pressure transducers have been developed. We described the ImPressure AAA Sac Pressure Sensor (the first implanted pressure sensor used in animal models and a small clinical trial), the EndoSure Wireless AAA Pressure Sensor (the only pressure sensor with FDA approval) and, the TPS Telemetric Pressure Sensor (based on a completely digital data-processing and transmitting unit). Finally, we introduced a novel flexible pressure sensor with passive telemetry that is underdevelopment.

ACKNOWLEDGMENTS

The first author wishes to thank FCT—Fundação para a Ciência e Tecnologia, in Portugal, for the financial support provided by the grant SFRH/BD/42967/2008.
This work is supported by FCT under the project MIT-Pt/EDAM-EMD/0007/2008.

REFERENCES

Baril, D.T., Kahn, R.A. et al. 2007. Endovascular abdominal aortic aneurysm repair: Emerging developments and anesthetic considerations. Journal of Cardiothoracic and Vascular Anesthesia 21(5): 730–742.
Bello, D., Hart, A.J. et al. 2008. Particle exposure levels during CVD growth and subsequent handling of vertically-aligned carbon nanotube films. Carbon 46(6): 974–977.
Carnero, L. & Milner, R. 2007. Advanced Endovascular Therapy of Aortic Disease. Blackwell Publishing.
Ellozy, SH., Carroccio, A. et al. 2004. First experience in human beings with a permanently implantable intrasac pressure transducer for monitoring endovascular repair of abdominal aortic aneurysms. Journal of Vascular Surgery 40(3): 405–412.
Johnston, K.W., Robert, B.R. et al. 1991. Suggested standards for reporting on arterial aneurysms. Journal of Vascular Surgery 13(3): 452–458.
Katzen, B.T. & MacLean, A.A. 2006. Complications of endovascular repair of abdominal aortic aneurysms: A review. CardioVascular and Interventional Radiology 29(6): 935–946.
Li, Z. & Kleinstreuer, C. 2006. Analysis of biomechanical factors affecting stent-graft migration in an abdominal aortic aneurysm model. Journal of Biomechanics 39(12): 2264–2273.
Milner, R., Kasirajan, K. et al. 2006. Future of endograft surveillance. Seminars in Vascular Surgery 19(2): 75–82.
Mita, T., Arita, T. et al. 2000. Complications of endovascular repair for thoracic and abdominal aortic aneurysm: An imaging spectrum. Radiographics 20(5): 1263–1278.
Mokwa, W. 2007. Medical implants based on microsystems. Measurement Science and Technology 18(5): R47.
Parodi, JC., Palmaz, JC. et al. 1991. Transfemoral intraluminal graft implantation for abdominal aortic aneurysms. Annals of Vascular Surgery 5(6): 491–499.
Receveur, R.A.M., Lindemans, F.W. et al. 2007. Microsystem technologies for implantable applications. Journal of Micromechanics and Microengineering 17(5): R50.
Ricotta II, J.J., Malgor, R.D. et al. 2009. Endovascular abdominal aortic aneurysm repair: Part I. Annals of Vascular Surgery 23(6): 799–812.

Silveira, P.G., Miller, C.W.T. et al. 2008. Correlation between intrasac pressure measurements of a pressure sensor and an angiographic catheter during endovascular repair of abdominal aortic aneurysm. *Clinics* 63: 59–66.

Springer, F., Günther, R.W. et al. 2007a. Aneurysm sac pressure measurement with minimally invasive implantable pressure sensors: An alternative to current surveillance regimes after EVAR? *CardioVascular and Interventional Radiology* 31(3): 460–467.

Springer, F., Schlierf, R. et al. 2007b. Detecting endoleaks after endovascular AAA repair with a minimally invasive, implantable, telemetric pressure sensor: an in vitro study. *European Radiology* 17(10): 2589–2597.

White, G.H. 2001. What Are the Causes of Endotension? *Journal of Endovascular Therapy* 8(5): 454–456.

Technology and Medical Sciences – Natal Jorge et al. (eds)
© 2011 Taylor & Francis Group, London, ISBN 978-0-415-66822-4

Development of an adaptable system for a stationary bike to convert mechanical energy into electric power applied in indoor cyclism training

João Batista Soldati Junior & Leszek Antoni Szmuchrowski
School of Physical Education, Physiotherapy and Occupational Therapy, Universidade Federal de Minas Gerais, Belo Horizonte (MG), Brazil

Daniel Neves Rocha, Fábio Lucio Corrêa Júnior, Tálita Saemi Payossim Sono,
Claysson Bruno Santos Vimieiro & Marcos Pinotti
Department of Mechanical Engineering, Universidade Federal de Minas Gerais, Belo Horizonte (MG), Brazil

Claysson Bruno Santos Vimieiro
Department of Mechanical Engineering, Pontifícia Universidade Católica de Minas Gerais and Universidade Federal de Minas Gerais, Belo Horizonte (MG), Brazil

ABSTRACT: The world today faces a crisis related to global warming result of years of environmental pollution, caused mainly by the use of non-renewable of energy sources. The consequence of this is the search by the government and the scientific community to develop renewable energy sources. Although in gyms, there is considerable expenditure of human energy, it is not characterized as an energy management model that can reflect in considerable economy in monthly electric energy consumption. This type of environment conception could be based on the use of energy alternative sources and work mainly as a way to harness the mechanical energy from the exercise. A devise of energy conversion has been developed in this study and engaged in the back of a stationary bike so the mechanical energy applied on pedal is transformed into electrical energy. The device consists of an induced magnetic field generator with its axis of rotation connected to the revolving wheel of the bicycle by a pulley. The energy generated is sent to a set of electrical resistances formed by lights switched gradually and progressively. In addition, an electric current sensor (shunt), a data acquisition board and LabVIEW 8.5 software allows constant monitoring of electric power output. Tests were performed to characterize the behavior of the system in relation to both variations in the rate of rotation (rpm) and the electrical resistance coupled to it. Data on the rate of rotation (rpm) and electric power output (W) were collected and later analyzed. The results showed that the system varies the amount of electrical power output in relation to electrical resistance concomitantly with the variation of resistive torque provided on the pedal of the bicycle, and the same is not true in relation to the cadence. Therefore, the developed device enables both the practice of physical exercise and a model of energy management that uses human action as source characterized by self-sustainability, working also as a way to combine the physical well being and the eco-friendly conscience.

Keywords: Exercise, Electromechanical converter, Stationary bike, Self-sustainability

1 GENERAL INSTRUCTIONS

1.1 *Cycle ergometer*

Since the second half of the nineteenth century (especially after the invention of the dynamo, which dates from mid 1860) the idea of generating electricity from the movement of pedaling is in the popular imagination (even in science).

A bicycle power generator is capable of providing electrical current while being used. Among the many ways to do it we can highlight those which use different types of power converters like dynamos and alternators.

Normally, when coupled to the bicycle, the dynamo saturates its conversion capacity and limits the amount of electrical energy output. For this reason, the alternators are the most used for this application (Silva, 2008).

Some electronic devices coupled to the alternator such as diodes, are used in order to convert alternating current into direct current, and depending on the application, it uses a voltage regulator that limits the output voltage of the converter around 14.8 V aiming to protect the circuit (battery) which the system is feeding.

1.2 *Power and human energy*

The human body is an energy store where only one gram of fat equals nine kilocalories. An average person weighing 68 kg with 15% body fat have stored in your body roughly equivalent to 384 MJ of energy (Starner e Paradiso, 2004).

Studies have shown the physical limits of the human body to produce work in short periods of time (Daams, 1994 e Starner, 1996). The next steps in research on human energy system are to model and quantify the relationship between product functionality, motivation and considerations regarding the discomfort associated with this system (Jansen e Stevels, 2006). It is known that the efficiency of the human body is around 20–30% for activities such as walking, running and stationary cycling, having fitness as dependent variables, as well as the technique, gender and body size of the individual. (Mcardle, et al, 1998). The average values for muscular efficiency, according to what Hansen and Sjogaard (2007) observed in their study were 26%, consistent with the values cited above. Mcardle calculates the mechanical efficiency of human through the relationship between external work done and the influx of energy.

1.3 *Energy quantification*

There are several methods for quantifying the energy expended by the human body when it performs a particular movement. These methods may use parameters such as metabolic energy, external work performed, kinematic or kineticmethods (Neptune e Bogert, 1997).

The current cycle ergometers are not able to quantify accurately the mechanical power exerted by the user during exercise, preventing the proper assessment of their training. Another shortcoming is the failure to measure the electrical power produced, which consequently does not allow the quantification of the electric energy produced during the training, as well as the system efficiency and economics of electric energy in the place which the stationary bike is being used.

The aim of this study was to develop a system for control and monitoring of energy production during exercise training in cycle ergometer exercise apparatus for measuring the parameters related to exercise, such as mechanical power supplied by the user and electric power generated by the system. This system allows you to precisely control the torque submitted to the rotating shaft to monitor the power generated by the user during exercise.

2 MATERIALS AND METHODS

2.1 *Cycle ergometer development*

The system consists of a metal support structure which was attached a bike (mountain bike). This structure allows the rotational movement of the rear wheel without its horizontal displacement. On it, was placed a massive metal wheel (thereby increasing its inertia moment) with the equivalent diameter of 50 cm and a 20 kg mass.

Stuck to the back of the structure, was inserted an induced magnetic field electric generator commonly used in automotive vehicles. Attached to it are three diodes that convert alternating current into direct current produced, as well as a voltage regulator which limits the output voltage at 14.2 V. The shaft of the alternator was aligned to the wheel in question so that a rubber belt would be able to connect them, and as the structure allows the alternator some freedom of horizontal displacement, before being properly secured to the structure by bolts and nuts, so the tension applied on the belt can then be adjusted to avoid possible efficiency loss by sliding. As the generator needs to induce electrical current in the rotor magnetic field, we used a battery.

2.2 *Acquisition system*

The variables measured were the rate of rotation of the pedals and the electric current output. For cadence spinning was used a magnetic sensor placed at a fixed point on the bike frame and a magnet attached to a rotating point of the system (the ring) so that the magnetic field of the magnet is able to reach the sensor in a particular point of rotation. Each time the magnet passes by the sensor closes a circuit that generates an output voltage of 1.5 V forming a series of pulses with equal frequency to the frequency of turns.

For the reading function of the electric current was inserted in series with the circuit output, a shunt with low resistance value (0.001 Ω) so that the total current flowing through the circuit also passes through it. Thus, measuring the voltage drop on the shunt and having known the resistance value, it is possible to calculate the value of electric current passing through the circuit.

For the acquisition of the two aforementioned variables, we used a data acquisition board USB, model 6008 (National Instruments).

2.3 Torque control

The electrical power produced by the generator feeds a system of electrical resistances consisting of nine lamps 12 V–100 W. These resistors are responsible for the variation of mechanical resistance resulting in a torque on the pedal of the bicycle which the volunteer overcomes during the test. The electrical resistance coupled to the system is proportional to the resultant mechanical torque on the pedal, which means the higher the electrical resistance the greater is the resultant torque.

The total electrical resistance (9 lamps) was divided and switched to allow finer control of submitted torque (Fig. 1).

Each key, when activated, adds on the system a corresponding value of total electrical resistance. This value depends on the resistance of the lamp (R), the number of lamps and how they are connected to the system (serial and/or parallel). This switch also allows the drive of two or more keys simultaneously. When this occurs, the values of the driven keys resistors are added (in parallel) decreasing the value of equivalent resistance. This allows the system a gradual progress in the variable in question and therefore a gradual progress in the mechanical strength that is applied on the pedal. All keys were positioned on the handlebars allowing the user to adjust itself the resistance (electrical and mechanical).

An electronic circuit was built to control the opening and closing of the system so that it works only when the minimum power required to drive the alternator is generated. This prevents the battery connected to the alternator, with the main

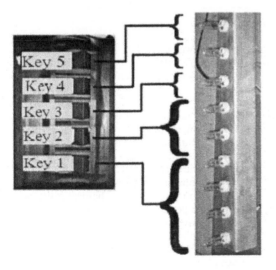

Figure 1. Electrical resistance switch. Key 1 composed of four lamps in series. Key 2 consists of two lamps in series. Keys 3, 4 and 5 consist of a single lamp.

function is to induce its field and feed the circuit. This control is done according to the speed of rotation of the pedal so that when the rotation of the generator is less than the minimum necessary for its proper drive, the system remains open and the lights are not lit. When the rotation is greater than this limit, the system is closed allowing the generator to supply the energy demand imposed by the lamps. This control is achieved through activation of relays.

The data acquisition of the magnetic sensor and the shunt, as well as the calculations of the pedal rotation, rotation of the alternator and the electric power generated was performed using a data acquisition board USB model 6008 and the LABVIEW 8.5 software, both by National Instruments brand. This software was also used to control actuation of the relay. The frequency of data acquisition was 80 Hz.

3 RESULTS

3.1 Torque control

The conversion system developed allows the user to adjust the exercise intensity during training, varying both the pedaling cadence and the value of electrical resistance that the system is connected.

Using as reference for the resistance value of a lamp (R), Table 1 shows the equivalent electrical resistance value for each form of switching.

3.2 Cadence characterization test

The results refer to the system characterization test carried out in order to know their behavior in relation to variation in pedaling cadence (angular velocity). In Figure 2 you can check the behavior of pedaling cadence as a function of time, ranging from 70 rpm to 120 rpm (range adopted in the

Table 1. Characterization of electrical resistances.

Resistance values	Key 1	Key 2	Key 3	Key 4
4 R	X			
2 R		X		
R			X	
3/4 R	X	X		
4/5 R	X		X	
2/3 R		X	X	
4/5 R	X	X	X	
1/2 R			X	X
4/9 R	X		X	X
2/5 R		X	X	X
4/11 R	X	X	X	X

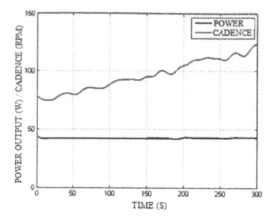

Figure 2. Test result on the characterization of cadence.

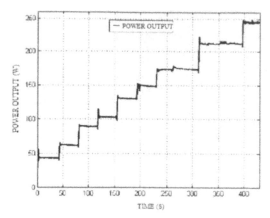

Figure 3. Test result on the characterization of electrical resistance.

simulation of an indoor cycle class), where the electrical power output of the system remained constant at around 42.3 ± 0.4 watts.

This shows that despite the elevation of the pedaling cadence represent an increase in caloric expenditure of the individual as well as the work done (energy produced), it has no influence on the electrical power output of the system in question. This is due to the use of the generator voltage regulator that limits the voltage output of around 14.2 V. Therefore, it was found that the minimum speed used in the training of this study was sufficient to saturate the voltage regulator. Angular not cause additional increases in value of the voltage output, and hence into electrical power. Some how this fact represents a disadvantage to the system since the energy expended to raise the pedaling cadence above this point is being missed, but then, so it is allowed a stable control of the mechanical resistance applied to the bicycle pedal which in turn allows you to control the intensity of sports training that is being performed.

3.3 Characterization test of electrical resistance

Figure 3 shows the test results of the characterization carried out in order to meet the system's behavior in relation to the variation of electrical resistance coupled to it.

The result shows that the system provides different electrical power output according to the resistance value that is being imposed on the circuit. Such resistances are composed of 100 W lamps switched so that their value might have increased gradually. Table 2 shows the value of power output for each stage of the test as well as the keys driven with its respective value of equivalent strength.

The influence that the electrical resistance has on the behavior of the system is explained by the

Table 2. Value of power output relative to activated key.

Resistance values	Activated key	Power output
4 R	1	42.9 ± 3.1
2 R	2	61.7 ± 1.4
R	3	88.4 ± 4.2
3/4 R	1 and 2	102.8 ± 2.9
4/5 R	1 and 3	129.4 ± 5.2
2/3 R	2 and 3	148.7 ± 3.2
4/5 R	1, 2 and 3	172.7 ± 2.8
1/2 R	3 and 4	174.5 ± 1.3
4/9 R	1, 3 and 4	211.8 ± 5.6
2/5 R	2, 3 and 4	213.3 ± 1.2
4/11 R	1, 2, 3 and 4	244.0 ± 4.8

fact that the lower the value, the lower is also the force that opposes the passage of electrons in the circuit that they comprise. Therefore a lower electrical resistance allows a higher electric current passes through the circuit. Therefore, a larger current, ultimately resulting in greater electrical power output (since the latter is the result of the product between the voltage and current).

Once the alternator has its voltage output constant, the electric current was the only variable free and it was responsible for both the variation of the electric power output as the mechanical resistance imposed on the pedal bike. Thus, when the volunteers switches the key that controls the electrical resistance, increase or decrease the torque applied on the pedal, but in contrast increased or decreased the amount of electrical current generated by it. The results also show the gradual increase of every key place in the electric power system output (around 20 W per key).

4 CONCLUSIONS

This study aimed to analyze the electrical energy behavior of an energy conversion system attached to a stationary bike of indoor cycling, using the electromechanical conversion system developed. The conversion system developed was able to transform the mechanical energy input from the user into electric power output as well as monitoring the electrical power produced. The system has varied inversely proportional to the amount of power produced in relation to changes in the amount of electrical resistance that was connected to the circuit, and directly proportional to the mechanical resistive torque applied to the pedal. Also, did not show variations in electrical power output when the alternating pedaling cadence (rpm), the restriction imposed by the voltage regulator electrical generator.

ACKNOWLEDGEMENTS

The authors wish to acknowledge the financial support of CNPq and CAPES.

REFERENCES

Daams, B.J. 1994. Human force exertion in use reproduct interaction, backgrounds for design, Series physical ergonomics nr. 2. Delft University Press.

Hansen, E.A. and Sjogaard, G. 2007. Relationship between efficiency and pedal rate in cycling: significance of internal power and muscle fiber type composition. Scand. J. Med. Sci. Sports, 17, 408–414.

Jansen, A. and Stevels, A. 2006. Combining eco-design and user benefits from human-powered energy systems, a win-win situation. Journal of Cleaner Production, 14, 1299–1306.

Mcardle, W.D., Katch, F.I. and Katch, V.L. 1998. Fisiologia do Exercício: Energia, Nutrição e Desempenho Humano. Rio de Janeiro. Ed. Guanabara.

Neptune, R.R. and Van den bogert, A.J. 1997. "Standard mechanical energy analyses do not correlate with muscle work in cycling." Journal of Biomechanics 31(3): 239–245.

Silva, L.P.S. 2008. Disponibilidade de Energia Produzida em Exercício Físico Realizado em Bicicleta Estacionária. Dissertação (Mestrado em Engenharia Mecânica) PPGMEC Universidade Federal de Minas Gerais. Belo Horizonte.

Starner, T. and Paradiso, J. 2004. "Human generated power for mobile electronics", C.(ed), Low-Power Electronics, CRC Press, Chapter 45.

Starner, T. 1996. Human-powered wearable computing. IBM Systems Journal; 35(3e4), 618e29.

Technology and Medical Sciences – Natal Jorge et al. (eds)
© 2011 Taylor & Francis Group, London, ISBN 978-0-415-66822-4

Development of computational model to analyze the influence of fiber direction in the Tympanic Membrane

C. Garbe, F. Gentil, M.P.L. Parente, P. Martins, A.J.M. Ferreira & R.M. Natal Jorge
IDMEC, Faculdade de Engenharia da Universidade do Porto, Porto, Portugal

ABSTRACT: The auditory system consists of the external ear, Middle Ear (ME) and inner ear. The ME consists of the ossicular chain (malleus, incus and stapes), ligaments, muscles and tendons. The sound energy perceived by the ear passes through the external auditory canal to the Tympanic Membrane (TM), where it is transformed into mechanical energy being transmitted to the ossicles. The objective of this study is to analyze the fibers directions effects of central layer of the TM in the dynamic analysis of the human ME. A digital model was constructed based on images extracted from Computed Tomography (CT). The discretization of the model was based on the Finite Element Method (FEM), using the ABAQUS software. The material properties were based on previous work. Distinct properties for each layer of the TM were considered, since they have different performance. The central layer was considered orthotropic (because of the concentration of fibers) while the others two were considered isotropic. The simulation was conducted focusing on the TM sound pressure level of 130 dB SPL, since this is the highest level of intensity of a sound wave that the human ear can perceive and interpret. The results were compared in the dynamic analysis of the ME for a frequency range of 100 Hz to 10 kHz. This led to the displacement of the four quadrants of the *pars tensa* of the TM. Varying only the predominance of the circular fibers, it is possible to verify the differences of the movements of the TM.

1 INTRODUCTION

1.1 *Middle ear and Tympanic Membrane*

The auditory system is divided into two parts: auditory peripheral and central auditory system. The peripheral auditory system is divided into the external ear, ME and inner ear and central auditory system is formed by the nerve and auditory cortex.

The external ear collects and channels the sound waves to the ME. TM, the movement of pressure and decompression, cause the sound energy is converted into mechanical energy is then communicated to the ossicular chain. The ME ossicles are articulated so that the displacements of one of them interfere indirectly in the displacement of others. The movement of the malleus/stapes also determines the displacement at the oval window, causing the vibration of the liquid of the inner ear by transforming mechanical energy into hydraulic. The vibrations, captured by the hair cells of the cochlea, are converted into impulses to the brain, resulting in sound sensations.

The human ear is the organ that allows us to perceive and interpret sound waves in a frequency range between 16 Hz and 20 kHz and intensities ranging from 0 dB to 130 dB [1].

The ME consists of the ossicular chain (malleus, incus and stapes), six ligaments, two muscles and their tendons. The sound energy pass external auditory canal to the TM, where it is transformed into mechanical energy, which in turn is communicated to the ME ossicles.

The TM is like a mirror of what is happening inside the ME, and knowledge of this structure is fundamental to understanding many diseases that affect the ME [2].

The TM is divided into two parts (Figure 1): *pars tensa* and *pars flaccida*.

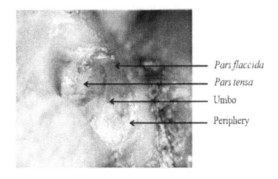

Figure 1. Tympanic Membrane.

The most prominent of the TM, corresponding to the end of the malleus umbo is called.

Topographically, the TM can be divided in six quadrants (Figure 2), four related to *pars tensa* and two related to *pars flaccida*.

The TM is formed by three layers of tissue: external, middle and inner. The external layer is skin and is linked to the external auditory canal. The middle layer is primarily responsible for the rigidity of the TM, with fibers radiating, circular, and parabolic issues. The inner layer is continuous with the mucous of the ME.

The external face of the TM is covered by a layer of epidermis that has similar characteristics to the skin epidermis with four layers, which are the depth to the surface, basal cells malpiguianas, granulosa cells and keratin.

The fibers of the TM middle layer an responsible for its rigidity. This layer has two planes of fibers: an external, located in contact with the epidermis, which is constituted by the radial arrangement of fibers, and another, displaced in contact with the mucosa consists of fibers of circular arrangement. The radial fibers are found throughout the surface of the *pars tensa*, the circular fibers are not found near the umbo [2].

A layer of radial fibers radiates its fibers, beginning with the malleus and then heading out afterwards to the periphery of the TM. There is no difference between sides regarding the distribution of radial fibers [2].

The layer of circular fibers has become available by in radial fibers. Joao Paço [2], examined the distribution of the range of circular fibers, which enabled him to distinguish two morphological types. Thus, in 55% of cases, the range of circular fibers had a sickle-shaped, wider in front and narrowing as they walked to the póstero-superior quadrant, and the remaining 45% of the full fiber move the same width across the tympanic ring.

Figure 3 shows the inside of the eardrum and demonstrates how the arrangement of circular fibers the central layer of the tympanic membrane, where A) occurs in 45% of cases and represents the

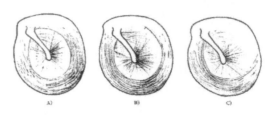

Figure 3.   Inner face of the TM.

band of circular fibers involving all quadrants of equally, B) represents 30% of cases in which the range of circular fibers decreases in thickness in subsequent quadrant, and C) shows the remaining 25% of cases, where there is a circular band of fibers in the póstero-superior quadrant.

1.2 *Objectives*

The objective of this study is to analyze the effects of directionality of the fibers of the central layer of the TM in ME dynamic analysis of the human ear. A digital model was constructed based on images extracted from the CT. The discretization of the model was based on the FEM using the ABAQUS software [3]. The properties of the materials were based on previous work. Attributed to different properties for each layer of the TM. The central layer was considered orthotropic (because of the concentration of fibers), while the other two were considered isotropic. The simulation was performed focusing on the sound pressure level of 130 dB SPL, since this is the highest level of intensity of a sound wave that the human ear can perceive and interprets. The results were compared to analyze the dynamics of the ME for a frequency range from 100 Hz to 10 kHz. Varying only the predominance of circular fibers, can you check the differences of the movements of the TM to the frequency range between 100 Hz to 1 kHz.

2   MATERIALS AND METHODS

2.1 *Construction of the model*

The digital model of the TM and ossicles of the ME was built up based on images extracted from CT [4], belonging to a woman of 65 years with normal hearing (Figure 4). The methodology was based on manual segmentation, using CAD software because of the difficult recognition of the outlines of images of ossicles by ME structure and reducing its size.

Methods were used solely for manual sectioning of images (slices) and delineation of boundaries of the area of interest. Once extracted all the contours of the cross sections, the reconstruction was

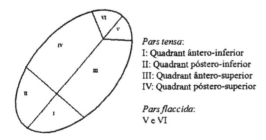

Pars tensa:
I: Quadrant ántero-inferior
II: Quadrant póstero-inferior
III: Quadrant ántero-superior
IV: Quadrant póstero-superior

Pars flaccida:
V e VI

Figure 2.   Topographical division of the TM.

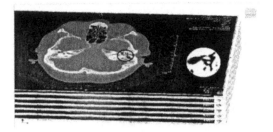

Figure 4. Axial 2D image obtained by CT of the ME.

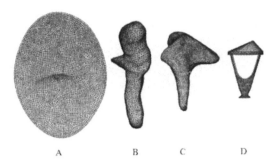

A   B   C   D

Figure 5. Representation of the geometry and finite element mesh.

made between them, and finally obtained the 3D geometric model.

2.2 *Discretization of the model*

Using the ABAQUS program [4] the discretization of the model was made, starting from the discretization of the TM and then to the ossicles. The TM was considered in two ways, one that had only one layer and another in which had three layers, and this point will be further detailed in this paper. Figure 5 shows the representation of the geometry and finite element mesh of the (A) TM, (B) malleus, (C) incus and (D) stapes.

The TM was discretized by using three-dimensional hexahedral elements with eight nodes and divided into two parts: the *pars flaccida* and *pars tensa* (membrane itself).

The TM is characterized as follows according to their anatomy: layer 1, known as external or skin or thin, layer 2, called intermediate or fibrous, layer 3, called the internal or mucous. The TM is composed of 11.165 hexahedral elements of type C3D8, with 15.295 nodes in the finite element mesh. For the ossicles were use tetrahedral elements of type C3D4 because the geometry is irregular. On the outskirts of the stapes footplate was placed 78 linear elements, the type T3D2, formed by nodes of platinum and many other exterior, simulating the annular ligament. In this work we used one-dimensional elements to the ligaments and tendons, to the extent that the state of tension (and/or strain) is uniaxial. Finally, we applied the two muscles, also the ones with linear elements. Table 1 presents in a succinct and brief characterization of the elements and nodes used for discretization of the main components used in this model.

2.3 *Material properties*

The properties of the material were based on previous works, and are specified in Table 2. The index of Young's modulus indicates tangential direction ($E_{(\theta)}$) and radial direction ($E_{(r)}$).

Table 1. Number of nodes and characterization of the elements of the TM and ossicles.

	MEF				
	Elements				Nodes
TM	Hexahedral	C3D8	11165		15295
Malleus	Tetrahedral	C3D4	18841		3932
Incus	Tetrahedral	C3D4	39228		8373
Stapes	Tetrahedral	C3D4	9218		2840

Table 2. Material properties for TM.

Material properties *Pars tensa*					
		Density (Kg/m^3)	Model	Young module (N/m^2)	
				E(θ)	E(r)
Layer 1		1.20E+03	Isotropic	1.00E+07	1.00E+07
LAYER 2	Outside	1.20E+03	Orthotropic	2.00E+07	3.20E+07
	Inside	1.20E+03	Orthotropic	0.50E+07	3.20E+07
Layer 3		1.20E+03	Isotropic	1.00E+07	1.00E+07

The ossicles were all considered with isotropic elastic behavior and the same coefficient of Poisson (0.3) and the Young's modulus of 1.41 E + 10 N/m^2.

The properties of layer 2 were set according to the discretization performed in this layer, which is characterized according to the fiber that has (Figure 6): (i) in 45% of cases the band of circular fibers involving all quadrants of equally, (ii) in 30% of cases, the range of circular fibers decreases in thickness in subsequent quarters, and (iii) the remaining 25% of cases, there is a band of circular fibers in the postero-superior quadrant.

Based on the Yeoh model, ligaments were considered as having a hyperelastic behavior. The energy function of deformation for this material model is given below:

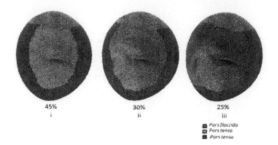

Figure 6.   External face—Representation circular fibers.

$$\psi = c_1(I_1-3) + c_2(I_1-3)^2 + c_3(I_1-3)^3 \qquad (1)$$

where I_1 is the first invariant of the right Cauchy-Green deformation tensor and c_1 c_2 and c_3 are material constants.

2.4   Boundary conditions

For boundary conditions, the TM and stapes footplate were fixed throughout its periphery, simulating, respectively, the tympanic *sulcus* and the annular ligament. The anterior, lateral and superior ligaments of malleus, superior and posterior ligaments of incus were also fixed. The links between the ossicles malleus/incus and incus/stapes were made through mathematical formulations representative of contact [4], with a friction coefficient equal to 0.9 [8].

These ligaments were considered as linear elements with two nodes of type T3D2.

3   RESULTS AND DISCUSSION

3.1   Numerical simulation

In order to understand the behavior of middle ear over a frequency range between 100 Hz and 10 kHz, simulations of the application of a uniform sound pressure level corresponding to 130 dB SPL were done. The sound pressure level is corresponding to pressure caused by vibration, measured at a certain point. The dB SPL scale defines sound levels comparing sound pressure, p, with a reference sound pressure, p_0, and is given by:

$$SPL = 20\log\left(\frac{p}{p_0}\right) \qquad (2)$$

where $p_0 = 20\ \mu Pa$ corresponds to the threshold of audibility.

To perform the analysis, the TM was divided in their respective quadrants (Figure 7). After this division, picked up a node of the finite element

1 – Postero-superior quadrant
2 – Postero-inferior quadrant
3 – Antero-inferior quadrant
4 – Antero-superior quadrant
5 and 6 – *Pars flaccida*

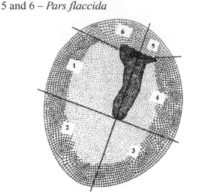

Figure 7.   External face—TM quadrants.

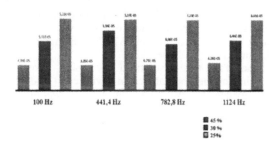

Figure 8.   Displacements postero-superior quadrant.

mesh for each quadrant were determined and the displacement of the TM for this node.

For the analysis of results, were chosen displacements obtained at four frequencies (100; 441,4; 782,8 and 1124 Hz) which are recorded the differences.

3.2   Results

It can be observed in Figure 8 shifts from a central point of the postero-superior quadrant of tympanic membrane. We analyzed the results of this quadrant, as it will have the difference in concentration of fibers.

The displacements obtained with the TM in the central layer do not have the range of circular fibers in the postero-superior quadrant (25% of cases) are larger than the displacement obtained with the TM of 30% of cases. It is also observed that the displacements of the TM with 30% of cases are greater than 45% of cases.

4 CONCLUSION

We can conclude that for the postero-superior quadrant, the displacements are greater, respectively, for the TM of 25% of cases, 30% of cases and 45% of cases. It is concluded that this occurs because the incidence of concentration of fibers in this quadrant.

ACKNOWLEDGEMENT

The authors acknowledge the funding provided by the Ministry of Science and Higher Education (FCT—Portugal), supported the project PTDC/EME-PME/81229/2006.

REFERENCES

[1] Henrique, L. (2002). *Acústica Musical*. Fundação Calouste Gulbenkian.
[2] Paço, J. *Doenças do Timpano*, Lidel, Lisboa, 2003.
[3] ABAQUS *Analyses User's Manual*, Version 6.5, 2005.
[4] Gentil, F. *Estudo Biomecânico do Ouvido Médio*. Tese de Doutoramento, Faculdade de Engenharia da Universidade do Porto, 2008.
[5] Anson, B. & Donaldson, J. (1976). The Surgical anatomy of the temporal bone and ear.
[6] Prendergast, P., Ferris, P., Rice, H. & Blayney, A. (1999). *Vibro-Acoustic Modelling of the Outer and Middle Ear Using the Finite-Element Method*. Audiology & Neuro-Otology.
[7] Sun, Q., Gan, R., Chang, K. & Dormer, K. (2002). Computer-integrated finite element modeling of human middle ear. *Biomechanics and Modeling in Mechanobiology*, 1, pp. 109–122.
[8] Gentil, F., Parente, M., Martins, P., Garbe, C., Jorge, R.N., Ferreira, A. & Tavares, J. (2010). The ifluence of the mechanical behavior of the middle ear ligaments: a finite element analysis. J. Engineering in Medicine. Vol. 224. Part H.

Technology and Medical Sciences – Natal Jorge et al. (eds)
© 2011 Taylor & Francis Group, London, ISBN 978-0-415-66822-4

Electronic device for temperature monitoring during the decompression surgery of the facial nerve

S.S.R.F. Rosa, M.L. Altoé, L.S. Santos, C.P. Silva & M.V.G. Morais
University of Brasilia—Gama College, Gama, Brazil

ABSTRACT: The facial nerve is a cranial pair of nerves more vulnerable to traumatic injuries. The surgical accidents are the most frequent causes of intratemporal complications of the facial nerve. Among the postoperative sequelae, the thermal injuries are common due to overheating of the ontological burr resulting in facial paralysis. For the prevention of thermal injuries in the facial nerve was designed a data acquisition board to obtain the temperature measured by sensor using a thermocouple and virtual instrumentation. Tests were realized in bovine bone to validation of the proposal. Futures tests will be *in vivo*.

1 INTRODUCTION

The facial nerve in its intratemporal course, despite its apparent protection being deeply located in the bony canal, is one of the cranial nerves most likely to suffer traumatic injuries and that causes more sequelae (Turner, 1944). When the nerve suffers some injury, trauma or infection, it swells. As the nerve is inside a bony canal, it is unable to swell and go into distress. To avoid this suffering and permanent loss of function, a surgery can be performed to the release of the bony canal for facial nerve decompression. This surgery is based on the surgical process called mastoidectomy.

In this surgery, the bone behind the ear is removed to improve the visualization of the facial nerve that lies within the temporal bone. The identification of the fallopian tube and exposure of the facial nerve are made through a small burr and a delicate curette. The lack of possible variations in the nerve anatomical distribution and the key elements of the surgical technique influence the risk of postoperative sequelae (Perez, 2002). The injury usually results of an accidental use of a curette, thermal injuries or penetration trauma by the skipping motion of the drill (Hoffbauer, 1973), (Salaverry, 1984). Between them, the most common surgical lesion is the thermal trauma committed by the burr heating during otologic surgery facial nerve decompression (Castañares, 1974), (Parra & Saad, 1987), (Goff, 2001).

Currently, hospital equipments used for mastoidectomy provide a source of irrigation to avoid this excessive accumulation of heat, but do not provide effective control of temperature variation. There is also the introduction of equipment for monitoring intra-operative facial nerve, but these are restricted to stimulate the facial nerve mechanically and electrically during surgery. This monitoring results in auditory and visual signals of a nerve branch that alert the surgeon about the proximity and facilitates nerve identification but does not include the thermal monitoring of the nerve.

As a result, falls to the surgeon the difficult task of total control of the burr when accessing the nerve to minimize the possibility of severe thermal injury occurrences. It is noticeable the need of temperature monitoring during surgical access to the facial nerve as the heating in the surgical procedure leads to different degrees of sequelae and, therefore, burns the nerve resulting in temporary or permanent paralysis of muscles innervated by the facial (Perez, 2002), (Schaitkin, 2000), (Call, 1978).

In order to evaluate the thermal variations in the facial nerve during the surgery is presented a new proposal for monitoring the facial nerve temperature. For that, it was designed an electronic device that performs the signal acquisition to capture temperature measurements using a thermocouple. The data are sent to Virtual Instrument (VI) created. And it is possible a graphic output of the temperature range.

The curves of temperature change permit to check the times of rising and falling temperature of the facial nerve during the surgical procedure steps.

2 MATERIAL AND METHODS

It was chosen a thermocouple Type K (Chromel/ Alumel) that is for general purpose. It is low cost and easy availability in the marketing. Sweep a range of –200°C to 1200°C, with a sensitivity of approximately 41μV/°C. It was covered with heat shrink tube.

The link between the thermocouple responsible for data acquisition of temperature and the computer is made through National Instruments device, the NI USB 9213. With the device does not necessary the amplification and conversion A/D of signal readied. The device has digital output and it is connected with computer via USB. The data are sent to Virtual Instrument (VI) created. So it is possible a graphic output of the temperature range.

The system instrumentation of temperature signal acquisition was executed by means of graphic interface. For this, was used LabVIEW of National Instruments based in the program language G.

First, it was created a front pane that is the interface with user. For this, it was insert control devices (input devices) and indicators (interactive terminal).

For the temperature control was used the *stop* button as control device. And the graphic was the indicator, in other words, the resources used to output information. After the construction of the front pane, the code is added in form of the block diagrams in the second workspace.

The system calibration was performed after measuring the temperature (T0) with a thermometer and using a table of the thermocouple readings to associate the corresponding correction Vo = V(T0). Then, the reading of the thermocouple (Vread) of an unknown temperature was corrected (Vcor) by the calibration algorithm according to the equation (1).

$$Vcor = \frac{(Vread + Vo)}{2} \qquad (1)$$

Tests was realized for observe the monitoring proposal. For this, it was used bovine bone and burr with 3 mm of the diameter and 3000 rpm. The bone temperature in environmental temperature was 27°C.

The method for data acquisition of the accumulation of the heat during the use of the burr was do one center hole to put the thermocouple and others four holes around the thermocouple, with 5 mm of the distance and at 11 mm depth, to measure temperature (Fig. 1). Thus, it was realized four tests.

3 RESULTS AND DISCUSSION

In Fig. 1 and can be see the block diagram of the virtual instrument created for the second proposal of electronic monitoring.

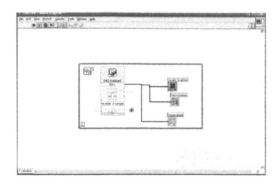

Figure 1. Block Diagram for the VI (Virtual Instrument) created.

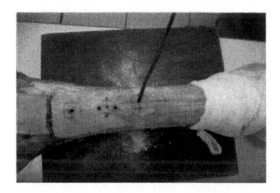

Figure 2. Demonstration of acquisition of temperature using thermocouple during the friction generated by the drill at a distance of 5 mm from the center point.

The method for temperature data acquisition in bovine bone is show in Fig. 2.

In Fig. 3 can be see the front panel with the graphic obtained in one test realized.

It was realized four tests with a burr of the 3 mm diameter and at 3.000 rpm. The results can be see in Table 1.

It was observed that there is an increase of temperature due to the energy transferred by the burr during the paring. The energy transferred to the facial nerve due to the friction is made in the form of heating and the remaining energy is transferred in the form of internal energy in the material that is removed by the burr. Therefore, it is believed that the sudden increase in temperature at the instant of removal of the burr is due to the portion of the energy transferred by friction, which no longer is removed by the action of the burr.

The experiment was realized with drill at 3000 rpm to verify and to test the proposed system. But now is necessary to use otologic burr, because in surgery facial nerve decompression the speed burr is 40.000 rpm.

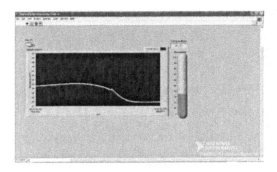

Figure 3. Output graphic of the block diagram for the VI (Virtual Instrument) created.

Table 1. Temperature registered during tests.

	Test 1	Test 2	Test 3	Test 4
The bone temperature in environmental temperature	27°C	27°C	27°C	27°C
Maximum temperature during reaming	36°C	32°C	33°C	29°C
Maximum temperature after reaming	42°C	34°C	36°C	34°C

4 CONCLUSION

In this paper was presented a electronic system for temperature monitoring during the Decompression Surgery of the Facial Nerve. For the prove system efficiency was proposed tests in bovine bone, but was used a burr at 3.000 rpm. It was observed that there is an increase of temperature due to the energy transferred by the burr during the paring. The future proposed is to realize tests with surgical burr at 40.000 rpm.

This study is important, because as previously described, one of the common surgical lesions in the facial nerve is the thermal trauma committed by the burr heating during otologic surgery facial nerve decompression. An electronic device for monitoring and control the temperature during the surgery could be used as a preventive action to minimize the risk of injuries in the facial nerve.

REFERENCES

Castañares, S. 1974. Facial nerve paralyses coincident with, or subsequent to, rhytidectomy. Plastic and Reconstructive Surgery. Vol. 54, Issue 6, pp. 637–643.

Call, W.H. 1978. Thermal injury from mastoid bone burrs. Ann Otol Rhinol Laryngol. Vol. 87, Issue 1 Pt 1, pp. 43–49.

Goffi, F.S., Tolosa, E.M.C., Guimarães, J.S., Margarido, N.F. and Lemos, P.C.P. 2001. Técnica cirúrgica: bases anatômicas, fisiopatológicas e técnicas da cirurgia. Atheneu, São Paulo—SP (in Portuguese).

Hoffbauer, H.H. 1973. Cirurgia descompressiva do nervo facial. Thesis presented in the competition for the post of professor of otorhinolaryngology at the Faculty of Medicine of the Federal University of Rio de Janeiro. Guanabara. pp. 09–14 (in Portuguese).

May, M. and Schaitkin, B.M. 2000. The facial nerve. 2nd Ed, Theime Medical Publishers, New York., pp. 376–607.

Perez, F.F.G. 2002. Avaliação do riscopotencial de lesão do nervo facial nas vias de acesso pré-auricular e submandibular no tratamento cirúrgico das fraturas do processo condilar da mandíbula. Masters dissertation in bucomaxilofacial surgery and traumatology, Faculty of dentistry, University of São Paulo—USP, São Paulo—SP, pp. 02–52 (in Portuguese).

Parra, O.M. and Saad, W.A. 1987. Técnica operatória fundamental: descrição das manobras operatórias básicas. Atheneu, Rio de Janeiro—RJ (in Portuguese).

Salaverry, M.A. 1984. Tratamento das paralisias faciais periféricas endotemporais. Caderno de Otorrinolaringologia. pp. 67–74 (in Portuguese).

Turner, J.W.A. 1944. Facial palsy in closed head injuries. Lancet. Vol. 246, pp. 756–757.

Technology and Medical Sciences – Natal Jorge et al. (eds)
© 2011 Taylor & Francis Group, London, ISBN 978-0-415-66822-4

Ethical aspects in the design of medical devices

J. Ferreira & F. Soares
Industrial Electronic Department, ALGORITM, University of Minho, Guimarães, Portugal

J. Machado
Mechanical Engineering Department, CT2M, University of Minho, Guimarães, Portugal

M. Curado
Institute of Letters and Human Sciences, University of Minho, Braga, Portugal

ABSTRACT: This work is part of a research and development project of a medical device to quantify Spasticity. As the project involves human trials, in order to validate the medical device to be developed, the first step is to obtain Informed Consent. Informed Consent is now an important element in engineering projects involving human trials. Currently a large percentage of engineering projects submitted to ethics communities, for approval, returns to the authors without approval, due to the absence or inadequacy of the Informed Consent term. This work presents the main concern in the preparation of the Informed Consent, according to the international guidelines, such as the historical context. The procedure to obtaining the Term of Informed Consent is described. It is intended that this approach is a valuable aid to researchers who wish to enhance the consistency and adequacy of their term of Informed Consent, when they project medical devices.

1 INTRODUCTION

One of the objective of Scientifics investigations is to increase the knowledge to improve our society. The safety of the humans evolving in these studies cannot be neglected (Parvizi *et al.*, 2008). All the projects involving trials with humans need approbation of ethical committees. Informed Consent is an important aspect to the approbation of the research, by the ethical committees and cannot be neglected. Currently, a large percentage of engineering projects submitted to ethics committees, for approval, returns to the authors without approval, due to the absence or inadequacy of the Informed Consent term. When a research project is being developed, the ethical issues and the project impact must be evaluated (Parvizi *et al.*, 2008). Research integrity is more than avoiding immoral acts. It requires a proactive and preventive approach. Professionalism is built upon foundation of trust, such that is foremost between the patient and the investigator. Obviously, honesty is crucial to such trust. The patient or client needs to be reassured that researchers can be trusted; trust is something that must be carefully cultivated. The "Guidelines for the protection of humans as subjects of research" consider treating people as research subjects and include: respect for persons; beneficence; and justice (Daniel, 2007). Much of

the modern framework for research and scientific ethics has grown out of negative acts. One example is the unquestionably immoral behaviour, in the second world war crimes of the Nazi "medical" experiments, when undertaken clinical trials with humans, without respect for human rights, elicited a bioethical response to the blatant mistreatment of person in experimentation (Daniel, 2007), (Eveline, 1998). The resulting Nuremberg Code set standards for research involving humans. The first rule of the Code states that: "The voluntary consent of the human subject is absolutely essential." The Nuremberg Code implied Informed Consent requirement and was latter formalized by the world Medical Association in its Declaration of Helsinki. It reiterated the need for voluntary Consent, but added that participants must be fully and completely informed before deciding to participate. The question is: what is the sufficient amount of information needed to make such a decision?. Informed Consent consists of both, the relevant information about the research and the actual consent (Daniel, 2007). The Informed Consent, actually, is a balance between respect for persons and advancing knowledge. It plays an important role in research involving trials with humans. it serves as a tool for participants in order to understand all the relevant aspects of the study. It also ensures that the investigator, during the trials, will ensure the rights and safety of participants. The Informed Consent seeks to ensure the ethical behaviour to be guaranteed during the research (Parvizi et al., 2008), (Daniel, 2007). The bioethical lesson for engineers is that there are unexpected consequences from even the most thoughtful decisions (Daniel, 2007).

This work presents the study on the ethical's aspects in research projects involving trials with humans, and takes into account the importance of the Informed Consent term. Special attention must be paid in obtaining the Informed Consent, when it is intended to project medical devices. This work is based on the international standards, accordingly to documents and internationals guidelines. This article is divided in four sections: the first section introduces the ethical aspects and the Informed Consent concept; section two presents the description, origin and motivation for the Informed Consent; section three refers to the precaution to obtaining the Informed Consentterm. Finally, section four resumes the conclusions.

2 INFORMED CONSENT

The target participants in a research project must explicitly and freely give their approval in a written, dated and signed declaration. If they do not have with the ability or capacity to give this consent they must have a legal representative. They must beduly informed of the nature, significance, implication and of the risks of the research receiving appropriate documentation. Exceptionally, if the participant is not able to give the written consent, it can be given orally, in the presence of two witnesses (Curado, 2008).

2.1 Historic context

Several situations occurred that require more regulation for research involving trials with humans. The beginning of the Informed Consent has origins with the Nuremberg Code, in 1945 (Parvizi et al., 2008). The tension between Hippocratic ethics and human rights is evident, in the origin of the Nuremberg Code. The Code was founded in August 1947 in Nuremberg, Germany, by judges during the judgement of 23 doctors and scientists accused of crimes and tortures in medical trials, in Nazi concentration fields. The Nuremberg Code was characterized as the most authoritative in defining standards for the protection of human's rights, of people who are participating in research trials. James McHamey, in his closing arguments on 14 July 1947, said "Consent of participant should be obtained without any form of pressure, and they should be previously informed about the risks." This is clearly the threshold between what can be considered or not a crime.

The Nuremberg judges understood the importance of Hippocratic ethics, to safeguard the life and heath of participants. But they conclude that it was not enough to protect them in research, because the decision only depends on the investigator opinion. So, articulate principles were based on the participants in researches instead of the investigator, including the Informed Consent, absolute and complete, and the participant right to their involvement in a trial. These principles are known as the Nuremberg Code (Declaration of Helsinki (DH), 1967). The main reason to combining the Hippocratic ethics and the rights of human is to resist to the temptation to subordinate the right of the participants to the researcher, benefiting the view of Hippocratic ethics. World Health Organization, created during the Second World War, based on the Informed Consent, the work "Recommendations Guiding Physicians in Biomedical Research Involving Human Subjects". The Declaration of Helsinki in its original version, in 1964, and in the subsequent revision, includes specific details of duties and obligations for investigators and participants: It is not legitimate to conduce trials whose importance and risks do not justify the incurred risks by participant in the research (Eveline, 1998). Investigation must be undertaken by qualified professionals and supervised by qualified entities (DH, 1967). It is the investigator duty to protect the life and health of the participant and respecting their rights; the participant must be informed of the nature, purpose, potentials risks and benefices of their participation in the research, adequately their cognitive and intellectual ability; no clinical trials with human can be undertaken without the free and Informed Consent of participant; the research is always responsibility of the researcher; even after having participants' Informed Consent; the participant or his legal representative are free at any time withdraw Informed Consent and withdraw from the research.In turn, the researchers must interrupt the research if he knows that it can be prejudicial to the patient (DH, 1967).

2.2 Informed Consent in contemporaneous investigation

The requirement of the Informed Consent is currently seen as an ethical necessity, not only in researches but also in medical treatments (Eveline, 1998). Contemporaneous research has many conflicts of interests, for example, investigators can be tempted to be less honest or not to be as diligent in pursuing research that does not serve their research purpose; these conflicts can be financial or ideological, and sometimes both (Daniel, 2007). Obtaining the Informed Consent is essential but not sufficient to undertake researches evolving trials with humans. This happen, for example, when developed countries perform trials in undeveloped countries that, in many cases, will not enjoy the results of the research. Even if the participant understands the complication associated with their participation in the research, he gives the Informed Consent, for receiving a medical treatment, which otherwise would not be guaranteed (Eveline, 1998).

3 OBTAINING INFORMED CONSENT

The process to obtaining the Informed Consent begins in the first contact with the participant in the research, and goes along the entire study duration. By informing the participant, by repetition and explanation, answering his questions, ensuring that each participant understands all procedures.. Each participant must have the necessary time to take his decision, including the time needed to consult his family, or other persons. (Council for International Organization of Medical Science, CIOMS, 2002).

3.1 *Research thatrequires Informed Consent*

For all biomedical researches involving trials with humans, the investigator must obtain the Informed Consent (CIOMS, 2002). It is not required for research involving minimal risks. Minimal risks are defined as a risk comparable to the risks of daily life. Also, Informed Consent is not necessary in studies where the obtaining process of Informed Consent can adversely affect the results. Sometimes to start an emergency treatment it is needed to waive the Informed Consent; in this situation the Consent can be given later, during the course of the study (Parvizi *et al.*, 2008). The exception must be approved by the Ethic Comities (CIOMS, 2002).

3.2 *Adequate language*

The investigator must give the information, orally or by writing, in a language adapted to the participant understanding. The investigator must pay attention to the capacity of the participant to understand the information to give their Informed Consent, depending on the nationality, intelligence and education. The capacity of the participant to understand the information depends on the capacity, sensibility and willingness of the researcher in communicating with patience (CIOMS, 2002).

3.3 *Inducement to participate*

The participants in the research may be reimbursed for: loss of benefices; expenses of travel and other expenses associated to the participation in a research; can also receive free medical assistance. The participants who did not receive direct profits of the study can also be paid or recompensed for the inconvenience and time spent. Payment or treatment cannot be such as to induce the participant to take part in the study, against his will. All payment reimbursements and medical treatment need to be approved by Ethical Communities (CIOMS, 2002).

3.4 *Essential information to support decision*

The key issue is to known what amount of information is sufficient for the participant. Before obtaining the Informed Consent the investigator must provide to the participant the following information:

- benefits of the research to the participant, societies or contribution for Scientifics communities;
- freedom to refuse to participate in the research, freedom to withdraw from the study at any time without loosing any benefits that were provided;
- the aim of the research, procedure undertaken by the investigator and how research differs from routines medicals cares;
- total duration, individual, expected to the participation, number of visits to the center of research and duration of each visit, and the possibilities to end the test in advance;
- if money or other form of property are available by the participants, gender and amount should be reimbursed;
- after finishing the study the participant will be informed of the general conclusion of the project and their individual finding related to their health;
- each participant has the right to access his data, even if the study is not yet complete (unless the Ethical Communities of Clinical Investigation has not delivered dissemination of data, temporarily or permanently; in this case the participant must be informed about the reason of confidentiality);
- possible risks, pain or discomfort, or inconvenient to the participant, associated with his participation in the research, including the risks for their health or welfare of spouse or partner of the participant; after the conclusion of the study if proved that the product or equipment can be beneficial to the participant this should be informed if it will be available and how much he needs to pay to have access to this product;
- alternatives available for interventions or procedures for treatment;

- measures to ensure confidentiality an anonymity, for the data obtained in his participation in the research. Participant should be informed about the terms existing for ensure the confidentiality, and possible consequences in case of breach of confidentiality;
- politics concerning the use of genetic tests, genetic information, measures implemented to prevent the disclosure of the results of genetic test, of the participant and their family members;
- fate of the biological sample collected in the research; the sample may be destroyed at the end of the research, or the details of this storage and possible future use, and who has the right to decide on the future use;
- if commercial product can be developed from biological sample, if the participant will received any monetary or other benefits by the product developed;
- researcher funders, institution with the investigator belong, motivation that origin the study;
- if the investigator only work as investigator or as a doctor of the patient too;
- the extent of liability of investigator to promote medical services to the participant;
- the treatment will be provided at no cost for certain injuries or complication associated with the participation in the study. The name of institution or individual that will ensure this treatment;
- how and by which organization the participant or their family member can be compensated by disability or death resulting from the study;
- if in the country where the participant is invited to participate in the research, the right to compensation is legalized;
- if it exists a protocol approved by the Ethical Communities for Clinical Investigation (CIOMS, 2002).

3.5 *Investigators and participants obligation*

The Investigators and participants should: avoid misunderstandings, influences or intimidations; take the Informed Consent only after verification that the participant has an adequate perspective of the relevant facts and consequences of participation and had sufficient opportunities to ponder his participation; as a general rule, obtain from the participant a written and signed document as an evidence of Informed Consent; the investigator should justify any exception and obtain approbation of the Ethical Communities; renew the Informed Consent document if it exceed the deadline initially defined, even if the initial protocol had not been changed (CIOMS, 2002).

4 CONCLUSION

Informed Consent is an important aspect that should be taken into account in medical devices design. Mechatronic Engineers who usually develop this kind of systems, do not often have sensibility for this important questions, mainly if the development of these systems implies, directly, the test and development of prototypes that must be tested before being commercialized in the market. The success, or not, of a project involving mechatronic devices frequently depends on Informed Consent of the patients that would be the first ones testing the equipment.

In the other hand, the Informed Consent is a crucial factor in project approval by ethic committees. Taking into account the importance of this document, this paper provides, in a synthetic form, a familiarity with the key caring for the preparation of a term of Informed Consent. To meet this objective, an historic context, description of Informed Consent and precaution to take, for obtaining such document was presented. This work is intended to provide a useful supporting tool as a reference to the investigator, who intends to build expertise in drafting the Informed Consent term, in order to ensure that projects submitted for approval, are not returned duo to lack or inadequate term. However, the development of an Informed Consent term relies on consultation and analyses of national and international standards and laws. Thus, the specifications of this text should be understood as a basic principle.

REFERENCES

Council for International Organization of Medical Science. 2002, *International Ethical Guidelines for Biomedical Research Involving Human Subjects*.

Curado, M. 2008. *Direito Biomedico, Colectânea de legislação e outros documentos*, QUID, 343–368 (in Portuguese).

Daniel, A.V. 2007. Biomedical Ethics for Engineers, Ethics and Decision Making in Biomedical and Biosystem Engineering, *Elsevier Inc*, 169–174.

Declaration of Helsinki, 19677. Recommendations Guiding Doctors in Clinical Research. *The journal of clinical investigation.* 46(6), 1140.

Eveline, S. 1998. The Nuremberg Code. Hippocratic ethics and human rights, *The Lancet*, 351, 977.

Parvizi, J., Chakrawarty, R., Bora & Rodrigez-Paez, A. 2008. Informed Consent is ti always necessary? *Injury, int. J. Care Injured*, 651–655.

Technology and Medical Sciences – Natal Jorge et al. (eds)
© *2011 Taylor & Francis Group, London, ISBN 978-0-415-66822-4*

Evaluation and implementation of technology in health care

R. Santos

Faculdade de Motricidade Humana, Universidade Técnica de Lisboa, Portugal

ABSTRACT: The implementation of technology in medicine besides all benefits known has brought new technological and organizational challenges. To overcome the problems resulting from a deficient human-technology interaction, this paper proposes a human factors methodology in order to improve work system performance and to support decision, based on user profile, task/activity analysis and usability evaluation methods.

1 INTRODUCTION

Technology is usually considered a workplace optimization element. With the increasing rhythm of technology implementation it is imperative that organizations understand how maximize technology benefits due to its very high costs of acquisition. A recent European Union study has emphasize that technology is the most important factor in the increasing costs of healthcare, and that Portugal will be in the five European countries that will spend more with health in the next years. Inversely to what happens in other society sectors, the great technological progress of health care tends to augment significantly its costs. With technology implementation health care organizations try to decrease the occurrence of human errors andimprove systems' efficiency.

2 PROBLEM

Patient safety has become a core issue for many modern health care systems. The goal of patient safety initiatives is to reduce the risk of injury or harm to patients. This can be accomplished by eliminating or minimizing unintended risks and hazards associated with the organization and process of care.

The report of the Institute of Medicine, "To Err is Human" (Kohn et al. 2000), stressed the importance of automated, repetitive, time-consuming and error prone tasks in the delivery of health care through the use of technology. But while automation holds substantial promises for improved patient safety and overall efficiency of the health care process, experts in the safety domain alert that any new technology also introduces the potential for different and unexpected risk hazards.

That is, technology implementation doesn't remove the human error potential—it only modifies it.

The introduction of technology in health care has provoked deep changes, not only on the technological level, but also on the organizational one. Technology changes the way tasks are performed and the way information is exchanged, it creates new demands for communication, adds complexity and creates new constraints for cooperation (Nyssen & Blavier, 2008). Recent literature (Nemeth, 2008) reports that, for example, at the "sharp end of the system", communication failures in operation rooms are the leading cause of inadvertent patient harm. One of the main root causes of these failed communications is the inappropriate design and use of the technology.

However, although most of the difficulties arise from the interactions between health care professionals and their technical environment, there is currently a lack of systematic consideration of human factors and organizational aspects. In the past ten years, the design and implementation of technologies in health care have repeatedly raised various cognitive ergonomics issues such as usability of medical devices and cognitive workload related with various types of information and communication technology (Beuscart-Zephir et al. 2007).

Additionally, equipment and supplies are configured ad hoc—assembled and adapted to fit the individual patient and specific procedures. There's no multidisciplinary approach to support decision. Decisions on the acquisition of highly sophisticated clinical equipment are routinely made by staff members who have no clinical experience and are advised by clinicians who have no experience in the technical evaluation of complex products or systems. And this situation has to change.

3 BACKGROUND

Studies in many countries have established that about 10% of patients admitted to hospital suffer adverse events, meaning that they experience some harm as a result of their health care (Vincent et al. 2001). Many of these events are preventable and therefore considered errors and about half are associated with a surgical procedure (Brennan et al. 1991). Sources of these errors can be contained in any of the work system elements or can be the product of interactions between these elements (Carayon et al. 2007). In this sense several authors like Healey & Vincent (2007) defend that a system approach to safety should be implemented in the surgical domain. This approach focuses heavily on interdependence and interaction among system components. They include such factors as equipments design and use, communication, team coordination and the environment in which the team operates.

According to Nyssen & Blavier (2008), during the past decade there have been two important developments in medical care relevant to the study of communications in hospital: a) the increased specialization of medical sciences, which has increased the division and distribution of tasks among experts from different disciplines and, thus, the need for coordination and communication between health care providers, and b) the development and introduction of new computer-based technology in hospitals, that requires practitioners to communicate with computers, introduces new forms of media and more distance between the operators and their tasks, as well as between task performers themselves. This author was one of the few that tried to integrate cognitive and collective aspects of work in technology evaluation (Nyssen, 2004) and tried to understand how technology, namely a surgical robot, changed the communication in the operating room (Nyssen & Blavier, 2008).

Until now, human machine interaction research has generally focused on the individual user and supporting individual operator performance through appropriate interface design. However, in reality, work is performed by teams of operators. And teams have different requirements than individuals. Teams rely heavily on communication, on a common overview of the situation, and on delegation of tasks so that team members share the workload. Thus the technology must be designed to support the teamwork, not simply to support an individual user. Consequently a particular kind of innovation is needed, the transformation of tools and applications supporting the work of individuals, to tools and applications supporting the work of teams.

Therefore, studying both the behavior of the system and the communication process provides markers of the systems' adaptation and inadequate adaptation, and, in turn, will help to develop adaptive technology that enhances coupling between agents and their environment. In order for new technologies to be truly effective and to be used safely, they must provide communication modes and interaction modalities that accommodate the diverse requirements of the user population, tasks and contexts.

The literature shows that human factors discipline can very much contribute to the safe design of health care systems by considering the various needs, abilities and limitations of people involved in those systems. The quality and safety of care provided by health care systems are obviously dependent on the patients' risk factors and on the technical skills and knowledge of the health care staff, but they are also very much influenced by non-technical skills and various characteristics of the work system that can be manipulated, changed and improved with the methods and principles of ergonomics/human factors.

Indeed the application of human factors/usability engineering to health care work situations is well documented in several studies by Beuscart-Zéphir et al. This approach proves useful to support the procurement process for new technological devices and applications in hospitals (Beuscart-Zephir et al. 2002), the design of evaluation studies integrated in the implementation process of Clinical Information Systems (Beuscart-Zephir et al. 2005), and the re-engineering process of complex IT applications to better fit the users needs and the constraints of clinical workflows (Beuscart-Zephir et al. 2009; Watbled et al. 2009; Beuscart-Zephir et al. 2008). It is also a powerful tool to identify how organizational and technical dimensions impact the patterns of communications between health care professionals and their efficiency in the care process (Pelayo et al. 2009; Beuscart-Zephir et al. 2006). However, the adaptation of the human factors engineering framework to new health care contexts always proves to be a scientific challenge.

4 OBJECTIVE

Thus, to avoid problems resulting from a deficient human-technology interaction, this paper proposes a human factors approach to evaluate and implement technology in health care.

On the one hand, to optimize the technology adequacy to the context and performed tasks, it is necessary to analyze health care professionals' activity: identify task constraints; consider the environment influence on task; analyze communication and cooperation modes; identify tasks that cause interruptions in the interaction and its consequences; and consider information processing with high levels of stress and fatigue. Moreover it is essential the analysis of tasks sequence, work flows and existent protocols.

On the other hand, to adequate the technology to the capacities, limitations, needs and expectations of operators and organizationsit is also necessary to evaluate its usability, observing the problems faced, the efficacy and efficiency, and the satisfaction of the user in the interaction with the system.

The context knowledge and usability evaluation are the base to support the decision in the technology evaluation and implementation phases.

5 METHODS

In order to provide a proof of concept of the efficiency of this approach in terms of improved efficiency and safety of the care process, this framework has started to be applied to a cardiac surgery work system, in a hospital of Lisbon. The objective is to demonstrate the contribution of the human factors approach to the optimization of system performance through the improvement of patient safety and system efficiency.

The objective is to analyze all interactions between humans and technology and between humans themselves in order to describe work activities and detect all problems involved. Considering the two main factors that literature refers to, as the most contributing to adverse events in this context, this study intends to analyze how the interaction with technologies/equipments influences the communications efficiency, how they integrate with each other and what are the resultant problems of this interaction.

In a first step, through observation and work system analysis we can identify technological, organizational and human problems and provide recommendations aiming at reduce the inefficiencies, unnecessary activities, performance obstacles and communication problems, not only in the operating room, but also for the entire surgery related care process starting with patient entry in the hospital and ending at patient discharge after surgery.

This information will provide guidance to the next step (usability inspection) identifying the equipments and aspects to evaluate and allowing the identification of all feasible evaluation criterions with application in this particular context.

Thus in a second step, through a usability evaluation of technology/equipment/medical devices, following the orientations indicated by international norms, we can identify specific usability problems that affect the interaction with the user and the communication with the rest of the surgical team.

Usability is based on principles that facilitate the three phases of the cognitive activity: perception, cognition and response. The usability evaluation is made through observation and register of user problems, interaction efficacy and efficiency quantification, and user satisfaction (Gosbee & Gosbee, 2007). The advantages of a good usability are obvious: higher speed performance increasing efficiency; error reduction increasing patient safety; less training needs because technology is easy to learn; increased user satisfaction aiding the adoption of new technologies; and an overall quality increment. The result of these advantages is a considerable cost reduction to the organization.

6 OUTCOMES

The expected outcomes of the project are: a) the identification of a set of technology functionalities needing improvement, b) a clear description of the users needs that could be integrated in the hospitals' calls for proposals, therefore guiding an adequate selection of technology in the future; c) a list of design recommendations to the manufacturers, and finally d) a list of recommendations for the work situation.

These recommendations will support a re-design process according to the system needs, ensuring the adaptation of the technology to the existent work flow and the interoperability with other technologies/equipments already in place. The expected optimization of the interactions should reduce the probability of error, therefore increasing patient safety, and will decrease the time needed for training and learning to use technologies.

So, one of the core goals of this approach is to help stake holders become aware of the health care teams' needs and support the dialogue between all parts, to propose and discuss the best solutions for the implementation of counter measures to solve the detected problems.

Health care authorities and stake holders must be aware of the opportunities that this approach can bring: for health care organizations managers and staff the benefits in terms of efficiency improvement and cost reduction; and for manufacturers, the evidence of the clients' needs and competitive opportunities that it holds. The initiative will also permit the recommendations validation assuring the best agreement between the interests, and possibilities of each stakeholder. At a larger scale, the results of this study could be generalized to other situations.

7 CONCLUSIONS

This paper doesn't talk about technology. It talks about the interaction with technology.

The introduction of technology in medicine besides all benefits known, have brought new technological and organizational challenges. It has developed the potential for new risk hazards that most of the times health care system is unable to address by itself. The consequences are negative to patient safety and systems' efficiency. In order to overcome these difficulties a human factors approach is proposed in order to improve work system performance, by identifying usability problems with technology and organizational problems within the system.

In conclusion the proposed human factors methodology aim to support decision based on user profile, task/activity analysis and usability evaluation methods. Consequently, support will be provided to develop needs specification and also identify indicators to compare the utilization before and after technology implementation. Regarding usability evaluation it can be provided a comparison between several options of purchase, an identification of problems and its gravity classification, a selection of features to ameliorate and recommendations to technology update. Regarding technology development this approach provides the functional requirements and concept validation to promote the user acceptance, namely in the development of software, medical devices, policies, guidelines and training.

More and more the evaluation and implementation of technology in health care must be a proactive approach,based on a multidisciplinary team integrating the core areas needed to optimize the system performance, each partner contributing with its specific knowledge and expertise to create the necessary synergies for the success of the project. And the human factors/ergonomics element must take part of that team.

REFERENCES

Beuscart-Zephir, M.C., Anceaux, F., Menu, H., Guerlinger, S., Watbled, L. & Evrard, F. 2005. User-centred, multidimensional assessment method of Clinical Information Systems: a case-study in anaesthesiology. *Int J Med Inform* 74(2–4): 179–189.

Beuscart-Zéphir, M.C., Elkin, P., Pelayo, S. & Beuscart, R. 2007. The human factors engineering approach to biomedical informatics projects: state of the art, results, benefits and challenges. *Yearb. Med. Inform*: 109–127.

Beuscart-Zephir, M.C., Pelayo, S., Anceaux, F., Maxwell, D. & Guerlinger, S. 2006. Cognitive analysis of physicians and nurses cooperation in the medication ordering and administration process. *Int J Med Inform* 76(1) Sup 1: S65–S77.

Beuscart-Zéphir, M.C., Pelayo, S. & Bernonville, S. 2009. Example of a Human Factors Engineering approach to a medication administration work system: Potential impact on patient safety. *Int J Med Inform* 79(4): e43–e57.

Beuscart-Zéphir, M.C., Pelayo, S. & Leroy, L. 2008. Optimization of a medication administration sociotechnical system: benefits of a Human Factors Engineering approach. *Proc. HEPS Symp.*, Strasbourg, 25–27 June.

Beuscart-Zephir, M.C., Watbled, L., Carpentier, A.M., Degroisse, M. & Alao, O. 2002. A rapid usability assessment methodology to support the choice of clinical information systems: a case study. *Proc. AMIA Symp.*: 46–50.

Brennan, T., Leape, L., Laird, N., Hebert, L., Localio, A., Lawthers, A., Newhouse, J., Weiler, P. & Hiatt, H. 1991. Incidence of adverse events and negligence in hospitalized patients.Results of the Harvard Medical Practice Study I. *New England Journal of Medicine* 324(6): 370–376.

Carayon, P., Alvarado, C. & Hundt, A. 2007. Work system design in health care. In P. Carayon (ed), *Handbook of Human Factors and Ergonomics in Health Care and Patient Safety*: 61–78. Lawrence Erlbaum Associates.

Gosbee, J. & Gosbee, L.L. 2007. Usability evaluation in health care. In P. Carayon (ed), *Handbook of human factors and ergonomics in health care and patient safety*: 679–692. Lawrence Erlbaum Associates.

Healey, A. & Vincent, C. 2007. The systems of surgery. *Theoretical Issues in Ergonomics Science* 8(5): 429–443.

Kohn, l., Corrigan, J. & Donaldson, M. 2000. *To err is human—Building a safer health system*. Institute of Medicine. National Academy Press.

Nemeth, C. 2008. The context for improving healthcare team communication. In C.P. Nemeth (ed), *Improving Healthcare Team Communication—Building on Lessons from Aviation and Aerospace*: 1–7. Ashgate.

Nyssen, A. 2004. Integrating cognitive and collective aspects of work in evaluating technology. *IEEE Transactions on Systems, Man, and Cybernetics—part A: Systems and Humans* 34(6): 743–748.

Nyssen, A. & Blavier, A. 2008. Communication as a sign of adaptation in socio-technical systems: the case of robotic surgery. In C.P. Nemeth (ed), *Improving Healthcare Team Communication*: 207–219. Ashgate.

Pelayo, S., Anceaux, F., Rogalski, J. & Beuscart-Zéphir, M.C. 2009. Organizational vs. technical variables: impact on the collective aspects of healthcare work situations. *Stud Health Technol Inform* 150: 307–11.

Vincent, C.A. Neale, G. & Wooloshynowych, M. 2001. Adverse events in British hospitals: preliminary retrospective record review. *Bristish Medical Journal* 322: 517–519.

Watbled, L., Marcilly, R. & Guerlinger, S. 2009. Intérêt de la démarche ergonomique dans la conception et l'implémentation d'un système informatique en santé: exemple du dossier d'anesthésie électronique. *Proc intern Ergonomie-Design*, Lyon, 8–10 Juin.

Technology and Medical Sciences – Natal Jorge et al. (eds)
© 2011 Taylor & Francis Group, London, ISBN 978-0-415-66822-4

Frequency domain validation of a tetrapolar bioimpedance spectroscopy system with tissue equivalent circuit

A.S. Paterno, V.C. Vincence & P. Bertemes-Filho
Department of Electrical Engineering, Santa Catarina State University, Joinville, Brazil

ABSTRACT: Bioimpedance Spectroscopy (BIS) Analysis is a method used to characterize biological materials. Many BIS systems consist of applying a multi-frequency sinusoidal current of constant amplitude in the material and measuring the resulting potential to calculate the transfer impedance. It is necessary to assure that the injecting current has constant amplitude over a wide frequency range. However, stray capacitances and other non-idealities present in the instrumentation reduce the current amplitude at higher and lower frequencies. Therefore, a complete circuit analysis of a voltage-controlled-current source for multi-frequency bioimpedance spectroscopy is reported using a SPICE representation of the whole tetrapolar spectroscopy system including the tissue bioimpedance. This full simulation procedure containing the bioimpedance circuit representation allows the development and optimization of application-oriented bioimpedance systems as demonstrated in the description of this technique.

1 INTRODUCTION

Bioimpedance Spectroscopy (BIS) has been widely used as a non-invasive technique for diagnostic, as, for example, in the detection of cancerous tissues. In addition, it is considered a fast, low cost, practical and efficient method of diagnostic (Bertemes-Filho 2002). This technique has shown reasonable results while detecting normal and cancerous skin tissues (Brown, Tidy, Boston, Blackett & Sharp 1998, Gonzlez-Correa, Brown, Smallwood, Kalia, Stoddard, Stephenson, Haggie, Slatter & Bardhan 1999). Many EIS systems consist of applying a multi-frequency sinusoidal current of constant amplitude in the tissue sample, measuring the resulting potential and then producing the transfer impedance (Zt) through the measurement of currents and voltages in the sample to be evaluated (Barsoukov & Macdonald 2005). From the impedance acquired data, the electrical properties of tissue under study can be obtained by fitting data to an equivalent electrical model. In order to identify associated pathologies it is of great interest that tissue electrical parameters can be calculated (Cole & Cole 1941), such as the intracellular and extracellular resistances, the capacitance of the cellular membrane and the electrical dispersion of the tissue. In order to get an accurate calculated transfer impedance with a relative error lower than 1%, there is a need to assure that the injecting current have a constant amplitude over a wide frequency range. This goal may be obtained by using a current source with high output impedance (Bertemes-Filho 2002). However, stray capacitances reduce the current amplitude at higher frequencies (Lu & Brown 1994). Therefore, the frequency response optimization of the BIS system is to be attained by adjusting the implemented current source. Several circuit simulations use computer SPICE modeling by assuming resistive load (Bertemes-Filho, Brown & Wilson 2000, Qureshi, Chatwin, Huber, Zarafshani, Tunstall & Wang 2010). If the target is to implement a system for bio-impedance measurements, a more realistic load should be used in simulations. Furthermore, the output impedance of the many current sources are frequency dependent and quite sensitive to load changes (Frounchi, Dehkhoda & Zarifi 2009), and this can be evaluated during the system simulations.

2 MATERIALS AND METHODS

Tissue impedance data from a post-mortem bovine kidney were collected by an implemented BIS system, which has its block diagram depicted in Fig. 1. The acquired data were compensated against a non-constant current along the used frquency interval and stray capacitances. The parameters that characterize the Cole-Cole function associated with the impedance were obtained from the acquired compensated data. In this case,

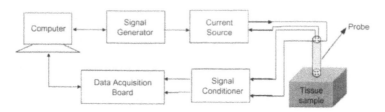

Figure 1. Block diagram of the implemented BIS system connected to a tetrapolar probe with total diameter of 4.5 mm. The electrodes have a diameter of 1 mm and a distance between them of 1.5 mm.

2.1 Data acquisition system

Basically, the BIS system may be divided into four parts: a signal generator controlling with frequency range from 0.5 to 1,000 kHz produced by a board PCI-5401 (National Instruments) with a resolution of 12 bits. This signal controls the current source which has a floating load (also called balanced current source) and it is based on the modified Howland structure (Bertemes-Filho, Brown & Wilson 2000, Stiz, Ramos, Bertemes-Filho & Vincence 2009). It generates an output current of 1 mApp over a frequency range 500 Hz to 1 MHz with a measured output impedance higher than 20 MΩ at 100 kHz (Stiz, Ramos, Bertemes-Filho & Vincence 2009). In practice, 33 sinusoidal signals at discrete frequencies within the range are generated. The measuring hardwar is a Data Acquisition (DAQ) Board of 16 bits (model PCI-6259-National Instruments). The board is set to work in a differential mode and one channel, performing a maximum sampling rate of 1.25 MS/s. A graphical interface in LabVIEW was implemented in order to visualize the measured voltages, calculate the real and imaginary part of the impedance, control the signal generator board (model PCI-5401) and sweep the frequency of the input signal. The amplitude of the measured signal was detected and all values were averaged. This amplitude detection method was used for each frequency and then the voltage spectrum was obtained. The impedance data were compensated against the errors in low and high frequency due to stray capacitances and due to intervals of frequency with a non-constant current. However, such compensation requires an additional computational burden, which may be avoided if the current source is properly optimized in low and high frequencies using the techniques of a simulated realistic load.

2.2 Tissue modeling

For the virtual evaluation of circuits for bioimpedance spectroscopy, a circuit whose impedance approximates a tissue bioimpedance is created containing a sufficient number of series RC parallel

circuits and is added to the circuit model in the system. This approximating circuit allows the spectral representation of a bioimpedance from which one knows the fundamental parameters, as the characteristic angular frequency, resistance at infinite and low frequencies and the constant exponent parameter associated with the constant-phase element. A direct approximation of a fractional Cole function by means of an expansion using ordinary first-order processes determines the parallel RC single-pole circuits in the representation associated in series. The Cole impedance function, which is usually used to fit experimental bioimpedance data, is simulated to evaluate the behavior of the algorithm. It can be obtained from a 2R1C circuit by the replacement of the ideal capacitor with a general Constant-Phase-Element (CPE) (Cole, 1940), as shown in Fig. 2 for a capacitor with C_{eq} taking the place of the constant phase element. The impedance function for the frequency dependence of tissue is then represented by (Grimnes & Martinsen 2008):

$$Z_{Cole}(\omega) = R_\infty + \frac{R - R_\infty}{1 + (j\omega\tau_0)^\alpha} \qquad (1)$$

where $R_\infty = RS/(R + S)$ is the resistance at very high frequencies, j is the imaginary unit, α describes a Cole-type distribution of relaxation times (McAdams & Jossinet 1996), and τ_0 is the characteristic relaxation time. The parameters used were measured for a bovine kidney tissue having the values of $\tau_0 = 1.4 \times 10^{-6}$, $R_\infty = 169.6\ \Omega$, R = 14.4 Ω and $\alpha = 0.62$. Such a function in eq.1 is approximated by a summation of 20 single-pole partial fractions corresponding to the same number of RC circuits in the simulation. The RC values were calculated using an algorithm developed for the approximation of Cole-Cole functions in electrochemistry impedance spectroscopy (Haschka & Krebs 2007) and are shown in Table 1.

The output impedance is calculated by measuring both Short-Circuit (SC) and load current. This is made in two steps: the short-circuit current is measured along the terminals a and b; and in a second

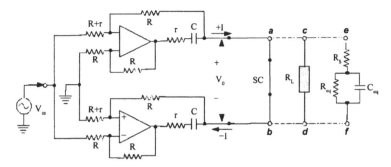

Figure 2. Schematic diagram of the simulated differential Howland current source with an 2R1C circuit as a load. R_{eq}, R and C_{eq}, which is the capacitor that would be substituted for a constant-phase element when the load is represented by a circuit associated with a Cole-Cole model.

Table 1. Resistors and capacitors calculated for the Cole-function approximation using a summation of single-pole partial fractions.

C(F)	R(Ω)
0.11×10^{-12}	0.068
0.39×10^{-12}	0.147
1.37×10^{-12}	0.313
4.75×10^{-12}	0.669
16.54×10^{-12}	1.421
58×10^{-12}	2.996
207.03×10^{-12}	6.203
771.4×10^{-12}	12.302
$3,187.8 \times 10^{-12}$	21.996
$16,491.1 \times 10^{-12}$	31.419
$121,854.3 \times 10^{-12}$	31.419
$1,286,074.4 \times 10^{-12}$	21.996
$16,991,416.7 \times 10^{-12}$	12.302
0.000248	6.203
0.003808	2.996
0.0593	1.421
0.9309	0.669
14.663	0.313
231.353	0.147
3652.9	0.068

step when the short-circuit is removed and resistive load (R_L) is connected between terminals c and d; the differential output impedance of the current source is then calculated. During this stage, the project of the current source can be adjusted in order to have a high output impedance and a constant output current within the desirable frequency range.

3 RESULTS AND DISCUSSION

In order to investigate the output current of the differential Howland current source in the frequency range from 100 Hz to 10 MHz, a resistive load of 1 kΩ was used. The output current was set to be 1 mApp, which can be defined by dividing the input voltage $Vin = 1$ Vpp to the resistor $r = 1$ kΩ as in Fig. 2. It can be seen that the modulus of the output current is lower than 1 mApp at low frequencies (less than 1 kHz) whereas it is constant in the frequency range from 1 kHz up to 1 MHz with a maximum error of approximately 0.6% at 1 kHz. The lower frequency behavior can be compensated by a tenfold increment in the capacitor C of the current source (see Fig. 2). This capacitor with the resistor r behaves like a high-pass filter, and it also blocks the direct current in the positive feedback of the amplifier preventing a direct current to the load. It can be seen in Fig. 3 that the current starts to increase above 2 MHz, and this can be explained by the frequency response of the operational amplifier OPA655 used in the simulations.

The frequency dependence of the current source upon load is obtained while evaluating the load voltage bandwidth when using an ideal current source from a SPICE model. An ideal current of 1 mApp in the frequency range from 100 Hz to 10 MHz was driven across the equivalent load impedance of the bovine kidney tissue. This is the reference spectrum of the load impedance with the non-idealities which were suppressed in this simulation and would be unavoidable in the instrumentation. Secondly, the current source was then loaded by the equivalent impedance. It can be seen in Fig. 4 that the spectrum of the load impedance is similar for both current source in the frequency range from 1 kHz to 10 MHz. However, at lower frequencies the load impedance decreases from 150 Ω to 118 Ω. This can be explained by the frequency response of the output current of the current source circuit, specially at lower frequencies. If the capacitor C of the current source is increased this non-ideality can be corrected and the order of this value may be estimated with this simulation. In addition, one may see that the actual impedance has a much lower modulus value at high frequencies, that may guide

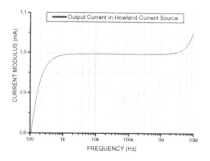

Figure 3.   Output current bandwidth of the fully differential Howland current source.

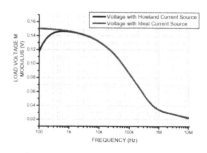

Figure 4.   Load voltage spectrum of a fully differential Howland source.

the determination of output impedances values in the instrumentation circuit design.

4   CONCLUSIONS

A tissue equivalent impedance circuit was used to optimize the current source project that is used in an electrical bioimpedance system. The current source had its capacitors changed to improve frequency response in low frequencies. The technique developed in this work allowed a guide to improve component values in hardware used for instrumentation in electrical bioimpedance systems. The approximation of the Cole-Cole impedance functions, which are non-rational functions in the frequency domain was implemented as a combination of single-pole series circuits with a combination of 20 circuits and it allowed the simulation of a complete BIS system including the circuit equivalent tissue. This technique is going to be used to optimize the voltage interrogation instrumentation for the BIS system at the Santa Catarina State University in a future work.

ACKNOWLEDGEMENTS

This work could not have succeeded without the support of the National Counsel of Technological and Scientific Development (CNPq) and the Santa Catarina State University (UDESC).

REFERENCES

Barsoukov, E. & Macdonald, J.R. (Eds.) (2005). *Impedance spectroscopy: theory, experiment and applications* (2nd ed.). New York: Wiley.

Bertemes-Filho, P. (2002). *Tissue Characterisation using an Impedance Spectroscopy Probe*. Phd Thesis, The University of Sheffield, UK.

Bertemes-Filho, P., Brown, B.H. & Wilson, A.J. (2000). A comparison of modified howland circuits as current generators with current mirror type circuits. *Physiological Measurement* 21(1), 1.

Brown, B., Tidy, J., Boston, K., Blackett, A. & Sharp, F. (1998, 29). Tetrapolar measurement of cervical tissue structure using impedance spectroscopy. In *Engineering in Medicine and Biology Society, 1998. Proceedings of the 20th Annual International Conference of the IEEE*, Volume 6, pp. 2886–2889.

Cole, K.S. (1940). Permeability and Impermeability of Cell Membranes for Ions. In *Proc. of the Cold Spring Harbor Symposia*, Volume 8, pp. 110–122.

Cole, K.S. & Cole, R.H. (1941). Dispersion and absorption in dielectrics: I. Alternating current characteristics. *J. Chem. Phys. 9*, 97–108.

Frounchi, J., Dehkhoda, F. & Zarifi, M.H. (2009). A low-distortion wideband integrated current source for tomography applications. *European Journal of Scientific Research* 27(1), 56–65.

Gonzlez-Correa, C.A., Brown, B.H., Smallwood, R.H., Kalia, N., Stoddard, C.J., Stephenson, T.J., Haggie, S.J., Slatter, D.N. & Bardhan, K.D. (1999). Virtual biopsies in Barrett's esophagus using an impedance probe. In *Annals of the New York Academy of Sciences*, Volume 873, pp. 313–321.

Grimnes, S. & Martinsen, O.G. (2008). *Bioimpedance and Bioelectricity: Basics* (2nd ed.). London: Academic Press.

Haschka, M. & Krebs, V. (2007). *Advances in Fractional Calculus Theoretical Developments and Applications in Physics and Engineering*, Chapter A Direct Approximation of Fractional Cole-Cole Systems by Ordinary First-Order Processes, pp. 257–270. Springer Netherlands.

Lu, L. & Brown, B.H. (1994). The electrode and electronic interface in an EIT spectroscopy system. *Innovation et technologie en biologie et mdecine* 15, 97–103.

McAdams, E.T. & Jossinet, J. (1996). Problems in Equivalent Circuit modelling of the Electrical Properties of Biological Tissues. *Bioelectrochem. Bioenerg.* 40, 147–152.

Qureshi, T.R., Chatwin, C.R., Huber, N., Zarafshani, A. Tunstall, B. & Wang, W. (2010). Comparison of howland and general impedance converter (gic) circuit based current sources for bio-impedance measurements. *Journal of Physics: Conference Series* 224(1), 012167.

Stiz, R.A., Ramos, A., Bertemes-Filho, P. & Vincence, V.C. (2009). Wide band Howland bipolar current source using AGC amplifier. *IEEE Latin Aamerica Transactions* 7(5), 514–517.

Technology and Medical Sciences – Natal Jorge et al. (eds)
© 2011 Taylor & Francis Group, London, ISBN 978-0-415-66822-4

Highly Focalized Thermotherapy: A minimally invasive technique for the treatment of solid tumours

A. Portela & M. Vasconcelos
Faculty of Dental Medicine, University of Porto, Porto, Portugal

J. Cavalheiro
INEB/Engineering Faculty, University of Porto, Porto, Portugal

ABSTRACT: The application of heat in the cancer treatment, the thermotherapy or hyperthermia, is a widely studied method, operating in the tumours cells, in the angiogenic vascular net and it may sometimes originate an immunologic response in the whole organism. The methods currently available to produce hyperthermia are generally limited by the inability to selectively target the tumour cells, with the subsequent risk of affecting adjacent healthy tissues. To overcome this limitation and in the context of the magnetically mediated hyperthermia, the Highly Focalized Thermotherapy (HFT) technique was developed, consisting in the direct injection of a material into the tumour and the subsequent exposition to an external high frequency magnetic field, that will heat the magnetic particles and subsequently, the tumour cells. Methods and materials: The material, a Ferrimagnetic silicate Cement (FC), is a fine powder which has a chemical composition in weight percent, based on oxides, corresponding to $10SiO_2$, $2Al2O_3$, $52Fe_2O_3$, $0,6MgO$, $33CaO$, $(SO_3 + K_2O)$ R. In this study it was determined the FC in vitro (SEM/EDS; XRD) and in vivo (histological evaluation) biocompatibility, its injectability and its capability to generate heat when placed within a high frequency magnetic field. Results: The in vitro and the in vivo studies suggest the FC biocompatibility, so it can remain in the organism during the treatment period without side effects. FC can be injected directly into the tumour, stays located at the injection site, allowing the repetition of treatments dispensing a repeat injection. Its temperature increases when exposed to a magnetic field, also increasing the tumour temperature. Conclusion: Based on the results, the FC seems to be a promising material for the heat of solid tumours in the hyperthermia context.

1 INTRODUCTION

The effects of hyperthermia at the cellular and tissue level have been extensively studied in a multitude of tumour models (Moyer, 2008). Hyperthermia acts in several fronts, in the tumour cells, in the angiogenic vascular net and it may sometimes originate an immunologic response in the whole organism (Shen, 1987; Dellian, 1994; Hildebrandt, 2002).

In the latest seventies, Overgaard J published an article reviewing the experimental observation on the hyperthemic effect on tumour cells (Overgaard, 1977).

Nowadays, the methods available to produce hyperthermia are generally limited by the inability to selectively target the tumour cells, with the subsequent risk of affecting adjacent healthy tissues (Field, 1987; Szasz, 2007). To overcome these limitations, many investigations are in course with the propose of develop a minimal invasive and local technique for the tumour treatment by hyperthermia.

One of those investigations lines is the magnetically mediated hyperthermia, a technique that consist of localizing magnetic particles or seeds within tumour tissue and then applying an external alternating magnetic field to cause them to heat. This heat then conducts into the surrounding tumour tissue (Moroz, 2002).

In this context, Cavalheiro J developed a new method of tumour treatment by hyperthermia, the Highly Focalized Thermotherapy (HFT). This method consist in the direct injection of a material into the tumour and the subsequent exposition to an external high frequency magnetic field that will heat the magnetic particles and subsequently, the tumour cells (Almeida, 2001). For this purpose, the same author developed a material in the form of an injectable paste. The composition of this new material, the Ferrimagnetic Cement (FC), is similar to the silicon–calcium cements but with a large amount of ferrimagnetic oxide.

Since FC will remain in the organism during the treatment period, is important to determine it's interaction with the surrounding medium, it's biocompatibility, capability to be injected in the tumour and generate heat when exposed to a high frequency magnetic field.

2 MATERIAL AND METHODS

The Ferrimagnetic Cement (FC), is a fine powder system which has a chemical composition in weight percent, based on oxides, corresponding to $10SiO_2$, $2Al_2O_3$, $52Fe_2O_3$, $0.6MgO$, $33CaO$, $(SO_3 + K_2O)$ R.

Samples were immersed in SBF Sr (SBF Sr in substitution of Ca) at 37°C, for 43 hours. The control samples were not immersed. The morphological analysis of the samples surface was performed using the SEM JEOL JSM-6301 (Joel Ltd., Japan) with an accelerating voltage of 15 kV and a working distance of 15 mm, at different magnifications (200×, 2000×). The qualitative and semi-quantitative microanalysis of the samples surface was accessed through EDS, using a Voyager system (Noran Instruments, Inc, USA).

X-Ray Diffraction (XRD) analysis of FC samples control and FC samples immersed in SBF Sr for 7 days, was performed by a X'Pert Philips diffractometer, using CuK_1 radiation, Generator Settings: 50 mA, 40 kV with identification software PANalytical. The start position was (°2Th.) 3,5221 and the end position (°2Th.) 106,4421.

The FC in vivo biocompatibility was accessed by the implantation of FC samples and a control material in the muscles of the animal's flank, on the left and right-hand side respectively, of nine female Wistar rats (with an average weight of 200–230 g). Short-term tests were performed at 1, 3, and 9 weeks.

After animals euthanasia the implanted material was removed along with the adjacent tissues. The collected samples were prepared for histological evaluation, stained with haematoxylin and eosin and observed under a LEICA Optical Microscope (LEICA DMLB, Q 500 IW) at 50× magnification.

To determine the injectable FC paste percentage it was calculated the difference between the volume of expelled paste and the volume of the paste that was initially in the syringe. Than, FC was injected in a tumour model (B16F10 melanoma in C57BL6 mouse) with approximately 10 mm in diameter and then observed with Rx.

The FC specific heating power (P) was calculated according to the following formula:

$$P = \Sigma(Cp_i \cdot m_i) \cdot \Delta T / 300,$$

where Cp_i and m_i are the specific heat capacity and the mass of each material (polyethylene, FC, water), respectively. Small discs of FC were placed in an isolated polyethylene tube with distilled water and exposed to a magnetic field (10 kHz) in a vertical coil (diameter 11 cm, 12 turns), using an induction system High Frequency Electronic Furnace K10/RV (CALAMARI and Milan, Italy). The variation of temperature was measured after 300 s of exposure to the magnetic field, using a digital thermometer.

The capability to generate heat in vivo was obtained through the image the animal's tumour injected with FC captured with a thermographic camera (FLIR ThermaCAM, 1998).

3 RESULTS AND DISCUSSION

When examining the images of the FC surface characterized by SEM and EDS, before and after immersion in SBF Sr significant alterations were detected in the samples' morphology and composition. The porous surface observed in the control samples (Figure 1) was covered by a layer of precipitates emerging from the initial surface (Figure 2). The EDS spectrum of the control surface (Graph 1) shows peaks of Fe, Ca and Si, as well as small percentages of Al and Mg, which are components of FC. The layer which covers the initial surface

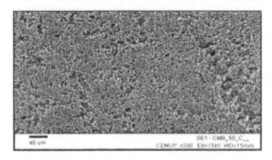

Figure 1. FC control samples after cement preparation at ×200.

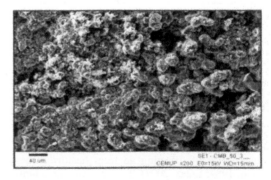

Figure 2. FC samples immersed for 43 h in SBF Sr, at ×200 magnification.

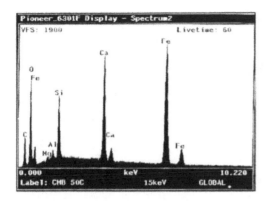

Graph 1. FC control surface spectrum.

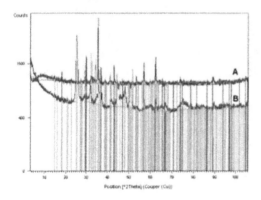

Graph 2. FC 43 h immersion spectrum.

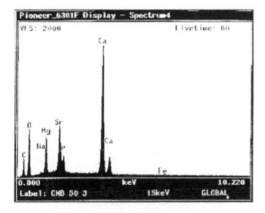

Graph 3. X-ray diffraction patterns of control samples (A) allow the identification of peaks of the two major compounds of the cement: magnetite (2 h = 35.48; 62.56) and calcium silicate Ca_3SiO_5 (2 h = 29.46; 32.26; 34.40), and samples immersed 7 days in SBF Sr (B).

(Graph 2) is composed of Ca, Mg and Sr associated to high peaks of C and P. Crossing the EDS results with XRD analysis (Graph 3) proves to be mainly crystalline $SrCO_2$ in association with amorphous

calcium compounds, because it was not possible to identify crystalline phases of phosphorus or carbonate calcium compounds. Due to the inexistence of Ca in the special SBF Sr medium, the existent Ca of the precipitate layer can only comes from the FC. Part of the cement will dissolve and the Ca will reprecipitate on the surface. Therefore, there was an ionic exchange between the initial cement sample and the surrounding environment.

The physical structure of a material and the properties of its surface are known to be indicative of a material's biocompatibility (Ratner, 1996). The FC samples quickly become coated with precipitates rich in calcium and phosphate, the initial surface is covered with a precipitates layer resulting from interaction with the surrounding medium allowing the conclusion that the FC exhibits a high bioactive behaviour.

In vivo studies are essential for the assessment of medical devices, given that, their approval requires that they must be tested on animals before being used in human (Stevens, 2000). The in vivo biocompatibility of FC was performed by its implantation in an animal model, which required a surgical procedure that causes lesions in the surrounding tissues. Inflammation, the wound scarring process and the foreign-body responses of the organism are generally considered as the tissues' physiological response to lesions (Andersan, 1994; Ryhanen, 1998). The histological data regarding the samples obtained 1 week after implantation of the control material (Figure 3a) are compatible with a chronic inflammatory process mainly consisting of lymphocytes and macrophages, among other less relevant inflammatory cells surrounding the material. During the first week after the implantation of FC (Figure 4a), a chronic foreign-body granulomatous inflammatory process was observed. Besides the inflammatory cells identified in the control material samples, a few foreign-body reactive multinucleate giant cells were found. The presence of foreign-body reactive multinucleate giant cells is important because it represents a specific inflammatory response triggered by the foreign substance (Thomsen, 1991). The giant cells are present in small numbers and display their characteristic ring of particle remnants. Depending on the size of the implanted material's particles, the organism reacts in a different manner. Larger particles cannot undergo phagocytosis, thus remaining inside of the giant cells, producing a relatively inert tissue response (Thomsen, 1991; Hallam, 2002). At the end of 3 weeks of implantation (Figure 3b), a cystic lesion was observed around the control material, surrounded by a fine layer of inflammatory cells, mostly composed of lymphocytes and macrophages. The FC samples (Figure 4b) were very similar to those obtained

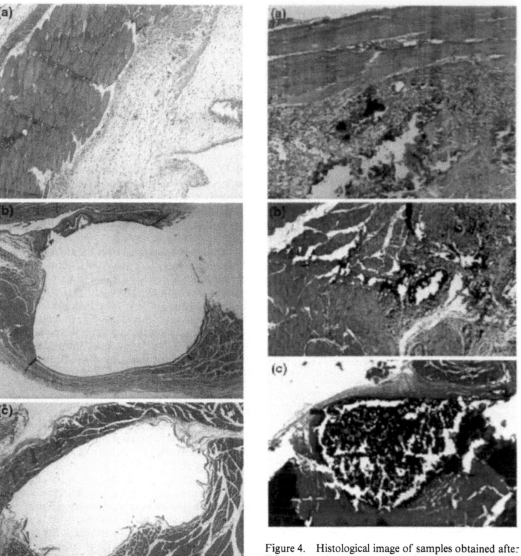

Figure 3. Histological image of samples obtained after implantation of the control material. (a) 1 week; (b) 3 weeks; (c) 9 weeks.

Figure 4. Histological image of samples obtained after FC implantation. (a) 1 week; (b) 3 weeks; (c) 9 weeks.

after 1 week of implantation, only displaying a slight decrease in the inflammation around the cement, thus reducing the presence of inflammatory cells in the adjacent muscle tissue. The images of the implanted samples after 9 weeks display a significant decrease in the inflammatory response. In the control material (Figure 3c), the cystic lesion surrounding it was coated with a fine layer of inflammatory cells, where only lymphocytes

were detected. The FC samples (Figure 4c) revealed a fine layer of inflammatory cells, with lymphocytes and macrophages surrounding part of the cement. Owing to the absence of giant cells in these images, FC may be considered well tolerated. The most significant finding was the presence of cement in direct contact with the muscle tissue, displaying no inflammatory infiltrate. If a material is very toxic, it induces an acute local response for an indefinite period of time, but this did not occur with FC.

The determined FC powder/water ratio is easy to mix. The paste obtained enabled the injection of a substantial percentage of the sample (90 ± 1%), which can be handled within a reasonable period of time (5 min) and with an adequate setting time.

The Rx image (Figure 5) of FC inside the tumour 1 week after injection shows that FC remains in the injection location, the tumour.

The treatment of tumours with hyperthermia, induced by magnetic materials and a magnetic field, has been developed by many researchers, with different approaches ((Moyer, 2008; Moroz, 2002; Suzuki, 2003; Ito, 2003; Kawashita, 2005; Sato, 2008; Ito, 2009). Since FC will be used in the treatment of solid tumours by this methodology, it's necessary that the FC has the capability to generate heat when exposed to a magnetic field. The in vitro evaluation of the specific heating power of FC, demonstrate a temperature increase in the FC sample environment (maximum heating power 2.11 W g-1).

The in vivo capability to generate heat (Figure 6) shows that in a short period of time (3–5 min) the tumour temperature increase 5°C.

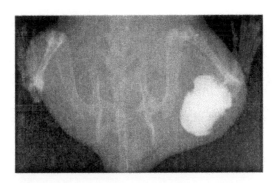

Figure 5. Rx image of FC injected in the tumour.

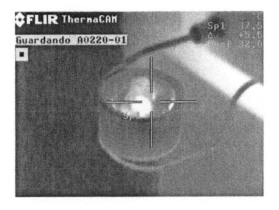

Figure 6. Thermographic camera image of the animal injected with FC, during the HFT treatment.

4 CONCLUSIONS

The HFT methodology will probably be considered a promising approach in the treatment of solid tumours through local hyperthermia.

The data obtained in this study allows us to conclude that FC can remain in the inject site, the tumour, during a period of time enough to give repeated hyperthermia treatments using high frequency magnetic fields, with a desirable biological response, interacting and stabilizing in the surrounding medium. The fluid paste obtained with FC can be directly injected into the solid tumours and it has the capability to generate heat when placed within a magnetic field, providing a minimally invasive technique to treat solid tumours with HFT.

ACKNOWLEDGEMENTS

The authors would like to thank to Fundação para a Ciência e Tecnologia (FCT), for the support of the project PTDC/EEA-ACR/75454/2006.

REFERENCES

Almeida T. Estudo in vivo de um Cerâmico Ferrimagnético com potencial em Oncoterapia. *Tese de Mestrado em Engenharia Biomédica pela Faculdade de Engenharia da Universidade do Porto*. 2001.

Anderson J.M. In vivo biocompatibility of implantable delivery systems and biomaterials. *Eur J Pharm Biopharm*. 1994;40:1–8.

Dellian, et al. High-energy shock waves enhance hyperthermia response of tumors: effects on blood flow, energy metabolism, and tumor growth. *J Natl Cancer Inst*. 1994;86(4):287–93.

Field S.B. *Physics and technology of hyperthermia*. In: Field S.B. Franconi C, editors. NATO ASI series, E: applied sciences. Dordrecht: Martinus Nijhoff Publisher; 1987. pp. 19–27.

Hallam J.B.P. The interaction of biomaterials with the body is a two way phenomenon-long. *Sci Today*, 2002;20:420–423.

Hildebrandt B., Wust P. & Ahlers O. The cellular and molecular basis of hyperthermia. *Crit Rev Oncol, Hematol*. 2002;43(1):33–56.

Ito A., Tanaka K., Honda H., Abe S., Yamaguchi H. & Kobayashi T. Complete regression of mouse mammary carcinoma with a size greater than 15 mm by frequent repeated hyperthermia using magnetic nanoparticles. *J Biosci Bioeng*, 2003;96(4):364–369.

Ito A., Saito H., Mitobe K., Minamiya Y., Takahashi N., Maruyama K., Motoyama S., Katayose Y. & Ogawa J. Inhibition of heat shock protein 90 sensitizes melanoma cells to thermosensitive ferromagnetic particle-mediated hyperthermia with low Curie temperature. *Cancer Sci*, 2009;100(3):558–564.

Kawashita M., Tanaka M., Kokubo T., Inoue Y., Yao T., Hamada S. & Shinjo T. Preparation of ferrimagnetic magnetite microspheres for in situ hyperthermic treatment of câncer. *Biomaterials*, 2005;26(15):2231–2238.

Moyer H.R. & Delman K.A. The role of huperthermia in optimizing tumor response to regional therapy. *Int J Hyperthermia*, 2008;24(3):251–261.

Moroz P., Jones S.K. & Gray B.N. Magnetically mediated hyperthermia: current status and future directions. *Int J Hyperthermia*, 2002;18(4):267–284.

Overgaard J. Effect of Hyperthermia on malignant cells in vivo: A review and hypothesis. *Cancer*, 1977;39:2637–2646.

Ratner B.D., Hoffman A., Schoen F.J. & Lemons J.L. *Biomaterials science: an introduction to materials in medicine.* 2nd ed. London: Academic Press; 1996. pp. 325–398.

Ryhanen J., Kallioinen M., Tuukkanen J., Junila J., Niemela E., Sandvik P. & Serlo W. In vivo biocompatibility evaluation of nickel–titanium shape memory metal alloy: muscle and perineural tissue responses and encapsule membrane thickness. *J Biomed Mater Res*, 1998;41:481–488.

Sato K., Watanabe Y., Horiuchi A., Yukumi S., Doi T., Yoshida M., Yamamoto Y., Tsunooka N. & Kawachi K. Feasibility of new heating method of hepatic parenchyma using a sintered $MgFe_2O_4$ needle under an alternating magnetic field. *J Surg Res*, 2008;146:110–116.

Shen R., Hornback N.B, Shidnia H., Shupe R.E. & Brahmi Z. Wholebody hyperthermia decreases lung metastases in lung tumor bearing mice, possibly via a mechanism involving natural killer cells. *J ClinImmunol*. 1987;7(3):246–253.

Stevens K. In vivo testing of biomaterials. *BME*, 2000;430(4):31–33.

Suzuki M., Shinkai M., Honda H., Kobayashi T. Anticancer effect and immune induction by hyperthermia of malignant melanoma using magnetite cationic liposomes. *Melanoma Res*, 2003;13(2):129–135.

Szasz A. Hyperthermia, a modality in the wings. *J Cancer Res Ther*, 2007;3(1):56–66.

Thomsen P., Ericson L.E. *Inflammatory cell response to bone implant surfaces.* In: Davis JE, editor. The bone biomaterial interface. Toronto: University of Toronto Press. 1991. pp. 153–164.

Technology and Medical Sciences – Natal Jorge et al. (eds)
© 2011 Taylor & Francis Group, London, ISBN 978-0-415-66822-4

Identification of rib boundaries in chest X-ray images using elliptical models

Luís Brás & Alípio M. Jorge
LIAAD-INESC Porto, LA, Portugal
DCC-FCUP, Porto, Portugal

Elsa Ferreira Gomes
GECAD, Portugal
ISEP-IPP, Portugal

Raquel Duarte
Centro Diagnóstico Pneumológico (Chest Disease Centre) V.N. Gaia, Portugal
FMUP, Portugal

ABSTRACT: We are developing a new method for the identification of rib boundaries in chest x-ray images. The identification of rib boundaries is important for radiologist diagnosis of lung diseases as TB. The radiologists use the ribs as reference for location and can be used to eliminate false positives in the detection of abnormalities. Our method automatically identifies rib boundaries from raw images through a sequence of steps using a combination of image processing techniques. Radiographs are still very relevant in practice because in Portugal and many other countries it is the first step for TB detection. We have access a large database of x-ray images provided by the pneumological screening centre (CDP) of Vila Nova de Gaia, in Portugal.

1 INTRODUCTION

Tuberculosis (TB) remains worldwide a serious problem. In Portugal, TB incidence is 29.9/100.000 inhabitants, higher than the European Union average. Radiographic (x-ray) screening as a means of detecting active disease can play an important role in the prevention of this disease. Due to different reasons, experienced radiologists may misinterpret x-rays in more than a marginal percentage of the abnormal cases (Yoshida, Keserci & Doi 1998). Work on Computer Aided Diagnosis (CAD) systems has been done in the last two decades, frequently involving image processing and image classification (Doi, MacMahon, Giger & Hoffmann 1999, Katsuragawa & Doi 2007).

This work is a part of a project where the main objective is to develop a novel x-ray image automatic multi-classification (tagging) approach to support medical diagnosis (to determinate the disease activity) for the detection, in chest radiograph images, of any abnormality. The x-ray images are provided by the pneumological screening centre of Vila Nova de Gaia, in Portugal.

2 PROBLEM DEFINITION

The specific work we are addressing in this paper is the rib boundary identification in x-ray images. The automatic delineation of rib borders is important in the detection of lung abnormalities. Frequently, the radiologists use the ribs as reference for location and can be used to eliminate false positives in the detection of abnormalities. This issue, despite being a subject of large study, is a hard problem (van Ginneken, ter Haar Romeny & Viergever 2001) and, as far as we know, is not satisfactorily solved for x-ray images.

2.1 Related work

In van Ginneken, ter Haar Romeny & Viergever 2001 and van Ginneken 2001 we find an overview of existing methods (up to 2001) to find rib boundaries. Those authors summarize what they call the classical approach as follows. Find the rib candidates using edge detection and fit geometrical models such as parabolas or ellipses (or a combination) to those candidates. The use of snakes and a modified Hough transform to detect candidates have also been used. Shoaib, Ghani, Shazia, K. & K. 2009 use the gray scale, histogram equalization, threshold finding, edge detection, and local average to detect ribs. Park, Jin & Wilson 2004 extracts the lung field to limit the region to be processed. This is done using a knowledge based lung field extraction. Rib shadow is also reduced, using filter combination methods. Our method follows the classical approach of combining rib boundary detection with geometrical model fitting. However, we propose specific solutions for some of the steps.

3 OUR APPROACH

In this section, we describe our image treatment approach from the original digitized x-ray

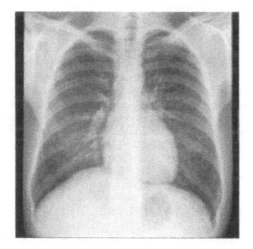

Figure 1. Original x-ray image.

(Figure 1) to the identified rib boundaries. This is done in several steps. First we equalize the image to increase contrast. Then smoothing is applied to obtain a high contrast black and white version. The lung field contour is then obtained with an extrapolation method. This contour can be superimposed on the original image to obtain the segments corresponding to the lung fields where the ribs are located. Before that, we take the original image again and look for possible rib boundaries.

Specifically for the rib boundary identification we start by using the Canny edge detection filter. After this step we have a set of candidate pixels which will be subject to further filtering.

Next, we try to match the high score boundary points to rib models stored in a database. The models in the database are manually obtained from real images.

3.1 Obtaining the lung field borders

We start by filtering and equalizing the raw x-ray image to obtain higher contrast. The next step is to smoothen the image by replacing each pixel with an average of neighboring pixels. This image is then thresholded into a black and white image (Figure 2, left). After that, white objects smaller then 3000 pixels are deleted (Figure 2, right).

Finally, we identify the lung field borders through an iterative process as follows.

We start with a given point of the border (e.g. the leftmost point) and use this point as centre of a rotating radius (see Figure 3). When the rotation finds a white pixel, this new point will be the new centre. The process repeats (separately for each lung) until the lung is fully surrounded. The lines between each pair of consecutive points are on the delimitation of the lung field. These borders

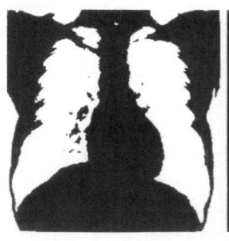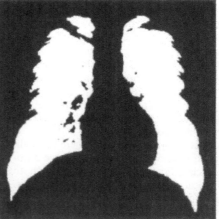

Figure 2. Thresholded image (left) and image without small white segments (right).

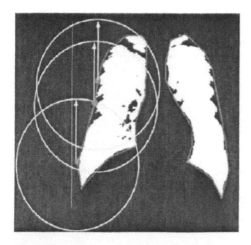

Figure 3. Lung field iterative delimitation process.

will be used to clip the images and enable focusing on the area of interest (the lung field).

3.2 *Obtaining the primary rib boundaries*

The aim of this process is to identify the pixels that are most likely associated with rib boundaries. We start again with the original image and after filtering the highest spatial frequencies we apply a derivative method for contour detection (Canny). The result on the example image can be seen in Figure 4. In Figure 5 (right) we can see the resulting image after being clipped with the previously found lung field borders.

With the Canny method we obtain a very large number of pixels. We have now to filter out the ones which are less likely to be on rib boundaries. Since we have a fairly good idea of the general drawing of the ribs we are looking for, we can measure the steepness of the lines found with Canny and eliminate unlikely segments.

For that we measure the gradient of the resulting lines. Then, for each pixel we calculate a score which takes into account the steepness of the line the pixel is in, as well as the side of the lung field. Each pixel is classified as belonging to a steep/soft ascent/descent or to an approximately horizontal arch.

This pixel classification is done by convolution using an appropriate mask for each pattern. Figure 6 shows an example of one of the convolution masks. With this procedure we determine a score for each pixel to find which ones have a higher likelihood of being on the rib boundary.

Score calculation for the left side (right side):

- score $P1$—not belonging to a steep ascent/descent;
- score $P2$—not belonging to a descent (ascent);

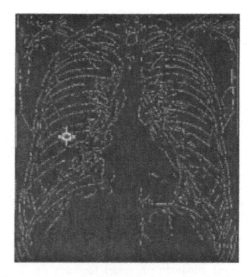

Figure 4. Contour image obtained with the Canny method.

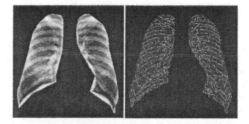

Figure 5. Frame for the lung fields superimposed on the original image (left) and on after using the Canny method (right).

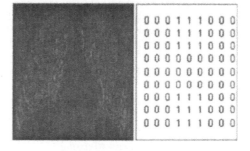

Figure 6. Candidate pixels are classified into soft ascents/descents or not using a convolution mask. On the left we see the resulting classification (blue or yellow pixels) and on the right we see the convolution mask.

- score $P3$—belonging to a soft arch or to an ascent (descent);
- score $P4$—the gradient direction is between 45° and 135° or between 225° and 315°.

The final score is calculated as $P = P1 + P2 + P3 + P4$. The pixels with a score above the

131

average are selected. The remaining ones are filtered out.

3.3 *Matching the rib boundaries with stored models*

We now find a frame for the lung fields using straight lines (Figure 4). Two horizontal lines, one vertical line on the inside, and one diagonal on the outside (the reference diagonal). These lines are determined from the lung fields previously obtained. Then, we find the operational diagonal, which is parallel to reference diagonal. The operational diagonal is the one that contains the pixels corresponding to the highest sum of scores. The high scoring pixels in the diagonal will be used to search for rib models in a rib model database.

The rib model database contains ellipse arches for different rib configurations. The task is to find the most adequate rib model for each rib. The search starts by (1) considering the steepness of the operational diagonal (the operational angle). This will help restrict the set of models to be considered, since different inclinations (operational angles) will correspond to different body structures. Then, (2) for each candidate pixel on the operational diagonal we consider its y coordinate (height), which indicates the ribs to model. This, once more, will restrict the search to the models corresponding to rib $n, n - 1$ or $n + 1$.

After focusing on a smaller set of models, we obtain the direction of the gradient of the candidate pixel. We restrict to models with a value of the normal to the tangent in a vicinity to the gradient of the pixel is chosen. Then, we also measure the degree of matching between the model and the suspected rib boundary in the processed image. For a given model we count the number of pixels that overlap with the suspected rib boundary (matching), and the number of missed pixels. This assesses the adequacy of the model. The most adequate model is the one which maximizes the *MatchingScore*.

$$MatchingScore = \frac{\#matching}{\#matching + \#missing} \quad (1)$$

In fact, this match count is made over a neighborhood of the model, as is shown in Figure 8. In our experiments the neighborhood includes all the points at most 6 pixels away from the model.

To simplify these procedures, the models must be adequately stored. In particular, each ellipse arch is stored with the value of the normal to the tangent for each pixel. To retrieve the most appropriate model from the database we proceed as follows for each candidate model.

1. Take the operational distance (label B in Figure 7) and consider the corresponding pixel of the model.
2. Compare the angle of the normal to the tangent on this pixel of the model with the angle of the gradient from the processed image. The model is accepted if the difference is below 10°.
3. Measure the *MatchingScore* for the selected models.
4. Choose the model which maximizes the *MatchingScore*.

In the end, we may not have identified all the ribs, or extra ribs may appear. This advices for a post-processing step.

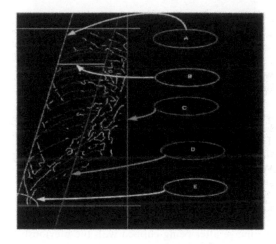

Figure 7. Straight line frame for the identification of the best diagonal for model retrieval. A–reference diagonal, B–operational distance, C–height, D–operational diagonal (automatically found), E–operational angle.

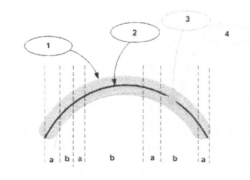

Figure 8. Matching process. 1–Matching neighborhood, 2–Model ellipse arch, 3–Overlapping pixel, 4–Image contour, a–Missing pixels, b–Matching pixels.

4 EVALUATION

We have performed a preliminary experimental evaluation of our procedure using five x-ray images. Although we have access to a large database of images, we have focused on these five images for now in order to obtain some early feedback.

For each of the five images, we have worked on one single rib (the fourth on the left lung field). In other words, we tried to solve the problem of selecting the most appropriate model for a given rib in each image in a given set. The set of models considered were manually built by adjusting an ellipse each to the rib on the original x-ray image.

Again, a full evaluation would require dealing with each one of the ribs. Focusing on one single rib per image helped focusing on the process. All the other ribs can be handled with a similar process.

The evaluation procedure is as follows. Given a set of images and a set of rib models, for each image, look for the appropriate model for the left fourth rib (Section 3.3). Analyze the matching scores of each model for each image (Section 3.2). The chosen model is also visually checked for a qualitative evaluation.

4.1 *Results*

Table 1 shows the calculated *MatchingScore* (Eq 1) for each image (except image 2) and for each model. Model *i* was obtained from image *i*. We can assume that, for each image, the process should retrieve the model which had been built from that image. In our five test images, this "correct" retrieval happens twice. In two other cases the "correct" model gets a high *MatchingScore*, but is not the best one. In the case of one image (image 2), the process failed to retrieve a model for the fourth rib because the operational diagonal did not find a pixel at the appropriate height. Such cases will be handle in a post-processing phase which is under development.

Although encouraging, these empirical results indicate that the process still requires further developments. Not retrieving the exact "correct" model is not necessarily bad, since other models may be very

Table 1. *MatchingScore* for each model on each test image. Highest values per image are shown in bold.

Models	Image 1	Image 3	Image 4	Image 5
1	0.42	0.39	0.20	0.36
2	**0.46**	0.38	0.24	0.22
3	0.32	**0.62**	**0.81**	0.41
4	0.23	0.44	0.74	0.47(5)
5	0.22	0.52	0.75	**0.48(4)**

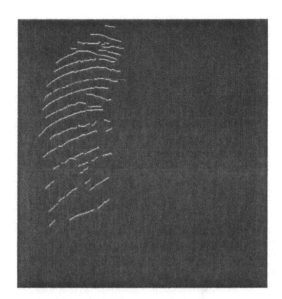

Figure 9. Visualization of the matching between model 3 and the fourth rib on image 4. The blue ellipse arch is the model, the yellow points are the pixels found by image processing and the red points are the matching pixels.

similar. As matter of fact, in table 1 we can see that some models obtain very similar results in all images (e.g. models 4 and 5). In Figure 9 we can qualitatively assess, for image 4, the matching between the chose model (3) and the identified contour.

5 SUBSEQUENT WORK

The process so far consists in the identification of an appropriate model for a given rib position. We still need to evaluate the ability of the process to successfully identify suspected rib positions. Moreover, other steps will be required to correctly model the whole ribcage. Further steps will use this process for automatic image segment tagging and classification.

5.1 *Post-processing*

After identifying the rib models, we will most likely need a post-processing step, since some false ribs may appear, as well as some ribs may be missing. Given that we have a fair idea of the position and the number of the ribs, we can try to infer these faults.

5.2 *Tagging and classification*

After optimizing rib segmentation we will proceed to the identification of other relevant parts of the x-ray image. The ultimate aim is to apply multi-label classification (tagging), possibly using association rules, for automatically tagging relevant occurrences in the x-ray. These labels will be used as support for a more efficient pneumological diagnosis by the expert.

6 CONCLUSIONS

In this paper we have presented a process for the identification of rib boundaries in chest radiographs. The process starts with a raw x-ray image, obtains the lung fields and the set of pixels most likely on the rib boundaries. Then the process retrieves, for each rib, the most adequate model from a database. The process has been evaluated on five images using a database of five models. We have focused on one particular rib. The empirical results obtained indicate that the process is able to retrieve adequate models. However, further evaluation of the process is required, which will lead to necessary refinements and extensions.

REFERENCES

Doi, K., MacMahon, H., Giger, M. & Hoffmann, K. (1999). Computer-aided diagnosis in medical imaging. In *Proc. of the First International Workshop on Computer-Aided Diagnosis*, Amsterdam: Elsevier Science, pp. 11–20.

Katsuragawa, S. & Doi, K. (2007). Computer-aided diagnosis in chest radiography. *Computerized medical Imaging and Graphics* 31, 212–223.

Park, M., Jin, J.S. & Wilson, L.S. (2004). Detection of abnormal texture in chest x-rays with reduction of ribs. In *Pan-Sydney Area Workshop on Visual Information Processing VIP2003, Sydney. Conferences in Research and Practice in Information Technology*, Volume 36, Sydney.

Shoaib, M., Ghani, U., Shazia, K.k. & S.K.K. (2009). Design and implementation of efficient information retrieval algorithm for chest x-ray images. *Journal of American Science* 5(4), 43–48.

van Ginneken, B. (2001). *Computer-Aided Diagnosis in Chest Radiography*. Ph.D. thesis, Utrecht University.

van Ginneken, B., ter Haar Romeny, B.M. & Viergever, M.A. (2001). Computer-aided diagnosis in chest radiography: A survey. *IEEE Trans. Med. Imaging* 20, 1228–1241.

Yoshida, H., Keserci, B. & Doi, K. (1998). Computer-aided diagnosis of pulmonary nodules in chest radiographs: Distinction of nodules from false positives based on wavelet snake and artificial neural network. In *11th IEEE Symposium on Computer-Based Medical Systems (CBMS'98)*, Lubbock, Texas, p. 258.

Technology and Medical Sciences – Natal Jorge et al. (eds)
© 2011 Taylor & Francis Group, London, ISBN 978-0-415-66822-4

Improving diagnosis processes through multidimensional analysis in medical institutions

Orlando Belo

Department of Informatics, School of Engineering, Universidade do Minho, Braga, Portugal

ABSTRACT: For many years, decision support mechanisms have been used on medical applications, providing knowledge and practical expertise on specific areas, as well ensuring a better support to medical staff do enhance their jobs. Nowadays, we haven't the need to prove once more their utility in clinical scenarios. Existing applications can easily show that. However, we can discuss some alternatives to improve some of the existing decision-support systems, especially at the data repositories level. We believe that a well designed and implemented data repository could make the difference in the effectiveness and in the quality of service provided by any decision support systems, and especially by an associated data warehousing system. A well organised multidimensional schema, containing every possible dimension of analysis and the necessary evaluation metrics, combined with an effective populating strategy, integrating specific domain oriented extraction, transformation and integration mechanisms, are basic ingredients to dispose a successful data warehouse for a conventional data warehousing system. In this paper, we discuss a possible schema for a data warehouse especially oriented to support medical diagnosis processes, presenting all its basic structures, including multidimensional schemas, fact-tables organization, dimensions of analysis, and some exploitation mechanisms. Moreover, we intend to demonstrate that it's possible to have more effective diagnosis processes if we take into consideration some multidimensional data design and populating aspects in the data structures, that receives diagnosis information, and use adequately an On-Line Analytical Processing system to explore them.

Keywords: Medical Decision Support Systems, Diagnosis and Treatments, Data Warehousing Systems, On-Line Analytical Processing, Multi-dimensional Data Structures

1 INTRODUCTION

Today's *Decision Support Systems* (DSS) application spectre is quite large, including areas such as retail, banking, telecommunications, and, of course, medicine, just to name a few. However, why people decide to implement them in their organizations stills, for many reasons, a very well closed "secret". We could speculate a little bit about it, but it's preferable focusing our attention in a area where we believe that DSS, and particularly *Data Warehousing Systems* (DWS) (Inmon 1996) (Kimball et al. 2008), are useful assets in conventional daily operations—basically, in things that people need to do currently. Medicine is clearly one of the areas where we easily find tasks owning such characteristics (Shams & Farishta 2001). From the beginning, DWS were seen as having an enormous potential to be applied in the medicine domain, supporting clinical data repositories in academic medical centers (Einbinder et al. 2001), providing architectures for clinical applications (Pedersen & Jensen 1998),

combinating analytical processing with geographic information for community health assessment data analysis (Scotch et al. 2008), supporting health care decision-making (Berndt et al. 2003), improving prescribing services (Lin et al. 2009), or just supporting decision-making platforms for Orthopedics (Lin et al. 2010). Medical diagnosis and treatments are two good examples of tasks where we believe that the use of DWS technology can be quite useful, contributing to increment the effectiveness of the diagnosis and treatment applications. These two well know activities to be well and correctly done require often, beyond the obvious clinicians knowledge and expertise, consulting patient records, analysing medical images, or studying biological analysis results, among other important things. Commonly, all this stuff is located in disparate heterogeneous sources, which keep data in so many formats that clinicians need to have additional skills to deal with it properly or need to appeal to outsourcing services.

The implementation of a DWS especially oriented to support decision making in medical diagnosis and treatment fields should be prepared to deal with such diversity of data, ensuring a single data repository with factual information (with the respective temporal tags) as well the mechanisms to explore it according the various diagnosis perspectives of analysis communicated previously by clinicians. In (Stolba & Tjoa 2006) authors approached the application of DWS and *Data Mining* (DM) (Fayyad et al. 1996) exposing a DWS architecture and services especially oriented to evidence-based medicine applications. Many of the aspects covered by those authors in the several scenarios discussed are essential for the success of a DWS in this area. However, our perspective is a little bit different.

In this paper we do not intend to discuss the viability of introducing a DWS in a medical institution, or to justify the importance of having sophisticated *On-Line Analytical Processing* (OLAP) tools for data exploitation (Baralis et al. 1997). We assumed the existence of a DWS for healthcare decision making in a medical institution, containing a set of multidimensional structures, exclusively designed for support diagnosis and treatment analysis—a specific multidimensional schema that keeps the institutions data patrimony about diagnosis. However, we propose another multidimensional model in order to provide a sustainable OLAP platform capable to provide different aggregation levels (with adequate metrics) for a more diversified set of variables—analytical dimensions (diseases, symptoms, causes, signs, etc.)—over time. We will present this multidimensional structure, its potentialities, and finally we demonstrate how an OLAP platform could help in their exploitation.

2 KEEPING DIAGNOSIS PROCESSES IN DATA WAREHOUSES

Diagnosis is one of the most relevant areas for many professional in the field of Medicine. Its importance is well recognised for everyone that fills the responsibility to apply the right and the best treatment for some medical episode. It's essential in Medicine. However, we do not intend here to discuss any aspect of medical diagnosis or confront any ideas about how a diagnosis process must be done or applied. We are only concerned about how to give a more effective support to such processes, in terms of diagnosis data storage and exploitation, proving better means to compare medical processes and facts, or to conciliate information from distinct medical sources clarifying or giving support to diagnosis paths, symptoms analysis or even exploring non regular diagnosis analysis dimensions. Basically, we will discuss the validity and adoption of a DWS to support medical diagnosis

tasks as regular decision-making activities and trying to contribute to the improvement of medical institutions' performance.

Usually, to be effective, a diagnosis process involves a lot of things (http://www.suite101. com/content/the-process-of-clinical-diagnosis-a90627). When doing it, doctors follow a set of basic analysis perspectives involving patient's clinical histories and their current physical status, physical examinations, and several other tests. They do all of this following some very well known medical classification procedures complemented with their knowledge, expertise and sensitivity for the case. From these processes, doctors gather a lot of data, which as we can see provided by different sources involving medical equipment, doctors' evaluations, or observation reports done by other medical staff—different sources, with disparate data formats. At the end, frequently, its the doctor that does the final conciliation of the data, accordingly to its current needs, status of the patient, and, of course, process's metadata. Imagine now, how many data repositories doctors maintain autonomously in a medical institution like a hospital in cases where there is no centralised way to receive all this disparate data. It's a huge problem, because doctors do not have the possibility to share in an immediate (automatic) way their processes, to compare notes or having different diagnosis perspectives from their colleagues about similar cases. So, we can conclude that, most of the times doctors don't use to get advantage of each others' experience and diagnosis process data.

However, in the last few years significant efforts have been done in the sense to create mechanisms to conciliate medical data inside institutions, increasing data exchange and experiences sharing. Part of this is due to the introduction of DWS in medical institutions, providing adequate means to gather, conciliate, adapt and integrate medical diagnosis data from disparate data sources into a single data repository, which can be accessed by anyone with enough credentials. Although, the creation of a unique and centralised data repository is not, by itself, the solution for sharing experiences and information about diagnosis processes. It must be organised accordingly all the possible analysis perspectives that doctors follow during a diagnosis process, and integrating large amounts of diagnosis facts collected in past processes for other patients. In fact, doing this, we are design and prepare a specialized subject oriented data repository—a data warehouse—to support decision making in diagnosis processes.

Disparate data conciliation is so a basic key aspect for the success of having a homogeneous data repository for diagnosis processes. To ensure that, we must provide effective gateways for every single information source identified that was been considered as essential to any diagnosis processes. Additionally, each information source must be profiled in order to identify eventual data anomalies (wrong formats, acronymous resolution, foreign keys validation, nulls treatments, etc.) and if necessary applying correctional measures accordingly to the anomalies that were verified. The populating tasks sequence (responsible to feed the data warehouse) demonstrates all the elementary steps to conduce data from its origin to its destiny: the data warehouse. The data warehouse populating process—usually known as ETL (Extract, Transform and Load) process—is often very difficult to accomplish, basically due to the heterogeneity of the data sources and consequently due to the high number of gateways and data bridges that we must implemented, and ensure that they perform data transformation tasks in the better way, filtering erroneous and ambiguous data and letting pass the "good" data to be loaded in the data warehouse. Before proceed to the design and implementation of populating process another important task must be referred: data source profiling. With it, we gather precious information about sources and its functioning, which means getting a complete characterisation about the sources, access and permission modes, operational availability status and, of course, the quality level of the data we want. After validating this information, we begin the design of the populating system, making a logical mapping plan, which will gives us all the correspondence among sources' and data warehouse's data objects and attributes.

3 THE USE OF MULTIDIMENSIONAL STRUCTURES

The significant increase of electronic health records usage in medical institutions brought new quests in the treatment and exploitation of medical data. At the same time, as a direct consequence, the volume of medical data also increased as well as the variety of medical metadata. Today we have better information resources that contribute surely for better medical processes appliance and decision making support. Medical institutions are investing in new equipment and information systems contributing to provide better data, more structured and detailed. However, the introduction of new technologies and systems in new areas of medical services is done not considering a full integration of data records and services, which contributes to create disparate information sources. The implementation of a DWS could be quite useful in these scenarios. When well designed DWS provides the necessary structures to conciliate and enrich disparate data in a single repository. Additionally its nature allows structuring and creating data storage repositories accordingly different points of view presented by doctors for a particular medical information process.

DWS are not operational systems neither any kind of substitutes for information process. They are analytical systems oriented to support decision-making activities. This means that we are not speaking about using them to support a specific diagnosis process execution, but to provide analytical data (factual information with temporal labels, subject oriented, and with no possibility to be updated) to decision making processes in which medical staff is involved with. These characteristics induced new ways to structure data in order to be more adequate to fast ad hoc queries answering.

A DWS keeps data inside a special repository: the data warehouse, which is frequently organised as a set of data marts structured accordingly their own dimensional schemas (Kimball & Ross 2002). Usually, the data warehouse is designed taking into consideration the different analysis perspectives of decision makers—the doctors in cases of medical diagnosis processes. During the DWS's requirement analysis phase those perspectives—the dimensions—are identified and characterized, being the main axis for cross analysis among them using the facts stored in the data warehouse. So, if we try to define a dimensional schema for a data mart designed to support medical diagnosis data analysis we need to know what are the dimensions and the facts that will be included in the schema. Taking into consideration the information usually used during a typical diagnosis process, and appealing to the four steps design process (Kimball et al., 2008) for a data warehouse, we can propose a multidimensional structure (equivalent to a data mart) for medical diagnosis support decision, having the following components.

- *Dimensions*, which receive data characterizing each analysis axle. Basically, they are the coordinates of a multidimensional space where we can find (if exists) a specific fact. We assumed that our medical diagnosis data mart include the following dimensions: 1) *Calendar*, it's a mandatory dimension; it supports all the temporal analysis about medical diagnosis processes allowing us to cross facts among different recognized periods of time (date, weekday, month, quarter, year, season, and so forth) with other dimensions in the schema; 2) *Health Institution*, includes a brief description about the institution where the diagnosis process was done; 3) *Patients*, that stores the most basic medical information about patients; it can have also some direct links to other data marts, especially the ones related to the patients' medical history—one important piece of information in any diagnosis process; 4) *Doctors*, this dimension has a set of attributes that indentifies and characterizes all the doctors involved with diagnosis processes, having properties like age, speciality, years of service, etc.; 5) *Symptoms*, where we could keep a complete list of all the symptoms known for diseases, as well their types and a list of provable causes; 6) *Signs*, that contains all the medical facts observed during the examination of patients; 7) *Tests*, all the test that were done during a diagnosis process are stored in this dimension, including a summary of their results; 8) *Causes*, which has a brief description of the causes that were responsible by the patient's diagnosis situation; and 9) *Diseases*, this receives the characterization of all known diseases, including data about the disease and its classification based, for instance, on the ICD-9 codes (e.g. icd9cm. chrisendres.com).

- *Measures*, that are usually numeric attributes used to process aggregates accordingly the dimensions' hierarchies. In our case we considered only two measures, namely: 1) *Diagnosis Time*, this additive measure represents the time spent by doctors to reach a final diagnosis; and 2) *Diagnosis Cost*, which receives the cost of the entire diagnosis process.

All the referred components—dimensions and measures—could be arranged in a single star-schema (Figure 1), a multi-dimensional structure where all the dimensions tables surround a single fact-table. This star-schema structure is recognized as one of the best database structures that provides the right conditions to combine easily facts with any of the dimensions that integrates the star-schema. The selected star-schema it's not complete. We don't have the possibility here to describe in a more detailed way all the possible attributes that we could define and integrate in the corresponding dimensions tables. Figure 1 only shows a scratch schema. However it was enough to support the main ideas presented in this paper. Due to the very simple organization of the star-schema, as you can notice, any ad hoc query could be easily satisfied through direct joins among dimensions tables and the fact table, which means that we can ask the star about any one of the elements of the diagnosis (calendar, doctors, signs, symptoms, etc.) and cross such information with other of the available dimensions, like we were positioned in a multidimensional space. For instance, a SQL query like the following:

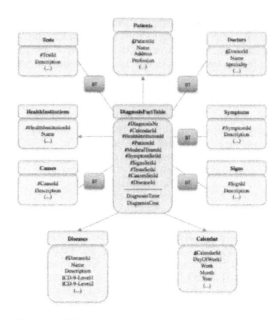

Figure 1.   The star-schema for medical diagnosis support.

```
SELECT DH.Name, COUNT(*)
    FROM DiagnosisFactTable AS FT
        JOIN HealthInstitutions AS DH
            ON DH.#HealthInstitutionId=FT.
            #HealthInstitutionId
        JOIN Calendar AS DC
            ON DC.#CalendarId=FT.
        #CalendarID
        JOIN Diseases AS DD
            ON DD.#DiseaseId=FT.
        #DiseaseID
    WHERE DC.Year=2009 AND
    DC.Month='December'
        AND DD.[ICD-9-Level1]=
        'Appendicitis'
    GROUP BY DH.Name;
```

provides us the number of diagnoses of 'Appendicitis' (ICD-9 classification, level2), a very well known disease of the Digestive System that occurred during 'December' of '2009' for each health institution categorized in the system. In this query we combine data from one fact table (where factual data is located) and three dimensions (Calendar, Diseases, and Health Institutions). As well we launched this query, we could require the execution of a lot more of queries approaching different dimensions and facts combination. To do that, we only need to know the organization of the data (the multidimensional schema), their characteristics and how to combine them. Today, we don't need to know a database language like SQL to post queries to a database, because the market of decision support systems an business intelligence supplies us with a large and diverse package of tools that establish a middle layer between the data warehouses and their users, which dispose high level interfaces to explore effectively and quite fast the information stored in any multidimensional schema. For now, it's important to say that this kind of queries support frequently reporting services, generating periodically pre defined reports, which are used in regular management tasks and daily decision making.

In spite of the recognised simplicity of star-schemas, sometimes we deal with some special cases that emerge from the own nature of the diagnosis process. In our case, we have a star-schema with five bridging situations among dimension tables and the fact table, basically due to the many-to-many relationships that exist among them and that cannot be represented in conventional relational databases. They need to be transformed in one-to-many relationships. Usually, in regular cases relationships represented in multidimensional schemas are one-to-many, which indicates that a single instance of a dimension could have zero or more corresponding instances in the fact table. For example, in a single day, which involves the dimension table 'Calendar', we could have recorded several diagnosis processes in the 'Diagnosis-FactTable' database object. But, when a bridging case appears relationships are, as we said, many-to-many, which imposes the creation of bridge tables (designated in the schema as BT), allowing us to transform them in one-to-many relationships. Lets then give an example of such kind of transformation. Considering the many-to-many relationship between 'Doctors' and 'DiagnosisFactTable'—one or more doctors could have participated in one or more diagnosis process –, to be possible to implemented it in relational databases we need to insert a new table in the schema that will act as a bridge between the referred objects and making possible to implement the relationship (Figure 2). The introduction of bridge tables affects querying performance once it makes join operations a little bit more complicated and demanding. However, it is one of the most ordinary ways to solve problems generated by the occurrence of many-to-many relationships. There are a few techniques to avoid bridges tables and the additional workload that they cause. Here, we decided to maintain a more conventional approach.

Taking into consideration the star-schema designed for medical diagnosis support (Figure 1), we believe that any user, and in particular doctors, easily understand the principles and the reasons to design and implemented multidimensional databases, as well understand the extreme advantages of cross-joins over a multidimensional space and, consequently, the results provided. If inside a medical institution we are able to develop the means and the facilities necessary to ensure that the data coming from diagnosis processes will be filtered and conciliated into a data warehouse accordingly the requisites of doctors and their quality requirements, we have the sufficient conditions to guarantee that such data warehouse will be a very useful instrument in the improvement and in the effectiveness of future diagnosis processes. To reinforce this, lets see another querying example. Suppose that a doctor wants to reduce its space of decision after recording the symptoms revealed by a patient. To help him, we can develop a query that provides all the diseases that were diagnosed in the past that had such list of symptoms. The query could be something like this:

```
SELECT DD.Name, DS.Description
    FROM DiagnosisFactTable AS FT
        JOIN Diseases AS DD
            ON DD.#DiseaseId=FT.
            #DiseaseId
        JOIN BridgeSDFTS AS BR
            ON BR.#SymptomSetId=FT.
            #SymptomSetID
        JOIN Simptoms AS DS ON
            DS.#SymptomId=BR.#SymptomID
    WHERE DS.Description IN
    ('Nauseas','Abdominal pain','Fever',
     'Loss of Appetite','Vomiting')
    ORDER BY DD.Name;
```

4 MULTIDIMENSIONAL ANALYSIS

At this point, it's time to see how we can make a better exploitation of the data stored inside the data warehouse in a multidimensional point of view. In a dimensional approach all the structures of a data warehouse were designed to provide fast answers to high demanding queries. The star-schema model organization reflects clearly such goals. However, in a conventional data warehouse we cannot find materialized all the possible aggregates that we

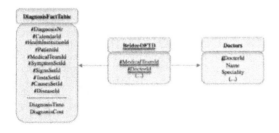

Figure 2. A bridge table ensuring the 'many-to-many' relationship between 'Doctors' and 'DiagnosisFactTable'.

are able to calculate based on the dimensions and measures that are present in a particular schema. There are a lot of reasons that justify such inexistence of aggregate values, ranging from high demanding processing and storage resources to the fact that most of times the aggregates are not used. Thus, to maintain in the data warehouse only the records that correspond to the grain it a good strategy. This saves a lot of data storage and simplifies the ETL processes. However, the time to satisfy a query involving aggregates calculations grow significantly when compared to the time of an answer based on pre materialized aggregates, obviously. A lot of research works have been done to deal with such problem. From the works of Codd et al. (1993) and Gray et al. (1997) to Morfonios et al. (2007) or Karayannidis & Sellis (2008) in recent days, many analytical processing techniques and systems were proposed and developed. All of them deal with one of the most sophisticated data structures: the hypercube, which is an ideal structure to support analytical processing and multidimensional data exploitation.

Currently, OLAP platforms are a natural evolution of a DWS. They bring to us a very diversified package of solutions to support multidimensional data exploitation. The data structures and data operators that they dispose, allow us to materialize almost everything. They have sophisticated processes to compute and materialize "all" the possible aggregates that a star-schema could provide, following its dimensions' hierarchies and calculating the aggregate values accordingly the measures defined in the fact-table. So, it's not very difficult to imagine how simple is to answer a query that have already an answer materialized. It's only a question of a click: we select the analysis axle we want (the dimensions), define filters we want apply, and the OLAP system shows us a cube view with the values that are the result of the query. To make this possible in the medical diagnosis area, we need to build a cube with a structure like the one presented before (Figure 1) and process it in a OLAP platform.

To get a more clear view of a cube application (and its exploitation) we can access to the site of the Australian Institute of Health and Welfare (http://www.aihw.gov.au/hospitals/datacubes/datacube_ pdx.cfm) and select one of the interactive cubes available there, about the diagnosis of patients in Australian hospitals. After selecting a data cube we can make a large variety of multidimensional queries just clicking on an attribute cell, filtering results by disease, year, age group, and many more properties used in the diagnosis processes, or changing the current data view selecting another dimension as a primary analysis axle. A few minutes are enough to see the potentialities of a cube in practical medical diagnosis decision-making.

5 CONCLUSIONS

In this paper it was discussed the use of data warehouses to support the process of medical diagnosis, presenting all the key factors and processes involve with, and referring the measures and cares in the implementation and exploitation of this kind of systems. The main goal was to show to medical staff the importance that a DWS could assume in medical institutions, and the kind of services that it provides in day-by-day activities. Moreover, we assume that a more effective explanation about the adoption and implementation of a DWS was necessary in order to give a more clear view about how things could be improved in clinical processes with the use of good planned and implemented decision support structures and processes. We believe that a well designed and planned DWS helps effectively the quality of service of any medical professional that use it to support its decision activities or any of the regular analysis or reporting task that he need to do. A significant part of this work was about the proposal of a dimensional model—a star-schema—especially oriented to support doctors in diagnosis activities. The schema was designed based on a set of the most important pieces of information that doctors use. It was also presented how to explore such dimensional structures retrieving useful information about past diagnosis processes that could reduce significantly the time of the diagnosis and improve its quality and effectiveness. Finally, we discuss the impact of OLAP tools as complementary exploitation means for conventional data warehouses, presenting some of the most relevant characteristics and data browsing mechanisms.

REFERENCES

Baralis, E., Paraboschi, S. and Teniente, E. 1997. Materialized Views Selection in a Multidimensional Database. In Proceedings of the 23rd international Conference on Very Large Data Bases (August 25–29, 1997). M. Jarke, M.J. Carey, K.R. Dittrich, F.H. Lochovsky, P. Loucopoulos and M.A. Jeusfeld, Eds. Very Large Data Bases. Morgan Kaufmann Publishers, San Francisco, CA, 156–165.

Berndt, D.J, Hevner, A.R. and Studnicki, J. The Catch Data Warehouse: Support for Community Health Care Decision-Making. Decision Support Systems. 2003; 35(3): 36784.

Codd, E.F., Codd, S.B. and Salley, C.T. "Providing OLAP (On-line Analytical Processing) to User-Analysts: An IT Mandate". Codd & Date, Inc 1993.

Einbinder, J., Scully, K., Pates, R., Schubart, J. and Reynolds, R. Case Study: A Data Warehouse for an Academic Medical Center, Journal of Healthcare Information Management, Vol. 15, no. 2, Summer, John Wiley & Sons, Inc., 2001.

Fayyad, U., Piatetsky-Shapiro, G. and Smyth, P. From Data Mining to Knowledge Discovery in Databases, AI Magazine, vol. 13, pp. 37–54, 1996.

Gray, J., Chaudhuri, S., Bosworth, A., Layman, A., Reichart, D., Venkatrao, M. Pellow, F. and Pirahesh, H., Data Cube: A Relational Aggregation Operator Generalizing Group-by, Cross-Tab, and Sub Totals, Data Mining and Knowledge Discovery 1(1), 1997, 29–53.

Inmon, W., Building the Data Warehouse, 2nd Edition, J. Wiley & Sons, New York, 1996.

Karayannidis, N. and Sellis, T. Hierarchical clustering for OLAP: the CUBE File approach. The VLDB Journal, Volume 17, Number 1, January 2008, 621–655.

Kimball, R. and Ross, M. The Data Warehouse Toolkit: The Complete Guide to Dimensional Modeling (Second Edition), Wiley, 2002.

Kimball, R., Ross, M., Thornthwaite, W., Mundy, J. and Becker, B. The Data Warehouse Lifecycle Toolkit, Wiley, 2nd ed. January, 2008.

Lin, S., Lee, Y. and Hsu, C. Data Warehouse Approach to Build a Decision-Support Platform for Orthopedics Based on Clinical and Academic Requirements, International Journal of Bio-Science and Bio-Technology, Vol. 2, No. 1, March, 2010.

Lin, C., Lin, C.M., Lin, B. and Yang, M. 2009. A decision support system for improving doctors' prescribing behavior. Expert Syst. Appl. 36, 4 (May. 2009), 7975–7984.

Morfonios, K., Konakas, S., Ioannidis, Y. and Kotsis, N. ROLAP Implementations of the Data Cube. ACM Computing Surveys 39:4 (2007): pp. 12:1–12:53.

Pedersen, T.B. and Jensen, C.S. 1998. Research Issues in Clinical Data Warehousing. In Proceedings of the 10th international Conference on Scientific and Statistical Database Management (July 01–03, 1998). Rafanelli M. and Jarke, M. Eds. SSDBM. IEEE Computer Society, Washington, DC, USA.

Podgorelec, V. and Kokol, P. Towards more optimal medical diagnosing with evolutionary algorithms, Journal of Medical Systems 25:3 (2001): 195–219.

Scotch, M., Parmanto, B. and Monaco, V. Evaluation of SOVAT: An OLAP-GIS decision support system for community health assessment data analysis, BMC Medical Informatics and Decision Making 2008, 8: 22.

Shams, K. and Farishta, M. Data Warehousing: Toward Knowledge Management, Topics in Health Information Management 21:3 (2001): 24–32.

Solomon, M. Ensuring a Successful Data Warehouse Initiative, Information Systems Management, 2005, Vol. 22 Iss. 1, 26–36.

Stolba, N. and Tjoa, A. The Relevance of Data Warehousing and Data Mining in the Field of Evidence-Based Medicine to Support Healthcare Decision Making, International Conference on Computer Science (ICCS 2006), Prague, Czech Republic, Enformatika: Volume 11, February 2006.

Technology and Medical Sciences – Natal Jorge et al. (eds)
© 2011 Taylor & Francis Group, London, ISBN 978-0-415-66822-4

In vivo measurement of skeletal muscle impedance from rest to fatigue

O.L. Silva, I.O. Hoffmann, J.C. Aya, S. Rodriguez, E.D.L.B. Camargo,
F.S. Moura, T.H.S. Sousa & R.G. Lima
*Departamento de Engenharia Mecânica, Escola Politécnica,
Universidade de São Paulo, São Paulo, Brasil*

A.R.C. Martins & D.T. Fantoni
*Departamento de Cirurgia, Faculdade de Medicina Veterinária e Zootecnia,
Universidade de São Paulo, São Paulo, Brasil*

ABSTRACT: Electrical Impedance Tomography (EIT) is a non-invasive method employed to estimate electrical impeditivity distribution maps of internal structures and tissues *in vivo*. Electrical impeditivity in living tissues is a function, among other factors, of the number of available charge carriers (ions). It is well known that muscle in the anaerobic regime produces an excess of lactic acid, a condition known as muscle fatigue, which is removed by blood flow once the exercise stops. This lactic acid dissociates into H^+ and lactate, and we hypothesize that this increased concentration of H^+ ions could be responsible for a decrease in impedance within the muscle. The aim of this study is to verify qualitatively and quantitatively how muscle impedance is affected by fatigue. For that an experiment was designed in which the musculo-cutaneous nerve of a swine was electrically stimulated in order to produce intense repeated contractions for 60 seconds. Electrical impedance was continuously measured with a probe directly inserted into biceps brachii muscle, parallel to its fibers, from 15 seconds before until 25 seconds after nerve stimulation. The experiment is repeated in the transverse direction and with direct muscle stimulation. Plots of impedance versus time are presented, and results are discussed from a physiological perspective and its implications for the design of an EIT device that images muscle contraction.

1 INTRODUCTION

Electrical Impedance Tomography (EIT) is a non-invasive technique used to estimate electrical impeditivity distribution maps within a subject or object. It can be used both in medical (Victorino, Borges, Okamoto, Matos, Tucci, Caramez, Tanaka, Sipmann, Santos, Barbas, Carvalho, C.R.R. & Amato 2004) and industrial applications (Heikkinen, Kourunen, Savolainen, Vauhkonen, Kaipio & M.Vauhkonen 2006). In the former case, an array of electrodes is attached to the skin, around the region to be imaged, which are used to inject current and to measure electrical potentials. Thus, it is possible to solve a non linear ill-posed inverse problem that estimates electrical impeditivity distribution inside a domain that best "explains" boundary measured potentials.

Monitoring lung function in Intensive Care Units (ICU) is one of the most successful medical applications of EIT. It is well known that lung,

muscle, fat, bone, blood and other biological tissues have different impeditivity properties. As long as air goes into the lungs it locally changes its electrical impeditivity because air impeditivity is several orders of magnitude greater than surrounding tissues. As a result, EIT image can unveil both ventilation and blood perfusion phenomena. Designing an EIT device tuned to produce muscle images in activity posses a big challenge because little is known about its impeditivity behavior during contraction (moderate or intense) and recovery. Some authors (Gielen, de Jorge & Boon 1984) and (Aaron, Huang & Shiffman 1997) have made *in vivo* conductivity measurements of the muscle at rest; however, we believe that a continuous impedance[1] measurement of a skeletal muscle from rest to fatigue performing repetitive contractions has not been made yet.

---

[1] While impeditivity is a property of material only, impedance also depends on geometry.

To consistently develop an EIT device focused on producing skeletal muscle images, several questions should be answered:

1. How much is the muscle impedance at rest?
2. Does muscle impedance changes when in activity?
3. If so, what are maximum and minimum expected values? In which conditions do they occur?
4. Does this change is related to some easily observable phenomena, for instance, contraction rate, heart beat or muscle fatigue?

Although the first question have already been addressed by several authors, for a review see (Gabriel, Gabriel & Corthout 1996), the others remain unanswered. However, there are several physiological evidences that muscle impeditivity property could change when performing contractions. For instance: (i) muscle is more irrigated by blood when in activity than at rest; (ii) there are many ions such as phosphate and calcium that play an important role in actin/myosin mechanism (Guyton & Hall 1992); (iii) there is a net accumulation of H^+ inside the muscle in intense excercise resulting a decrease in cellular pH related to lactic acid production (Robergs, Ghiasvand & Parker 2004). These are enough to believe that muscle activity and impeditivity are intimately related as long as electrical impeditivity in electrolytes is determined by concentration, valence number and mobility of dissolved ion, and well as temperature.

Thus, an experiment was designed in which a swine biceps brachii muscle was made to contract several times for 60 seconds through both direct and nerve stimulation and impedance was measured with a probe directly inserted into the muscle, parallel to its fibers, from 15 seconds before until 25 seconds after nerve stimulation. The experiment was repeated measuring impedance in the transverse direction relative to muscle fibers. The plots presented in this work are the results of a pilot study we believe can shed some light to questions 2 to 4.

2 METHODOLOGY

2.1 Data acquisition system

Our impedance measurement device is in fact a system composed by a probe, a sine wave generator, a voltage to current converter and an acquisition board connected to a computer. The probe has four needles in line, spaced 2.0 mm apart, 12.2 mm length and 0.7 mm in diameter. The current source is designed to produce a sine wave of 1.4 mA at 125 kHz. Each acquisition board channel measures the potential difference between the respective needle and the ground. There is a sensing resistor

R between needle 4 and the ground, needed to capture the current signal.

2.2 Data processing

Each impedance measurement is calculated from Eq. 1, where V_1 and V_4 are phasors (complex variables) representing the sinusoidal signal measured by needles 1 and 4, respectively and $R = 198.3\ \Omega$. Phasors are computed from a vector of 36864 voltage measurements sampled at 10 Mhz by a demodulation procedure.

$$Z = \frac{V_1 - V_4}{V_4/R} \tag{1}$$

2.3 Experimental protocol

A 6–month old domestic swine was adequately sedated according to the protocol approved by Comissão de Bioética da Faculdade de Medicina Veterinária e Zootecnia da Universidade de São Paulo. An incision was made to expose right biceps brachii muscle and musculo-cutaneous nerve. The probe was inserted transversely to muscle fibers direction for impedance measurement. Then two stimulation needle-electrodes connected to a neuromuscular electrotherapy device (model FES VIF 995, QUARK, Piracicaba, Brasil) were inserted into proximal and distal sites of the same muscle. The equipment was set in "burst" mode where trains of pulses were delivered at a frequency of 2 Hz, each pulse with a period of 100 µs with a frequency of 100 Hz inside each train. Current intensity was adjusted to produce visually observable muscle fatigue. Data collection was triggered with muscle initially at rest; after 15 seconds, the electrotherapy device was turned on. Stimulation was kept for 60 seconds and data collection was maintained for additional 25 seconds. The experiment was repeated varying the direction of the probe and the site of stimulation, according to Table 1. For musculo-cutaneous nerve stimulation we used tweezers electrodes instead of needles. A period of 5 minutes elapsed between each measurement to allow muscle recovery from fatigue.

3 RESULTS

Figure 1 shows the absolute value of muscle impedance, computed through Eq. 1, for all measurements that the muscle was directly stimulated. On the other hand, Figure 2 exhibits the absolute value of the impedance, computed in the same way, for the measurements that the nerve was stimulated. Figure 3 is a plot of the curves shown at Figures 1

Table 1. Experiments description.

#	Name	Meas. direction	Stim. site	Stim. intensity (mA)	Max. imped. variation (Ω)	Imped. percent variation	Moment when contraction stops (s)
1	BT1	Trans	None	0	4.7	–	–
2	MT1	Trans	muscle	22	21.3	7.8%	42
3	MT2	Trans	muscle	22	16.7	7.0%	35
4	MT3	Trans	muscle	50	18.5	8.9%	38
5	ML1	Long	muscle	50	5.1	4.4%	29
6	ML2	Long	muscle	50	9.4	6.6%	27
7	NL1	Long	nerve	20 to 38	5.8	3.8%	75
8	NL2	Long	nerve	46	7.0	12.6%	75
9	NL3	Long	nerve	46	13.6	10.2%	56
10	NT1	Trans	nerve	56	17.6	4.4%	75
11	NT2	Trans	nerve	56	13.3	7.8%	51

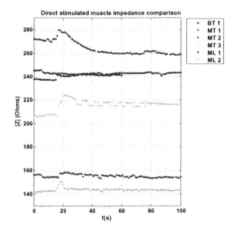

Figure 1. Absolute value of muscle complex impedance with direct muscle stimulation.

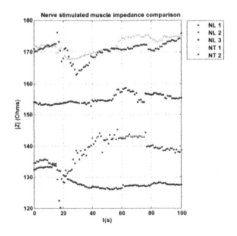

Figure 2. Absolute value of muscle complex impedance with nerve stimulation.

and 2 displayed in a chronological way for the ease of comparison and to reveal how muscle impedance behaved along the hole experiment.

Maximum impedance variation of each curve displayed at Figures 1 and 2 are shown in Table 1. It is also shown a percent impedance variation with respect to the mean impedance of the first 15 seconds of each trial, period the muscle had no stimulation. Evaluating the experiment video recordings it was possible to indentify the moment when muscle contraction no longer was observed (Table 1, last column) indicating that the muscle was in complete fatigue.

4 DISCUSSION

In all experiments with direct muscle stimulation a sudden rise in impedance was observed as soon as stimulation started, as shown in Figure 1. Conversely, impedance seems to drop when nerve stimulation starts and then begins a slow rise. The difference suggest that there are different biochemical or vascular behaviors depending on direct or nerve stimulation.

In all measurements the impedance remained almost constant after second 75, when stimulation was removed. In some cases, namely NT 1 and NL 2, the impedance reached, by the end of the measurement, a level higher than in the first 15 seconds. Curiously, in these two situations muscle movement did not ceased at all, except when stimulator was turned off. Although the same behavior is present in case NL 1, it can not be used because the initial stimulation current was insufficient to produce an observable contraction and thus the current was increased during data collection.

There was a noticeable decrease in impedance during the first four experiments as shown in Figure 3.

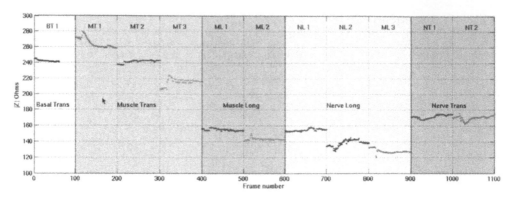

Figure 3. Overview of all measurements presented in chronological order. The figure is plotted against number of frames. There is an interval of 1 s between each frame except between frames 100 and 101, 200 and 201, etc., when an interval of 5 min. has elapsed.

Notice also that impedances of experiments 1 to 4 are above 200 Ω and from experiments 5 to 11 are below 180 Ω. It suggests that there is slow decrease of impedence with muscular activity.

5   FINAL COMMENTS

Although this was a pilot study and data was collected from a single animal, these results suggest that muscle impedance does change with contractions, which can be a preliminary answer to question number 2, Section 1. The percentages shown in Table 1 state that this change is about 8% of resting impedance. Variations of impedance of 8% are likely to be detected by Electrical Impedance Tomography. Therefore, it may be possible to distinguish muscles that suffered a sequence of contractions from muscles that did not contracted using Electrical Impedance Tomography.

No light was brought to questions 3 and 4, as well as about the underling biochemical mechanism that govern muscle impedance during a sequence of contractions. The methodology of the present work does not allow further analysis concerning questions 3 and 4 as well as to explain the observed impedance changes.

ACKNOWLEDGMENTS

The authors would like to thank CNPq, and FAPESP for financial support and express their gratitude to Caio Biasi (FMVZ-USP), Denise Aya Otsuki (LIM/08-FMUSP), Denise Vaz de Macedo (IB-UNICAMP), Gilberto (LIM/08-FMUSP), Jessica Noel-Morgan (LIM/08-FMUSP), Francisco Javier Hernandez Blazquez (FMVZ-USP), Marcos Duarte (EEFE-USP), Natasha Garofalo (FMVZ-USP), and Rudolf de Almeida Prado Hellmuth (Poli-USP), for their help in planning, preparing and executing this work.

REFERENCES

Aaron, R., Huang, M. & Shiffman, C. (1997). Anisotropy of human muscle via non-invasive impedance measurements. *Physics in Medicine and Biology* 42.

Gabriel, C., Gabriel, S. & Corthout, E. (1996). The dielectric properties of biological tissues: I. literature survey. *Physics in Medicine and Biology* 41.

Gielen, F., de Jorge, W.W. & Boon, K. (1984). Electrical conductivity of skeletal muscle tissue: experimental results from different muscles in vivo. *Medical and Biological Engineering and Computing* 22.

Guyton, A. & Hall, J. (1992). *Textbook of Medical Phisiology*. Elsevier Saunders.

Heikkinen, L., Kourunen, J., Savolainen, T., Vauhkonen, P. Kaipio, J. & Vauhkonen, M. (2006). Real time three-dimensional electrical impedance tomography applied in multiphase flow imaging. *Meas. Sci. Technol.* 17, 2083–2087.

Robergs, R., Ghiasvand, F. & Parker, D. (2004). Biochemistry of exercise-induced metabolic acidosis. *Am J Physiol Regulatory Integrative Comp Physiol* 287.

Victorino, J., Borges, J., Okamoto, V., Matos, G., Tucci, M., Caramez, M., Tanaka, H., Sipmann, F.S., Santos, D., Barbas, C., Carvalho, C.R.R. & Amato, M. (2004). Imbalances in regional lung ventilation, a validation study on electrical impedance tomography. *Am. J. Crit. Care. Med.* 169, 791–800.

Technology and Medical Sciences – Natal Jorge et al. (eds)
© 2011 Taylor & Francis Group, London, ISBN 978-0-415-66822-4

Influence on the mandible and on a condyle implant of the distribution of the fixation surgical screws

A. Ramos
Department of Mechanical Engineering, University of Aveiro, Aveiro, Portugal

M. Mesnard
Laboratoire de Mécanique Physique, CNRS UMR 5469, Université de Bordeaux, Bordeaux, France

C. Relvas, A. Completo & J.A. Simões
Department of Mechanical Engineering, University of Aveiro, Aveiro, Portugal

ABSTRACT: Temporomandibular Joint (TMJ) reconstruction was developed to improve mandibular function and to reduce disability. Replacement of the mandible condyle involves the local resection of the bone and the fixation of an artificial condyle. Most of the condyle implants are rigid plates fixed using surgical screws. This study aims to describe the influence of the distribution of the screwson the strain pattern in the mandible and particularly near these screws.

3D Finite Element Models (FEM) of an intact and of an implanted mandible were analyzed. The mandible geometry was obtained using a laser scan process. The FEM and the implant were positioned in a CAD model. The loads were applied including the five more important muscular loads.

Numerical results were successfully obtained for different screw positions. If materials and geometry play an important key role in enhancing the long-term life of the implant, it was observed that the last screw positions influence mainly the success of thecondyle implant.

1 INTRODUCTION

1.1 *Context*

Several diseases can affect the human TMJ among which we highlight cancer, trauma or fracture, congenital malformation and osteochondritis [1]. In the USA TMJ diseases may affect 30 million people; a large majority of these patients can be treated without surgery but a small group requires surgery [2]. Pain relief and partial functional recovery of the joint are the more frequent objectives of a TMJ arthroplasty [3].

TMJ reconstruction was developed to improve mandibular function and to reduce disability [4]. Although implants have records of short-term successes widely documented, the recent arrival of failures and complications related to placement of such implants again feed the discussions [2,5]. In the UK three current available systems are implanted in 60 to 65 patients annually [6]. Total replacement of the TMJ involves the removal of the non functional joint and placing an artificial one [7]. Most of the used TMJ implants are plates that are flat and rigid; surgeons must bend the plates and spend a too long time to fit it to the contours of patient bones [6].

1.2 *Prosthesis design*

The design of TMJ prostheses presupposes the use of numerical tools like finite element analysis [8,9]. The application of these must be carefully made and it is prudent that they are calibrated by some experimental model [10].

The mandible bone presents a complex geometry and boundary conditions need to be correctly specified, otherwise these conditions can undermine the reality of results. For this reason, the numerical models have to be tested and validated experimentally [11,12].

Finite element and experimental models have been used to determine stresses and strains on the surface of bone structures [13,14,15]. These models can be used for different biomechanical analyses and to predict the performance of implants.

TMJ reconstruction with metallic materials modifies the physiological behavior of the mandible (stress and strain patterns, condyle displacements). The changing of the bone strains imposes an adaptation of the TMJ and of the articular contacts.

Some problems related to TMJ implants concern the mandible implant fracture or the initial fixation and the stability of the implant [4]. Some solutions exist to improve the TMJ survival rate; the most frequently used consist in an initial fixation of the plate using surgical screws [4, 5, 16].

1.3 Objective

The objective of this study was to assess the biomechanical performance of a condyle implant using finite element models experimentally validated. To determine the strain patterns around the surgical screws, finite element models of a left condyle were built. For the purpose of the study finite element models of a fractured left condyle were developed.

2 MATERIALS AND METHOD

2.1 Geometry of the Finit Element Models (FEM)

The model of the mandible was based on a polymeric replica of a human mandible from Sawbones* (model 1337). This model has adequate geometric accuracy for the experiments and is similar to the one presented by other authors [10]. The geometry of the model was obtained using a 3D laser scanning device (Roland LPX 250 machine). The resolution of the scans was 0.2×0.2 mm and the final geometry is represented in Figure 1.

The final model of the mandible was obtained with dedicated CAD software (CATIA, Dassault Systems). A solid homogeneous polymeric model was considered. Ichim et al. [13] concluded that the thickness of the mandible cortical bone does not have any significant influence on the strain distribution. The CAD model of the implant was copied from a commercial implant represented in Figure 2. This implant has a straight geometry and seven holes aligned to receive the surgical screws.

2.2 Boundary conditions and loads

The boundary conditions have been chosen as follow: the incisive tooth was fixed in the three directions but it could rotate and the condyle could slide on the plane surface of the "support" as shown in Figure 3. The variations of parameters as the mandible size, the mandible shape, the bone properties, the bite forces could undetermined the quantitative stress and strain data in a real situation. One of the reasons to use a polymeric mandible as opposed to cadaveric ones is to minimize the impact of these variations.

There are reported failures of this implant. The load conditions, the fatigue situations, the geometry of the holes and the fact that the top hole is not always used have provoked some fractures. The implant material was a titanium alloy.

The loads are included in Table 1 for a mouth opening of 5 mm on the incisive tooth which is the condition that causes the most critical situation on the condyle [17]. The muscular actions applied

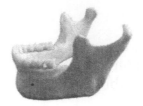

Figure 1.   Polymeric mandible model (Sawbones).

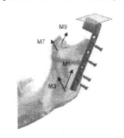

Figure 2.   Normal screw positions.

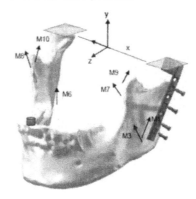

Figure 3.   Boundary conditions and loads.

were similar to the ones presented in Iwasaki et al. [18]. Five principal muscles were included in the loading configuration: deep and superficial masseter, medial pterygoid, anterior temporal and medial temporal. The insertions have been observed through MRI images by Mesnard et al. [17] and were defined on the FEM.

2.3 Convergence and validation

The FEM had been previously validated [17]. The FEM is composed of 71280 tetrahedral linear elements with 4 nodes and 51245 degrees of freedom DOF (Fig. 4). The teeth are considered to have marginal influence on the mandible biomechanics and, particularly, on the behavior of the condyles. Ta et al. [15] use the same hypothesis.

For the convergence tests, the maximal displacements and the maximal equivalent strains were assessed. The convergence rate for the displacements and the equivalent strains was reached for a

148

Table 1. Muscular forces

Muscles actions	Ref.	Load (N)		
		x	y	z
Deep masseter	M1, 2	7,776	127,23	22,68
Superficial masseter	M3, 4	12,873	183,5	12,11
Medial pterygoid	M5, 6	140,38	237,8	–77,3
Temporalis	M7, 8	0,064	0,37	–0,13
Medial temporal	M9, 10	0,97	5,68	–7,44

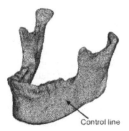

Figure 4. FEM and external control line.

mesh of more or less 40 000 DOF. Hart et al. [19] considered the convergence for 25000 DOF. The FEM was built with Hyperworks® 10RS1 and runs were performed with MSc MARC™ solver.

2.4 Simulations

The simulations took into account the mandible mechanical properties. The cortical bone was considered to have a Young modulus of 14700 MPa and a Poisson coefficient of 0.3.

The implant was fixed on the left side of the mandible with four screws as in a real clinical situation (Figures 2 & 3); the implant position with respect to the mandible was defined by the surgeon. Very often, due to the bone resection, there is no screw in the top hole. The Young modulus and the Poisson coefficient of the implant and of the screws were 110 GPa and 0.3 respectively as a Titanium material.

The goal was to analyze the behavior of the condyle. In these simulations, the screws were completely bounded to the cortical bone. A touching contact was considered for the screw-implant contact. A coefficient of friction (0.3) was introduced for the implant-bone contact. The stresses and the strains were analyzed on the external surface of the mandible as defined in Figure 4.

3 RESULTS AND DISCUSSION

3.1 Minimal principal strain on the bone

Figure 5 presents the minimal principal strain on the external surface of the mandible for the intact mandible and for the mandible equipped with the implant and four screws. One can observe that the mandible was manly submitted to compression and that the implant increased the strain level in the condyle area (33%). The minimum principal strain distribution increased also the strain level in the right condyle area (16%).

Previously in the area of the implant fixation a diminution of the strain level had been observed [20]. This was explained by the too high rigidity of the condyle implant.

3.2 Principal strains near the screws

Considering the same four screws, the distribution of the maximum principal strains near these screws is presented in Figure 6. The top screw was near the condyle centre. Results reveal two different remarks.

Analyzing the influence of the screws one can observe that the first and last screws present high solicitation; the values were over 4000 μ strain. This situation seems favorable to a hypotrophy, and in a short time these screws can be unable to ensure their function.

The last screw presents the most critical solicitation and this fact points out that it is important to ensure the contact between the implant and the bone. The second screw presents a lower strain level; then it can be pre-loaded to under load the first screw.

The distribution of the minimum principal strains near the four screws is presented in Figure 7. The results present a lower strain value near the two first screws.

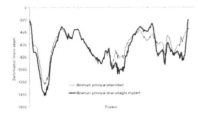

Figure 5. Distribution of the minimum principal strain.

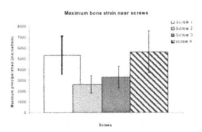

Figure 6. Maximum principal strains in the mandible near the four screws.

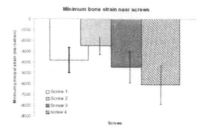

Figure 7. Minimum principal strains in the mandible near the four screws.

Considering the strain distribution for the bone growth as [21], a strain level over 4000 μ strain may generate a hypotrophy. This point underlines the necessity of putting more screws in the lowest part of the condyle implant. If the implant presents parallel holes in the fourth position the problem should be solved.

For the two first screws the deformation remains under 4000 μ strain; this situation is favorable to the bone adaptation and integration.

4 CONCLUSIONS

The implant affected the behavior of the mandible and of the two condyles. The mandible was mainly solicited by compression on the exterior lateral surface. The screws in the extreme positions ensure an important function on the implant fixation.

The results revealed that it will be important to reconsider the plate geometry to limit the strain near the extreme screws and to enhance bone integration.

ACKNOWLEDGEMENTS

To the Portuguese Science and Technology Foundation, funding project PTDC/EME-PME/65749/2006 and to the Ministère des Affaires Etrangères of France, project PESSOA 14630 YA.

REFERENCES

[1] Merrill, RG. (1986). Historical perspectives and comparisons of TMJ surgery for internal disk derangement and arthropathy, J Craniomandib Pract, 4, 74–83.

[2] Wolford, L.M, et al., (2003). TMJ Concepts/Techmedica custom-made TMJ total joint prosthesis: 5-year follow-up study, Int J Oral Maxillofac Surg, 32, 3, 268–74.

[3] Silver, CM. (1985). Long-term results of meniscectomy of the temporomandibular joint, J Craniomandibular Prac, 3, 47.

[4] Mercuri, L.G. (2009). Temporomandibular joint Reconstruction, Alpha Omegan, 102, 2, 51–54.

[5] Mercuri, L.G. et al., (2007). Fourteen-year follow-up of a patient-fitted total temporomandibular joint reconstruction system, JOM Surg, 65, 6, 1140–1148.

[6] Speculand, B., Hensher, R. & Powell, D. (2000). Total prosthetic replacement of the TMJ: experience with two systems 1988–1997, BrJO Max Surg., 38, 4, 360–369.

[7] Guarda-Nardini, L. et al., (2008). Temporomandibular joint total replacement prosthesis: current knowledge and considerations for the future, Int. J of Oral & M Surgery, 37, 2, 103–110.

[8] Tanne, K., et al., (1996). Stress distribution in the temporomandibular joint produced by orthopedic chincup forces applied in varying directions: a three-dimensional analytic approach with the finite element method, Am J Orthod Dent Orthop, 110, 502–7.

[9] Al-Sukhun, J. et al., (2007). Development of a three-dimensional finite element model of a human mandible containing endosseous dental implants I. Mathematical validation and experimental verification, J B. Mater Res A., 80, 1, 234–246.

[10] De Santis, R. et al., (2005). An experimental and theoretical composite model of the human mandible, J. of Mat Sc: Materials in Medicine, 16, 1191–1197.

[11] DeVocht, J.W. et al., (2001), Experimental Validation of a Finite Element Model of the Temporomandibular Joint, J Oral Max Surg, 59, 775–778.

[12] Maurer, P., Holweg, S. & Schubert, J. (1999). Finite-element-analysis of different screw-diameters in the sagittal split osteotomy of the mandible, Journal of Cranio-Max Surgery, 27, 365–372.

[13] Ichim, J.A., Kieser, M,V. and Swain, M, (2007). Functional significance of strain distribution in the human mandible under masticatory load: Numerical predictions, Arch of Oral Biology, 52, 5, 465–473.

[14] Field, C. et al., (2009). Mechanical response to orthodontic loading, A 3 dimensional finite element multi-tooth model, Am J of Orth and D Orhop 135, 2, 174–181.

[15] Korioth, T.W. et al., (1992). Three-dimensional finite element stress analysis of the dentate human mandible, Am J Phys Anthropol, 88, 69–96.

[16] Ta, E.L. et al., (2002). Clinical evaluation of Patients with temporomandibular joint implants, Journal of Oral Maxillofacial Surgery, 60, 1389–1399.

[17] Mesnard, M. et al., (2006). Numerical-experimental models to study the tem-poromandibular joint, 5th World Congress of Biomechanics & 15th Conference of the European Society of Biomechanics, Munich, De., J of Biomec, 39, 1, 458.

[18] Iwasaki, L.R. et al., (2003). Muscle and temporomandibular joint forces associated with chincup loading predicted by numerical modeling, American J of Orth and Dent Orthopedics, 124, 5, 530–540.

[19] Hart, T.R. et al., (1992). Modeling the biomechanics of the mandible: A three-dimensional finite element study, J of Biomec., 25, 3, 261–286.

[20] Mesnard, M. et al., Biomechanical analysis comparing natural and alloplastic TMJ replacement using a finite element model, Journal of Oral and Maxillofacial Surgery, in press.

[21] Roberts, W., Huja, S. & Roberts, J. (2004). Bone modeling: biomechanics, molecular mechanisms and clinical perspectives, Sem. Orthodontics, 10(2), 123–161.

Technology and Medical Sciences – Natal Jorge et al. (eds)
© *2011 Taylor & Francis Group, London, ISBN 978-0-415-66822-4*

Intensity inhomogeneity corrections in MRI simulated images for segmentation

R. Lavrador
Siemens S.A. Healthcare Sector, Matosinhos, Portugal
FCT University of Coimbra, Coimbra, Portugal

L. Caldeira
Siemens S.A. Healthcare Sector, Matosinhos, Portugal
Instituto de Biofísica e Engenharia Biomédica, Faculty of Sciences of University of Lisbon, Lisbon, Portugal

N.F. Lori
Faculty of Medicine of the University of Coimbra, Coimbra, Portugal
Brain Imaging Network, Portugal

F. Janela
Siemens S.A. Healthcare Sector, Matosinhos, Portugal

ABSTRACT: In this work four known algorithms were used to correct intensity inhomogeneities in order to find optimal method and parameters that improve automatic segmentation in T1-weighted MRI simulated images, generated with similar sequence parameters of real acquisitions. The resulting segmentation was measured by several features and the results are similar for both gray matter and white matter and for different applied bias fields. The intensity inhomogeneity correction algorithm that shows to be more stable was the one present in SPM8, but it was not found an algorithm that overcomes all the others in all aspects. With higher noise levels (9%) the correcting algorithms fail to improve segmentation. It was also found that the segmentation with a better relationship between sensitivity and specificity in the majority of the cases corresponds to a higher Dice coefficient.

1 INTRODUCTION

Magnetic Resonance Imaging (MRI) is a powerful non invasive technique that allows great contrast on soft tissues, high spatial resolution, and has both anatomical and functional information. The automatic extraction of clinical relevant information has become mandatory to efficiently deal with the large amount of data generated using this modality.

The vast amounts of image data presently used in many studies leads to an increased interest in computer-aided image analysis methods. The segmentation of clinical images helps physicians to differentiate between tissues, providing a unique insight into morphometric changes in the brain; they are particularly useful in monitoring neurodegenerative diseases such as Alzheimer's disease, or the effect of possible treatments (Boyes et al. 2008; de Boer et al. 2010). If these procedures were assisted by an automatic segmentation algorithm, it could simplify and reduce the cost of image analysis (Duncan & Ayache 2000; Kaus et al. 2001). However, several artifacts can degrade

the quality of acquired data, namely the Intensity Inhomogeneity (IIH) (Duncan & Ayache 2000, Hendee 2002, Vovk, Pernus & Likar 2007).

The IIH is mainly caused by unwanted local flip angle variations that happen due to inhomogeneous Radio-Frequency (RF) excitation, non-uniform reception sensitivity and electrodynamic interactions with the object often described as RF penetration, and standing wave effects. This results in a smooth undesirable variation of intensity levels of a tissue across the image. Thus the same tissue has different intensities according to its location. This distortion, in many cases, is hardly noticeable to a human observer but can influence many medical image analysis methods such as segmentation and registration (Zhang, Brady & Smith 2001; Vovk, Pernus & Likar 2007; Ashburner & Friston 2005).

In the literature the most common model assumes that the IIH is multiplicative, that means that the inhomogeneity field (b) is multiplied to the image (u). This model is frequently used due to its consistency with the inhomogeneous sensibility of the reception coil. In addition a high-frequency noise (*n*), typically with a Rician distribution, should be incorporated to the MR image formation model (*v*), Equation 1.

$$v = ub + n \qquad (1)$$

IIH correction is often a necessary preprocessing step to enable a better segmentation, yet it is unknown which are the IIH correction algorithms that improve segmentation and if it stands for several acquisition protocols, levels of noise and of IIH.

T1-weighted images are commonly used for segmentation, because they have good contrast between white matter and gray matter and high resolution in the usual neuroimaging protocols.

This work is intended to segment T1-weighted images that were corrected with four known IIH correction algorithms and find the IIH correction algorithm and parameters that improve segmentation of T1-weighted data the most. It is also important to observe if the results for the two sequence protocols are identical.

2 METHODS

2.1 *Images*

In order to have ground truth images, in this work we used MRI simulated images of the brain obtained using BrainWeb (Cocosco et al. 1997), with parameters, for FLASH (fl) and Inversion Recovery (IR) pulse sequences, identical to the parameters usually used to perform scans on patients (Table 1). The image size was maintained constant and equal to $217 \times 181 \times 60$. We used two levels of noise (no), 3% and 9%. For the 3% noise level we simulated an image with no inhomogeneities (control image) and images with 3 different bias fields, A, B and C, provided by the simulator. The 3 bias fields were applied with also 3 levels of inhomogeneities (rf), 20%, 40% and 100%, which means that, as an example for 20%, the multiplicative field has a range of values of 0.90 to 1.10 over the brain area.

For the 9% noise level it was simulated an image with no inhomogeneities and three more images, one for each inhomogeneity level of field A.

The images with no inhomogeneity applied and 3% noise are shown on Table 1.

2.2 *IIH correction algorithms*

The IIH in the simulated images was corrected by four well known algorithms: the N3 developed by Sled et al. (Sled, Zijdenbos & Evans 2002) with minor changes (http://hdl.handle.net/10380/3053) and the parametric bias field correction (PABIC)

Table 1. Simulated images, 3% noise and no bias field applied.

Custom designation	Sequence parameters	Simulated images
T1_fl_no3_rf0	FLASH TR: 250 ms TE: 2,46 ms Flip angle: 70°	
T1_IR_no3_rf0	INVERSION RECOVERY TR: 2300 ms TE: 2.28 ms Flip angle: 90° IR: 900ms	

developed by Styner et al. (Styner et al. 2000), both algorithms are implemented on Insight Segmentation and Registration Toolkit (ITK) (Ibanez et al. 2003); the algorithm developed by Guillemaud and Brady (Guillemaud & Brady 1997) that is integrated on a segmentation framework developed by Zhang et al. (Zhang, Brady & Smith 2001) and implemented on FMRIB Software Library (FSL) software; and the last algorithm was developed by Ashburner and Friston (Ashburner & Friston 2005) and implemented on Statistical Parametric Mapping (SPM8).

N3 is described as a non-uniform intensity normalization method that finds the smooth, slowly varying, multiplicative field that maximizes the frequency content of the intensity distribution of the uncorrected image. The N3 proceeds by estimating a Gaussian distribution of an ideal uncorrupted image by deconvolution, and then uses this distribution and the distribution of the original corrupted image to estimate the non-uniform field. This field is smoothed by a B-spline curve. The resulting bias field is then removed from the original image and this process iterates until reaching a convergence threshold (Sled, Zijdenbos & Evans 2002).

The second algorithm is called PABIC. It assumes that each pixel of the image is associated to a small number of categories with *a priori* known statistics and that the bias field can be modeled by smooth functions, which in this case are Legendre polynomials. The estimation of the bias is formulated as a nonlinear energy minimization problem using an evolution strategy (Styner, Brechbuhler, Szckely & Gerig 2000). The starting mean values for each class were obtained with k-means classifier using MATLAB.

The algorithm proposed by Guillemaud & Brady (1997) is a modification of Wells et al. algorithm for IIH correction (Wells et al. 1996), introducing a new class "others" with a non-Gaussian probability distribution. On the FSL software the method is integrated in a hidden Markov random field model that uses an estimation-maximization algorithm

(HMRF-EM), so as to use the information about spatial connectedness of neighboring pixels of the same class (Zhang, Brady & Smith 2001).

In the algorithm proposed in SPM8 it is used an iterative framework that interleaves segmentation, registration and IIH correction. The model is based in a finite Gaussians mixture and is extended to incorporate a smooth intensity variation and nonlinear registration with tissue probability maps. For optimization of the objective function it is used an iterated conditional modes approach, using the EM to find the mixture-classification parameters and Levenberg-Marquardt optimization for inhomogeneity field and registration step.

The algorithms were used as automatically as possible and for each algorithm several parameters were chosen, considering those with greater potential impact on the algorithm performance.

In N3 we chose to vary the Full Width at Half Maximum (FWHM), the shrink factor, and the number of fitting levels. For the FSL algorithm it was changed the number of classes and the FWHM. The FWHM was the only parameter changed on the IIH correction algorithm present in SPM8. In PABIC it was changed the number of classes.

2.3 *Segmentation*

After correcting the images for inhomogeneities, the segmentation was performed using the segmentation framework developed by Zhang et al. (Zhang, Brady & Smith 2001) and implemented on FSL software, using 3 classes, the default parameters and with no additional IIH correction.

As said before the segmentation algorithm implemented on FSL incorporates a hidden Markov random field and in this method the segmentation is treated as a statistical model-based problem with 3 steps: model selection, model fitting and classification. The HMRF-EM enables an adaptive and reliable automatic segmentation (Zhang, Brady & Smith 2001).

2.4 *Evaluation parameters*

The effects in the performance of the segmentation were quantitatively evaluated calculating the dice coefficient, the specificity and sensitivity of each segmented image.

Dice coefficient, Equation 2, is used to compare the similarity between sample sets, in this case, between the obtained segmentation and the gold standard segmentation. In this work it has been used a discrete anatomical model, available on BrainWeb as gold standard segmentation.

$$Dice(S_1, S_2) = \frac{2|S_1 \cap S_2|}{|S_1| + |S_2|} \quad (2)$$

where the S_1 and S_2 sets are, respectively, the obtained and the gold standard segmentations.

Sensitivity, Equation 3, is intended to evaluate the ability of the segmentation to correctly classify the tissues, and it gives the probability of deciding if a tissue was well classified, when it belongs to that class.

$$sensitivity = \frac{TP}{TP + FN} \quad (3)$$

where TP is true positives and FN is false negatives.

The sensitivity, by itself, does not give us if the other tissues were well classified, for that it is necessary to calculate the specificity. The specificity, Equation 4, intends to evaluate the ability of the segmentation to correctly exclude the tissues that do not belong to a given class. So it gives the probability of deciding if the tissue in question was excluded of a class, when it actually does not belong to it.

$$specificity = \frac{TN}{TN + FP} \quad (4)$$

where TN is true negatives and FN is false negatives.

After obtaining the specificity and the sensitivity, a Receiver Operator Characteristic (ROC) space was built for each image with the four correcting algorithms. All evaluation parameters were calculated for Grey Matter (GM) and White Matter (WM).

In order to evaluate the significance of changes in the Dice coefficients in relation to the IIH correction method an ANOVA of repeated measures was performed. The multiple comparisons were made using contrasts and having the uncorrected image as reference. All analysis was performed on SPSS software.

3 RESULTS

The Dice coefficient for each image, with different bias field and noise was obtained. The values of the Dice coefficient, for GM and WM, could be considered similar for all bias fields and noise levels, except in few situations. The identical results for GM and WM show that the IIH correction acts equally in all tissues. Some representative results are shown in Table 2–5.

Table 6 shows the influence of a higher noise level in the correction and segmentation of GM in a T1_fl image.

The sigma values resulting of a test from the ANOVA analysis are shown in Table 7.

Table 2. Dice coefficient for T1_fl images with 3% noise, bias field A, 3 different rf levels and for GM.

	Parameters			Images		
				rf20	rf40	rf100
Uncorrected				0.7641	0.7086	0.5742
N3	a	b	c			
	0.1	2	4	0.7561	0.7564	0.7297
	0.3	2	4	0.7349	0.7365	0.7414
	0.15	2	2	0.7579	0.7192	0.5786
	0.15	2	4	0.7688	0.7505	0.7451
FSL algorithm		d	c			
		2	20	0.6980	0.7368	0.7451
		3	10	0.6883	0.7491	0.7343
		3	20	0.7632	0.7753	0.7629
		3	30	0.7884	0.7801	0.7524
		4	20	**0.8009**	0.7745	0.7188
SPM algorithm			c			
			60	0.7577	0.7615	0.7441
			90	0.7771	**0.8061**	**0.8061**
PABIC			c			
			2	0.7811	0.7247	0.6797
			3	0.7709	0.7492	0.6878

Backgrounds: no background = worse than the uncorrected image, = better than the uncorrected image, = best value for this algorithm, bold = best value
Parameters: a = shrink factor; b = number of fitting levels, c = full width at half maximum, d = number of classes

Table 4. Dice coefficient for T1_fl images with 3% noise, bias field B, 3 different rf levels and for WM.

	Parameters			Images		
				rf20	rf40	rf100
Uncorrected				0.8297	0.7847	0.6772
N3	a	b	c			
	0.1	2	4	0.8215	0.8266	0.8077
	0.3	2	4	0.8027	0.8028	0.8120
	0.15	2	2	0.8341	0.7931	0.6808
	0.15	2	4	0.8239	0.8128	0.8022
FSL algorithm		d	c			
		2	20	0.8016	0.8067	0.8128
		3	10	0.8203	0.8087	0.7928
		3	20	0.8396	0.8363	0.8157
		3	30	0.8443	0.8402	0.8009
		4	20	0.8424	0.8373	0.7734
SPM algorithm			c			
			60	0.8250	0.8276	0.8302
			90	**0.8577**	**0.8575**	**0.8553**
PABIC			c			
			2	0.8419	0.7995	0.7578
			3	0.8306	0.8203	0.7360

Backgrounds: no background = worse than the uncorrected image, = better than the uncorrected image, = best value for this algorithm, bold = best value
Parameters: a = shrink factor; b = number of fitting levels, c = full width at half maximum, d = number of classes

Table 3. Dice coefficient for T1_IR images with 3% noise, bias field A, 3 different rf levels and for GM.

	Parameters			Images		
				rf20	rf40	rf100
Uncorrected				0.8003	0.7891	0.7004
N3	a	b	c			
	0.1	2	4	0.8046	0.8048	0.7769
	0.3	2	4	0.8039	0.8041	0.7948
	0.15	2	2	**0.8055**	0.7916	0.7046
	0.15	2	4	0.8022	**0.8056**	0.7925
FSL algorithm		d	c			
		2	20	0.7655	0.7679	0.7728
		3	10	0.8002	0.8001	0.7905
		3	20	0.8033	0.8037	0.8009
		3	30	0.8048	0.8051	0.8004
		4	20	0.8040	0.8043	0.7897
SPM algorithm			c			
			60	0.8031	0.8033	**0.8033**
			90	0.8047	0.7784	0.7651
PABIC			c			
			2	0.8013	0.8010	0.7806
			3	0.7998	0.7934	0.7637

Backgrounds: no background = worse than the uncorrected image, = better than the uncorrected image, = best value for this algorithm, bold = best value
Parameters: a = shrink factor; b = number of fitting levels, c = full width at half maximum, d = number of classes

Table 5. Dice coefficient for T1_IR images with 3% noise, bias field B, 3 different rf levels and for WM.

	Parameters			Images		
				rf20	rf40	rf100
Uncorrected				0.8532	0.8456	0.7617
N3	a	b	c			
	0.1	2	4	0.8573	0.8569	0.8233
	0.3	2	4	0.8574	0.8575	0.8486
	0.15	2	2	0.8543	0.8476	0.7650
	0.15	2	4	**0.8579**	0.8574	0.8417
FSL algorithm		d	c			
		2	20	0.8306	0.8340	0.8352
		3	10	0.8544	0.8546	0.8392
		3	20	0.8565	0.8566	0.8498
		3	30	0.8578	**0.8579**	0.8479
		4	20	0.8565	0.8564	0.8304
SPM algorithm			c			
			60	0.8566	0.8568	**0.8553**
			90	0.8430	0.8440	0.8423
PABIC			c			
			2	0.8546	0.8547	0.8315
			3	0.8547	0.8521	0.8154

Backgrounds: no background = worse than the uncorrected image, = better than the uncorrected image, = best value for this algorithm, bold = best value
Parameters: a = shrink factor; b = number of fitting levels, c = full width at half maximum, d = number of classes

Table 6. Dice coefficient for T1_fl images with 9% noise, bias field A, 3 different rf levels and for GM.

	Parameters			Images		
				rf20	rf40	rf100
Uncorrected				0.6275	0.6180	0.5539
N3	a	b	c			
	0.1	2	4	0.6102	0.6170	0.6074
	0.3	2	4	0.6016	0.6063	0.6023
	0.15	2	2	0.6280	0.6199	0.5570
	0.15	2	4	0.6077	0.6119	0.6092
FSL algorithm		d	c			
		2	20	0.5825	0.5862	0.5942
		3	10	0.5543	0.5560	0.5636
		3	20	0.5949	0.5991	0.6061
		3	30	0.6106	0.6164	0.6190
		4	20	0.6059	0.6110	0.6089
SPM algorithm			c			
			60	0.5976	0.6021	0.6038
			90	**0.6941**	**0.7003**	**0.7026**
PABIC			c			
			2	0.6162	0.6253	0.5918
			3	0.6051	0.6065	0.5814

Backgrounds: no background = worse than the uncorrected image, ▨ = better than the uncorrected image, ▨ = best value for this algorithm, bold = best value

Parameters: a = shrink factor; b = number of fitting levels, c = full width at half maximum, d = number of classes

Table 7. Sigma values of the tests of within-subjects contrasts (ANOVA test) of the Dice Coefficients.

	Parameters			Images			
				T1 fl		T1 IR	
				GM	WM	GM	WM
N3	a	b	c				
	0.1	2	4	0.024	0.048	0.012	0.008
	0.3	2	4	0.095	0.229	0.021	0.018
	0.15	2	2	0.007	0.03	7E-05	2E-04
	0.15	2	4	0.027	0.633	0.016	0.341
FSL algorithm		d	c				
		2	20	0.18	0.453	0.883	0.96
		3	10	0.227	0.746	0.386	0.558
		3	20	0.018	0.048	0.055	0.066
		3	30	0.005	0.012	0.023	0.023
		4	20	0.004	0.012	0.029	0.036
SPM algorithm			c				
			60	0.038	0.048	0.044	0.044
			90	4E-04	3E-04	0.656	0.887
PABIC			c			0.556	
			2	0.012	0.043	0.326	0.34
			3	0.019	0.060	0.012	0.683

Parameters: a = shrink factor; b = number of fitting levels, c = full width at half maximum, d = number of classes.

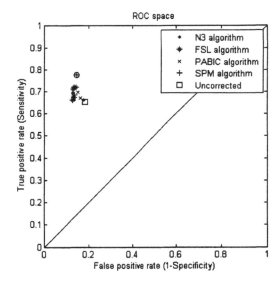

Figure 1. ROC space considering the sensitivity and specificity of the segmentation of the GM in the T1_IR image, with 3% noise, B bias field and 40% inhomogeneity.

In each figure we represent the ROC points for the four algorithms and the best relation between the sensitivity and specificity (point closer to the coordinates (0,1) is marked with a circle). An example of a Roc space is shown in Figure 1.

4 DISCUSSION

It can be observed that the IIH corrections improve the subsequent segmentation of most images.

In the N3 algorithm, it is unclear what are the parameters which allow for higher Dice coefficients, and it works well for higher rf's. N3 is the algorithm that appears to deal better with images that have high noise levels and/or high rf. For the IR image the best parameters seem to be a FWHM of 0.15, with shrink factor of 2 and fitting levels of 4. For the T1_fl image the parameters are not so clear. Some other experiences showed that a higher fitting level gives a worse segmentation and it was also observed that using a greater shrink factor, e.g. 4, the results do not vary much and the time necessary for correction decreases.

In FSL the parameters that allow a greater Dice coefficient, are number of classes equal to 3; and for a rf20 and rf40 a FWHM of 30 mm, whereas for a rf100 a 20 mm FWHM is better. This occurs because the variation is more abrupt for higher rf values and a smaller FWHM fits those cases better.

The IIH correction algorithm present on SPM is considered to be the most regular of the algorithms. The best parameter for T1_fl images is to use a FWHM of 90 mm, and for the T1_IR images is to use a FWHM of 60 mm. A FWHM of 30 mm was also used, but the results of the segmentations show it is worse than for the uncorrected image.

The analysis of the PABIC and SPM is quite limited, since we only have changed two parameters. However, it can be observed that for rf20 the use of 2 classes is adequate for T1_fl images, while the use of 3 classes is adequate for T1_IR images. For higher rf's, the opposite happens.

It can be seen that the algorithm used for the segmentation does not perform as well in 9% noise images. However, the correction algorithms still fail to improve segmentation. An analysis of the coefficient of variation is likely to provide better answers.

With the analysis of the Table 7 it is possible to say that the increase of the Dice coefficients with the corrections is statistically significant for most of the correction methods, sigma lower than 0.05.

A typical problem of segmentation methods was observed: a higher sensitivity corresponds normally to a lower specificity and vice versa. However, observing the ROC space it is possible to find the best relationship, and often this relationship corresponds to a higher Dice coefficient.

5 CONCLUSION

It is unquestionable that the IIH corrections improve the segmentation of MRI brain images, especially for higher rf, as long as the noise level is not too high. However it was not found an IIH correction algorithm or set of parameters that performs well for all analyzed images. Besides that, it can be said that the algorithm that shows to be the most stable and offers the best evaluation parameters for the majority of images is the one present on SPM8 software.

With these results we reinforce the utility and the need of using a preprocessing method for IIH correction, before applying a segmentation algorithm.

REFERENCES

Ashburner, J. & Friston, K.J. 2005, "Unified segmentation." *NeuroImage*, vol. 26, no. 3, pp. 839–851.

Boyes, R., Gunter, J., Frost, C., Janke, A. et al. 2008, "Intensity non-uniformity correction using N3 on 3-T scanners with multichannel phased array coils." *NeuroImage*, vol. 39, no. 4, pp. 1752–1762.

Cocosco, C., Kollokian, V., Kwan, R., Pike, B. & Evans, A. 1997, "BrainWeb: Online Interface to a 3D MRI Simulated Brain Database." *NeuroImage*, vol. 5.

de Boer, R., Vrooman, H.A., Ikram, M.A., Vernooij, M.W. et al. 2010, "Accuracy and reproducibility study of automatic MRI brain tissue segmentation methods." *NeuroImage*, vol. 51, no. 3, pp. 1047–1056.

Duncan, J. & Ayache, N. 2000, "Medical image analysis: progress over two decades and the challenges ahead." *IEEE Transactions on Pattern Analysis and Machine Intelligence*, vol. 22, no. 1, pp. 85–106.

Guillemaud, R. & Brady, M. 1997, "Estimating the bias field of MR images." *IEEE Transactions on Medical Imaging*, vol. 16, no. 3, pp. 238–251.

Hendee, W. 2002, *Medical imaging physics* 4th ed., New York; Wiley-Liss.

Ibanez, L, Schroeder, W., Ng, L. & Cates, J. 2003, *The ITK Software Guide: The Insight Segmentation and Registration Toolkit*, Kitware Inc.

Kaus, M.R., Warfield, S.K., Nabavi, A., Black, P.M. et al. 2001, "Automated Segmentation of MR Images of Brain Tumors1." *Radiology*, vol. 218, no. 2, pp. 586–591.

Sled, J., Zijdenbos, A. & Evans, A. 2002, "A nonparametric method for automatic correction of intensity nonuniformity in MRI data." *Medical Imaging, IEEE Transactions on*, vol. 17, no. 1, p. 97, 87.

Styner, M., Brechbuhler, C., Szckely, G. & Gerig, G. 2000, "Parametric estimate of intensity inhomogeneities applied to MRI." *Medical Imaging, IEEE Transactions on*, vol. 19, no. 3, pp. 153–165.

Vovk, U., Pernus, F. & Likar, B. 2007, "A review of methods for correction of intensity inhomogeneity in MRI." *IEEE Trans Med Imaging*, vol. 26, no. 3, pp. 421, 405.

Wells, W.M., Grimson, W.L., Kikinis, R. & Jolesz, F.A. 1996, "Adaptive segmentation of MRI data." *IEEE Transactions on Medical Imaging*, vol. 15, no. 4, pp. 429–442.

Zhang, Y., Brady, M. & Smith, S. 2001, "Segmentation of brain MR images through a hidden Markov random field model and the expectation-maximization algorithm." *IEEE Transactions on Medical Imaging*, vol. 20, no. 1, pp. 45–57.

Technology and Medical Sciences – Natal Jorge et al. (eds)
© *2011 Taylor & Francis Group, London, ISBN 978-0-415-66822-4*

Interactive collaboration for Virtual Reality systems related to medical education and training

B.R.A. Sales & L.S. Machado
Department of Informatics of Federal University of Paraíba, Paraíba, Brazil

R.M. Moraes
Department of Statistics of Federal University of Paraíba, Paraíba, Brazil

ABSTRACT: Virtual Reality (VR) systems have a recent story from the social and practical applications point of view. The main idea related to this area refers to the use of three-dimensional environments in which users can explore and interact in virtual worlds and feel immersed and involved in this process. Nowadays the state of art in VR researches includes collaborative VR environments for medical training and teaching. The use of such collaborative environments allows students to share their knowledge or to be assisted by a tutor during a simulation. This paper presents the development process of a module for interactive collaboration to CyberMed, a framework available since 2004 to speed up the building of medical simulations based on VR technologies. The module for collaboration that was integrated to this framework was used to develop test applications.

1 INTRODUCTION

Virtual Reality (VR) has been established as an area that provides an effective and motivating way to help teaching in several fields (Kim & Park 2006, Riva 2003). It allows multi-sensory experiments by user interaction with Virtual Environments (VE) generated by computer. In the medical area, VR applications have become an alternative tool for training of medical procedures and a tool to support the implementation of laboratory practices.

Some factors like the cost of training, as well as ethical issues, have contributed to the search of new training methods of medical procedures. In this context, VR systems can simulate and also improve the traditional training methods. Thus, the use of VE permits the student to interact and improve their skills in environments that simulate real activities. The environments may be developed by focusing on key-points of a procedure or even points at which medical errors are often noticed. Moreover, there is the possibility for repeat the procedure as many as desired, until the student is able to perform it on a real situation. However, there are procedures that are performed not only by one person, but by a team of professionals together. In these cases, it is necessary to add collaborative features in the VE in order to allow simulating real-world situations. Thus, it becomes possible interaction of multiple participants in

what is called Collaborative Virtual Environment (CVE) (Benford et al. 2001).

In this work the collaboration in Virtual Environments is discussed as a way to help students and professionals in the training of medical procedures, independently of their geographical location. The paper describes the design and development of a Collaboration module to be integrated into the framework CyberMed. The framework integrated with the module was used to design a case study on a collaborative virtual environment for bone marrow harvest.

2 COLLABORATION FOR EDUCATIONAL VIRTUAL ENVIRONMENTS

The collaboration concept has various definitions in literature. In this work, collaboration is considered as the information exchange by user interaction in a shared environment, i.e., there is collaboration when two or more users are included in a shared space performing some task together.

Virtual Environments have been used in educational context in several areas of knowledge (Youngblut 1998), including medicine (Riva 2003). In general, these environments are designed to allow the acquisition of specific knowledge through the use of computer applications.

The educational VEs can be explored to develop an environment that allows the presence of multiple users. Therefore, it is necessary to use techniques to allow people in different locations feel immersed in a common environment (Singhal & Zyda 1999). Thus, the use of network VE makes possible to replicate situations in which participants work together for a common goal. In this context, the participants of such environments can be able to learn and, at the same time, contribute for other users learning. The use of such environments in medicine context brings benefits to student learning. For example, collaborative simulations can be used to overcome distance problems and provide remotely monitored training in regions without specialists. In this case, a specialist can perform techniques through simulations or interactions in the VE and users can experience and follow the procedure. Furthermore, collaboration in VR environments also enables students to be a part of simulations with others situated in distant locations, promoting the exchange of knowledge.

3 VIRTUAL REALITY IN MEDICINE

As a flexible tool, Virtual Environments have been designed to simulate several real world problems and used with different purposes, approaches or objectives. In medicine, VR can be applied joined to other technologies to help students in the learning process. Applications of human structures three-dimensional (3D) visualization and simulations of medical procedures have been analyzed by researcher groups as tools for teaching and training.

The study of anatomy, as example, is often made by static image visualization. In this context, the VR tools can be used to generate 3D visualization of anatomy structures. Thus students are able to interact with these structures and visualize them from different points of view. Moreover, the Virtual Environments are a way to replace some methods that are frequently questioned about financial and ethical issues, as the use of human corpse or live animals.

The simulations of medical procedures enable users to perceive sensorial cues, into a VE, similarly to real procedures. This is important to prepare students technically and psychologically to deal with real situations. The current VR medical simulations provide high resolution graphics, haptic interaction and a diversity of functionalities that improve the training efficacy (Sung et al. 2003, Friedl et al. 2002).

3.1 Collaborative Virtual Environments for medical training

Dev (2002) developed two simulation-based learning environments, one for teaching anatomy and other

for practicing basic surgical maneuvers like probing, cutting, and suturing. The first environment contains a three-dimensional model of the hand which has interactive rotating view. The hand can be viewed in stereoscopic visualization at different depths of dissection. The second environment contains models of pelvic anatomy and surgical tools to enable the medical training, even collaboratively. Figure 1 illustrates the two learning environments developed. The left image (Fig. 1a) shows the 3D hand model used by the anatomical learning environment. The others two images (Fig. 1b) show the virtual environment for practicing basic surgical maneuvers.

Another use of Collaborative Virtual Environments in medicine is the remotely conduction of classes through haptic interaction. In this case, an instructor performs a task while students follow the movements remotely. Gunn (2005) built an environment to simulate the gall bladder removal with instructor and student working in the same virtual space on a 3D model of body organs (Fig. 2).

There are several virtual environments that provide alternative ways to perform medical training. However, the development of these applications requests a lot of time and hard work. Frequently, a framework is used to support the development of medical training virtual environments.

3.2 Frameworks for medical training simulations development

A framework is an abstract project and implementation that provides a set of services to be used

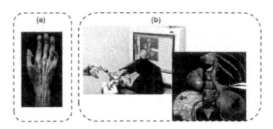

Figure 1. Learning environments developed by Dev (2002).

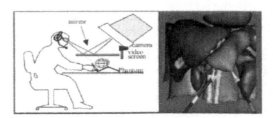

Figure 2. Collaborative virtual environment to conduct a remote surgical master class using haptic device (Gunn et al. 2005).

in application development (Bosh & Mattsson 1999). Frameworks allow decreasing development time and offer several functionalities that can be selected by the programmer, allowing the reuse of components. The tendency to reuse services encourages researcher groups to spend their time on frameworks development. To support the development of medical training virtual environments, the frameworks have to deal with some requirements, such as: different visualization modes, complex modeling, haptic feedback, etc.

Recently, some solutions were proposed and developed to help the design and implementation of simulators for medicine. Examples include frameworks as SOFA (Allard et al. 2007), ViMeT (Oliveira et al. 2006), Spring (Montgomery et al. 2002), GiPSi (Goktekin et al. 2004). Although the same goal, they do not include a tool that assess the simulation performed in the applications developed with them. Furthermore, to allow the representation of scenarios in which there are two or more people working together, the frameworks have to provide collaboration functionalities. Some of these frameworks provide features to create simulations with collaborative tasks. Nevertheless, they generally allow collaboration activities in only one or few modes. Some aspects like collaborative object manipulation and remote mentoring were not addressed yet.

4 CONCEPTION

The development of a collaboration module to be integrated to the CyberMed framework came up as purpose of framework functionalities increase. It was intended to enhance the framework power by providing activities related to collaboration among users. This module aims to provide multi-user collaboration to medical simulation VEs in several ways, such as two different object manipulation modes, interaction devices, etc. The module was designed to let the developers free to choose what way would best fit into their specific case. The collaboration module, called CybCollaboration, is a set of services at a high level that deals with network communication and devices requirements. In this way, the user need to be focused only on the specific characteristics of the desired collaboration scenario.

CyberMed was chosen as the framework to contain the collaboration module because it is a free and stable development tool with a large diversity of features compared to others with similar purposes (Machado et al. 2009). CyberMed contains packages for visualization, collision, deformation, assessment, support for haptic and tracker devices, etc. The CybCollaboration module aims to enable all the features already available on CyberMed and also the building collaborative medical simulations.

The research related to this work aims to examine ways in which users could collaborate in medicine VEs. To improve the usability of the module, it was decided to support collaboration across conventional and unconventional devices such as mouse, haptic and tracker devices.

5 DEVELOPMENT

This section describes the development of the Cyb-Collaboration module. Initially, requirements analysis was done to elucidate the needs of the module. The development was divided in three parts: architecture definitions, CyberMed modifications and; CybCollaboration design and implementation.

5.1 Architecture

The CybCollaboration has direct dependency on CybNetwork, which consists in a set of classes implemented in C++ using sockets, designed to be the CyberMed communication module. The Cyb-Network was developed and tested, but had not yet been integrated into CyberMed architecture. To integrate these two modules to the framework, it was done changes in the CyberMed Application Engine layer. This layer provides services that are used directly by the CyberMed user, such as visualization, collision, deformation, assessment and haptic interaction. Figure 3 allows the observation of the CyberMed architecture after the insertion of CybCollaboration and CybCommunication modules.

5.2 CyberMed modifications

The integration of CybCollaboration module forced some changes on CyberMed modules. During a collaborative simulation, avatars (devices representations on VE) of remote users must be

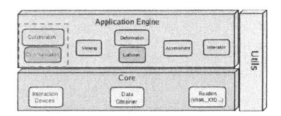

Figure 3. General architecture of CyberMed with communication and collaboration modules (Machado et al. 2009).

presented in the environment together with the local user avatar, in a way that every user can realize the presence of the others. Since this multiple avatar presentation was not possible in CyberMed, it was necessary to reformulate the structure of some Interator Management classes.

Some changes were made on CybView (visualization module) and also on CybCollision (module that treats with collision events). They were adapted to deal with multiple users' avatars.

5.3 *Design and implementation*

The design of CybCollaboration module aimed at simplifies the development of collaborative applications. Moreover, it is also possible to the user the implementation of new collaboration methods and the addition of these methods in CyberMed.

The class diagram shown in Figure 4 is a simplified illustration of how the CybCollaboration module is defined. The main class, also named CybCollaboration, contains generic operations common to all collaboration methods. The other classes were divided according to the device type used in collaboration. The main properties of collaboration are stored in class CybCollaborationProperties. It also contains operations to choose the type of desired object manipulation at the collaboration scenario. As a particular behavior, the class CybAssistedHapticCollab is sponsor for assisted haptic collaboration, i.e. a mode of collaboration in which the participants are guided by a tutor during a task.

The implemented classes have increased CyberMed framework with a set of features related to collaborative activities. The main features referred to:

Number of users: Methods to support collaboration with different numbers of users (one-to-one, one-to-many, many-to-many);

Object manipulation: There are two different ways implemented to manage the user interaction

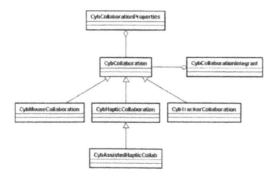

Figure 4. General class diagram of CyberMed collaboration module.

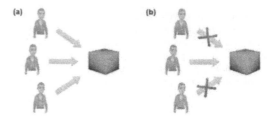

Figure 5. Two different approaches for object manipulation. In (a) the interactions performed by users are applied to the object like a resultant interaction. In (b) only one user is able to interact with the object, while the others have to wait.

with objects in the VE. The first one allows users to interact with the same object simultaneously (Fig. 5a). The users' interactions are unified and the result is applied to the object. The other approach, blocks the object for other users, when it already been interacted by a user (Fig. 5b);

Devices: Collaboration through the use of conventional devices like mouse, and unconventional, like haptic systems (that provides force feedback), or tracker systems;

Remote Mentoring: Determination of a participant to tutor the others within the environment. This mentoring can be done at different levels. With the use of haptic systems, for example, it is possible to determine if users shall be restricted to movements performed by the tutor or if only a visual representation of the tutor device will appear in the user environment to guide him in the activity.

6 RESULTS

After the development and integration of the Cyb-Collaboration module, applications were built to test the module. In particular, a simulation of a bone marrow harvest procedure was adapted to provide collaboration with touch and force feedback among remote users. In this application a user was selected as a tutor and guided all other users connected.

The bone marrow harvest consists of a procedure in which the doctor interacts with the patient in order to extract material for donation. During the procedure, the doctor has no visual information from inside the patient. He must touch the patient externally to determine the correct location to insert the needle. Then he must pierce the layers of tissue to reach the interior of the bone where the marrow is collected. Two important things are: the site of needle insertion and the force that the doctor will apply to reach the desired location. The correct site of needle insertion is the iliac bone which contains the correct width and hardness to the procedure realization. If this force is applied in excess, it can be harmful for the patient and may cause sequel (Machado et al. 2002, 2003).

The simulation of bone marrow harvest (Fig. 6) is divided into three modules: Observation, Location and Harvest. In the three modules, users will be able to interact with the system by the use of a haptic device (Phantom Omni). The interactions performed by the guide user are perceived in real-time by all users connected to the simulation. Then, they are able to feel sensory impressions and experience the movements and forces presented in the procedure.

In the tests were used two computers connected to a Gigabit LAN. Both computers were equipped with haptic devices and one user was defined as the tutor while the others were tutored, perceiving only the tutor interactions. Two other tests were also conducted with three computers equipped with haptic devices of different models and five computers with interaction through mouse (Fig. 7), respectively. In all experiments, the information send and receive occurred in real-time.

Other experiments performed consisted on the free manipulation of devices by every user present in the virtual environment. The experiments were made with the same number of computers and devices of the previous tests. All participants were able to observe the position of self-avatar as well as the other participants avatars.

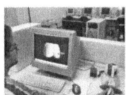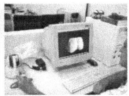

Figure 6. Collaborative simulation of the bone marrow harvest procedure. Haptic device Phantom was used to interact with models.

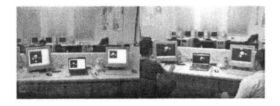

Figure 7. Application to test mouse collaboration scenario.

7 CONCLUSIONS

The results pointed out the potential of using collaborative virtual environments for education, particularly in medicine. The possibility of share knowledge in VR supported medical simulations is a promising alternative in medical training field. Moreover, the collaborative simulations enable professionals to demonstrate, through tactile interactions, how students must proceed during a specific medical procedure. This possibility allows students of remote places to increase your medical skills by sharing and receiving knowledge from experts.

In this work it was detailed three applications to test and validate the CybCollaboration module functionalities. Also, a complete simulation of the bone marrow harvest procedure was adapted to be performed collaboratively. In this sense, this research suggests discussions on validation of collaborative applications to medicine. It is also important to highlight that, whereas the use of collaboration for training is not limited to medical field, researches can be conducted to examine how collaboration can be inserted to assist training in other areas.

Future work includes the expansion of the collaboration features to the addition of object manipulation specific techniques, providing means to participants, in addition to handling, also interactively modify objects of the VE. Ruddle and colleagues describe some techniques for manipulating objects in collaborative virtual environments (Ruddle et al. 2002a, b). It can be analyzed to be added to the collaboration module according to its relevance in medical environments. It is important to mention that the basis for implementation of such expansion is already available in the module presented in this work.

The implemented module is available on version 2.0 of CyberMed (CyberMed 2010). The framework can be obtained freely on the project page on the Internet (http://cybermed.sourceforge.net/).

REFERENCES

Allard, J., Cotin, S., Faure, F., Bensoussan, P.J., Poyer, F., Duriez, C. et al. 2007. SOFA—an Open Source Framework for Medical Simulation. *Medicine Meets Virtual Reality* 15:1–6.

Benford, S., Greenhalgh, C., Rodden, T. & Pycock, J. 2001. Collaborative virtual environments. *Communications of the ACM* 44(7):79–85.

Bosh, J. & Mattsson, M. 1999. Framework Problems and Experiences. In M. Fayad, R. Johnson, D. Schmidt, *Building Application Frameworks: Object-Oriented Foundations of Framework Design*: 55–82. New York: John Willey and Sons.

CyberMed. 2010. Online: http://cybermed.sourceforge.net/

Dev, P., Montgomery, K., Senger, S., Heinrichs, W.L., Srivastava, S. & Waldron, K. 2002. Simulated Medical Learning Environments on the Internet. *Journal of the American Medical Informatics Association* 9(5):437–447.

Friedl, R., Preisack, M.B., Klas, W., Rose, T., Stracke, S. & Quast, K.J. et al. 2002. Vritual Reality and 3D Visualizations in Heart Surgery Education, *Heart Surg Forum* 5(3):17–21.

Goktekin, T., Cavusoglu, M.C., Tendick, F. & Sastry, S. 2004. GiPSi: An Open Source/Open Architecture Software Development Framework for Surgical Simulation. *In Proceedings of the International Symposium on Medical Simulation*, Cambridge.

Gunn, C., Hutchins, M., Stevenson, D., Adcock, M. & Youngblood, P. 2005. Using collaborative haptics in remote surgical training. *Eurohaptics Conference and Symposium on Haptic Interfaces for Virtual Environment and Teleoperator Systems (WHC'05)*, Italy.

Kim, L. & Park, S.H. 2006. Haptic interaction and volume modeling techniques for realistic dental simulation. *The Visual Computer: International Journal of Computer Graphics* 22:90–98.

Machado, L.S., Mello, A.N., Odone Filho, V. & Zuffo, M.K. 2002. Virtual Reality Simulation of Pediatric Bone Marrow Harvest for Transplant. *Medical and Pediatric Oncology.* 39(4):282.

Machado, L.S., Moraes, R.M., Souza, D.F.L., Souza, L.C. & Cunha, I.L.L. 2009. A Framework for Development of Virtual Reality-Based Training Simulators. *Studies in Health Technology and Informatics* 142:174–176.

Machado, L.S. & Zuffo, M.K. 2003. Development and Evaluation of a Simulator of Invasive Procedures in Pediatric Bone Marrow Transplant. *Studies In Health Technology And Informatics.* 94:193–195.

Montgomery, K. et al. 2002. Spring: A general framework for collaborative, real-time surgical simulation, *Proceedings of Medicine Meets Virtual Reality*, IOS Press, pp. 23–26.

Oliveira, A.C.M.T.G., Botega, L.C., Pavarini, L., Rossatto, D.J., Nunes, F.L.S. & Bezerra, A. 2006. Virtual Reality Framework for Medical Training: Implementation of a deformation class using Java. *In Proceedings of the SIGGRAPH International Conference on Virtual-Reality Continuum and its Applications in Industry (SIGGRAPH '06)*:347–351, Hong Kong.

Riva, G. 2003. Applications of Virtual Environments in Medicine. *Methods of Information in Medicine* 42(5):524–534.

Ruddle, R.A., Savage, J.C.D. & Jones, D.M. 2002a. Implementing flexible rules of interaction for object manipulation in cluttered virtual environments. *In Proceedings of the ACM Symposium on Virtual Reality Software and Technology (VRST'02)*: 89–96.

Ruddle, R.A., Savage, J.C.D. & Jones, D.M. 2002b. Symmetric and asymmetric action integration during cooperative object manipulation in virtual environments. *ACM Transactions on Computer-Human Interaction* 9(6):285–308.

Singhal, S. & Zyda, M. 1999. *Networked virtual environments: design and implementation*, New York: ACM Press/Addison-Wesley Publishing Co.

Sung, W.H., Fung, C.P., Chen, A.C., Yuan, C.C., Ng, H.T. & Doong, J.L. 2003. The assessment of stability and reliability of a virtual reality-based laparoscopic gynecology simulation system. *Eur J Ginaecol Oncol.* 24(2):143–146.

Youngblut, C. 1998. Educational Uses of V R Technology. *Technical Report IDA Document D-2128*, Institute for Defense Analyses, Alexandria.

Technology and Medical Sciences – Natal Jorge et al. (eds)
© *2011 Taylor & Francis Group, London, ISBN 978-0-415-66822-4*

Lissajous scanning pattern simulation, for development of a FLO

Pedro Nunes
Faculdade de Ciências e Tecnologia-UNL, Lisboa, Portugal
Escola Superior de Tecnologia e Gestão-IPL, Leiria, Portugal
Instituto de Biofísica e Engenharia Biomédica-UL, Lisboa, Portugal

Pedro Vieira
Faculdade de Ciências e Tecnologia-UNL, Lisboa, Portugal
Instituto de Biofísica e Engenharia Biomédica-UL, Lisboa, Portugal

ABSTRACT: Reflection and fluorescence imaging of the ocular fund us, using a Scanning Laser Ophthalmoscope (SLO), is an established tool of diagnosing several eye diseases. Fluorescence lifetime imaging (FLIM) is considered a potential technique for identifying different fluorophores which cannot be clearly separated in intensity images. We're currently developing a Fluorescence Lifetime Ophthal moscope (FLO), integrating frequency domain FLIM technique with a SLO. The first attempt to make this integration, conducted by us, shown the need for slower scanning system and frame grabber reprogram. We've then setup a test protocol to analyze the operating conditions of a couple of galvanic mirrors and have developed a Matlab program to simulate and analyze several scanning pattern characteristics. The results of our simulations show that a 2 img/sec acquisition rate is a possibility and that a uniform distribution of energy is obtained using a Lissajous pattern, avoiding mirror inertia and high speed horizontal raster problems.

1 INTRODUCTION

1.1 *FLIM*

Far-field fluorescence imaging techniques are some of the most adequate methods for non-invasive and rapid investigation of biological systems, allowing intravital microscopy in real-time, and providing information on a molecular basis (Niesner et al. 2008). Among these fluorescence techniques is Fluorescence Lifetime Imaging Microscopy (FLIM), which allows mapping the spatial distribution of nanosecond excited state lifetimes within microscopic images, and that has been used for numerous applications (Niesner et al. 2008) (Castleman et al. 2005), some of them with important clinical implications (Munro et al. 2005). These studies have shown images with good contrast between different types or states of a tissue, while the traditional fluorescence intensity images have shown none.

1.2 *Time domain versus frequency domain FLIM*

FLIM systems have been implemented both in the frequency domain, using sinusoidal intensity modulated excitation light and modulated detectors, and in the time domain, using pulsed excitation sources and time-correlated or time-gated detection (van Munster et al. 2005).

FLIM in time-domain provides a direct measurement of the fluorescence decay and thus, a direct access to the parameter/parameters of interest which allows it to reach time-resolutions in the low ps-range or even fs-range (Castleman et al. 2005). To achieve it, although, very high energy density is used, which may be hazardous for biological samples, due to the low exposure limits allowed, and therefore difficult to apply to in-vivo situations (ICNIRP, 2005). In frequency-domain FLIM, the intensity of the excitation light is continuously modulated. Due to the (non-instant) fluorescence decay, the fluorescence emission will display a phase shift and a decrease in modulation. Thus, it is possible to determine the lifetime from the observed phase shift or from the decrease in modulation depth of the emitted fluorescent relative to the excitation signal (van Munster et al. 2005). This may be done at a much higher image acquisition rate that the one time-domain FLIM allows to and lower energy density is needed (ICNIRP ,2005), both of which are very important factors in ophthalmology and give good perspective for FLO human use.

1.3 *FLIM as ophthalmic tool*

Reflection and fluorescence imaging of the ocular fundus is an established tool of diagnosing eye diseases such as diabetes, hypertension, glaucoma and age-related macular degeneration (Hammer et al. 2008) (Hammer et al. 2009). There are also studies indicating that time-resolved fluorescence of biological tissues can be used in tissue discrimination and oxygenation measurements, and contain much more information than that resulting from conventional steady-state fluorescence (Schweitzer et al. 2007) (Niesner et al. 2008). As functional alterations are the first signs of a starting pathological process, a device that measures parameter associated with metabolic changes of the human eye-ground, and therefore could identify those alterations, would be a helpful tool for early diagnostics in stages when alterations are yet reversible. The new technique of auto-fluorescence lifetime measurement (FLIM) opens in combination with selected excitation and emission ranges the possibility for that metabolic mapping (Schweitzer et al. 2007). FLIM not only adds an additional discrimination parameter to distinguish different fluorophores but also resolves different quenching states of the same fluorophore (Schweitzer et al. 2007). A laser scanning ophthalmoscope (SLO) can relatively easily be combined with the FLIM technique to produce such a device.

The integration of the SLO with the FLIM techniques, in order to achieve a FLO has been recently tried by others (Schweitzer et al. 2007) and by us (Barbosa et al. 2006). The two approaches are quite different in terms of how the excitation laser is used. In the first one time-domain FLIM is used while the second one uses frequency-domain FLIM that, as stated before, yields a better compromise between laser power and image rate. Preliminary studies made with the FLIM prototype, developed by us in CEFITEC/FCT/UNL, together with the SLO of Aberdeen University—UK, had shown very promising results in the fusion of these two technologies (Barbosa et al. 2006). Figure 1 shows the schematics of the SLO and FLIM integration.

The results from this first integration attempt have shown the system has sufficient sensitivity for in-vivo imaging, that fluorescence time of decay

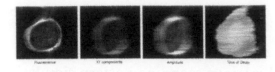

Figure 2. Raster blur evidence on results from Aberdeen SLO tests. Human nail image acquisition with several techniques: Fluorescence, XY components, Amplitude, time of decay.

is accurately measured and that an acquisition rate of two images per second (2 img/sec) should be possible based on the LockIn SR844 processing velocity upper limit. The Aberdeen SLO uses a scanning system based on polygon mirrors, built to acquire 25 img/sec, which we adjusted to the slowest acquisition rate we found possible with this system (5 img/sec).

Despite this adjustment a raster blur due to high speed horizontal scan was detected on the acquired data, as can be seen on Figure 2, making us realize the need for a system with slower scanning mirrors and a frame grabber reprogram.

A new dedicated scanning system is than being developed, based on galvanic mirrors instead of polygon mirrors, due to the higher versatility and lower oscillating frequency that the first often present compared to the second ones.

2 MATERIALS & METHODS

2.1 *Galvanic mirrors analysis*

Galvanic mirrors are a high performance, high accuracy and compact positioning system designed for a specific range of inertial loads that allow for mirrors with different inertia to be precisely controlled. We're currently working with a couple of galvanic mirrors from MicroMax™ Series 671, consisting on single-channel servo amplifiers coupled to high performance scanners. Each scanner is designed for a specific range of inertial loads allowing mirrors with inertias from less than 0.001 g.cm^2 to greater than 100,000 g.cm^2 to be precisely controlled.

Galvanic mirrors technical specifications state the possibility to use analog or digital command input for mirror positioning. Analog input maximum range is ±10V that relates to mirror position trough an adjustable input scale factor ranging from 0.5V/° to 2.0V/°. Digital input consists of 16 bit word converted to the above analog scale via AD7846 DAC. A position output is also available at a scale factor of 0.5V/° and will be used to evaluate system performance in the subsequent analysis.

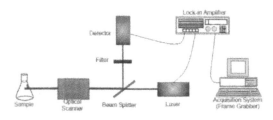

Figure 1. Schematics of SLO integration with FLIM.

In order to evaluate system limitations we've set up a test protocol to determine parameters that could, by any way, influence or limit the use of this mirrors on FLO scanning system development. The evaluated parameters were: maximum oscillating amplitude vs. input frequency, for several input amplitudes; maximum operating frequency, without output amplitude loss, for several input amplitude corresponding to specific oscillating angles required for FLO implementation, namely those which makes it possible to have a FOV of 20° to 25°; input amplitude needed for maintaining required output amplitude, at different oscillating frequencies.

The above tests we're performed on both mirrors of the system, using adjustable analog inputs and defining input scale factor for 0.5V/° to achieve maximum oscillating angle of ±20° at input ±10 V. The output signals we're acquired trough the position output port available at the 671 board and its amplitude compared to input signal via digital oscilloscope. Input and output signal frequencies we're also determined via the same digital oscilloscope.

2.2 Pattern analysis

Raster pattern is the most commonly used pattern in scanning systems due to the fact that it guarantees 100% pixel coverage of the defined Field Of View (FOV). Despite this advantage, overshoot and damping problems due to mirror inertia are common in this kind of apparatus and for that reason raster scan may not be the best approach to accomplish our purposes. To overcome those limitations we have than developed a Matlab program to simulate and analyze several pattern characteristics obtained by the use of sinusoidal signals, arranged to produce a Lissajous pattern. Comparison between raster and Lissajous pattern production sequence is presented in Figure 3.

Lissajous figures are graphical representation of a mathematical system of parametric equations which describe complex harmonic motion. The equations used to define a 2D pattern are:

$$x = A \sin(at + \delta)$$
$$y = B \sin(bt)$$
$$(1)$$

The appearance of the pattern is highly dependent on the ratio a/b that in our case represents the ratio between the oscillating frequency of each mirror. The δ parameter represents the phase shift between the two sinusoids and affects the Lissajous pattern in terms of eccentricity. A phase shift of $\pm\pi/2$ corresponds to an eccentricity of 1 and produces a circular pattern. A phase shift of 0 or $\pm\pi$ corresponds to an eccentricity of ∞ and produces a linear pattern. In order to obtain maximum coverage of the FOV an eccentricity of 1 is preferable so we've used $\delta = \pi/2$ in all the subsequent described implementation.

The developed program generates two, time dependent, vector arrays according to the parametric equations (1) with a and b being variables that represent the possible oscillating frequencies of the scanning mirrors. The two vector arrays are then matched together to form a XY pair that points out the, virtual, laser center position over time on a 512×512 matrix representing the scanned retina.

2.2.1 Frequency optimization

As pattern coverage depends mainly on the ratio a/b, a program function was created to analyze all the possible frequency combinations in a specified range, being the upper limit of this range defined from the galvanic mirrors analysis results. This simple function makes a laser energy distribution, according to the subsequently defined protocol, over the 512×512 matrix for every pair of frequency combination and analyzes the energy distribution homogeneity and the number of zero-energy pixels (matrix cells). The best homogeneity distribution of energy is determined as the minimum value of average energy distribution over the pixels covered by the laser. Frequency pair with the minimum zero-energy pixels gives back the best FOV coverage. The function then returns the frequency pair that held the most homogeneous energy distribution for the maximum FOV coverage.

2.2.2 Energy distribution analysis

Energy distribution over the FOV is a key issue to evaluate the performance of the scanning system using the Lissajous pattern. The program function that makes such energy distribution has to take into account some physical constrictions of the system such as: retinal FOV size; focal spot size of the laser; laser power at retina.

The retinal FOV size is a function of the laser entrance angle at pupil which, in turn, is equal to the oscillating angle present at the galvanic mirror. All calculus was then made for the maximum oscillating angle in order to obtain the maximum retinal

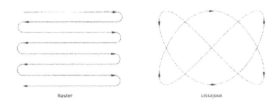

Figure 3. Raster pattern production sequence Vs Lissajous pattern production sequence.

FOV size possible. Mean eye diameter measured from pupil is 1.5 cm which combined with the ±20° entrance angle results in a square retinal FOV of approximately 10.92 mm. If the FOV is a 512 × 512 matrix then pixel size is 21.33 μm².

Assuming that the quality of the eye optics is a perfect one, the resolution at retina is only limited by physical factors such as focal length, wavelength of incident radiation, size of aperture, etc. (Hecht 2001). Assuming a laser with λ wavelength incident on pupil with a aperture radius R and focal length f, being the refractive index of the vitreous humour n, the Focal spot is a circle (Airy disc) who's radius is given by equation 2.

$$y_0 = 0.61 \times \frac{\lambda \cdot f}{n \cdot R} \qquad (2)$$

Using as physical characteristics of the eye the parameters given by the Gulstrand eye (Fulton 2000) with a pupil radius of 1.5 mm and a laser wavelength of 437 nm, corresponding to the available laser head in our institute, we determine the focal spot size as 4.51 μm. This focal spot size was then used to determine a unitary proportion to the pixel size by finding the ratio between them with the focal spot size being 0.2 of the pixel size. This ratio was used to simplify the implementation of the energy percentage distribution over the pixels, which is determined based on area percentage of focal spot over the covered pixels in each time sample (Figure 4).

In order to obtain a laser energy distribution as close as possible to a continuous motion of the scanning system we've used sequential time intervals of 0.1 μs to perform a 1 s or 2 s analysis. The laser head available in our institute has a maximum output power of 2.5 mW. For retina scan, power output is adjusted to insure values of about 150 μW at cornea, which corresponds to 15 pJ of energy deposited in each 0.1 μs on a circular area of $\pi \cdot 0 \cdot 1^2$ pixel unit. For the different situations shown in Figure 2 this energy is then divided on corresponding percentage by the covered pixels

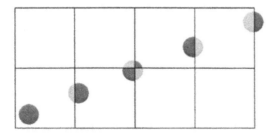

Figure 4. Laser focal spot for percentage energy distribution in different possible hitting situations over time.

and summed to the already deposited energy values on early interactions, if any.

2.2.3 Image acquisition rate

Image acquisition rate is an important parameter to evaluate as it must be high enough so that image won't be compromised by rapid eye movement. In raster pattern, image acquisition rate is easily determined as this pattern has inline sequential pixel by pixel coverage and subsequent line by line coverage, and hence an image is obtained as soon as all pixels in the FOV are covered by the laser. In Lissajous pattern scan we've decided to use a similar base of analysis to determine the image acquisition rate.

As in raster pattern, a laser hit on any point of a pixel determines that the pixel has been laser covered. Despite the fact that more theoretical calculation was used to evaluate the energy distribution, empirical results show that a laser hit will produce energy dispersion over the entire pixel, making it possible to state that one hit corresponds to a total pixel irradiation. For image acquisition rate determination we will use this second approach. In parallel to the energy distribution function, the program generates a second 512 × 512 matrix that accumulates the counts of laser hits per pixel. We then assume, as in raster pattern, that an image is obtained as soon as all pixels in the FOV have at least one hit, being the image acquisition rate determined by the ratio between the minimum hit counts present in this matrix and the time needed to obtain it. For better discrimination on this minimum, a histogram representation of the percentage of pixels in the matrix vs. the number of laser hits is plotted and used for calculus.

3 RESULTS

3.1 Galvanic mirrors

Table 1 shows the output amplitude measured for maximum input condition (±10 V) as function of increasing frequency values for horizontal oscillation (H) and for vertical oscillation. It's easily realized a decrease in amplitude for both oscillations but with different cutoff frequencies. The vertical oscillation as more sudden decrease at about 700 Hz, while the horizontal oscillation as a progressive decrease starting at only 200 Hz.

Table 1. Output amplitude as function of frequency for maximum input.

	100 Hz	200 Hz	400 Hz	600 Hz	700 Hz	800 Hz	1000 Hz
Ver	10 V	10 V	9.8 V	9.6 V	8.6 V	0.0 V	0.0 V
Hor	10 V	9.4 V	8.0 V	6.0 V	4.8 V	4.0 V	2.6 V

Table 2. Output amplitude as function of frequency for ±6.25 V input.

	100 Hz	200 Hz	400 Hz	600 Hz	700 Hz	800 Hz	1000 Hz
Ver	6.25 V	6.25 V	6.00 V	5.80 V	5.70 V	5.60 V	0.00 V
Hor	6.25 V	6.00 V	5.00 V	3.80 V	3.20 V	2.60 V	1.80 V

Table 3. Input amplitude needed, as function of frequency, to obtain an output amplitude of ±6.25 V.

	100 Hz	200 Hz	400 Hz	600 Hz	700 Hz	800 Hz	1000 Hz
Ver	6.25 V	6.25 V	6.30 V	6.65 V	6.70V	–	–
Hor	6.25 V	6.65 V	7.80 V	10.6 V	–	–	–

This result is an important physical limitation to the operating frequency of the mirrors, we can't impose oscillating frequencies above 600 Hz.

The pupil entrance angle needed for correct retinal analysis is of about ±12.5° which corresponds to an input amplitude of ±6.25 V. Table 2 shows the results obtained for an analysis similar to the previous one but using a ±6.25 V input. The behavior of the mirrors oscillating amplitude is identical to the previous one, which reinforces the 600 Hz operating limit.

In order to evaluate the possibility to use the galvanic mirrors close to the above limit, without amplitude loss, Table 3 shows the results from input compensation in order to maintain the desired output amplitude of ±6.25 V. As seen from this table the 600 Hz use is a possibility with some input compensation, being this compensation much larger on the horizontal mirror.

3.2 Frequency optimization

From the galvanic mirrors analysis it's clear that the frequency range to test in our pattern analysis program must not go above 600 Hz. In order to maintain the input compensation as low as possible we've tested all pairs of frequencies till 500 Hz only, having saved the highest pair of values possible, as this would be the one to give the better image acquisition rate.

Tests have shown that the highest frequency pair, till 500 Hz, that optimizes FOV coverage with the best energy distribution homogeneity is the 413 Hz by 423 Hz pair.

3.3 Energy distribution

Figure 5 shows the energy distribution over the 512 × 512 matrix revealing the homogeneity of this distribution and total coverage of the FOV.

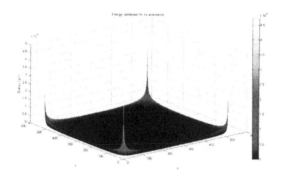

Figure 5. Energy distribution over the 512 × 512 matrix for 1 s time simulation.

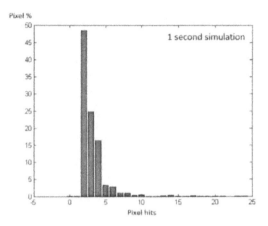

Figure 6. Histogram of the percentage of pixels in matrix vs. number of laser hits per pixel for 1 second simulation.

This results were obtained using the optimized frequency pair (413 Hz–423 Hz) for a 1 s time simulation with incremental intervals of 0.1 µs. It is evident, from figure, an energy accumulation at matrix corner pixels. This kind of pattern was expected, as the Lissajous figures present a velocity reduction on both axes at those pixels. Physical implementation of this pattern will require the use of system collimation or of energy modulation to avoid this energy peaks that could be hazardous to the retina.

3.4 Image acquisition rate

Image acquisition rates were determined for simulation times of 1 s, 2 s and 4 s. Figure 6 shows the histogram representation of the percentage of pixels in the matrix as a function of the number of hits for the 1 s simulation. It is seen from the figure that 100% of the pixels have 2 or more laser hits in 1 s which held a 2 img/sec acquisition rate. Similar and proportional results were obtained for the 2 s and 4 s simulation revealing redundancy on the intended calculus with 100% of the pixels with a minimum of 4 and 8 laser hits respectively and acquisition rates of 2 img/sec.

4 CONCLUSIONS

Raster pattern is the most used scanning pattern technique but has mirror inertia and high speed horizontal raster problems. Our study shows that the use of a Lissajous pattern to perform laser scanning is a possibility, by this way avoiding the above mentioned problems. Not only have we proved that this pattern performs a total coverage of the FOV as we've also proved that energy distribution is homogeneous and adequate to FLO development. The application of Lissajous pattern to other scanning systems is, by this way, also a possibility but relies dependent on the physical limitations of the system as happened with our galvanic mirrors whose oscillating limit is around 600 Hz, and even so with input compensation.

An acquisition rate of 2 img/sec was determined, in agreement with LockIn capabilities determined at first integration attempt in Aberdeen. A collimation system or an energy modulation is in need to avid retina damage, as corner pixels evidence peak energy accumulation.

REFERENCES

Barbosa, A., Manivannan, A. & Vieira, P. 2006. Development of a fluorescent lifetime image ophthalmoscope. *EVER 2006*. Vilamoura, Portugal.

Castleman, A.W., Toennies, J.P. & Zinth, W. 2005. Advanced time-correlated single photon counting techniques. *Springer*. Berlin Heidelberg.

Fulton, J.T. 2000. Processes in biological vision. *Vision Concepts*.

Hammer, M. *et al.* 2008. Ocular fundus auto-fluorescence observations at different wavelengths in patients with age-related macular degeneration and diabetic retinopathy. *Graefes Arch Clin Exp Ophtalmol* 246:105–114.

Hammer, M. *et al.* 2009. Diabetic patients with retinopathy show increased retinal venous oxygen saturation. *Graefes Arch Clin Exp Ophtalmol* 247:1025–1030.

Hecht, E. 2001. Optics 4th edition. *Addison Wesley*.

ICNIRP (International Commission on Non-Ionizing Radiation Protection) 2005. Revision of guidelines on limits of exposure to laser radiation of wavelengths between 400 nm and 1.4 (micro)m.

Munro, I., McGinty, J., Gallety, N. & Requejo, J. 2005. Toward the clinical application of time-domain fluorescence lifetime imaging. *Journal of Biomedical Optics*.

Niesner, R. & Gericke, H. 2008. Fluorescence lifetime imaging in biosciences: technologies and applications. *Front.Phys. China* 3(1):88–104.

Schweitzer, D. *et al.* 2007. Towards metabolic mapping of human retina. *Microscopy research and technique* 70:410–419.

van Munster, E.B. & Gadella, T. 2005. Fluorescence Lifetime Imaging Microscopy (FLIM). *Adv Biochem Engin/Biotechnol* 95:143–175.

Vieira, P. 1999. Tomographic imaging with a scanning laser ophthalmoscope. *PhD thesis, University of Aberdeen, Scotland.*

Technology and Medical Sciences – Natal Jorge et al. (eds)
© *2011 Taylor & Francis Group, London, ISBN 978-0-415-66822-4*

Measuring the pressure in a laryngoscope blade

A. Silva
Faculty of Engineering, University of Porto, Porto, Portugal

J. Teixeira
Instituto de Ciências Biomédicas Abel Salazar, University of Porto, Porto, Portugal

P. Amorim
Hospital Geral de Santo António, Porto, Portugal
Instituto de Ciências Biomédicas Abel Salazar, Porto, Portugal

J. Gabriel, M. Quintas & R.M. Natal Jorge
IDMEC—Polo FEUP, Faculty of Engineering, University of Porto, Porto, Portugal

ABSTRACT: A laryngoscope is a medical device used to facilitate endotracheal intubation during general anesthesia or mechanical ventilation. Usually, a laryngoscopy can be performed in less than a minute, but requires very precise movements and force control abilities; otherwise, it may result in serious damages to the patient incisors, larynx, spinal column, or significant changes of the vital signals like heart rate and/or blood pressure.

For this study, a laryngoscope blade was covered by a spray ink which is naturally removed in the areas where the contact is more intense, while remaining untouched in the other areas; giving this way a basic picture of the contact pattern.

This paper evaluates the pressure distribution on a Macintosh laryngoscope blade, when a laryngoscopy is performed by experienced doctors and medical students. This technique may be useful to improve the students intubation performance and to diminishing the risk factors of upper-airway patient damages.

Keywords: Laryngoscopy, pressure measurement, endotracheal intubation, anesthesia

1 INTRODUCTION

Usually surgeries are performed under local or general anesthesia, which intend to reach three main objectives: block the muscular activity (to prevent inadequate movement or involuntary spasms that may result in serious injuries for the patient or for the medical staff), the unconsciousness (achieved by an hypnotic drug) and analgesia (to avoid the sense of pain). However, under general anesthesia, one loses his muscular control, and therefore is not anymore able to breathe without assistance, being necessary to receive mechanical ventilation. In general, during a chirurgical procedure, the patient ventilation is achieved using an endotracheal tube that conducts the air directly to his lungs.

The laryngoscope is, in its basic configuration, a simple mechanical device, like the one shown in Figure 1 that helps the introduction of the ventilation tube, by opening the endotracheal cavity. During the Laryngoscopy, the anesthetist places the laryngoscope blade over the patient's tongue,

and slides it back and downwards while forcing the aperture of the throat; then carefully inserts the endotracheal tube that will supply the air and other internal sensing devices.

Usually, a laryngoscopy is a task that can be performed quickly; however it does require very precise movement and force control abilities, which needs well trained professionals. The objective of this work is to introduce a new method that can be used to improve the medical students' skills, by evaluating the pressure distribution applied to the laryngoscope blade. This method consists on the application of an ink film over the lower surface of the blade.

1.1 *Laryngoscopy problems*

During the insertion of the endotracheal tube, the laryngoscope blade subjects the patient internal organs to significant pressure that may cause local mild mucosal edema and problems related with the cardiovascular system, Heiden et al. (1976).

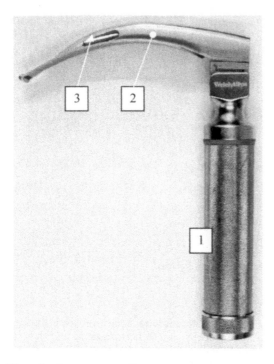

Figure 1. Laryngoscope (Truphatek).

One of the most common claims against intubators' laryngoscope providers are tooth break (Waner et al. 1999, Owen 2000), however only 20% of such cases are reported as "difficult intubation", Tolan et al. (2004). Palatopharyngeal wall perforation during intubation with a laryngoscope is also reported as a problem, Leong et al. (2008). The use of unnecessary force during the Laryngoscopy intervention, excessive large laryngoscope blade and a rigid stylet, have been contributory factors to these complications (Waner et al. 1999, Leong et al. 2008).

In order to reduce risk of such injuries, several approaches have been described in clinical practice as the use of extension position, Lee et al. (2008) video-laryngoscopy, Nishikawa et al. (2009) or face-mask ventilation, Ortega et al. (2007). Despite the presumed safety and efficacy of video-laryngoscopy and disposable laryngoscopes, conventional techniques are still the most used.

1.2 *Proposed approach*

This paper proposes the analysis of the pressure distribution pattern to minimize the above referred problems. This method is not part of the laryngoscope it-self, but can be put in the place quickly and easily and can be used whether in training or in a real situation.

Evaluating the pressure distribution applied to the blade during laryngoscopy in a manikin, can improve trainees' intubation skills curricula. During intubation, inexperienced professionals tend to generate higher force, or taking longer, than experienced intubators (anesthetists and residents) (Bucx et al. 1996; Waddington et al. 2009). In fact, the applied force pulse (force × duration) has shown to be higher for the inexperienced group, largely because of the duration of intubation, Bishop et al. (1992).

Next chapter describes the laryngoscope device and the protocol used for the tests. Chapter three analyses the main results. Finally, chapter four summarizes the main ideas of this work.

2 MATERIALS AND METHODS

2.1 *Laryngoscope*

A laryngoscope is a medical instrument used to perform oral intubation during general anesthesia. It is normally used to facilitate the mechanical ventilation.

For this study, it was used a laryngoscope equipped with a Macintosh blade type, size 3, produced by Truphatek, Figure 1. This instrument is usually composed of two stainless steel parts: a handle (1) and an interchangeable blade (2). The handler incorporates a small white bulb and the respective power batteries. The blade usually includes an optical fiber protected by a stainless steel pipe, to conduct the light to the intervention area (3).

There are several types of blades: Macintosh, Miller, Bullard, Easy Scope, with articulated tip, articulated blade, etc. However, Macintosh type blades are still probably the most commonly used. This blade is characterized by a curved shaped that intends to give more space to the endotracheal tube and better adapt to the thong. In addition, this blade may cause less damage to the teeth, and has fewer tendencies to induce cough. The blade size came in three standard sizes 1, 2 and 3, which should be selected according with the patient physical characteristics.

A direct laryngoscopy is performed with the patient lying down on the surgery bed, while inserting the laryngoscope into the oral cavity. The laryngoscope blade presses downwards the base of the tongue against the lower jaw. With the blade positioned anterior to the epiglottis, the professional should apply a firm moment and force to the handle in order to open the airways path. When applying the force, the laryngoscope handle should be in a position 45° degree from the horizontal, corresponding to the patient body. This task requires a precise combination of upwards and inwards movements in order to produce the desired opening of the oral cavity. Usually, it is necessary less than a minute to place the laryngoscope in the target position and to proceed with the intubation. However, sometimes the patient's physical characteristics may make this task hard to accomplish.

The airways difficulty of the intubation should be previously evaluated in order to minimize possible accidents. One of the common classifications is based on Mallampati scale, which defines four classes (I to IV). In this classification, class III and IV may present an increased intubation difficulty.

Unsuccessful laryngoscopy is normally associated with an high force level and/or a large duration may cause serious damages to the patient incisive teeth, larynx, bruised thong and throat, spinal column or changes in the heart rate and blood-pressure.

2.2 Evaluation procedure

The laryngoscope blade was pulverized with a thin layer of a colored film in order to determine the contact area and the pressure distribution. For this purpose, it was used the Arti-Spray® BK287 (blue color) from Bausch. This is a universal color indicator commonly used in dental medicine to test the oclusal contacts.

After each test, the color layer was firstly removed using simple tap water, and secondly the blade was cleaned and sterilizing, as usually.

2.3 Protocol used with manikin

The protocol established for the laryngoscopy train with manikin was similar to the one used in surgery room situations.

Following the protocol, the blade was connected to the handle and then put in place by rotating 90 degrees. The batteries were placed inside the handler and the bulb light intensity checked.

Before the intubation starts, the lower surface of the blade was pulverized with the Arti-Spray. The pulverization was performed carefully, according to the manufacture instructions (3–5 cm from the surface), this way it was obtained a smooth, thin and uniform layer. In some cases, due to the very good smoothness of the surface, it was necessary to clean the blade and start the process again.

The laryngoscopy was performed with the manikin Laerda® Airway Management Trainer life, upper torso, lying down, and a 7.5 endotracheal tube, as in the surgery room.

3 MAIN RESULTS

During this study, several intubations were performed, some by experienced anesthetists and the others by medical students.

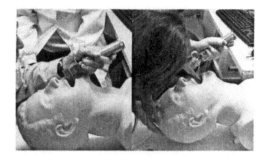

Figure 2. Laryngoscopy intubations: on the left performed by anesthetists, on the right by inexperienced students.

Figure 2 shows a combined picture of a laryngoscopy performed by an anesthetist, on the left side, and an inexperienced student on the right side.

By looking at Figure 2 (left, experienced laryngoscope user), it is visible that the blade is completely inside the patient, letting the bottom surface of the blade contacts in all length with the patient thong. This is the right procedure to achieve the best aperture and easier intubation.

On the other hand, it can be seen on Figure 2 (right, inexperienced user) that the laryngoscope is placed slightly out of the mouth. This position is usually not appropriated. Only the tip of the blade is in contact with the thong which may cause serious damages to the patient. Also, it does not produce the intended result, by reducing the aperture of the throat and making the intubation difficult. Thus, a new attempted has to be taken in order to get a better position which will eventually extends the duration of the laryngoscopy.

After the laryngoscopy, the laryngoscope blade was carefully inspected and photographed to determine the pressure distribution. This was achieved by direct observation of the surface of the blade. Due to the Arti-Spray characteristics, the area with higher friction and pressure had its color removed, while the one with less interaction with the patient is still blue.

Figure 3 bottom surface of the laryngoscope blade after use. It can be seen that the tip of the blade was the most important contact area. In fact, the color film in this area was completely removed, indicating the strongest stress.

In the remaining surface, only the area close to the borders got its color faded, symmetrically, on both sides. Therefore, the pressure was located in the middle of the blade, and well balanced.

A manikin is a good platform that allows medical students to train without risk, which can be complemented with the presented spray technique. This way the laryngoscopy is recorded in the blade surface allowing the comparison with professionals.

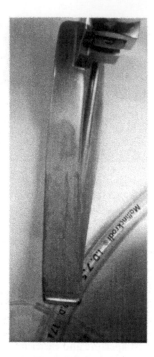

Figure 3. Laryngoscope blade after the laryngoscopy.

4 CONCLUSIONS

A laryngoscope is a stainless steel medical device intended to facilitate the intubation, by opening the oral air-ways path. However, if not well used, it can be responsible for damages in internal organs, namely the throat and the tongue, and also to originate cardiovascular problems.

The aim of the present study was to identify the area of the laryngoscope blade subjected to the maximum pressure, and also its distribution along the blade. For this purpose it was used the spray Arti-Spray, commonly used in dental medicine for oclusal contact check. Although this spray was designed for a completed different use, it showed to be a practical, cheap and useful mean for this purpose. It indicates if the intubation was performed properly, as it shows a different pattern of the spray removed areas, for the two groups: experienced and inexperienced users. With this technique it may be possible to improve the intubation skills of the trainees and diminish the risk factors of the patient upper-airway damage.

It was also clear that in a laryngoscope the pressure is mainly applied closed to the tip, and therefore it confirms the importance of selecting the blade size that matches the patient physical characteristics.

In future, it is planned to conduct tests with different laryngoscope blades and shapes to complement the actual results.

ACKNOWLEDGEMENTS

The authors would like to thank to Fundação para a Ciência e Tecnologia (FCT), for the support given by the project PTDC/EEA-ACR/75454/2006, and also to the University of Porto/Santander Totta by the program "Projectos de Iniciação à Investigação".

A special thanks also to Eng. Jorge Reis, for his collaboration in this project.

REFERENCES

Bucx, M.J., Van der Vegt, M.H., Snijders, C.J. et al. 1996. Transverse forces exerted on the maxillary incisors during laryngoscopy. *Can J Anaesth*, 43(7): 665–671.

Bucx, M.J., Snijders, C.J., Van Geel, R.T.M. et al. 2007. Forces acting on the maxillary incisor teeth during laryngoscopy using Macintosh. *Anaesthesia*, 49(12): 1064–1070.

Bishop, M.J., Harrington, R.M. & Tencer, A.F. 1992. Force applied during tracheal intubation. *Anesth Analg*, 74(3): 411–414.

Heiden, C., Westhues, M. & Kornmesser, H.J. 1976. Side effects and complications following suspension laryngoscopy. *Laryng Rhinol Otol (Stuttgart)*, 55(4): 299–302.

Lee, L. & Weightman, W.M. 2008. Laryngoscopy force in the sniffing position compared to the extension-extension position. *Anaesthesia*, 63(4): 375–378.

Leong, W.L., Lim, Y. & Sia, A.T. 2008. Palatopharyngeal wall perforation during Glidescope intubation. *Anaesth Intensive Care*, 36(6): 870–874.

Nishikawa, K., Matsuoka, H. & Saito, S. 2009. Tracheal Intubation with the Pentax-AWS (Airway Scope) reduces changes of hemodynamic responses and bispectral index scores compared with Macintosh laryngoscope. *J Neurosurg Anaesthesiol*, 21(4): 292–296.

Ortega, F., Mehio, A.K., Woo, A. & Hafez, D.H. 2007. Positive-Pressure ventilation with a face mask and a bag-valve device. *NEJM*, 357, e4, videos in clinical medicine.

Owen, H. & Wadell-Smith, I. 2000. Dental trauma associated with anaesthesia. *Anaesth Intensive Care*, 28: 133–145.

Panacek, E.A., Laurin, E.G. & Bair, A.E. 2009. Fracture of a GlidesScop® Cobalt GVL® Stat disposable blade during an emergency intubation. *J Emerg Med*, (epub a head of print).

Tolan, T.F., Westerfield, S., Irvine, D. & Clark, T. 2004. Dental injuries in anesthesia. Incidence and preventive strategies. ASA annual meeting, Las Vegas, NV, October 2004, *ASA meeting abstract* 2004: A1256.

Waddington, M.S., Paech, M.J., Kurowski, I.H. et al. 2009. The influence of gender and experience on intubation ability and technique: a manikin study. *Anaesth Intensive Care*, 37(5): 791–801.

Waner, M.E., Benenfield, S.M., Mark, A. et al. 1999. Perianesthetic dental injuries. Frequency, outcomes and risc factors. *Anaesthesiology*, 90: 1302–1325.

Technology and Medical Sciences – Natal Jorge et al. (eds)
© 2011 Taylor & Francis Group, London, ISBN 978-0-415-66822-4

Mechanical properties of temporalis muscle: A preliminary study

V.L.A. Trindade, S. Santos, M.P.L. Parente, P. Martins & R.M. Natal Jorge
IDMEC—Faculty of Engineering, University of Porto, Porto, Portugal

A. Santos, L. Santos & J. Fernandes
INML—Instituto Nacional de Medicina Legal, Porto, Portugal

ABSTRACT: The act of chewing involves the use of the four pairs of mastication muscles, the temporalis, masseter and the external and of the pterigoideus. The temporalis integration occurs in the temporal fossa and ends on the anterior mandibular ramus and coronoid apophysis, thus is main function to elevate and retract the mandible [Gray, et al. 1995]. Studying the mastication muscles such as the temporal, it is an important step on understanding the bruxism pathology, which is responsible for many symptoms such as chronic headache, insomnia and sore or painful jaw that affect the patient's life quality. It is an oral parafunctional activity, characterized by the grinding of the teeth and is typically accompanied by the clenching of the jaw occurring mostly during sleep ultimately leading to temporomandibular joint dysfunction [Jadidi, et al. 2007]. This biomechanical study of the temporalis aims to characterize the chosen muscle's behavior by means of the Neo-Hookean constitutive equation and it constant. The method we used was uniaxial tension testes performed on samples collected from a cadaver donor at the National Institute of Legal Medicine (INML). The *Marquart-Leven's* algorithm, presented at [Martins, 2009], was employed to compute the constants associated with each stress-strain graphic to the chosen constitutive model. Afterwards we compared constants by some plotting work in order to determine what would the differences be, between the three samples taken from different areas of the muscle. The conclusions will eventually lead to the recognition of the temporalis importance on the mastication muscles' group and on oral health disorders such as bruxism and temporomandibular joint pathologies.

1 INTRODUCTION

Muscle tissue is highly specialized [Junqueira, et al. 2005]. It has four functional elements: Contractility, excitability, Extensibility and Elasticity. Contractility which is the ability of producing a given muscle twitch force. Excitability which is the muscle's ability to respond to stimuli sent by the nervous system for the skeletal muscles, or by the combination of hormones and nervous system in the case of smooth and cardiac muscle. Extensibility it's the ability of the muscle to be stretched and finally elasticity means that after being stretched, muscles return to their resting length.

1.1 *Types of muscle*

Muscle tissue is comprised of three types according to their morphological and functional characteristics: the skeletal muscle is capable of rapid and vigorous contraction, subject to voluntary control, the heart muscle whose contraction is involuntary, vigorous and rhythmic and the smooth muscle which contraction is subjected to slow and involuntary control.

1.2 *Skeletal muscle*

Skeletal muscle is composed of an orderly arrangement of connective tissue and contractile cells. It is surrounded by an external connective tissue wrapping called the epimysium and it is organized in fascicles, which are bundles of individual muscle cells, each fascicle surrounded also by a tissue layer called the perimysium, as shown in Figure 1.

Within the fascicle, the third connective layer, the endomysium separates an electrically insulates the muscle cells from each other.

1.3 *The temporalis*

The four pairs of mastication muscles are the temporalis, masseter and the external and internal pterigoideus. The temporalis' integration occurs in the temporal fossa and ends on the anterior mandibular ramus and coronoid apophysis, as shown

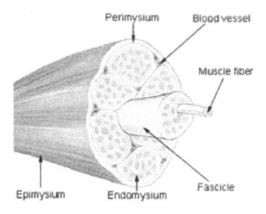

Figure 1. Schematic illustrating revealing the organization of the skeletal muscle. Adapted from [Netter, 2001].

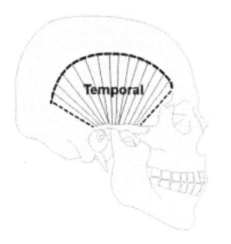

Figure 2. A temporalis after masseter withdrawal.

in the following picture, thus elevating and retracting the mandible.

2 CONSTITUTIVE MODELS

The constitutive models allow the demonstration of the behavior observed in a real material under specific conditions making use of mathematical models. Constitutive equations are a discipline of non-linear mechanics which determines the stress condition of any point for different types of solid bodies. The authors asserted that this material behaves as an incompressible non isotropic one best fitted by the hyperelastic model theory. For hyperelastic materials the constitutive equations are based on Helmholtz's equation of strain energy per unit volume [Lai, et al. 1993].

2.1 Neo-Hookean model

The Neo-Hookean model is acutally an Ogden's reduced version with different boundary conditions with $N = 1$ and $\alpha_1 = 2$ [Ogden, 1984].

The energy function in terms of the stretches is represented in eq. 1,

$$W = c_1(\lambda_1^2 + \lambda_2^2 + \lambda_3^2 - 3) \tag{1}$$

And eq. 2 is the same energy function expressed in terms of the invariants, in this case we only have one invariant,

$$W = c_1(I_1^c - 3) \text{ with } c_1 = \frac{\mu_1}{2} \tag{2}$$

The shear modulusis $\mu_1 = \mu$.

The final Cauchy stress expression given for the uni-axial extension is given by eq. 3, as a function of the uni-axial stretch and the constant c_1,

$$\sigma_{Neo-Hooke} = 2\left(\lambda^2 - \frac{1}{\lambda}\right)c_1 \tag{3}$$

The strain-energy function involves a single parameter only and provides a mathematically simple and reliable constitutive equation for the non-linear deformation behavior of isotropic rubber-like materials. It relies on phenomenological considerations and includes typical effects known from non-linear elasticity within the small strain domain [Holzappfel, 2004].

3 EXPERIMENTAL PROCEDURE

A temporal musclewas harvested from a cadaver donor at the INML (National institute of Legal Medicine) and contained on saline solution at 11°C for no more than 6 hours, after autopsy. The muscle was collected form a twenty years old, male patient not expired from traumatic head injury.

The state of dentition was thoroughly listed and presented itself on Figure 3.

The nomenclature used to distinguish the teething is based on the model used by INML professionals. From numbers 11 to 18 and 41 to 48 it's considered the left side of the mouth; as such the remaining numbers belong to the right side of the mouth. The present donor lacked 14, 47 and 48 teeth, as such most of the mouth teething was complete.

Before testing the muscle had to undergo dissection of the fascia and tendon structures form the actual muscle. Each of the three samples was carefully cut into a rectangular shape parallel to the fibers, avoiding as much as possible unnecessary

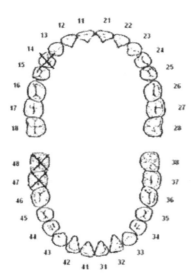

Figure 3.   Dental disposition's draft.

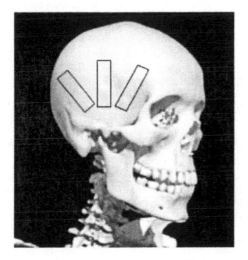

Figure 4.   The rectangles lying on the skull represent the samples' direction and approximate geometry although not at scale [McMinn, 2002].

indentations, from posterior, central and anterior areas of the muscle.

3.1   *The uni-axial tensile tests*

The BM laboratory is equipped with a uni-axial tensile testing machine monitored with a Linear Variable Differential Transformer (LVDT) a displacement measuring instrument.

All data and observations were collected and registered at the time. Subsequently an algorithm presented at [Martins, 2009], was employed to compute the constants associated with each

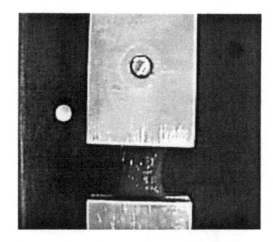

Figure 5.   Picture of one sample taken before the test.

stress-strain graphic to the Neo-Hookean constitutive model.

4   RESULTS

The calculated constants based on *Neo-Hooke* material model and on the experimental data resulted on Table 1.

According to equation 3, we can calculate the stress in the body once you have the constant c_1, hence we have done the necessary plotting of the stress-strain graphics resulting from the calculated constants.

Comparing different stress values reached at the maximum computed stretch, it is noticeable that central sample is the stiffer of all three samples which according to the numbers is a correct assumption as its maximum stress value is 60% higher than the anterior sample. The posterior sample coincides with the mean plot and has about 30% lower maximum stress values when compared to the central sample. Apparently the temporal muscle not only has got different morphological characteristics, like dissimilar thickness throughout it, but also has different levels of stiffness.

Apparently the temporal muscle not only has got different morphological characteristics, like dissimilar thickness throughout it, but also has different levels of stiffness.

The maximum stress reachable at a stretch of 1,5 points is of 0,1332 MPa, for this set of computed samples.

Observing Figure 7, we can see that that Neo-Hookean model does fit's poorly the experimental data curve because of its clear convex shape in contrast to the linearity of the Hookean based plot. The maximum stresses recorded for each of

175

Table 1. The computed constants for each sample. Number 1 is referred to the anterior, number 2 was taken from the central area and number 3 is from the posterior part of the muscle.

Sample	c_1	Area
1	0,0412	Anterior
2	0,0736	Central
3	0,0554	Posterior
Mean	0,05673	–

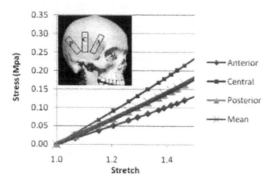

Figure 6. The constant plots and the mean of the constants plot.The letter A stands for anterior, C for central and P for posterior in the skull drawing.

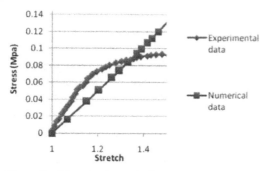

Figure 7. The experimental plot and the numerically obtained plot using the Neo-Hookean model.

the cases are dissimilar, as the numerical results are 18% higher than the experimental ones.

5 CONCLUSIONS

In conclusion the temporal muscle is a morphologically complex structure with different thicknesses and different stiffness throughout the entire system.

Applying the Neo-Hookean model to this non-linear biological tissue may not be a good idea as it didn't behave as well as expected in comparison with the experimental results. There are differences in stiffness within this muscle between the three considered areas. The central area is for this case the stiffer followed by the posterior and finally by the anterior area.

Future work will consist in revalidate this experimental procedure for multiple samples, using this model and others like the Mooney—Rivlin Model and the Yeoh model for hyperelastic materials, for example.

REFERENCES

Holzappfel, G.A. 2004. *Non-linear Solid Mechanics*. John Wiley & Sons, Ltd.
Junqueira, L.C. & Carneiro, J. 2005. *Histologia Básica*. Guanabara Koogan 10ª edição.
Lai, M.W., Rubin, D. Krempl, E., 1993. *Introduction to Continuum Mechanics*. Butterworth Heinmann, 3th Edition.
Martins, P., Peña, E., Calvo, B. Doblaré, M., Mascarenhas, T., Natal Jorge, R.M. & Ferreira, A.J.M. 2009. "Desenvolvimento de software interactivo para optimizar os parâmetros de modelos materiais hiperelásticos. *Congreso de Métodos Numéricos en Ingeniería 2009*, A. Huerta *et al.* (Eds), Livro de Resumos 379.
McMinn, 2002. *McMinn's Color Atlas of Human Anatomy*. Elsevier Science.
Netter, F.H., 2001. *Atlas de Anatomia Humana*. Icon Learning Systems.
Ogden, R.W., 1984. *Non-linear Elastic Deformations*. Dover Publication, Inc.

Technology and Medical Sciences – Natal Jorge et al. (eds)
© 2011 Taylor & Francis Group, London, ISBN 978-0-415-66822-4

Medial-lateral CoP-rearfoot relation during stance

T.J.V. Atalaia
Portuguese Red Cross Health School, Lisbon, Portugal

J.M.C.S. Abrantes
MovLab / CICANT / Lusófona University of Humanities and Technology, Lisbon, Portugal

ABSTRACT: *Objective:* The objective of this study is to find out synchronized Center of Pressure (CoP) and Rearfoot Angle (RA) data specifically related to the subject's gender and their left and right walking stance phase. *Subjects:* 15 masculine ($21{,}87 \pm 2{,}83$ years) and 15 feminine ($21{,}87 \pm 3{,}29$) with no lower limb injuries or injury past history. *Methods:* The gait cycle stance phase CoP in three different instants of Ground Reaction Force (RsScan pressure plate) and the synchronized RA data have been computed. Each performer replicated 10 trials for each left and right walking stance phase. Inter- and intra-individual data were statistically analyzed. *Results:* A significant relation was found between CoP and RA ($p < 0{,}05$ and $p < 0{,}01$), with different behaviors between left and right walking stance phase and gender. *Conclusions:* Different left and right stance behavior linking CoP, RA and gender should be considered in assessment procedures. Technology associated to the Biomechanics of Human Movement is a contribution for clinicians.

Keywords: Center of Pressure, Rearfoot Angle, Biomechanics, Gender differences

1 INTRODUCTION

Global functional analysis helps functional diagnosis and the understanding of patient/environment interaction and adaptation. Clinical Biomechanics allow this analysis, not by applyinglaws of physicsto the human body, but by assessing the motor strategy output in order to achieve the motor task objective. By combining kinematic and kinetic data, one can study joint stability and calculate how the system *had* controlled observed movement, thus assuming Biomechanicsan important complementary exam resource for clinicians (Abrantes, 2008). Joint stability can be defined as the joint's active component ability to control angular displacement along a path during a task, allowing the system to produce and dissipate muscle power towards intersegment energy transfer during locomotion (Abrantes, 2008; Gabriel, *et al.*, 2008). This ability depends on the subject's movement history upon which movement experience is compared towards feedback and feedfoward anticipatory behaviors production (Docherty, Arnold, Zinder, Granata & Gansneder, 2004). This is usually called dynamic joint stiffness as defined by (Davis & DeLuca, 1996), which reflects the joint stability process and its neurophysiologic control mechanism, allowing the study of co-contraction

contribution to joint stability (Houdijk, Doets, van Middelkoop & Dirkjan Veeger, 2008), and giving relevance to the believes of Von Holst & Mittelstaedt (1950 & 1973) and Bernstein (1967), as mentioned by Ostry & Feldman(2003), that mechanical language is not enough to explain and comprehend neuromuscular systems.

In addition, the gender influence strategy outcome in motor pattern, with female subjects less effective in dynamic stiffness control attributed to increase range of motion due to decrease of passive joint stability, which means that active joint response and passive joint response are interdependent (Gabriel, 1999; Gabriel, *et al.*, 2001; Granata, Padua & Wilson, 2002). On the other hand, human anticipatory behavior suggest a neural representation of limb dynamics and task environment equipped with motor commands suitable to adequate kinematic output (Dounskaia, 2005).

Changes in joint stability are caused by mechanical and functional reasons, in respect to the ankle joint, where mechanics refer to a decrease of joint position sense and function to decrease of effectiveness of active response, allowing dysfunctional motor patterns to develop and be learned (O'Loughlin, Hodgkins & Kennedy, 2008).

In summary, joint stability can be measured by dynamic joint stiffness, which reflects the ability of active control of joint position along a determinate path, defined by motor task objective and by considering the task environment. The increase in joint angular velocity can be seen as joint ineffective control that leads to different adaptation strategies to allow task achievement. The measure of this dysfunction or its control level gives the clinician objective data of therapeutic effectiveness.

The Center of Pressure (CoP) behavior during stance or gait is used to study the joint control strategy in normal subjects, as with different types of movement dysfunctions that have different etiologies (Fernandes & Abrantes, 2004; Hallemans, De Clercq, Van Dongen & Aerts, 2006; Robain, Valentini, Renard-Deniel, Chennevelle & Piera, 2006; Schweigart & Mergner, 2008; Termoz, et al., 2008; Winter, 2005). Since its description by Roos et al., in 1977, the Rearfoot Angle (RA) is used to classify foot types (Donatelli, et al., 1999) by relating rearfoot to tibia. Dynamically, it can be used to describe frontal angular variations during gait stance of subtalar joint inversion and eversion movements (Razeghi & Batt, 2002). To measure RA, a four mark protocol is described by some authors (Donatelli, et al., 1999; Razeghi & Batt, 2002). Figure 1 shows the location of the four markers.

There are some doubts over the clinical relevance of this measure. Some authors point out a weak relation between static and dynamic measures of RA (Cornwall & McPoil, 2004), but in our opinion, they didn't take into consideration the non deterministic behavior of human movement or the difference in motor planning to execute or maintain the given tasks. By omitting the performer in their analysis, the individual specificity of the motor behavior wasn't included, which can lead to an incomplete interpretation of performance outputs.

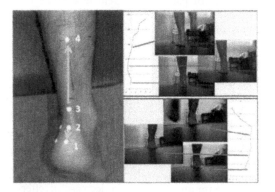

Figure 1. Location of the segment markers do define Rearfoot Angle and CoP pathway and related reafoot markers in three selected instants of walking stance phase.

To the 6th International Conference on Technology and Medical Sciences, we propose a simple and objective study about the medial-lateral relationship between Center of Pressure (CoP) and Rearfoot Angle (RA) during stance phase, showing the importance of knowing the neuromuscular system strategy in a specific motor task. This study within this Conference is a contribution to the technology meaning demonstration of how a very simple tool can simplify Clinical Biomechanics analysis. The objective of this study is to find out synchronized Center of Pressure (CoP) and RA data specifically related to the subject's gender and their left and right walking stance phase.

2 MATERIALS AND METHODS

In this study, 30 normal subjects participated, 15 males (21,87 ± 2,83 years old) and 15 females (21,87 ± 3,29 years old). Subjects with a history of ankle injury (present or past) weren't included.

The data of gait cycle stance phase Center of Pressure (CoP) and the vertical component of the Ground Reaction Force (GRF) was recorded at 100 Hz by the 1 meter *Footscan® 3D Gait Scientific System* 3D (RsScan® International- Belgium), placed in the middle of a 8 meter gait corridor. The same system was used to determinate the CoP's coordinates on GRF of heel contact (F0), foot contact (F1) and mid stance (F2). Those data has been synchronized with the RA 25 Hz data recorded by a small size wireless video camera (model 34426, Chacon) located at the beginning of the pressure plate. The video was later transformed into photogram's (*Kinovea®* freeware software). The segment markers coordinates were obtained by digitalization (*DigitizeXY* 3.0ᴷ freeware software). The markers located on the rearfoot defined the spatial coordinates in each picture as showed in Figure 1 were the CoP path coordinates F0, F1 and F2 is presented with the synchronized video of the rearfoot view for each of the instants observed. The RA was computed by scalar product of the two vectors delimited by the markers defined above, as shown in Figure 1. Polar coordinates of CoP position were used to correlate with RA, giving attention to the "Phi" value, where the increase or decrease corresponds to CoP medial or lateral displacement.

Each subject performed 20 trials, 10 for each foot. To decrease the target behavior upon subjects, a three steps protocol was used (Bus & de Lange, 2005).

A relation between leg and rearfoot was needed to study the rearfoot angle. This relation can occur in different scenarios concerning leg and rearfoot position and its relation to the ground surface.

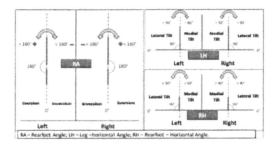

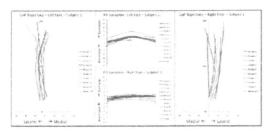

Figure 2. Relations between RA and leg/horizontal (LH) and rearfoot/horizontal (RH) angles.

Figure 4. Example of CoP and RA behavior for each foot on measured positions.

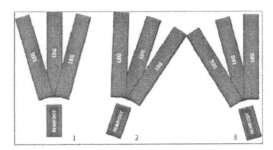

Figure 3. Relation leg/rearfoot at the three spatial rearfoot orientation possibilities.

Because CoP is a measure conducted on the surface, to fully understand RA behavior, two more angles were considered: Leg—Horizontal (LH) and Rearfoot—Horizontal (RH). These angles describe the leg or rearfoot segment position related to horizontal plane. As it can be observed in the angles relation presented in Figure 2, the same position of RA can occur in three different position of leg and rearfoot in the space as explicit in Figure 3, meaning that this should be take into consideration when analyzing CoP behavior. Statistically the data was analyzed inter and intra individual using Pearson Correlation Coefficient.

3 RESULTS

In Figure 4, an example of all trials for a single subject, considering CoP and RA behavior, can be observed. We verify that in each trial, the same subject presents different behaviors of CoP and RA. Each trial then, reflects a different strategy. Because of this, mean values of this behavior lead to different relations between CoP behavior and RA behavior, more if we consider the different positions present in both leg and rearfoot as explicit in Figure 3, all trials were considered as single strategies towards goal achievement and therefore isolated behaviors.

Pearson correlation used to verify the relation between CoP medial-lateral displacement and RA (plus LH and RH angles) angular variation in the three defined points find outsignificant correlations ($p < 0,05$ and $p < 0,01$) as we can see in Table 1, referring to right and left stance of all subjects, and the correlation in order to subjects gender.

In Table 2, the strength of correlation between CoP and RH and LH angles can be observed.

Considering male subjects' right foot stance, it show's at F0 a CoP in a lateral position related to angular behavior, consisting in a medial tilt of LH and RH. The same angular tendency shows that stability strategy seems to maintain angular position more than by changing RA using inversion-eversion movements at the Subtalar Joint (SJ).

In F1, this tendency changes. To CoP lateral displacement, RH responds with a medial tilt and LH with a lateral tilt, conducting to an inversion tendency in RA. In F2, no relations were found between CoP and angular displacement.

Male subjects' left foot stance shows at F0 a CoP lateral position to which a medial tilt of LH and CH (maintaining RA position) was associated. This behavior continues during F1 and changes at F2 with LH and RH adopting a lateral tilt behavior. This leads to a strategy in which maintenance of RA position is pretended.

Female subjects' right foot stance at F0 associate CoP lateral position to a lateral tilt of LH and RH angles, turning into medial tilt LH and RH angles in F1 and keeping the same behavior during F2, showing a strategy to maintain RA positioned during the stance.

Female subjects' left foot stance at F0 show lateral tilt LH and medial tilt RH, meaning a tendency to RA eversion. In F1, the tendency changes to medial tilt LH and lateral RH, conducting to a RA inversion. In F2, the system returns to F0 behavior.

4 DISCUSSION

In normal subjects, the non deterministic behavior is the first aspect to be given relevance. The CoP

Table 1. Pearson Coeficient between CoP medial-l ateral displacement and RA. Accessory angles RH and LH also shown.

	All Trials						Male Subjects						Female Subjects					
	Left Ankle			Right Ankle			Left Ankle			Right Ankle			Left Ankle			Right Ankle		
	RA	RH	LH	RA	RH	LH	RA	RH	LH	RA	RH	LH	RA	RH	LH	RA	RH	LH
Phi	s/r	s/r	p≤0,05	s/r	p≤0,05	s/r	s/r	p≤0,05	p≤0,05	s/r	p≤0,01	s/r	s/r	s/r	p≤0,01	s/r	p≤0,05	p≤0,01
F0 RA		s/r	p≤0,01		p≤0,01	p≤0,01		p≤0,01	p≤0,01		p≤0,01	p≤0,01		p≤0,05	p≤0,05		p≤0,05	p≤0,01
RH			p≤0,01			p≤0,01			p≤0,01			p≤0,01			s/r			p≤0,05
Phi	s/r	s/r	s/r	p≤0,05	s/r	p≤0,05	s/r	s/r	s/r	s/r	p≤0,05	p≤0,05	p≤0,01	s/r	p≤0,01	s/r	p≤0,01	s/r
F1 RA		p≤0,01	p≤0,01		p≤0,01	p≤0,01		p≤0,01	p≤0,05		p≤0,01	p≤0,01		p≤0,01	p≤0,01		p≤0,01	s/r
RH			p≤0,01			p≤0,01			p≤0,01			p≤0,01			s/r			p≤0,01
Phi	s/r	s/r	s/r	p≤0,05	s/r	p≤0,05	s/r	p≤0,05	s/r	s/r	s/r	s/r	p≤0,05	s/r	p≤0,01	p≤0,05	s/r	s/r
F2 RA		p≤0,01	p≤0,01		p≤0,01	p≤0,01		p≤0,01	p≤0,01		p≤0,01	p≤0,01		p≤0,01	p≤0,01		p≤0,01	s/r
RH			p≤0,01			p≤0,01			p≤0,01			p≤0,01			s/r			p≤0,01

Table 2. Strenght of correlation between Phi CoP value and angular variation.

Stance	Instant	Male	Female
Right	F0	Phi↓RH↑LH↑	Phi↓RH↓LH↓
	F1	Phi↓RH↓LH↑	Phi↓RH↑LH↑
	F2	s/r	Phi↓RH↓LH↑
Left	F0	Phi↑RH↓LH↓	Phi↑RH↓LH↑
	F1	Phi↑RH↓LH↓	Phi↑RH↑LH↓
	F2	Phi↑RH↑LH↑	Phi↑RH↓LH↑

and angles variation were different between trials in each subject and between subjects. Because of this variation and inter dependence between CoP and angles, the mean value of CoP and angles could not reflect the real association between them nor their behavior.

This is supported by (Abrantes, 2006, 2008) and makesit difficult to accept studies where human motor behavior is considered only in its mean value. Depending on the variables that were considered in this assumption, cold leads to a lack of real movement representation. For some authors, the most frequent behavior tendency should be the best value to take from data analysis. This tendency reflects a common behavior, more precisely, a group of movements that are similar and repeated along time—the basic definition of movement pattern. In Table 1, the Phi polar coordinate of CoP behavior appearsrelated to the angles studied when the data was analyzed by gender. This supports the believes of(Granata, et al., 2002), who say that changes in movement occur between gender with increase angular variation to female subjects. Considering by gender analysis, in F2, there is a small relation, possibly due to anterior load transfer as described by (Cote, Brunet, Gansneder, & Shultz, 2005), which is controlled through an anterior-posterior strategy with less participation of subtalar joint medial-lateral variation. If the observed behavior is considered, the RA can give significant information, not bycomparison between static and dynamic tasks like (Cornwall & McPoil, 2004) did, but by observing it during the performance of adefined task. Static and dynamic behaviors have different motor programs and strategies, as referred by several authors (Gabriel, 1999; Patla, Ishac & Winter, 2002; Schweigart & Mergner, 2008; Winter, 1995; Winter & Eng, 1995; Winter, Patla, Ishac & Gage, 2003; Winter, Patla, Prince, Ishac & Gielo-Perczak, 1998; Winter, Patla, Rietdyk & Ishac, 2001). By other hand, the no significant correlation genders behavior it is in accordance with other previous joint stability studies (Gabriel, et al., 2008; Granata, et al., 2002).

5 CONCLUSION

Human Movement is a non deterministic phenomenon emerging from a motor behavior that is unique in association with joint stability strategy. This motor behavior seems to be different between male and female subjects.

Independently of gender difference, we must point out that each subject performed different solutions in order to achieve the same motor task. Frontal kinematic changes at the ankle joint seem to be used as an adjustment strategy to control movement disturbance.

The existence of different left and right stance behavior linking CoP, RA and gender should be considered in assessment procedures.

Technology associated to the Biomechanics of Human Movement is a contribution for clinicians.

REFERENCES

Abrantes, J. (2006). Biomecânica da Estabilidade Articular. Rev. Bras. Educ. Fis. Esporte, 20, 87–90.

Abrantes, J. (2008). *Fundamentos e Elementos de Análise em Biomecânica do Movimento Humano*. MovLab—Universidade Lusófona de Humanidadese Tecnologias Lisboa. Avaiable online at: http://movlab.ulusofona. pt/cms/index.php?option=com_content & view=article&id=159&Itemid=196&lang=pt

Bus, S.A. & de Lange, A. (2005). A comparison of the 1-step, 2-step, and 3-step protocols for obtaining barefoot plantar pressure data in the diabetic neuropathic foot. Clin Biomech (Bristol, Avon), 20(9), 892–899.

Cornwall, M. & McPoil, T. (2004). Influence of rearfoot postural alignment on rearfoot motion during walking. The Foot(14), 133–138.

Cote, K.P., Brunet, M.E., Gansneder, B.M. & Shultz, S.J. (2005). Effects of Pronated and Supinated Foot Postures on Static and Dynamic Postural Stability. J Athl Train, 40(1), 41–46.

Davis, R. & DeLuca, P. (1996). Gait Characterization via Dynamic Joint Stiffness. Gait Posture, 4, 224–231.

Docherty, C.L., Arnold, B.L., Zinder, S.M., Granata, K. & Gansneder, B.M. (2004). Relationship between two proprioceptive measures and stiffness at the ankle. J Electromyogr Kinesiol, 14(3), 317–324.

Donatelli, R., Wooden, M., Ekedahl, S.R., Wilkes, J.S., Cooper, J. & Bush, A.J. (1999). Relationship between static and dynamic foot postures in professional baseball players. J Orthop Sports Phys Ther, 29(6), 316–325; discussion 326–330.

Dounskaia, N. (2005). The internal model and the leading joint hypothesis: implications for control of multi-joint movements. Exp Brain Res, 166(1), 1–16.

Fernandes, O. & Abrantes, J. (2004). Centro de Pressão como Indicador da Estabilidade Articular. Revista Portuguesa de Ciências do Desporto(4), 280.

Gabriel, R. (1999). *Biomecânica da Estabilidade Articular.* Universidade de Trás-os-Montes e Alto Douro, Vila Real.

Gabriel, R., Abrantes, J., Mourão, A., Filipe, V., Melo-Pinto, P. & Bulas-Cruz, J. (2001). Dynamic Joint Stiffness of the Ankle During Walking Displacement Plane Change (pp. 28–29). Zurich—Switzerland: XVIII Congress of the International Society of Biomechanics.

Gabriel, R.C., Abrantes, J., Granata, K., Bulas-Cruz, J., Melo-Pinto, P. & Filipe, V. (2008). Dynamic joint stiffness of the ankle during walking: gender-related differences. Phys Ther Sport, 9(1), 16–24.

Granata, K.P., Padua, D.A. & Wilson, S.E. (2002). Gender differences in active musculoskeletal stiffness. Part II. Quantification of leg stiffness during functional hopping tasks. J Electromyogr Kinesiol, 12(2), 127–135.

Hallemans, A., De Clercq, D., Van Dongen, S. & Aerts, P. (2006). Changes in foot-function parameters during the first 5 months after the onset of independent walking: a longitudinal follow-up study. Gait Posture, 23(2), 142–148.

Houdijk, H., Doets, H.C., van Middelkoop, M. & Dirkjan Veeger, H.E. (2008). Joint stiffness of the ankle during walking after successful mobile-bearing total ankle replacement. Gait Posture, 27(1), 115–119.

O'Loughlin, P.F., Hodgkins, C.W. & Kennedy, J.G. (2008). Ankle sprains and instability in dancers. Clin Sports Med, 27(2), 247–262.

Ostry, D.J. & Feldman, A.G. (2003). A critical evaluation of the force control hypothesis in motor control. Exp Brain Res, 153(3), 275–288.

Patla, A.E., Ishac, M.G. & Winter, D.A. (2002). Anticipatory control of center of mass and joint stability during voluntary arm movement from a standing posture: interplay between active and passive control. Exp Brain Res, 143(3), 318–327.

Razeghi, M., & Batt, M.E. (2002). Foot type classification: a critical review of current methods. Gait Posture, 15(3), 282–291.

Robain, G., Valentini, F., Renard-Deniel, S., Chennevelle, J.M. & Piera, J.B. (2006). [A baropodometric parameter to analyze the gait of hemiparetic patients: the path of center of pressure]. Ann Readapt Med Phys, 49(8), 609–613.

Schweigart, G. & Mergner, T. (2008). Human stance control beyond steady state response and inverted pendulum simplification. Exp Brain Res, 185, 635–653.

Termoz, N., Halliday, S.E., Winter, D.A., Frank, J.S., Patla, A.E. & Prince, F. (2008). The control of upright stance in young, elderly and persons with Parkinson's disease. Gait Posture, 27(3), 463–470.

Winter, D.A. (1995). Human balance and posture control during standing and walking. Gait Posture, 3, 193–214.

Winter, D.A. (2005). *Biomechanics and Motor Control of Human Movement* (3ª Ed ed.). New Jersey: John Wiley and Sons, Inc.

Winter, D.A. & Eng, P. (1995). Kinetics: our window into the goals and strategies of the central nervous system. Behav Brain Res, 67(2), 111–120.

Winter, D.A., Patla, A.E., Ishac, M. & Gage, W.H. (2003). Motor mechanisms of balance during quiet standing. J Electromyogr Kinesiol, 13(1), 49–56.

Winter, D.A., Patla, A.E., Prince, F., Ishac, M., & Gielo-Perczak, K. (1998). Stiffness control of balance in quiet standing. J Neurophysiol, 80(3), 1211–1221.

Winter, D.A., Patla, A.E., Rietdyk, S. & Ishac, M.G. (2001). Ankle muscle stiffness in the control of balance during quiet standing. J Neurophysiol, 85(6), 2630–2633.

Technology and Medical Sciences – Natal Jorge et al. (eds)
© *2011 Taylor & Francis Group, London, ISBN 978-0-415-66822-4*

Multidisciplinary interactions for the development of medical devices

Ricardo Simoes

Polytechnic Institute of Cávado and Ave, School of Technology, Campus do IPCA, Barcelos, Portugal
Institute for Polymers and Composites IPC / I3N, University of Minho, Guimarães, Portugal

ABSTRACT: The development of medical devices is becoming increasingly complex, with the advent of information technologies and continuous advances in micro and nanotechnologies. Moreover, the demands in terms of performance, costs and other requisites of these devices have also become stricter. If, on the one hand, the results are clearly positive for society in terms of better health services (and the arguable improvement of the quality of life), on the other hand, there is the need to involve people from a variety of fields in the development process, and the tasks of planning and coordinating the implementation of a development strategy are ever more paramount. This paper presents some considerations about the product development cycle and the need for multidisciplinary teams in the product design and development processes of medical devices. Subsequently, the work methods and communication channels within the team, and the organization and coordination of that team are analyzed. Finally, a case-study is presented of a university-industry project, involving healthcare providers, for the development of a new health support system comprised of different types of medical devices. This project encompassed all the stages of PDD up to the laboratory-stage and establishing the main requisites for industrial productification. The developed system was implemented and is currently being field-tested.

Keywords: medical devices, multidisciplinary development, product design and development

1 INTRODUCTION

As products are becoming increasingly complex, the Product Design and Development (PDD) processes are also evolving into collaborative multidisciplinary team processes. This creates new challenges, both for product development, but also in project management. In the case of medical devices, this is further complicated by rigorous specifications and regulatory requirements (Zenios et al. 2009), as well as the fact that the development process requires strong interaction with multiple individuals, with the concept of end-user depending on the specific device. It is this important to understand how the PDD process can be planned for and managed in the case of medical devices, whether they are a single biometric device or a complex information coordination system (Alexander et al. 2002). This paper follows previous studies on product design specifications (Simoes, 2009), wireless networks for health monitoring (Lopez et al. 2010), communication platforms for medical data (Pereira et al. 2010), embedded microelectronics (Sampaio et al. 2009), and performance evaluation of ZigBee networks (Lopez et al. 2009).

This paper starts by describing the life cycle of novel medical devices in the current context of increased complexity and performance demands.

The second chapter focuses on the laboratory development stage, with the goal of obtaining a fully functional product, although typically not optimized for production and not sufficiently competitive for the market. The actors and their respective roles are described, namely in the framework of user-centered design, with emphasis on the development team. In fact, for a successful outcome, a plethora of different people have to become involved in the project.

It is also important to establish how to get from user wants and needs to partial Product Design Specifications (PDS). These need to be understood by people from different areas, requiring agile and effective communication among team members. The PDS are partial due to the fact that many specifications only need to be defined (and in fact, can only be defined due to insufficient knowledge) at the industrial productification stage.

Some specifications must even be jointly specified by team members of different expertise. Thus, an analysis is provided in the third section on the multidisciplinary integration within the development team and communication between this team and the different other actors that are essential for a successful product development process.

In large projects, and particularly when multidisciplinary teams are involved, the role of coordination becomes pivotal, and it is very important to understand some of the characteristics of how that can be effectively achieved. This is the goal of section 4.

In the fifth chapter, a case-study is succinctly described, where several different areas of expertise were brought together in a multidisciplinary team, working closely together with different healthcare professionals, resulting in a health support system that includes biometric devices, communication networks, and information systems technology.

2 LIFE CYCLE OF NOVEL PRODUCTS

2.1 Main phases

Medical devices are typically developed either by:

- companies within the scope of their business plan;
- research teams at Universities or R&D Centers within the scope of their ongoing research activities on healthcare or a specific research project.

These two cases may appear very different at first sight. However, in both cases there are, almost inevitably, two different development stages; see Figure 1. The first stage results in a fully functional device but not optimized to be market competitive. A second stage is required, where many specifications and product features are revised, and several aspects which could (or had to) be left openare defined.

The difference between these two stages being conducted wholly within a single company or the first stage in a research unit and the second in a company (either through patenting or through a spin-off or a start-up) pertains essentially to:

- The extent of communication between the teams intervening in those two stages;
- Agility of the transfer process;
- Ability to retain members of the first stage team in the second stage team.

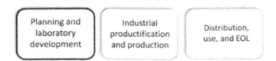

Figure 1. Stages in the life cycle of novel medical devices.

After the industrial productification stage, come all other stages of a product life cycle, such as distribution, end-of-life handling, etc, undoubtedly important, but outside the scope of this paper. Obviously, these later stages may have a large impact into decisions made for the development of subsequent versions of the product or future related products.

2.2 Focus of this study

This work focuses on the first development stage, conducted by a research team, with a fully functional, albeit laboratory-state prototype, being pursued.

3 THE LABORATORY DEVELOPMENT PROCESS

3.1 Actors and roles

One of the key features of current development practices in the field of medical devices is the involvement of health professionals from the start. This type of collaborative development, following widespread approaches such as living labs, translational research, or the most traditional subcontracting the advice of expert healthcare professionals, is currently regarded as most effective and followed by the major companies in the field.

Independently of the degree of interaction between the development team and the end-users, these two main groups are vital elements of the process, as shown in Figure 2.

Thus, on one side, we have the development team, responsible for the scientific development and technical implementation of the prototype solution.

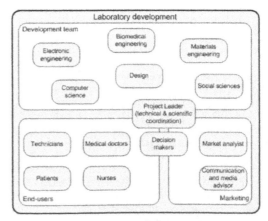

Figure 2. Typical actors involved in the laboratory-stage product development cycle of novel medical devices.

For most medical devices, development teams have to incorporate researchers from a variety of fields, such as electronic engineering, computer science, biomedical engineering, materials engineering, design, and social sciences. The formation and inner working of these teams is further explored in §3.2.

On the other side, we have end-users (various healthcare professionals and patients), marketing professionals, and decision makers (e.g. health provider facilities administrators):

- *Medical doctors*: They are the key interface between scientific research and field practice. Thus, they must be an integral part of the development, from concept development and selection, setting PDS (including technical and non-technical requirements), and product validation (including field trials). Their opinions will be collected by decision makers and thus they must find added value in the new products compared to previous solutions (if they exist). Their level of involvement and contribution to the project will naturally affect their opinion of the product.
- *Nurses*: Very often they will be the ones using the device. Even if not, they will be responsible for one of the following: setting it up, making it available to doctors, or giving it to patients. Their role is pivotal and their opinions should be collected from early development stages. It is important for them to validate the device.
- *Technicians*: Important to establish the physical placement/embedding of devices and equipment in the facility, interacting with existing computer networks and communication grids. Any changes required on the existing infrastructure or service practices will be difficult (due to the strict requisites and certifications in healthcare) and should be planned well in advance.
- *Patients*: It is vital to develop medical devices in a user-centered approach. In many cases, users are doctors or nurses, but often they are patients. In these cases, they should be involved from the earliest development stages.
- *Market analysts*: They should provide detailed information about current and upcoming technologies and solutions, trends in the specific field of the product being developed, and should also be involved in setting some PDS (e.g. cost).
- *Communication and media advisors*: Not only should they be involved in planning dissemination and advertising of the developed product, but they should create a plan for enticing the media, particularly for highly innovative devices.

On the end-user side, all these professionals are coordinated essentially by a few decision makers, such as hospital administrators (or board), or private healthcare facilities owners. These decision makers often have a technical or medical background, but will collect advice from their key staff on most decisions about the selection of health technologies or investing in new products. The bridge between the development team and all other actors, including the decision makers, marketing, and healthcare professionals, has to be coordinated by the project leader.

3.2 *The development team*

As previously stated, development teams have to incorporate researchers from a variety of fields:

- *Electronic engineering*: sensors, actuators, communication hardware/protocols, data processing.
- *Computer science/Information Systems*: data communication, data storage, data mining, security protocols, user interfaces.
- *Biomedical engineering*: usability, hardware, medical data acquisition and interpretation.
- *Materials engineering*: materials selection, device housing/casing, user interfaces.
- *Design*: user profiles, concept development, ergonomics, aesthetics, interfaces, device housing.
- *Social sciences*: user-perception of devices, user needs, questionnaires and interpretation, epidemiological aspects.

Obviously, the composition of the team is highly dependent on the specific device, but currently most devices will require tackling at least some of the competences listed for each of the fields of expertise above. It is thus not surprising to find teams will be based on the above listed competences, in some cases complemented by others with specific expertise.

One should notice that the only reason the development team roster above does not include clinical staff and medical doctors is because this discussion assumes the team is working cooperatively in close collaboration with those professionals, following the development approaches listed in §3.1.

3.3 *Understanding wants and needs*

On the earlier stages of the development process, methods such as Ethnographic Research and Voice of the Costumer can be employed to assess and understand user wants and user needs. These methods can help translating the 'needs and wants' of the user into product requirements and features. If the project is planned and implemented following a user-centered approach, identifying the best methods to be used for this purpose should not be a problem.

3.4 Product Design Specifications (PDS)

Pugh is one of the few authors dealing with this issue in some depth (Pugh, 1991). He compiled a comprehensive list of types of specifications, in a wide range of aspects of the product development process. In this work, namely in §4, we analyze and classify the PDS, based on Pugh's list, which we believe helps in selecting specifications for a particular project. A better understanding of specifications and their role on the product development process is required, particularly in the current trend of faster obsolescence and increasing complexity of products (Simoes and Sampaio, 2008).

The team will have to define a set of PDS at the early laboratory development stage. However, this will only be a partial PDS, since: a) the team does not have sufficient understanding of the problem and sufficient definition of the solution to set some of the specifications at this stage, and b) there is no need to establish specifications that will not affect the final output of the laboratory development process.

During the laboratory development stage, the key PDS to set are those that have a direct impact on the selection of concepts and solutions, selection of technologies (such as a communication standard), or usability. This is shown schematically in Figure 3.

In Figure 3, PDS are represented with respect to when they are set along the development process, considering two large stages: laboratory development and industrial productification. A bold PDS border implies a primary PDS, whereas dashed lines imply secondary PDS. Also, some PDS are shown stretching between phases, which implies they are either: 1) set in the first stage and revised in the second, or 2) preliminarily considered in the first stage, but only fully defined in the second stage.

As an example, while ergonomics is important at an early stage, since it will come into play in concept selection and in the validation of the conceptual solution with end-users, aesthetics and finish can only be specified when materials, manufacturing processes, and cost are being defined.

Note that although the assessment in Figure 3 categorizes PDS as being of primary or secondary importance in the specific framework of medical devices, this is quite subjective and dependent on the specific product. It also does not mean the secondary PDS do not require considerable attention. The assessment was essentially based on personal interpretation of current trends in development of medical devices from the analysis of multiple recent and ongoing projects in the area (Cunha et al. 2010).

From the analysis of Figure 3, one can state that the majority of what were labeled the most important PDS are set during the first stage of development, even though a little over half of them have to be revised in the second stage. Conversely, only a couple of the most important PDS are set in the second stage. It is also interesting that only about one third of second phase PDS can be left open during the first stage, while the others must be at least preliminarily considered in the first stage. Finally, about three fifths (circa 60%) of the PDS fall in the second phase, which means they can only be fully set during that stage of the development process.

3.5 The product development cycle

Within the laboratory development stage, a full product development cyclewill take place. In the framework of this paper, the important aspects to consider are the involvement of end-users early and throughout the process, as represented in Figure 4.

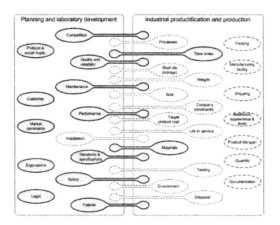

Figure 3. Setting product design specifications at different development process stages. See text for legend and discussion.

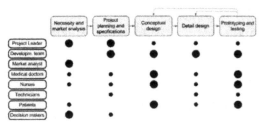

Figure 4. Simplified product development cycle for the laboratory-stage development of medical devices and involvement of different actors along the development cycle. Circle size represents the level of involvement in each stage.

4 MULTIDISCIPLINARITY

4.1 *Multidisciplinary integration within the development team*

Working in multidisciplinary teams offers several advantages to the researcher. One of these is the quick access to expertise in complementary areas of knowledge. Another is the possibility to debate decisions with colleagues that have different perspectives (and possibly, conflicting opinions). Equally important is the ability to tackle much more complex challenges than those which could be handled by a single individual, even if highly gifted.

However, such teams do not always work well, and it is frequent to observe personal incompatibilities develop between team members, often creating the need to replace individuals. As previously mentioned, communication among team members is a key factor. Aside from personality traits which can inexorably lead to conflicts, the main pitfalls have to do with team coordination, namely the need to:

- Clearly establish roles/responsibilities in the team;
- State the expertise each member adds to the team;
- Have team members frequently describe their individual work in (also frequent) team meetings.

One of the important aspects of multidisciplinary team interaction is language. Here we consider essentially technical terminology. It is vital to ensure that all team members are aware of specific technical terminology used by others. Also, some consensus must be reached regarding adoption of technical terms which might vary among scientific areas. It can be mitigated by frequent meetings and formally setting the terminology to be used by the team.

4.2 *Tasking and scheduling*

Stating that tasking and scheduling is important in this type of development projects is redundant. However, having multidisciplinary teams increases the complexity of the planning effort. First, as previously described, tasks must be very well defined and the role of each individual explicitly set for each task. Second, responsibilities must be assigned for every task, and it falls on the project leader to monitor task progress and intervene when necessary. Team members should not have to police each other. Last, while some tasks can be developed simultaneously, many will require input from other tasks. Almost any delay may cause other tasks to be put on-hold, possibly affecting the overall project schedule, and consequently, the predicted time to market.

Thus, compared to traditional project tasking and scheduling efforts, multidisciplinary teams for development of medical devices require additional care both in initial planning and in workflow monitoring.

4.3 *Communication with actors outside the development team*

There are clearly two different levels of communication here. On the one hand, multiple channels of communication are beneficial for the development process, namely between researchers and end-users. Examples are frequent meetings between the people responsible for collecting medical data (electronics or biomedical engineers) and doctors. Similarly, researchers working on devices with which healthcare professionals have to physically interact, need to meet with nurses, conduct brainstorming sessions, and perform preliminary tests with nurses, doctors, and possibly patients. These communication channels must work very effectively, and thus should be formally established jointly by the project leader and decision makers (e.g. hospital administrators).

On the other hand, the project leader is also responsible for communicating with the decision makers, market analysts, and media advisors. By having an overall view of the development project and being able to decide which information to release at each moment, the project leader has a pivotal role in lubricating the flow of information, simultaneously ensuring that confidential or sensitive information is not released untimely or unintentionally. There should be no direct independent communication between researchers and the decision makers and media advisors. Otherwise, their incomplete knowledge of the overall project, coupled with the fact that they are usually not aware of the long-term plans and strategy behind the development process, can lead to complicated communication mishaps.

4.4 *Coordinating the development team*

Following the discussion in §4.1 through §4.3, it becomes obvious that coordination of the development team requires a particular profile. The project leader has to supervise the development work, which makes a technical background highly desirable so he can articulate with the researchers and make decisions when necessary. He should be actively engaged in the development, but not supervise any of the tasks himself (e.g. brainstorming, field tests).

One of his main activities is coordination of the development team. This implies monitoring progress, but more importantly establishing boundaries, rules, roles, and responsibilities. He should assume a little more than his share of the blame for delays or the inability to fully reach intended development goals, and accept a little less than his share of the credits, recognizing the researchers' effort and congratulating individual achievements.

He must ensure team members learn to value the input of others, that they work cooperatively rather than competitively, and to be humble in their work. He should ensure no team member leaves questions unasked simply for fear of appearing ignorant.

Finally, it is often possible to delegate coordination of specific aspects of the development to the second most senior researcher (with extreme care to ensure that roles and responsibilities are understood by all), freeing the project leader for other tasks.

4.5 Coordinating the overall project

The role of coordinating the overall project is not trivial. This essentially includes:

– Monitor individual task progress, making swift changes to the workplan or redefining goals;
– Coordinate the research team, ensuring effective and efficient cooperation and communication channels (within the team and also external);
– Balance laboratory-stage development with the need to move on to productification to achieve a useful product time-to-market;
– Maintain frequent contact with decision makers and, when appropriate, with media advisors;
– Solve the plethora of problems that unexpectedly appear during development of medical devices (many common to any engineering project).

In the case of medical devices, the two main challenges relate to obtaining results within useful timeframes and usability issues (whether the device is employed by medical doctors, nurses, or patients).

5 CASE-STUDY

Although the discussion above follows from personal experience through the involvement in several projects related to medical devices, with varying degrees of complexity (and ambition), as well as team size, a case-study project is useful to illustrate it.

From 2007 through 2010 a new concept for mobile health was explored in the scope of the Mobile Health Living Lab project in Guimarães,

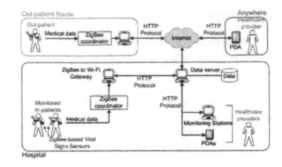

Figure 5. Simplified view of the system architecture developed and implemented in the case-study project.

Portugal. It aimed at increasing mobility of patients in hospitals and their homes through continuous remote monitoring of vital signals. The need was initially identified through discussions between decision makers and doctors at a healthcare provider and researchers from a university research center. It initially conceived the use of several support technologies and multiple support devices. It evolved along the first few months to a specific conceptual system design, including the need to develop hardware and software applications, narrowing the aims and goals, and defining project boundaries. During these 3 years, it involved researchers from all areas described in §3.2 (and others), and the different healthcare professionals and end-users in the roles described in §3.1. The system architecture is represented in Figure 5.

The developed sensors, network gateways, applications, user interfaces, etc, are being field tested at the Guimarães Private Hospital and have been recently showcased in many media sources, including national television. This project paves the way for future innovation in the area, highlighting the advantages of user-centered development and synergic cooperation between universities and companies, and will have practical effect on the quality of healthcare for many patients.

6 CONCLUDING REMARKS

This paper presents some considerations about the coordination of multidisciplinary teams for the development of medical devices, which can be further explored in a future expanded paper.

Vital aspects which could not be discussed here include medical device certification, and the different paradigms of developing medical devices within companies or in a university setting.

At the conference, the case-study will be further analyzed and used to illustrate each aspect of the described multidisciplinary development process.

ACKNOWLEDGEMENTS

Colleagues involved in the case-study, namely José A. Afonso, Higino Correia, Adriano Moreira, Joaquim Mendes, and students Helena Fernandez-López, Ana C. Matos, Duarte Pereira, and Bruno Fernandes. Financial support for the case-study has been provided by Casa de Saúde de Guimarães, Portugal, and the MIT-Portugal program. The author acknowledges the Foundation for Science and Technology, Lisbon, through the 3° Quadro Comunitário de Apoio and the POCTI and FEDER programs.

REFERENCES

Alexander, K., Clarkson, J., Bishop, D. & Fox, S. Good Design Practice for Medical Devices and Equipment: Requirements Capture. Engineering Design Centre. Cambridge University, 2002.

Cruz-Cunha, M.M., Tavares, A.J. & Simões, R. (Eds.). (2010). Handbook of Research on Developments in e-Health and Telemedicine: Technological and Social Perspectives. Hershey, PA: Information Science Reference.

Fernandez-Lopez, H., Macedo, P., Afonso, J.A., Correia, J.H. Simões R. Evaluation of the Impact of the Topology and Hidden Nodes in the Performance of a ZigBee Network, in: Lecture Notes of the Institute for Computer Sciences, Social-Informatics and Telecommunications Engineering 24 (S-Cube 2009), Pisa, Italy, pp. 256–271, 2009.

Fernandez-Lopez, H., Afonso, J.A., Correia, J.H., Simões, R. HM4 All: A Vital Signs Monitoring System based in Spatially Distributed ZigBee Networks, in: Proc. Pervasive Health2010–4th International Conference on Pervasive Computing Technologies for Healthcare, Munich, Germany, 22–25 March, 2010.

Pereira, D., Moreira, A., Simoes, R. Challenges on real-time monitoring of patients through the Internet, in: Proc. CISTI 2010, Santiago de Compostela – Spain, 16–19 June, 2010.

Pugh, S., Total Design – Integrated methods for successful product engineering. Addison-Wesley Pub Co., 1991.

Sampaio, M., Pontes, A.J., Simoes, R. Analysis of product design and development methodologies towards a specific implementation for embedded microelectronics, in: Proc. IDEMI09, Porto – Portugal, 14–15 September, 2009.

Simoes, R., Sampaio, A.M. Exceeding problem solving expectations in industrial design under severely restricted specifications, IRF – Integrity, Reliability and Failure: Challenges and Opportunities, 2009, p. 445, ISBN 978-972-8826-22-2.

Zenios, S., et al. Biodesign: The process of Innovating New Medical Technologies. Cambridge University Press, 2009.

Technology and Medical Sciences – Natal Jorge et al. (eds)
© *2011 Taylor & Francis Group, London, ISBN 978-0-415-66822-4*

Multi-objective optimization of bypass grafts in arteries

C.F. Castro, C.C. António & L.C. Sousa
IDMEC -FEUP, University of Porto, Porto, Portugal

ABSTRACT: Bypass grafts yield excellent results and remain the modern standard care for treatment of stenosed arteries in the vascular system. Geometry configuration of grafts and anastomosis has profound influences on the hemodynamics, such as flow patterns, pressure distribution and shear stress. Blood flow from the grafts strongly strikes the wall vessel, resulting in flow stagnation and reversed flow which are correlated with postoperative possibility of restenosis. The main goal of the present work is to develop a computational tool that enables the design of optimal geometries improving graft longevity. The optimization methodology considers the weight coefficients approach combining multiple objectives into one. A developed computer program models blood flow in artery and grafting the finite element method. A coupled genetic algorithm searches optimal graft geometries. Solutions exhibit the benefits of numerical shape optimization in achieving grafts inducing small gradient hemodynamic flows and minimizing reversed flow and residence times.

1 INTRODUCTION

Simulation of blood flow is of great importance for understanding the function of the vascular system under normal and abnormal conditions, designing cardiovascular devices, and diagnosing and treating diseases. Bypass grafts yield excellent results and remains the modern standard care for treatment of stenosed arteries in the vascular system. Geometry configuration of anastomosis has profound influences on the hemodynamics, such as flow patterns, pressure distribution and shear stress which are correlated with postoperative occlusion pathogenesis of bypass graft. It has been also suggested that high shear stress gradient and long residence times might be responsible for the localization of anastomotic intimal hyperplasia.

In order to show the application of the finite element method approach in biomedical engineering, numerical simulations of blood flow in arteries, such as hemodynamics of bypass grafts for stenosed arteries are addressed here. Kute & Vorp (2001) examined the effect of the proximal artery flow (prograde, zero, and retrograde) on the distal anastomosis, and suggested that the flow condition in the proximal artery affects the local hemodynamics at the distal anastomosis site and thus should be considered. Various configurations, such as patched, cuffed, and side-to-side anastomosis have been under consideration in the numerical simulation and clinical application (Bonert et al. 2002; Cole et al. 2002; Longest et al. 2003; Sankaranarayanan et al. 2006, Qiau & Liu 2008). In these studies, the bifurcating flow rate

into bypass graft is not a major concern since the fully occluded host artery is assumed and 100% flow issuing from the host artery entrance bifurcates into the bypass graft. The anastomotic angle, i.e., the angle between the host artery and implanted bypass graft, is a very important factor responsible for intimal hyperplasia. Su et al. (2005) have investigated the complexity of blood flow in the complete model of arterial bypass. Five types of stenosis models were presented: no stenosis, full-yoccluded, axisymmetric constriction stenosis with either 56% or 75% area reduction at the throat, and asymmetric stenosis with 75% area reduction. For the case of an asymmetric stenosis, three different locations of the asymmetric thrombus with respect to the bypass graft are considered: top, bottom and side. They found that the flow in the bypass graft is greatly dependent on the area reduction in the host artery. As the area reduction increases, higher stress concentration and larger recirculation zones are formed at the distal corner of the bifurcation as well as at the toe and heel of the distal anastomosis that could be damaging to the artery-graft junctions. Prior to bypass surgeries computer simulations can become a powerful tool since the location of the thrombus or plaque formation with respect to the anastomosis plays a nonnegligible role in the hemodynamics of the bypass system.

In the work presented here a genetic algorithm is considered in order to reach optimal graft geometries. Numerical results show the benefits of numerical shape optimization in achieving design improvements before a bypass surgery, minimizing recirculation zones formed at the distal corner of the bifurcation as well as at the toe and heel of the distal anastomosis that could be damaging to the artery-graft junctions.

2 COMPUTATIONAL STRATEGY

In shape optimization, the goal is to minimize an objective function that typically depends on a state vector v, over a domain that depends on a design vector b. The state vector and the design parameters are coupled by a partial differential equation that can be written in a generic form as

$$c(v, b) = 0 \qquad (1)$$

This so-called state equation forms the constraint of the minimization problem

Minimize $\Phi(v, b)$ $\qquad (2)$
subject to $c(v, b) = 0$ $\qquad (3)$

Furthermore, the problem can be recast using the reduced form of the objective function

Minimize $\Pi(v(b), b)$ $\qquad (4)$

where $v(b)$ is the solution of Equation (1). This form allows decoupling the solution of the state equation and the optimization problem. This shape optimization problem requires an efficient and accurate solver for the state equation. Plus, the objective function needs to be carefully chosen to capture the physics of the underlying problem.

2.1 Blood flow simulation

In the present study, the numerical analysis of the blood flow phenomena uses the finite element method approach and a geometrical model of the artery. Fluid is incompressible and governed by the continuity and the Navier-Stokes equations whose viscosity may not be constant. The simulation is carried out under steady flow conditions. In diseased vessels the wall motion is reduced and the assumption of zero wall motion is utilized in most approximations. So in the present work, biochemical and mechanical interactions between blood and vascular tissue are neglected, considering boundary conditions similar to physiological circumstances.

The continuity equation is given by

$$\nabla \cdot v = 0 \qquad (5)$$

and the momentum balance equation

$$\frac{\partial v}{\partial t} + (\nabla \cdot v)v = -\frac{1}{\rho}\nabla p + v\nabla^2 v \qquad (6)$$

where v is the velocity field, v the kinematic viscosity, ρ the blood density and p the pressure.

In the numerical simulation, considering the pseudo-constitutive relation for the incompressibility constraint (Babuska 1973; Babuska et al. 1980), the continuity equation is replaced by

$$p = -\alpha(\nabla \cdot v) \qquad (7)$$

where 10^{-8} or 10^{-9} are generally assigned values to the penalty parameter α. The Navier-Stokes equations become:

$$\rho\left(\frac{\partial v}{\partial t} + (\nabla \cdot v)v\right) = \alpha\nabla(\nabla \cdot v) + \mu\nabla^2 v \qquad (8)$$

with μ the dynamic viscosity.

If the standard Galerkin formulation is applied it is necessary to use compatible spaces for the velocity and the pressure in order to satisfy the Babuska-Brezzi stability (Babuska 1973; Babuska et al. 1980; Sousa et al. 2002; Sousa et al. 2009).

A non-Newtonian viscosity model is adopted in this work, where viscosity is empirically obtained using Casson law for the shear stress relation (Perktold et al. 1991)

$$\sqrt{\tau} = k_0(c) + k_1(c)\sqrt{\dot{\gamma}} \qquad (9)$$

where τ and $\dot{\gamma}$ denote shear stress and shear strain rate and c the red cell concentration. For generalized 2-D flow, this relation is modified using D_{II} the second invariant of the strain rate tensor. The shear stress τ given by the generalized Casson relation is

$$\sqrt{\tau} = k_0(c) + k_1(c)\sqrt{\sqrt[2]{D_{II}}} \qquad (10)$$

and the apparent viscosity $\mu = \mu(c, D_{II})$ a function of the red cell concentration is,

$$\mu = \frac{1}{2\sqrt{D_{II}}}\left(k_0(c) + k_1(c)\sqrt{\sqrt[2]{D_{II}}}\right)^2 \qquad (11)$$

where parameters $k_0(c)$ and $k_1(c)$ were obtained fitting experimental data, $c = 45\%$, $k_0(45\%) = 0.6125$ and $k_1(45\%) = 0.174$ (Perktold et al. 1991).

2.2 Multi-objective optimization approach

A general multi-objective optimization seeks to optimize the components of a vector-valued objective function mathematically formulated as

Minimize $F(b) = (f_1(b), ..., f_m(b))$ $\qquad (12)$

subject to

$$b_i^{lower} \le b_i \le b_i^{upper}, i=1,...,n$$
$$g_k(b) \le 0, \qquad k=1,...,p \tag{13}$$

where $b = (b_1, ..., b_n)$ is the design vector, b_i^{lower} and b_i^{upper} represent the lower and upper boundary of the ith design variable b_i, $f_j(b)$ is the jth objective function and $g_k(b)$ the kth constraint.

Unlike single objective optimization approaches, the solution to this problem is not a single point, but a family of points known as the Pareto-optimal set. Typically, there are infinitely many Pareto optimal solutionsfor a multi-objective problem. Thus, it is often necessary to incorporate user preferences for various objectives inorder to determine a single suitable solution.

The weighted sum method for multi-objective optimization problems (Marler & Arora 2010) continues to be used extensivelynotonly to provide multiple solution points by varying theweights consistently, but also to provide a single solutionpoint that reflects preferences presumably incorporatedin the selection of a single set of weights. Using the weighted sum methodto solve the optimization problem as given in Equation (12) entails selecting scalar weights w_j and minimizing the following composite objective function:

$$\mathscr{F}(b) = \sum_{j=1}^{m} w_j f_j(b) \tag{14}$$

If all of the weights are positive, as assumed in this study, then minimizing Equation (14) provides a sufficient conditionfor Pareto optimality, which means that its minimum is always Pareto optimal.

Regarding the choice of suitable objective function for the graft optimization problem, several different approaches have been pursued in the literature. The most frequently considered quantities in the context of blood flow are based on either shear stress and its gradient or the flow rate. Many authors choose to minimize the integral of the squared shear rate also called dissipation integral because it measures the dissipation of energy due to viscous effects, expressed in terms of the rate of strain tensor,

$$\frac{1}{2} \int_{\Omega(b)} \dot{\gamma}^2 \, dx \tag{15}$$

The minimization of this function is related to flow efficiency. Flow efficiency can be obtained by computing the maximum pressure variation in the domain. In this project we chose to minimize the flow efficiency quantified as

$$f_1(b) = \Delta p = |p_{max} - p_{min}| \tag{16}$$

The second chosen objective function is related to the minimization of regions presenting reversed flows and long residence timesalong the arterial bypass system. For eachidealized bypass graft geometry configurationa domain Ω^* is identified indicating where reversed flow and long residence times are enhanced. Being v_x the longitudinal velocity in that critical domain, the following objective functionis considered for the optimization problem investigated in this work,

$$f_2(b) = \sum_{\Omega^*(b)} v_x \tag{17}$$

Evolutionary algorithms are well suited to multi-objective optimization problems as they are fundamentally based on biological processes which are inherentlymulti-objective.

2.3 Genetic search

A Genetic Algorithm (GA) is a stochastic search method based on evolution and genetics exploiting the concept of survival of the fittest. For a given problem or design domain there exists a multitude of possible solutions that form a solution space. In a genetic algorithm, a highly effective search of the solution space is performed, allowing a population of strings representing possible design vectors to evolve through basic genetic operators. The goal of these operators is to progressively reduce the space design driving the process into more promising regions. Specific featuresof good solutions found in the GA optimization can also be used to initializeanother GA optimization.

The adopted genetic algorithmscheme (António et al. 2005; Castro et al. 2004) is based on four operators supported by an elitist strategy that always preserves a core of best individuals of the population whose genetic material is transferred into the next generations. A new population of solutions P^{t+1} is generated from the previous P^t using the genetic operators: Selection, Crossover, Mutation and Deletion.

The optimization scheme includes the following steps:

Coding: the design variables expressed by real number are converted to binary number, and each binary string is looked as an individual;

Initializing: the individuals which consist of an initial population P^0 are produced randomly;

Evaluation: the fitness of each individual is evaluated using objective function given in Equation (17), to determine the fitness value and individuals are ranked according to the fitness value;

Selection: definition of the elite group that includes individuals highly fitted. Selection of the progenitors: one from the best—fitted group (elite) and another from the least fitted one. This selection is done randomly with an equal probability distribution for each solution. Transfer of the whole population P^t to an intermediate step where they will join the offspring determined by the crossover operator;

Crossover: The crossover operator transforms two chromosomes (progenitors) into a new chromosome (offspring) having genes from both progenitors by a multipoint combination technique applied to the binary string of two selected chromosomes. The new individuals created by crossover will join to the original population.

Mutation: the implemented mutation is characterized by changing a set of bits of the binary string corresponding to one variable of a randomly selected chromosome from the elite group making possible the exploitation of previously unmapped space design regions and guaranteeing the diversity of the generated population.

Deletion: After mutation, new ranking of the enlarged population according to their fitness. Then, it follows the deletion of the worst solutions with low fitness simulating the natural death of low fitted and old individuals. The original size population is recovered and the new population P^{t+1} is obtained; the evolutionary process will continue until the stopping criterionis reached.

Termination: checking the termination condition. If it is satisfied, the GA is terminated. Otherwise, the process returns to step Selection.

As a compromise between computer time and population diversity, parameters for the genetic algorithm were taken as $N_{pop} = 12$ and $N_e = 5$ for the population and elite group size, respectively. The number of bits in binary codifying for the design variables was $N_{bit} = 5$. The evolutionary process stops when convergence is achieved, that is when the mean fitness of the elite group does not change during five consecutive generations.

3 NUMERICAL RESULTS

Research on the optimization of the geometry of an idealized arterial bypass system with fully occluded host artery is addressed here. The artery is simulated using a diameter tube of 10 mm. Design parameters are considered for the coupled graft presenting a sinusoidal geometry. The graft mesh does not maintain the same width along its whole length. At the centre line of the graft, nodes move in the radial direction preserving their distance to the deforming centreline. The graft is properly connected to the artery always in the same region. The boundary conditions for the flow field are parabolic inlet velocity, no-slip boundary conditions

including the graft and a parallel flow condition at the outlet.

The developed computer program (Sousa et al. 2002; Sousa et al. 2009) modelled blood flow in artery and graft using 2261 nodes and 2024 four-node linear elements for a two-dimensional finite element approximation and Reynolds number 300. Figure 1 presents the geometry and finite element mesh considered for the idealized arterial bypass system simulation.

For the optimization problem the graft/artery ratio diameter varies from 0.6 to 1.2 and the anastomosis varies accordingly. Since the search space is not known in absolute terms, simulations of 100 random possible graft geometries described by design vector b have been conducted in order to get an indication of the objective space distribution.

Figure 2 presents the calculations for maximum pressure variation in the whole domain $\Omega(b)$ and the longitudinal velocity in the critical domain $\Omega^*(b)$ where reversed flow and residence times are enhanced.

The optimal solutions in the decision spaceare in general denoted as the Pareto set and its image in the objective space as Pareto front. Results shown in Figure 2 allow identifying the likely presence of a Pareto front in the design problem.

Based on the visualization of the objective space the following composite function as been considered for the minimization problem:

$$\mathcal{F}(b) = 10^2 * f_1(b) - f_2(b) \qquad (18)$$

This way equal importance is given to both contributions. The coupling of the genetic algorithm with the finite element simulation (António et al. 2005; Castro et al. 2004) found an optimal solution. The design parameters for the optimal bypass systemare graft diameter of 11.7 mm and height 18.7 mm.

Figure 3 presents the pressure distribution along bypass and host arterywhich can be analysed in three parts. In the first part the flow is still undisturbed and therefore the pressure is quite uniform.

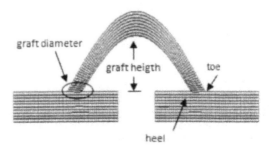

Figure 1. Geometry and finite element mesh for the arterial bypass system optimization problem.

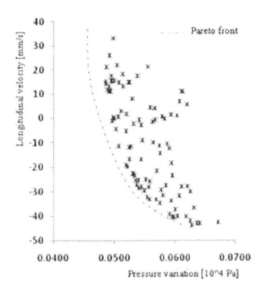

Figure 2. Summation of longitudinal velocities in $\Omega^*(b)$ and maximum pressure variation in $\Omega(b)$ for one hundred randomly chosen b designs.

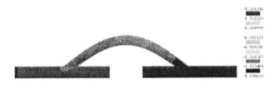

Figure 3. Pressure distribution [10⁴ Pa] for the optimal shape.

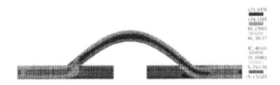

Figure 4. Longitudinal velocity distribution [mm/s] for the optimal shape.

In the second part the flow is within the graft area where the pressure raises as the flow moves along the graft. The pressure increases as the flow exits the graft. In the third part the flow is sufficiently far from the graft and therefore it exhibits a uniform distribution. After the artery-graft junction, the pressure values variation is rather smooth.

The simulated longitudinal velocity values for the optimal graft solution are given in Figure 4. It is interesting to notice that although the abrupt connection between artery and graft induces large velocity variations, the observable reverse flow is quite small. Long residence times usually

observable immediately after the toe of the distal anastomosis is also quite undetectable.

4 CONCLUSIONS

The present work addresses the complex blood flowstructure induced by a bypass graft. Numerical calculations simulate a graft/artery system including both proximal and distal anastomosis in a fully obstructed artery. An optimization algorithm is developed aiming the design of optimal geometries in order to improve graft longevity. The computational method considersa genetic search built around a developed finite element solver with added routines to evaluate suitable objectives functions. Consideringa design vector-defining the variable graft/artery configuration an optimal solution has been reached. The simulated optimal graft exhibits smoothed flow gradients with minimized reversed flows and residence times. These models will enable to predict temporary physiologic changes due to the vascular interventions or to replicate changes in physiologic conditions automatically.

ACKNOWLEDGEMENTS

The authors acknowledge the financial support by FCT, Portugal, projectPTDC/SAU-BEB/102547/2008. We thank Bernardo Relvas, IDMEC-FEUP, Portugal, for his help developing the finite element meshes.

REFERENCES

António, C.C., Castro, C.F. & Sousa, L.C. 2005. Eliminating forging defects using genetic algorithms, *Materials and Manufacturing Processes* 20: 509–522.

Babuska, I. 1973. The finite element method with Lagrangian multipliers, *Numerische Mathematik* 20: 179–192.

Babuska, I., Osborn, J. & Pitkaranta, J. 1980. Analysis of mixed methods usingmesh dependent norms. *Mathematics of Computation* 35: 1039–1062.

Bonert, M., Myers, J.G., Fremes, S., Williams, J. & Ethier, C.R. 2002. A numerical study of blood flow in coronary artery bypass graft side-to side anastomosis. *Ann. Biomed. Eng.* 30: 599–611.

Castro, C.F., António, C.A.C. & Sousa, L.C. 2004. Optimisation of shape and process parameters in metal forging using genetic algorithms. *Journal of Materials Processing Technology* 146: 356–364.

Cole, J.S., Watterson, J.K. & O'Reilly, M.J.G. 2002. Numerical investigation of the hemodynamics at a patched arterial bypass anastomosis. *Med. Eng. Phys.* 24: 393–401.

Kute, S.M. & Vorp, D.A. 2001. The Effect of Proximal Artery Flow onthe Hemodynamics at the

Distal Anastomosis of a Vascular Bypass Graft: Computational Study. *ASME J. Biomech. Eng.* 123: 277–283.

Longest, P.W., Kleinstreuer, C. & Archie Jr., J.P. 2003. Particle hemodynamics analysis of Miller cuff arterial anastomosis. *J. Vasc. Surg.* 38: 1353–1362.

Marler, R.T. & Arora, J.S. 2009. The weighted sum method for multi-objective optimization: new insights. *Struct. Multidisc. Optim.* DOI 10.1007/s00158-009-0460-7.

Perktold, K., Peter, R.O., Resch, M. & Langs, G. 1991. Pulsatile non-Newtonian flow in three-dimensional carotid bifurcation models: A numerical study of flow phenomena under different bifurcation angles. *J. Biomedical Eng.* 13: 507–515.

Qiao, A. & Liu, Y. 2008. Medical application oriented blood flow simulation. *Clinical Biomechanics* 23: S130–S136.

Sankaranarayanan, M., Ghista, D.N., Poh, C.L., Seng, T.Y. & Kassab, G.S. 2006. Analysis of blood flow in an out-of-plane CABG model. *Am. J. Physiol. Heart Circ. Physiol.* 291: 283–295.

Sousa, L.C., Castro, C.F., António, C.A.C. & Santos, A.D. 2002. Inverse methods in design of industrial forging processes. *Journal of Materials Processing Technology* 128(1–3): 266–273.

Sousa, L.C., Castro, C.F. & António, C.A.C. 2009. Numerical simulation of blood flow, *VipIMAGE 2009 - II ECCOMAS Thematic Conference on Computational Vision and Medical Image Processing*: 15–18.

Su, C.M., Lee, D., Tran-Son-Tay, R. & Shyy, W. 2005. Fluid flow structure in arterial bypass anastomosis. *J Biomech Eng.* 127(4):611–618.

Technology and Medical Sciences – Natal Jorge et al. (eds)
© 2011 Taylor & Francis Group, London, ISBN 978-0-415-66822-4

Multiple Sclerosis subjects plantar pressure—A new tool for postural instability diagnosis

Luis F.F. Santos
Department of Physical and Medicine Rehabilitation of SAMS, Lisbon, Portugal
ADFisio—Rehabilitation Center, Lisbon, Portugal

João M.C.S. Abrantes
MovLab, CICANT, Universidade Lusófona de Humanidades e Tecnologias, Lisbon, Portugal

ABSTRACT: Multiple Sclerosis (MS) is a chronic inflammatory, demyelinating disease of the Central Nervous System (CNS), and is the most common progressive neurological disease in young adults. Debilitating motor and sensory function are the major features of the disease. Balance disorders are associated with ambulation difficulties, sustaining an upright posture, and performing functional activities such as turning. Those skills predispose people with MS to loss the balance control and fall. An adequate evaluation of postural instability is essential for monitoring the various stages of disease. Sometimes clinical balance tests may not detect subtle deficits in adults with MS who are not yet experiencing functional limitations or disability. It's important to develop new instruments that could identify subtle impairments before they lead to functional decline. The purpose of this study was to determine if Center Of Pressure (COP) displacement assessed by plantar pressure could be a useful performance-based evaluative measure for adults with MS comparing with a clinical examination using the Berg Balance Scale (BBS). Twenty-nine subjects with MS were compared with 28 healthy adults. Subjects with MS performed a plantar pressure assessment in upright standing position and in the stance phase of gait (1-step protocol) and were also tested with the BBS. Control subjects performed the same test that MS group. COP measures show clear differences when comparing healthy adults with adults with MS. We found cinematic alterations of COP properties in all positions in multiple sclerosis group. A clinical approach that usually tests postural Stability (BBS) is ineffective in small postural disturbances.

1 INTRODUCTION

Multiple Sclerosis (MS) is the most common progressive neurological disease in young adults and is a chronic inflammatory, demyelinating disease of the Central Nervous System (CNS) (Waxman, 2005) (Palace, 2001). Debilitating motor and sensory function are the major features of the disease (Palace, 2001). Balance control is know to be a complex motor skills, that involves the integration of many types of sensory information and the planning and execution of flexible movement patterns, in order to achieve many potential postural goals (Horak, 1997). Adequate balance relies on input from de visual, somatosensory and vestibular system, which are frequently impaired in people with MS. Muscle weakness and spasticity further compromise the ability to balance by affecting the sequencing and force of muscle contraction(Kelleher et al., 2009).Various

measures of instability or body adaptation, to prevent instability, have been reported. Measures include, body Center Of Mass (COM) position, COM position relative to the COP under the foot, or measures that combine COM position and velocity (Buckley et al., 2005; Hahn & Chou, 2004; Hof et al., 2005). Another measure that has been widely used is COP (Winter et al., 1996). Médio-Lateral (ML) and Anterior-Posterior (AP) COP displacement has been used directly as stability measures (Ienaga et al., 2006; Schmid et al., 2005). Karst et al, studied the COP displacement in standing tasks in adults with MS who has minimal or no balance deficits, and concluded that COP measures show clearly differences when comparing healthy adults with minimally impaired adults with MS (Karst et al., 2005). An assessment of balance that could identify subtle impairments before they lead to functional decline could promote earlier intervention and possibly prevent or delay functional limitation and disability. Several studies evaluated balance impairment in MS patients but only with the use of force platforms (Daley & Swank, 1981; Rougier et al., 2007).

Plantar pressure measurement is being increasingly used in both research and clinical practice to compare static and gait patterns of different clinical groups and to evaluate the effects of footwear, orthotic, surgical procedures and physical therapy interventions (Taylor et al., 2004). Measurements of plantar pressure provide an indication of foot and ankle function in upright standing position, during gait and other functional activities, because the foot and ankle provide both the necessary support and flexibility for weight bearing and weight shifting, while performing these actions (Orlin & McPoil, 2000). Although plantar pressure data have been recognized as an important element in the assessment of patients with diabetes and peripheral neuropathy (Smith et al., 2000). The information derived from plantar pressure data can also assist, in determining and managing the impairments associated with various musculoskeletal and neurological disorders (Robain et al., 2006). Few studies to date have used a plantar pressure platform to assess postural stability in subjects with MS in upright standing position.

The aim of the present study was to find out if compared to the normal pattern, the patients with multiple sclerosis, when in quiet standing position and in the stance phase of gait, has changes in displacement pattern associated to the Centre Of Pressure (COP) recorded by a appropriate equipment.

2 METHODS

2.1 Subjects

The study was conducted with support from Portuguese Society of Multiple Sclerosis. Inclusion criteria for participation were: (1) clinical diagnosis of MS, conducted by a neurologist; (2) aged between 18 and 65; (3) ability to maintained upright standing position for 60 seconds. Exclusion criteria were: (1) other neurological conditions such stroke or brain trauma; (2) cardiovascular diseases or other causes that interfere with the implementation of the evaluation protocol; (3) cognitive deficits; (4) included in another study of MS. The verification of inclusion criteria, a questionnaire was sent by email, to each subject with MS, who intended to participate. Before test procedures, each subject performed an interview to collect demographic, anthropometric and clinical characteristics including age, gender, foot size, type of MS and disease duration.

Twenty-nine subjects with MS, 12 male and 17 female, mean age $43,24 \pm 12,08$, were included in the study. Control subjects were eligible to participate if they met the same inclusion criteria as the subjects with MS, with the exception of having a diagnosis of MS and were recruited from a variety of sources of convenience. The same exclusion criteria also applied to the control group. Twenty-eight control subjects, 9 male; 19 female, mean age $36,79 \pm 8,96$, met the criteria for the study and were tested. All subjects provided written informed consent prior to test procedures and the study was approved by ethic commission of Portuguese Catholic University were the study was presented. All subjects participated in one testing session which included plantar pressure assessment and clinical test. The study was conducted in accordance to recommendations guiding biomedical research involving human subjects (Helsinki Declaration).

2.2 Berg Balance Scale

The Berg Balance Scale (BBS) consists of 14 standardized sub-tests scored on five-point scales (0–4), with a maximum (best) score of 56 (Berg, K. et al., 1992). Reliability and validity have been demonstrated in elderly people (Berg, K et al., 1995), and scores below 45 may indicate increased risk of falling for elderly people (Maki et al., 1994). Reliability and validity of the BBS have not been established in persons with MS. However, the BBS has been found to change in response to rehabilitation in adults with clinically stable MS (Lord et al., 1998) and many studies included this scale to evaluate postural stability in MS (Cattaneo, D. et al., 2002; Cattaneo, D et al., 2007; Smedal et al., 2006). A recent systematic review (Tyson & Connell, 2009) to identify measurement tools of balance activity in people with neurological conditions, concluded that BBS is psychometrically robust and feasible to use in neurological disorders and clinical practice.

2.3 Plantar pressure assessment

Plantar pressure assessment was performed with Footscan 1 m—3D Gait Scientific System (RsScan® International—Belgium). The platform consists of 2 units of 0.5 m × 0.5 m installed in carbon mat and synchronized with each other. Each unit has dimensions: length 578 mm × width 418 mm × height 12 mm, and 4096 sensors (5.08 mm × 7.62 mm). Thus, it is possible to operate as a unit of 1 meter to gait analyses, or only using one unit of 0.5 meters to balance evaluation. The 1 m plantar pressure platform use resistive technology using 8192 sensors (5.08 mm by 7.62 mm). The dimensions are, 1068 mm, length by 418 mm width and 12 mm height. The actual study used the left unit. The platform was connected to analog-digital unit (Footscan® interface 3D Box) to synchronize the entire system and convert the signal in digital values of pressure data. The software provided by the manufacturer (Footscan 7.7 Balance 2nd Generation) was installed in one computer system to collect and store pressure data. The 100 Hz sample frequency was used to collect data from upright standing position (10 seconds) and 250 Hz sample frequency for the stance phase of gait (4 seconds).

2.4 Protocol

The platform was placed on the ground at a distance of 1.5 meters from front wall and calibrated by manufacturer's specifications. For upright standing position, each subject performed 3 repeated trials, each one with 10 seconds. The subjects stood on platform, barefoot (to reduce variability in performance that may occur due to differences in footwear and other clothing), in natural position and placed themselves in position that they considered more stable. They were instructed to stay more stable as possible during the trial. To avoid disturbing effects due to eye movements over postural control, the subjects were required, during the trial, to stare at a target. This target consisted in a blue circle (diameter = 0.16 m) drawn on a white sheet, positioned in the front wall at 1.6 m of the ground. During the trials, an assistance stay close to subjects to prevent instability and fall risk. Trial, in which the feet were not contacted with the whole platform, was not saved for data analysis and was repeated. If necessary, between trials, subjects with greater postural instability were allowed to sit for two minutes.

For gait stance phase the study used the 1-step protocol (Bus & Lange, 2005). Each subject performed 3 times with right foot and 3 times with left foot. The subjects stood in upright standing position behind the platform, and were instructed to perform a step moving inside the platform just with

one foot, and place the other foot out of platform. If the first test was performed with the right foot, then the other two tests were also conducted with the same foot. After the pressure assessment, subjects were evaluated by a clinical test (Berg Balance Scale—BBS) based on a qualified scale and applied by a specialist. The assessment is done by the visual direct observation of the balance behavior characteristics.

Testing for control subjects involved the same instruments and protocol as that described for subjects with MS.

2.5 Stability parameters

Based on previous studies (Chernikova et al., 2005; Doyle et al., 2007; Karst et al., 2005; Zabjek et al., 2005) the present study used five COP parameters sensitive to postural balance and MS postural changes: Medial-Lateral COP displacement (ML); Anterior-Posterior COP displacement (AP); Total COP displacement (TD); Ellipse Area (EA) and Total Contac Time (CT).

2.6 Statistical analysis

Statistical analysis was performed using the software Statistical Package for the Social Sciences (SPSS), version 17.0 software for Windows XP SP2 (SPSS, Chicago, IL, USA) and Microsoft® Excel 2003. We calculated Spearman correlation coefficients to evaluate the validity of the postural stabilization parameters for the considered population of MS subjects.

3 RESULTS

Demographic, anthropometric and clinical characteristics (mean, standard deviation and range) for all subjects are listed in Table 1. Fourteen of 28 MS subjects scored ≥51 points in BBS (maximum 56), with higher scores indicating better performance.

Table 1. Demographic, anthropometric and clinical characteristics of study population.

Variable	Mean ± S.D. (range)	
	MS subjects N = 29	Healthy subjects N = 28
Age (years)	43,2 ± 12,1 (20–63)	36,8 ± 8,96 (19–62)
Gender	17 females; 12 males	19 females; 9 males
Ratio	1.4:1	2.1:1
Foot size*	39,2 ± 2,48 (35–43)	38,5 ± 2,57 (35–44)
Berg Balance Scale (BBS)	46,6 ± 9,97 (21–56)	55,7 ± 0,47 (55–56)
Disease duration (years)	8,72 ± 6,18 (0,17–22)	–

* Foot size in continental European system (adults).

However the average BBS score in MS group is approximately 9 points less than the average score in healthy group. Ten MS subjects scored <44, below the score (45) from which increases the risk of falls and corresponds to 34.48% of total group. Nine healthy subjects scored 55 points, remaining subjects reached the maximum score.

3.1 Upright standing position

Results for upright standing position are shown in Table 2. In MS group, medio-lateral and anterior-posterior data demonstrate a substantially displacement than control group. A similar behavior is observed in total displacement and ellipse area values.

For each trial, an ellipse area is calculated. All the centre of pressure points within 1 standard deviation is represented in this ellipse, so the ellipse is a representation of the spreading of the centre of pressure line. Lower values correspond to stable measurements. Medio-lateral COP displacement in MS subjects is the triple value than verified in healthy subjects. Similarly the anterior-posterior COP displacement in MS subjects has a triple value too, compared to the other group. Comparing the results for ellipse area, the results demonstrate that the difference is even greater, and the result is five times higher in MS subjects.

These results identified impairments in balance and greater postural instability in MS group. To verify the behavior of the upright standing position stability parameters in individuals with little impairment, we constitute another MS group, with subjects who have BBS score ≥52 points. Table 3 shows the results of this new group. Unlike what happened with the initial group of MS, when compared healthy subjects with this restricted group of 12 MS Subjects, there are no statistical differences between BBS averages scores. However, the upright standing position stability parameters of this new MS group continue to demonstrate a substantially displacement than control group. The value for ellipse area is four times higher than

Table 3. Results for MS group with BBS ≥ 52.

| Subject | BBS | Mean of 3 trials | | | |
		ML	AP	DT	AE
1	54	4,0	9,0	99,0	5,5
2	55	3,3	9,7	88,3	3,6
3	52	2,7	7,0	113,7	3,3
4	55	2,7	4,0	88,0	2,4
5	54	2,0	5,3	86,3	1,4
6	56	6,7	11,7	108,0	13,8
7	55	3,0	8,3	117,3	3,6
8	55	3,3	3,0	112,7	1,5
9	56	1,7	3,0	84,0	0,7
10	56	6,3	13,3	106,0	10,4
11	56	2,3	3,7	90,7	0,7
12	54	3,3	4,3	94,3	4,4
Mean*	54,8	3,4	6,9	99,0	4,3

Values are the mean* of 3 trials for 29 MS subjects and 28 healthy subjects in millimetres
ML—Medio-Lateral COP displacement
AP—Anterior-Posterior COP displacement
TD—Total COP displacement
EA—Ellipse Area (mm 2)

verified in healthy subjects. As expected we found that disease duration positively correlated with age and impairments. There was a moderately negative correlation between BBS and ML, AP, TD ($p < 0,05$), indicating that high values of BBS are associated with low values of ML, AP and TD. The ML displacement has strongly positive correlation with the AP displacement ($rs = 0.835$), EA ($rs = 0,763$) and also a positive moderate intensity with TD ($rs = 0,555$).

3.2 Support phase of gait (1-step protocol)

Results for plantar pressure assessments in support phase of gait (1-step protocol) are listed in Table 4. In 1-step protocol, ML, TD and CT values for both feet are higher compared to control group. In both groups (MS and healthy) the ML COP displacement for left foot is inferior than registered in right foot. We also observed in MS group that the AP COP displacement is lower than they were assessed in the control group. This is because some subjects did not perform the initial contact with the heel but with metatarsal region. This difference in first contact area, decreased the AP COP displacement, contrary to what would be expected. In total displacement we assisted to opposite behavior to that seen in ML parameter. For both groups (MS and healthy) the TD value is superior than registered in right foot. Another interesting finding is the result of CT value in MS group, is equal in both foot and superior to

Table 2. Upright standing position—Results.

| MS subjects | | | | Healthy subjects | | | |
ML	AP	TD	EA	ML	AP	TD	EA
6,7	11,1	145,0	5,5	2,0	3,3	85,3	0,9

Values are the mean of 3 trials for 29 MS subjects and 28 healthy subjects in millimetres
ML—Medio-Lateral COP displacement
AP—Anterior-Posterior COP displacement
TD—Total COP displacement
EA—Ellipse Area (mm 2)

Table 4. Support phase of gait—Results.

	MS subjects			
	ML	AP	TD	CT
Right foot	37,73	209,28	369,63	1,35
Left foot	35,45	215,37	370,91	1,35
	Healthy subjects			
	ML	AP	TD	CT
Right foot	34,12	226,54	334,00	1,03
Left foot	29,08	228,26	342,36	1,01

Values are the mean of 3 trials for 29 MS subjects and 28 healthy subjects in millimetres
ML—Medio-Lateral COP displacement
AP—Anterior-Posterior COP displacement
TD—Total COP displacement
CT—Contact Time (s)

healthy group, more 31% in right foot and 33% in left foot. The disease duration has a positive correlation and moderate intensity with CT in both feet (rs = 0.472), indicating that the higher disease duration tend to be associated with higher CT. The BBS has a negative correlation and moderate intensity with the TD (rs = −0.585) indicating that high values of BBS tend to be related to low values of DT.

4 DISCUSSION

The main aim of this study was to investigate, if patients with multiple sclerosis, when in upright standing position and in the stance phase of gait, have cinematic changes associated to COP when compared with a healthy group. To perform this study we compare plantar pressure assessment with a clinical test. The primary limitation of the investigation is related to the disease itself. Multiple sclerosis is a chronic, inflammatory autoimmune central nervous system, causing motor and sensory changes. The disease course is variable and is related to changes in the inflammatory process, causing changes in symptoms over time (Kelleher et al., 2009). So it's very difficult to recruit subjects with the same characteristics and the same evolutionary stage of the disease. In this sense and in order to achieve the greatest number of subjects, we considered all patients with MS which satisfied the inclusion criteria, regardless the type and stage of MS evolution. Also, the study did not compare balance performance between subcategories of people with MS, such as those with spasticity, ataxia or sensory loss. These factors increased the group variability in the MS sample.

An important factor in data collection of plantar pressure is the test time. Test periods with short time may lead to results that aren't representative of postural stability. On the other hand long periods, in certain clinical situations, might influence the results due to increased fatigue. However it's necessary to establish what the optimum testing time, allowing the collection of data with confidence, without developing factors that may influence the results. A study with MS patients, to obtain the offset AP with eyes open and closed in upright standing position, used 3 trials with time 10 s (Daley & Swank, 1981).The validity and confidence in gait assessment with plantar pressure in this population is unknown. There are however studies on plantar pressure in subjects with MS, who used a first step protocol (Abdurakhmanov et al., 2006; Tsvetkova et al., 2008). In our study, we used the same protocol based on the subject safety and to minimize any effects of fatigue.

The analysis of test results in MS group shows that the variables are higher when compared to control group. In standing position an increase of ML is strongly correlated with increased AP, TD, and EA. In our study the statistical correlation between BBS and data obtained in the platform are not linear, showing large variations. BBS maintains the relationship with ML, AP and TD. A high value on BBS tends to be related to reduced values of ML, AP and TD. In 1-step protocol the correlation shows that a high value of BBS tends to be associated with a reduced value of the CT and TD, but with high value of AP. A major advantage of plantar pressure assessment is the ability to visualize the whole course of COP during foot contact. Thus it is possible to analyze and determine whether or not a stable support, and also visualize areas of the foot contact. This is particularly important when we are dealing with subjects with high scores in BBS. The relation between BBS and COP is more evident in standing position. There are situations in which BBS identifies increased instability, but tests on the platform indicate the maintenance of stability. Moreover, in some situations of maximum score in the BBS, this instrument is unable to detect the real situation of stability, because, as a compensatory response to postural instability, subjects can adopt a position or a more conservative gait pattern, to increasing security, reducing the risk of falls and reducing the variability of position and gait.

5 CONCLUSION

COP measures show clear differences when comparing healthy adults with adults with MS. The study found kinematic alterations on COP properties in all positions in multiple sclerosis group. As show, a clinical approach that usually tests postural stability (BBS) is ineffective in small postural disturbances. Specific and accurate analysis of postural stability in subjects with MS in upright standing position can be a useful tool to monitorize MS evolution and can be used to advise target oriented rehabilitative management of MS patients. Information obtained from pressure systems is also useful from a research perspective to address many questions regarding the relationship between plantar pressure and lower-extremity posture. The instrumented measures used here may be more sensitive than common clinical tests for objectively documenting both deficits and improvements in balance. With pressure technology becoming more common in physical therapy clinics, these parameters would be easy to capture as part of a physical therapy assessment. Because MS is a progressive disease, tools to measure balance impairments during early stages of the disease may lead to identification of people at risk for future decline. Specific and accurate analysis of postural stability in subjects with MS in upright standing position and support phase of gait can be a useful tool to monitorize MS evolution and can be used to advise target oriented rehabilitative management in these patients.

ACKNOWLEDGEMENTS

We would like to thank Elisabete Carolino (MSc) for statistical analysis; Cecilia Vaz Pinto (MD), for recruitment support and Pedro Portugal (PT), the blinded assessor in clinical test.

REFERENCES

Abdurakhmanov, M., Stolyarov, I., Il'vesa, A., Tsvetkova, T. & Lebedev, V. (2006). Measuring the distribution of plantar pressures during walking in patients with multiple sclerosis to evaluate treatment efficiency. Human Physiology, 32 (2), 154–156.

Berg, K., Wood-Dauphinee, S., Williams, J. & e Maki, B. (1992). Measuring balance in the elderly: validation of an instrument. Can J Public Health, 83 Suppl 2 S7–11.

Berg, K., Wood-Dauphinee, S. & Williams, J. (1995). The Balance Scale: reliability assessment with elderly residents and patients with an acute stroke. Scandinavian Journal of Rehabilitation Medicine, 27 (1), 27.

Buckley, J., Heasley, K., Scally, A. & Elliott, D. (2005). The effects of blurring vision on medio-lateral balance during stepping up or down to a new level in the elderly. Gait & Posture, (22), 146–153.

Bus, S. & Lange, A. (2005). A comparison of the 1-step, 2-step, and 3-step protocols for obtaining barefoot plantar pressure data in the diabetic neuropathic foot. Clinical Biomechanics, 20 (9), 892–899.

Cattaneo, D., De Nuzzo, C., Teresa Fascia, T., Macalli, M., Pisoni, I. & Cardini, R. (2002). Risks of Falls in Subjects With Multiple Sclerosis. Arch Phys Med Rehabil, 83 864–867.

Cattaneo, D., Jonsdottir, J., Zocchi, M. & Regola, A. (2007). Effects of balance exercises on people with multiple sclerosis: a pilot study. Clinical rehabilitation, 21 (9), 771.

Chernikova, L., Peressedova, A. & e Zavahshin, I. (2005). Postural disturbances in multiple sclerosis. Gait & Posture, 21 S128–S129.

Daley, M. & Swank, R. (1981). Quantitative Posturography: Use in Multiple Sclerosis. IEEE Transactions on Biomedical Engineering, 28 (9), 668–671.

Doyle, R., Hsiao-Wecksler, E., Ragan, B. & Rosengren, K. (2007). Generalizability of center of pressure measures of quiet standing. Gait & Posture, 25 166–171.

Hahn, M. & Chou, L.S. (2004). Age-related reduction in sagittal place center of mass motion during obstacle crossing. Journal of Biomechanics, (37), 837–844.

Hof, A., Gazendam, M. & Sinke, W. (2005). The condition for dynamic stability. Journal of Biomechanics (38,), 1–8.

Horak, F. (1997). Clinical assessment of balance disorders. Gait & Posture, (6), 76–84.

Ienaga, Y., Mitoma, H., Kubota, K., Morita, S. & Mizusawa, H. (2006). Dynamic imbalance in gait ataxia. Characteristics of plantar pressure measurements. Journal of the Neurological Sciences, (246), 53–57.

Karst, G.M., Venema, D.M., Roehrs, T.G. & Tyler, A.E. (2005). Center of pressure measures during standing tasks in minimally impaired persons with multiple sclerosis. J Neurol Phys Ther, 29 (4), 170–80.

Kelleher, K.J., Spence, W., Solomonidis, S. & Apatsidis, D. (2009). Ambulatory rehabilitation in multiple sclerosis. Disabil Rehabil, 1–8.

Lord, S., Wade, D. & Halligan, P. (1998). A comparison of two physiotherapy treatment approaches to improve walking in multiple sclerosis: a pilot randomized controlled study. Clinical rehabilitation, 12 (6), 477.

Maki, B.E., Holliday, P.J. & Topper, A.K. (1994). A prospective study of postural balance and risk of falling in an ambulatory and independent elderly population. J Gerontol, 49 (2), M72–84.

Orlin, M. & McPoil, T. (2000). Plantar pressure assessment. Phys Ther, 80 (4), 399–409.

Palace, J. (2001). Making the diagnosis of multiple sclerosis. J Neurol Neurosurg Psychiatry, 71 Suppl 2 ii3–8.

Robain, G., alentini, F., Renard-Deniel, S., Chennevelle, J. & Piera, J.B. (2006). A baropodometric parameter to analyze the gait of hemiparetic patients: the path of center of pressure. Ann Readapt Med Phys, 49 (8), 609–613.

Rougier, P., Faucher, M., Cantalloube, S., Lamotte, D., Vinti, M. & Thoumie, P. (2007). How proprioceptive impairments affect quiet standing in patients with multiple sclerosis. Somatosensory and Motor Research, (24), 41–51.

Schmid, M., Beltrami, G., Zambarbieri, D. & Verni, G. (2005). Centre of pressure displacements in trans-femoral amputees during gait. Gait & Posture 21 (255–262).

Smedal, T., Lygren, H., Myhr, K., Moe-Nilssen, R., Gjelsvik, B., Gjelsvik, O. & Strand, L. (2006). Balance and gait improved in patients with MS after physiotherapy based on the Bobath concept. Physiotherapy Research International, 11 (2), 104–116.

Smith, K., Commean, P., Mueller, M., Robertson, D., Pilgram, T. & Johnson, J. (2000). Assessment of the diabetic foot using spiral computed tomography imaging and plantar pressure measurements: a technical report. J Rehabil Res Dev, 37 (1), 31–40.

Taylor, A., Menz, H. & Keenan, A. (2004). The influence of walking speed on plantar pressure measurements using the two-step gait initiation protocol. 14 (1), 49–55.

Tsvetkova, T., Stoliarov, I., Ivko, O., Ilves, A., Abdurahmanov, M., Prakhova, L., Nikiforova, I. & Lebedev, V. (2008). Dynamic plantar pressure distribution in multiple sclerosis patients with different neurological status. Clinical Biomechanics, 23 (5), 691.

Tyson, S. & Connell, L. (2009). How to measure balance activity in clinical practice? A systematic review of the psychometric properties and clinical utility of measurement tools in neurological conditions. Clinical rehabilitation, 23 (9), 824–840.

Waxman, S. (2005). Multiple Sclerosis as a Neuronal Disease California USA: Elsevier Academic Press.

Winter, D., Prince, F. & e Patla, A. (1996). Interpretation of COM and COP balance control during quiet standing. Gait & posture, 4 (2), 174–175.

Zabjek, K., Hill, S., Gage, W., Danells, C., Closson, V., Maki, B. & e McIlroy, W. (2005). Gait and standing posture in patients with multiple sclerosis. Gait & Posture, 21 (Supplement 1), S136.

Technology and Medical Sciences – Natal Jorge et al. (eds)
© 2011 Taylor & Francis Group, London, ISBN 978-0-415-66822-4

Neurom: A motor treatment system for chronic stroke patients

Fábio Lucio Corrêa Junior
Universidade Federal de Minas Gerais—Brazil

Rodrigo Cappato de Araújo
Universidade Federal de Minas Gerais—Brazil
Universidade de Pernambuco—Brazil

Daniel Neves Rocha
Universidade Federal de Minas Gerais—Brazil
Instituto Federal de Minas Gerais—Brazil

Tálita Saemi Payossim Sono, Leandro Rodrigues dos Santos,
Adriana Maria Valladão N. Van Petten & Marcos Pinotti
Universidade Federal de Minas Gerais—Brazil

ABSTRACT: This paper describes a functional design of an active-assisted treatment system, which was developed at the Bioengineering Laboratory (LabBio) of the Universidade Federal de Minas Gerais (UFMG), for the upper limbs motor rehabilitation in patients with chronic stroke. This system consists of an exoskeleton and a functional glove to perform movements of the elbow and hand, respectively. It is based on the capture of myoelectric signals of the flexor and extensor muscles of the elbow and hand, which produce an intentional action and further drive the bio-mechanical their members, provided that the patient is able to partially control the movements of the affected limb. The system design brings together various aspects, such as low cost, low power consumption and most importantly, allows the realization of functional tasks during treatment, returning as soon as possible, the functionality and independence for these patients.

1 INTRODUCTION

Stroke is one of the main causes of mortality and functional disability in the worldwide. Recent research have shown that in Europe there are 200 to 300 new stroke cases per 100,000 every year (Muntner et al., 2002; Massiero et al., 2007). Moreover, World Health Organization (WHO) estimates that the incident of stroke in developed countries should increase 30% by the year 2025 (Truelsen et al., 2006).

Current data estimate that worldwide there are about forty-nine million people who survived the stroke and living with a sequel or functional disability (Feigin, 2005), which may cause the decrease in quality of life of survivors and an increase in burden on health centers.

Therefore, it is justified the search for more effective therapy for the treatment of motor sequel resulting from stroke, especially when it comes to the rehabilitation of upper limb, which still has low rates to recover the function and especially low pleased by the patients (Stein et al., 2007).

Studies report about 5% to 20% of patients affected by the stroke restore upper limb function (Gowland, 1982; Kwakkel et al., 1999; Kwakkell et al., 2003; Kwakkel et al., 2008), and that only 6% of these patients are satisfied with the level of functionality of the affected upper limb (Broeks et al., 1999).

Due to the unsuccessful of traditional rehabilitation programs to restore upper limb function after stroke, researchers have sought new technologies. Robotic devices have been developed to assist in recovery from motor function (Prange et al., 2006).

Robotic devices allow to perform specific tasks repeatedly in a controlled and reliable way, which has been demonstrated in the literature as a determinant factor to facilitate the cortical reorganization, with a concomitant increase in motor skills and improves the performance of functional activities (Liepert et al., 2001).

Some studies (Krebs et al., 1999; Lum et al., 2002; Song et al., 2006) have developed robotic systems to assist treatments of motor sequel resulting from stroke. These studies showed significant improvement in motor function of upper limb, especially the proximal joints, after treatment program using the aid of robots. However, few studies developed and evaluated the use of robotic devices applied to the rehabilitation of the joints of the wrist and hand. Moreover, these robots are fixed and don't allow reproduce functional tasks of daily life, limiting its application.

According to this information, it is necessary the developing of new therapeutic alternatives that are more effective and allow the execution of daily functional activities during the treatment, recovering as soon as possible the functionality and independence to these individuals.

Neuron is a proposed rehabilitation system designed for stroke patients to help them and train the movement of the elbow joint. This system consists of an elbow orthosis, actuator module and a control module.

2 NEURON PROTOTYPE

The Neuron was developed into functional modules described below.

2.1 Elbow orthosis

The elbow orthosis is constituted by two static parts fixed in an exoskeleton by screws (Fig. 1).

The static parts are made in thermoplastic material molded separately and fixed on the arm and forearm of each patient. They stabilize and position the arm and forearm in the functional position of the elbow joint. Specifically, the forearm is fixed in neutral position.

The exoskeleton consists of two structures connected by a joint which coincide with the rotation axis of the elbow. The structures of the exoskeleton are made of segments located at the side of the arm and forearm separated by metal spacers. These spacers are made according to the thickness of the patient's arm (Fig. 2).

The exoskeleton is responsible for flexion and extension of the elbow joint, which Range Of Motion (ROM) from 10 to 110 degrees. This range represents the elbow functional ROM

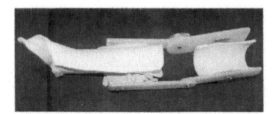

Figure 1. Elbow orthosis.

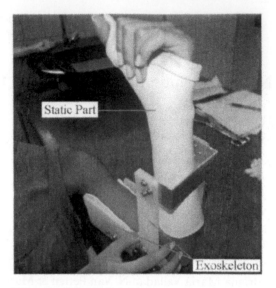

Figure 2. Patient using elbow orthosis.

(Lockard, 2006). These limitations are performed physically by stop mechanism to ensure patient safety.

2.2 Actuator module

The actuator module is responsible for flexion and extension of the elbow. It was positioned at static part of the arm of the elbow orthosis, and it is composed of an electro-mechanical actuator, a traction system and a pulley (Fig. 3).

The electro-mechanical actuator corresponds to a Direct Current (DC) motor drive by a control module. The DC motor is coupled to the shaft traction system.

The pulley was fixed to the mechanical structures of exoskeleton related to the forearm with its center coincident to the rotation axis of the elbow joint. The pulley diameter was calculated in function of motor speed and time required for the flexion and extension movements.

The traction system has a shaft suspended by bearing bushing. Two cables were connected to this shaft which their direction of winding are opposite, that is, when the shaft rotates in a direction, one of these cables is would while the other is unwinding. The ends of the cables were connected to the pulley.

The rotation action of the pulley produced by the traction system moves the elbow joint and, consequently, the patient's forearm. Therefore, the position of the pulley determines the angle position of elbow joint of the patient. The control of the angle or motion of the pulley is accomplished by the voluntary activation of muscle groups of

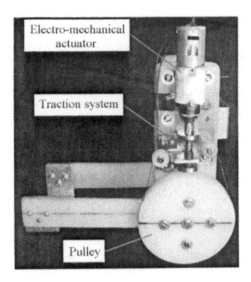

Figure 3. Actuator module.

the patient's arm. Normally, the biceps and triceps EMG are chosen to control this angle.

2.3 Control module

The control module is responsible by the acquisition, treatment and processing of electromyographic signals (EMG) from two preserved muscles groups. EMG data were collected using surface differential electrodes (two Ag-AgCl bars, $10 \times 2 \times 1$ mm, with 10 mm interelectrode distance, gain of 20, input impedance of 10 GΩ and common mode rejection ratio of 130 dB).

The action of EMG from one of these muscles activates the mechanism to flexion, while the other is responsible for extension of the elbow joint. The elbow orthosis has cutouts to facilitate housing and connection of electrodes in the patient's skin. Thus, a voluntary muscle contraction performed by the patient is converted to the movement the elbow joint.

3 DISCUSSION AND CONCLUSION

This research resulted in the development of a prototype for rehabilitation system for stroke patients called Neuron.

The elbow orthosis was built using lightweight and tough materials presenting a few adjustable pieces to simplify its manufacture and its adaptation.

The actuation module was tested at the laboratory and was able to simulate the function of elbow moving a weight equivalent to the forearm during the specified time.

In the laboratory tests, Neuron showed that can be used in different rehabilitation programs. Further more, this system allows both the performance of functional training in rehabilitation centers and its use as orthosis to assist in daily activities, which differs from other systems described in the literature. However clinical studies are needed to evaluate and demonstrate its efficacy.

ACKNOWLEDGEMENT

The authors gratefully acknowledge the Capes, CNPq and Fapemig for financial support.

REFERENCES

Broeks, J.G., Lankhorst, G.J., Rumping, K. & Prevo, A.J. 1999. The long-term outcome of arm function after stroke: results of a follow-up study. *Disability and Rehabilitation* 21(8): 357–364.

Feigin, V.L. 2005. Stroke epidemiology in the developing world. *Lancet* 365(9478): 2160–1.

Gowland, C. 1982. Recovery of motor function following stroke: profile and predictors. *Physiotherapy* 34: 77–84.

Krebs, H.I., Hogan, N., Aisen, M.L. & Volpe B.T. 1998. Robot-aided neurorehabilitation. *IEEE transactions on rehabilitation engineering* 6(1): 75–87.

Kwakkel, G., Kollen, B.J. & Wagenaar, R.C. 1999. Therapy impact on functional recovery in stroke rehabilitation: a critical review of the literature. *Physiotherapy* 13: 457–70.

Kwakkel, G., Kollen, B.J., Van der Grond, J. & Prevo, A.J. 2003. Probability of regaining dexterity in the flaccid upper limb: impact of severity of paresis and time since onset in acute stroke. *Stroke* Sep;34(9): 2181–6.

Kwakkel, G., Kollen, B.J. & Krebs, H.I. 2008. Effects of robot-assisted therapy on upper limb recovery after stroke: a systematic review. *Neurorehabilitation Neural Repair* 22: 111–121.

Liepert, J., Uhde, I., Graf, S., Leidner, O. & Weiller, C. 2001. Motor cortex plasticity during forced-use therapy in stroke patients: a preliminary study. *Journal of Neurology* 248(4): 315–321.

Lockard, M. 2006. Clinical Biomechanics of the elbow. *Journal of Hand Therapy* 19(2): 72–80.

Lum, P.S., Burgar, C.G., Shor, P.C., Majmundar, M. & Van der Loos, M. 2002. Robot-assisted movement training compared with conventional therapy techniques for rehabilitation of upper limb motor function after stroke. *Archives of physical medicine and rehabilitation* 83: 952–59.

Masiero, S., Celia, A., Rosati, G. & Armani, M. 2007. Robotic-assisted rehabilitation of the upper limb after acute stroke. *Archives of physical medicine and rehabilitation* 88(2): 142–149.

Muntner, P., Garret, E., Klag, M.J. & Coresh, J. 2002. Trends in stroke prevalence between 1973 and 1991 in the US population 25 to 74 years of age. *Stroke* 33: 1209–1213.

Prange, G.B., Jannink, M.J., Groothuis-oudshoorn, C.G., Hermens, H.J & Ijzerman, M.J. 2006. Systematic review of the effect of robot-aided therapy on recovery of the hemiparetic arm after stroke. *Journal of rehabilitation research and development* 2006, 43(2):171–184.

Song, R., Tong, K.Y., Hu, X.L., Tsang, S.F. & Li, L. 2006. The therapeutic effects of myoelectrically controlled robotic system for persons after stroke—a piloty study. *IEEE-EMBS Annual International Conference* 4945–48.

Stein, J., Narendran, K., Mcbean, J., Krebs, K. & Hughes, R. 2007. Electromyography controlled exoskeletal upper-limb-powered orthosis for exercise training after stroke. *American Journal of Physical Medicine Rehabilitation* 86: 255–261.

Truelsen, T., Piechowski-jozwiak, B., Bonita, R., Mathers, C., Bogousslavsky, J. & Boysen, G. 2006. Stroke incidence and prevalence in Europe: a review of available data. *European Journal of Neurology* 13(6): 581–598.

Technology and Medical Sciences – Natal Jorge et al. (eds)
© 2011 Taylor & Francis Group, London, ISBN 978-0-415-66822-4

Non-invasive diagnosis and monitoring of Cystic Fibrosis by mass spectrometry of the exhaled breath

S. Gramacho, M. Piñeiro, A.A.C.C. Pais & A.M.d'A Rocha Gonsalves
Departamento de Química, Faculdade de Ciências e Tecnologia, Universidade de Coimbra, Coimbra, Portugal

F. Gambôa & C. Robalo Cordeiro
Centro de Pneumologia da Faculdade de Medicina de Coimbra, Universidade de Coimbra, Coimbra, Portugal

ABSTRACT: Cystic Fibrosis is one of the most common lethal genetic diseases in Caucasians, in which the highermorbidity is associated with the pulmonary manifestation. As in many other cases, the increase of the life expectancy of CF patients is closely related with an adequate following and monitoring of the evolution of the disease, which is currently mostly based in spirometric test. The analysis of volatile organic compounds presents in exhaled breath using Solid Phase Micro-Extraction and Gas Chromatography with Mass Spectrometry detection, shows that FC patients exhibit a distinctconcentration of chlorinated compounds (dichloromethane, chloroform, bromochloromethane) and non-chlorinated compounds (acetonitrile, isopropanol, pentane/isoprene and toluene), allowing the differentiation from the healthy subjects.

1 INTRODUCTION

Cystic Fibrosis is one of the most common lethal genetic diseases in Caucasians. The gene defective in cystic fibrosis patients (Cystic Fibrosis transmenbrane conductance regulator—CFTR) causes the absence of the formation of nonfunctional CFTR protein, which is responsible for the transport of chlorine ions out of the cell. The anomalous concentration of chlorine ions leads to the transport of sodium ions into the cell, in order to keep the electrochemical equilibrium. The flow of water is affected by this abnormal concentration of chlorine and sodium atoms, increasing the transport of water into the cell through osmosis. The CFTR protein is in high concentration in the membrane of epithelial cells, lining the internal surface of pancreas, sweat and salivary glands, intestine, reproductive organs and in the submucosal glands of the airways. Consequently the clinical manifestations of the disease vary; the pulmonary manifestation of the Cystic Fibrosis is associated with the higher morbidity, being the cause of death in more than 90% of the patients.

The disease can be diagnosed by the determination of the mutation in the CF gene, through a genetic test that is highly specific but expensive, and/or by the sweat test, standardized by Gibson & Cooke in 1959 (Gibson & Cooke, 1989), that is still extensively used. Once diagnosed and without gene therapy, the CF is a chronicledisease. In their lifetime, the patients suffer from inflammatory processes and different types of pulmonary infections, among others problems. The development of methodologies to monitor the clinical stage of the patients that allows the implementation of the most adequate therapies for each patient at each moment, can increase the lifetime expectancy of these patients.

Any tool to monitor the disease has to take into consideration several aspects:it has to be non-invasive, require minimal or no effort from the patient, because some of them may be in a very critical stage or be very young infants (ideally it has to be possible to be used without the active collaboration of the patient), be repeatable in short time intervals without any damage for the patient, determine (or take into consideration) as many variables as possible, and the analysis has to be as little time consuming as possible andresortto equipment already present or in the analysis laboratory, or easily available commercially.

The most interesting matrix for monitoring the CF in a non-invasive way is the exhaled breath, having been in direct contact with the respiratory system, and being external to the patient. A few studies of the exhaled breath of patients with cystic fibrosis have been done. The analysis of exhaled breath condensate (Horváth et al. 2005) was used to measure inflammatory and oxidative stress biomarkers (Kharitonov & Barnes, 2001, Jobsin et al. 2000, Montuschi et al. 1999) and to determine the levels of Leukotriene B_4 and Interleukin-6related to the acute infective exarcebation

(Capagnano et al. 2003). The analysis of the condensate is easy to perform, repeatable andhas low costs associatedbut does not allow the analysis of highly volatile components and requires a respiratory effort from the patients.

The analysis of Volatile Organic Compounds (VOCs) of exhaled breath has been used in diverse applications, such as environmental characterization and occupational exposure to chemical pollutants, development of electronic nose system (Penza & Cassano, 2003) or the identification of biomarkers of different diseases (Cao & Duan, 2006, Di Francesco et al. 2005) such as lung cancer (Poli et al. 2005) or chronic obstructive pulmonary disease (Ibrahim et al. 2010). Breath gas analysis is difficult to perform mainly because of the low VOC concentrations in breath air, but these difficulties having partly been overcome by improvements in sampling and analytical techniques. Pre-concentrating of the breath Gas, Cryogenic cooling systems and thermodesorption systems combined with Mass Spectrometry (GC/MS) constitute reliable and sensitive methods for VOC analysis (Cao & Duan, 2007, Kharitinov & Barnes 2001).

High levels of ethane have been determined in the exhaled breath of patients with CF, and correlated with exhaled CO and airway obstruction (Paredi et al. 2000). In 2006, Barker and coworkers (Barker et al. 2006), evaluated the levels of volatile organic compounds in patients with cystic fibrosis using a sampling system involving canisters and equipment modification to allow for the pre-concentration and introduction of the sample. The author analyzed 12 VOCs, (ethane, propane, n-pentane, methanol, ethanol, 2-propanol, acetone, isoprene, benzene, toluene, dimethyl sulphide and limonene) in the samples of exhaled breath collected from 20 CF patients and 20 healthy controls concluding, among other findings, that "group comparison yielded no differences for ethane, isoprene, limonene and several other VOC".

In this study we present the analysis of VOCs of exhaled breath samples from 17 cystic fibrosis patients and 16 healthy, non-smoker subjects, using Solid Phase Micro-Extraction and Gas Chromatography with Mass Spectrometry detection (SPME-GC-MS). The chemometrics analysis of the results allows the both the identification of the compounds that are related to the disease, and to discriminate the severity of the manifestations.

2 METHODS

2.1 Subjects

The group of patients was composed of 17 subjects, five males and twelve females with ages between 15 and 35.

Patients were recruited in the Centro de Pneumologia dos Hospitais da Universidade de Coimbra. The diagnosis of their condition was performed by genetic testor the sweat test, in most cases during the period of adolescence. Patients 1, 8 and 12 are in the critical stage of the disease, patient 1 was submitted to lung transplant, patient 8 unfortunately passed away and patient 12 was recommended for lung transplant. Patient 13 suffered from frequent inflammation processes and subject 18 presented bacterial infection. The teams of Clinicians and chemists agreed to incorporate a healthy person into the group of patients, keeping the identity of the subject unknown to the team of chemists.

The control group was composed of 16 elements, four males and twelve females with ages between 22 and 45. Details on their medical history, current status and environmental exposure were registered in a structured interview, prior to sample collection.

All subjects are Caucasian. The distribution of age and height was compatible among the groups; however, the members of the patients' group have a much smaller body weight.

The characteristics of the study groups are presented in Table 1.

2.2 Lung function

Pulmonary function was evaluated by spirometric tests performed by the group of cardiopneumology of the Hospitais da Universidade de Coimbra. All the tests were performed on the same day of breath sampling.

2.3 Exhaled NO

Exhaled NO was measured using a Chemilunescence analyzer, NioxMino from Aerocrine.

Table 1. Characteristic of the study groups.

	CF subjects (n = 17)	Healthy subjects (n = 16)
Age, yr	25 ± 6	23 ± 6
Weight, Kg	57 ± 12.2	63 ± 12.5
Height, cm	160.9 ± 6.1	165.5 ± 9.5
Sex male/female	5/12	4/12
Sweat test, mEq/L	119 ± 18.6	–
FEV_1, % predicted	134	–
FVC, % predicted	202	–
Tiffeneau index	24	–
Tidal volume, % predited	146.6 ± 47.9	–
Rf, % predicted	101.4 ± 32.4	–
NO, ppb	10.4 ± 2.5	17.6 ± 9.8

2.4 Breath sampling

Before each sampling, the subject didengagein any physical activity or eat for at least 30 minutes. The volume of the collected samples was in a single respiratory act and during one minute on tidal volume.

Collection equipment was designed with the requirements that follow. Resistance to the passage of the exhaled airflow must be absent, and the risk of infection between individuals prevented, by elimination of salivary contamination. Also, the absorption of the analyte to the sample container must be minimal and the equipment should be portable, easy to operate, free of leaks and allow for sample storage. The equipment consists of a mouthpiece connected to a unidirectional valve, which fits perfectly in a glass vial where the air sample is captured. To avoid dilution of the sample due to dead space, a tube was inserted into the sampling bottle and connected to the outside, allowing excess airto exit. In order to circumventthe critical problem of the adsorption of VOCs to the walls of the container sample, glass was used, Scheme 1. So as to prevent nasal inhalation, tweezers on the nose are used. The sampling device consists of disposable components or components which can be washed and sterilized.

During the sampling period, the collection container is placed in an isothermal container with a mixture of ice/sodium chloride, providing a temperature below $-18°C$ to ensure efficient capture and storage of the more volatile metabolites. The collections were made in Centro de Pneumologia dos Hospitais da Universidade de Coimbra. The quality of the air of the room in which the collection took place was evaluated on each day of sampling. The samples were stored at $-18°C$ until the analyses were performed.

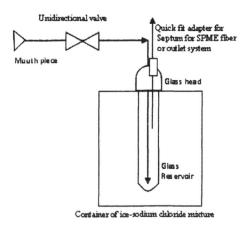

Scheme 1. Home-made equipment for breath sampling.

2.5 Sample preparation and analysis

The compounds were extracted with SPME technique using a combined fiber-coating Carboxen-PDMS, with thickness of 75 μm. The fiber was inserted into the sampling bottle through a septum for 30 minutes at room temperature ($22°C$). Then the sample was thermally desorbed for 5 minutes into the GC injector at $275°C$. Subsequently, the compounds were separated with a capillary column Hewlett Packard (HP) 1—Mass Spectrometry (MS), (30 m, 0.25 mm id., 0.25 μm film). After injection, the column was maintained isothermal at $30°C$ for 10 minutes and then heated to $200°C$ with an increment of $20°C/min$. The interface temperature was $280°C$. The equipment used for the chromatographic analysis was an Agilent 6890 seriesgas chromatograph, with a Hewlett Packard (HP) Selecive Mass Detector (MSD) 5973 withscanning mode of acquisition, in the mass range of 20 to 550 Da. The identification of the compounds present in the exhaled air samples under study was confirmed by comparison of retention times of each compound with pure standards and fragmentation characteristics of their ions. The measures include an internal chromatographic standard, fluorobenzene with 40 ppm concentration.

2.6 Data analysis

Demographic and clinical data were expressed as means ± SD.

Data analysis resorted to standard chemometrics techniques, including Hierarchical Cluster Analysis (HCA), with average linkage, for exploratory assessment of the data structure (Almeida et al. 2007), Principal Component Analysis (PCA) on both the variance-covariance and correlation matrices (Breretron, 2003) and varimax rotation of the main PCA axis (Abdi, 2003). Decision rules were created with a PCA/LDA approach (Massart, 1988), in which only the selected principal components are used for the discriminant function. The software code was developed by the authors in Octave.

In the exploratory data analysis we resorted to Hierarchical Cluster Analysis (HCA), for which a recent review can be found in reference Almeida et al. (Almeida et al. 2007). Briefly, scattered objects are joined in decreasing order of similarity i.e., increasing distance. Our results will be presented in terms of Euclidean distance. The first (and most significant) group is made up from the two most similar samples. The subsequent steps test not only the distance between samples, but also between a specific sample and a group of samples, or two groups already formed. To define the latter two distances, one must establish a linkage scheme. One of the usual linkage approaches is average-linkage, in which the distance between objects or groups is based on averaging over the members of the clusters. Another common scheme is single-linkage, in which distances are established in terms of the nearest-neighbors. This scheme will be followed in the present work, because it favors the growth of groups with inclusion of nearby objects, contrasting with the initial split of objects in various compact groups promoted by average linkage. The HCA procedure is graphically represented by a dendrogram.

Principal Component Analysis (PCA) is an appropriate technique for extracting underlying factors from a multivariate dataset. Based on an orthogonal linear transformation, PCA defines a lower dimensionality system, such that the highest variance of the data comes projected on the first Principal Component (PC1), the second largest on the second coordinate (PC2), and so on (Brereton, 2003). PCA is usually performed after centering the data, and is based on the solution of an eigenvalue problem, either based on the correlation or variance/covariance matrix of the original variables. In this work we present results based on both. We have also subjected the data to Varimax searches for a rotation (i.e., a linear combination) of the PCA axis (Abdi, 2003), such that the variance of the loadings, i.e., the weights of the original variables, are maximized. It facilitates the inspection of groups of variables present in the axis considered, allowing to rationalise the PCA results and determine the underlying factors.

Finally, the classification used Linear Discriminant Analysis (LDA), resorting only to the PCA variables on the main components. LDA maximizes the ratio of between-class variance to the within-class variance in any particular data set so as to ensure maximal separability. The objective is to find a decision rule to assign further, unclassified objects to the given classes (Brereton, 2003).

3 RESULTS AND DISCUSSION

The chromatogram of one sample of exhaled breath collected during 1 minute with tidal volume is presented in Figure 1. Excepting 4-methyl-2-pentanone, all the compounds detected in the analysis of 1 minute of tidal volume were also detected in the samples of one respiratory act but, as expected, in low concentrations. Heptane was only present in two of the samples analyzed and excluded from the data analysis procedures. In this study, the analysis of the data corresponding to the sampling of one minute of tidal volume is presented. In Table 2 the retention time and the mass of the molecular ion for each of the metabolites identified in the chromatograms are presented.

The chromatographic area determined for each VOC in each subject constitutes the set of data to perform the analysis. The main difference observed

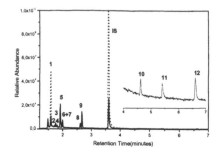

Figure 1. Typical chromatographic assay of exhaled breath during 1 minute with tidal volume in patient (solid line) and healthy subject (dot line).

Table 2. Identification of the chromatographic peaks.

Peak number	Retention time (min)	Molecular ion (Da)	Metabolite
1	1.73	46	Ethanol
2	1.77	41	Acetonitrile
3	1.82	58	Acetone
4	1.87	60	Isopropanol
5	1.93	72	n-Pentane
6	1.94	68	Isoprene
7	2.00	85	Dichloromethane
8	2.62	129	Bromochloromethane
9	2.67	119	Chloroform
10	4.62	100	Heptane
11	5.40	100	4-methyl-2-pentanone
12	6.61	92	Toluene
IS	3.61	96	Fluorobenzene

in the analysis of the VOCs of the patients' and control group is not the nature of the exhaled VOCs, but their quantity, the chromatographic area. None of the 11 VOCs alone discriminate the study groups, suggesting that there is no one VOC that could be a biomarker of the disease. The biomarkers of CF are the difference in the concentration of compounds that are usually present in the breath. The first approximation in the attempt of interpretation of the large amount of data obtained was the calculation of the mean of the chromatographic area of each VOC in the group of patients and healthy subjects.

With this calculation, the difference between the groups is diluted and a large quantity of information is missing. Therefore, the data base was subjected to HCA, based on Euclidean distance with single-linkage. Figure 2 depicts the corresponding dendrogram. It shows the formation of two coherent groups, one delimited by samples 18 and 26, corresponding to a total of 17 subjects, and the other by samples 10 and 7, totaling 8 subjects. The latter are, in general, less similar than in the other cluster. The structure is completed by

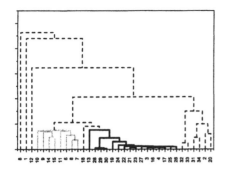

Figure 2. Dendrogram resulting from HCA analysis.

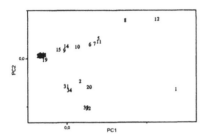

Figure 3. PCA scores plot from the variance-covariance matrixin two components.

6 samples in a less coherent cluster, delimited by samples 32 and 20, and by 3 clear outliers, 1, 8 and 12, that join the remaining subjects at a very late stage, with Euclidean distances above 1.5×10^7.

The whole set of results was also subjected to PCA, using both the variance-covariance and correlation matrices. The results from the first approach are depicted in Figure 3, and Table 3. Inspection of the Figure clearly reveals that two components are sufficient to promote the segregation of patient and control groups. The latter are, to a large extent, overlapping for low values of the scores in PC1. Patients are essentially disposed along a line, for higher values of PC2. Two exceptions are patients 1 and 2 that are situated at lower values of PC2. Healthy subjects 20 and 31–34 are also located at lower values of PC2.

Similar results are obtained resorting to the correlation matrix, Figure 4, which, as will be shown later, provides a slightly better discrimination. Recall, however, that three components should be used in the correlation analysis, that will be used in what follows.

Figure 3 is decomposed in two for the representations in panels (a) and (b) of Figure 5 and panel (c) is the representation of the PC3. This allowed decoupling of the superimposed results, and also facilitates the analysis in each of the components. It is seen, panel (a), that healthy subjects suggest a reference value for PC1 and PC2 while PC3 do not differentiate the groups. Also, PC1 and PC2 classify patient

Table 3. Loadings associated to each VOC in the corresponding PC.

| VOC | Eigenvalue Variance/Covariance | | Correlation | | |
	PC1	PC2	PC1	PC2	PC3
Ethanol	−6.8(−3)	−3.2(−3)	0.11	0.10	0.83
Acetonitrile	1.7(−1)	−1.9(−2)	−0.46	−0.07	0.07
Acetone	−1.4(−2)	6.9(−2)	0.04	0.40	0.44
Isopropanol	1.2(−2)	−9.9(−3)	−0.35	−0.26	0.06
Pentane-isoprene	5.2(−1)	−8.4(−1)	−0.32	−0.42	0.19
Dichloro-methane	3.0(−1)	1.7(−1)	−0.42	0.29	−0.04
Bromochloro methane	3.0(−1)	2.4(−1)	−0.29	0.24	−0.07
Chloroform	7.2(−1)	4.4(−1)	−0.41	0.33	−0.05
4-Methyl-2-pentanone	2.1(−2)	1.1(−2)	−0.27	0.25	−0.01
Toulene	2.1(−2)	−5.5(−2)	−0.22	−0.51	0.23

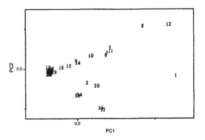

Figure 4. Same as Figure 3, form the correlation matrix.

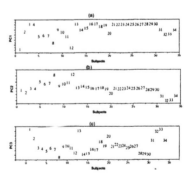

Figure 5. PCA analysis using the correlation matrix.

13, the healthy person included in the patient group as a blain test, as an healthy subject. Non direct correspondences were found between the PCs and the values of the NO or spirometrics test. If we further inspect the loadings depicted in Table 3, it can be seen that this first component is related to chlorinated compounds. Such observations are reinforced after Varimax rotation (Table 4) in which it is seen that the three groups of variables identified

Table 4. Varimax loadings.

VOC	Varimax loading			Group
Ethanol	0.121	−0.130	0.828	3
Acetonitrile	−0.305	−0.362	−0.010	2
Acetone	−0.166	0.170	0.553	3
Isopropanol	−0.098	−0.422	−0.071	2
Pentane-isoprene	−0.064	−0.554	0.008	2
Dichloromethane	−0.509	−0.043	0.011	1
Bromochloromethane	−0.385	0.015	−0.018	1
Chloroform	−0.532	−0.004	0.015	1
4-Methyl-2-pentanone	−0.366	0.016	0.045	1
Toulene	0.173	−0.579	0.026	2

comprise, respectively, dichloromethane, chloroform, bromochloromethane, and 4-methylpentanone in one of the groups and acetonitrile, isopropanol, pentane/isoprene and toluene in another and, finally, ethanol and acetone in the third group.

4 CONCLUSION

The developed methodology for the sampling and analysis of exhaled breath using a home-made sample-collector, easy to manufacture and reproduce, and SPME-GC-MS, proved to be efficient. The time required for the collection of the sample is about 35 minutes, without any additional effort from the patient, allowing for easy use in infants and even in patients with assisted ventilation. The methodology for theanalysis of exhaled breath samples avoids previous preparation of the samples or modification on the commercial GC-MS equipment, with a total analysis time of less than one hour.

The analysis of the VOCs, using PCA analysis allows the differentiation of healthy and CF patients and also discriminates the severity of the manifestations of the disease. While the compounds represented in PC2 (non-chlorinated compounds) separate the healthy and FC patients, the compounds in PC1 (chlorinated compounds) give information about the severity of the manifestation of the disease separating patients 1, 8 and 12 from the patients' group.

After diagnosisof cystic fibrosis, most of the treatment decisions remain based on clinical judgment and secondary parameters derived from pulmonary function testing, chest radiology or blood analysis. The non-invasive analysis of VOCs in exhaled breath could be a very useful tool for monitoring the disease activity and progression.

ACKNOWLEDGEMENTS

The authors thank Chymiotechnon and the Centro de Pneumologia dos Hospitais da Universidade de Coimbra and all the persons that agreed to take part in this study.

REFERENCES

Abdi, 2003. *Factor rotations.* In M. Lewis Beck, A. Bryman & T. Futing. Encyclopedia for research methods for social sciences. CA: Thousand Oaks.

Almeida, J. et al. 2007. Improving hierarchical cluster analysis: A new method with outlier detection and automatic clustering. *Chemometrics and Intelligent Systems.* 87: 208–217.

Barker, M. et al. 2006. Volatile organic compounds in the exhaled breath of young patients with cystic fibrosis. *Eur. Respir. J.* 27: 929–936.

Brereton, 2003. Chemometrics: *Data analysis for the laboratory and chemical plant.* Chichester: Wiley.

Capagnano, G.E. et al. 2003. Increased Leukotriene B4 and Interleukin-6 in exhaled breath condencatein-cistyc fibrosis. *Am. J. Respir. Crit. Care Med.* 167: 1109–1112.

Cao, W. & Duan, Y. 2006. Breath analysis: potential for clinic Diagnosis and exposure assessment. *Clinical Chem.* 52(5): 800–811.

Cao, W. & Duan, Y. 2007. Current status of methods and techniques for breath analysis. *Crit. Rev. Anal. Chem.* 37: 3–13.

Di Francesco, F. et al. 2005. Breath analysis: trends in techniques and clinical applications. *Microchem. J.* 79: 405–410.

Gibson & Cooke, 1989. A test for Concentration of electrolytes in sweat in cystic fibrosis of pancreas utilizing pilocarpineiontophoresis. *Pediatrics* 24: 545–549.

Horváth, I. et al. 2005. Exhaled breath condensate: methodological recommendations and unresolved questions. *Eur. Respir. J.* 26: 523–548.

Ibrahim, et al. 2010. Exhaled volatile organic compounds as potentional biomarkers in chronic obstructive pulmonary disease. *Am. J. Respir. Crit. Care Med.* 181: A 1012.

Jobsin, Q. et al. 2000. Hydrogen Peroxide and nitric oxide in exhaled air of children with cystic fibrosis during antibiotic treatment. *Eur. Respir. J* 16: 95–100.

Kharitonov, S.A. & Barnesm, P.J. 2001. Exhaled markers of pulmonary disease. *Am. J. Respir. Crit. Care Med.* 163: 1693–1722.

Montuschi, P. et al. 1999. Increased 8-isoprotane, a biomarker of oxidative stress, in exhaled condensate of asthma patients. *Am. J. Respir. Crit. Care Med.* 160: 216–220.

Massart, et al. 1998. Chemometrics a textbook. Elsevier Science Publishing Company Inc. Penza & Cassano 2003. Sensors and Actuators. *Chemical* 89: 269–284.

Paredi, P. et al. 2000. Exhaled ethane is elevated in cystic fibrosis and correlates with CO levels and airway obstruction. *Am. J. Respir. Crit. Care Med.* 161: 1247–1251.

Poli, D. et al. 2005. Exhaled volatile organic compounds in patients with non-small cell lung cancer: cross sectional and nested short-term follow-up study. *Respir. Res.* 6: 71–81.

Technology and Medical Sciences – Natal Jorge et al. (eds)
© 2011 Taylor & Francis Group, London, ISBN 978-0-415-66822-4

Noninvasive assessment of Blood-Retinal Barrier function by High-Definition Optical Coherence Tomography

T. Santos
Association for Innovation and Biomedical Research on Light and Image (AIBILI), Coimbra, Portugal
Institute of Biomedical Research on Light and Image (IBILI), Coimbra, Portugal

R. Bernardes
Association for Innovation and Biomedical Research on Light and Image (AIBILI), Coimbra, Portugal
Institute of Biomedical Research on Light and Image (IBILI), Coimbra, Portugal
Faculty of Medicine, University of Coimbra, Coimbra, Portugal

A. Santos & J. Cunha-Vaz
Association for Innovation and Biomedical Research on Light and Image (AIBILI), Coimbra, Portugal
Institute of Biomedical Research on Light and Image (IBILI), Coimbra, Portugal

ABSTRACT: The work herein presented aims to demonstrate the possibility of using a noninvasive technique, the High-Definition Optical Coherence Tomography (HD-OCT), as a surrogate technique for detection of Blood-Retinal Barrier (BRB) breakdown. New generation HD-OCT devices resort to spectral analysis to achieve higher acquisition rates and provide unprecedented detailed images of the retina's structure. Besides structural information of the retina in HD-OCT images, this work demonstrates that information on BRB function is also present and therefore opens a new perspective for a noninvasive imaging device to assess BRB function which aims to prevent harmful substances from the blood stream to enter the retina.

Keywords: blood-retinal barrier, functional imaging, optical coherence tomography, retinal leakage analyzer, diabetic retinopathy

1 INTRODUCTION

According to the International Diabetes Federation, [http://www.diabetesatlas.org/content/regional-overview, 14/July/2010] the estimate number of people with diabetes in the age range of 20–79 years will rise from 284.6 millions (in 2010) to 438.4 millions (in 2030) worldwide, representing a prevalence of 6.4% and 7.7%, respectively. One of the complications associated to diabetes mellitus is Diabetic Retinopathy (DR), being the main cause of vision loss in the active working population in the western countries and responsible for 10% of the new blinds each year (Alfaro, 2006). Countries such as Norway and Sweden have very distinct values for prevalence of blindness related to type 2 diabetes, 9% and 0.35% respectively, which makes this multifactorial disease a large global problem (Cunha-Vaz, 2006).

In healthy retinas the Blood-Retinal Barrier (BRB), composed by the tight junctions of the Retinal Pigment Epithelium (RPE) and by the tight junctions of the endothelial cells of the capillary networks, outer and inner BRB respectively, prevents toxic molecules present in the blood stream to enter the retina.

Fluorescein angiography is the most frequently used imaging technique to document the changes of the BRB function related to DR. It uses sodium fluorescein (NaFl) as an intravenous injected dye and images its presence in the retina and vitreous, requiring dedicated instrumentation operated by well trained personnel. Because of the intravenous dye administration, minimal adverse reactions occur in 5% of the cases as well as other sever complications. Death may still occur in the first 24 to 48 hours for each 220.000 cases (Alfaro, 2006).

For a precise location and mapping of BRB breakdown of the human retina, with special emphasis on diabetic patients, our research group developed the Retinal Leakage Analyzer (RLA), (Lobo, 1999, Bernardes, 2005), an in vivo BRB functional imaging technique which also resorts to NaFl to act as a dye.

The aim of the work presented in this paper is to demonstrate the possibility of using a noninvasive imaging technique, the spectral domain High-Definition Optical Coherence Tomography (HD-OCT), as a surrogate detector for BRB breakdown.

2 MATERIALS AND METHODS

2.1 Retinal leakage analyzer

Bernardes et al. (2005) were able to modify a confocal scanning laser ophthalmoscope in order to collect the 3-dimensional distribution of fluorescein, within the retina and vitreous, after the intravenous dye administration. Following these changes, software was developed to compute the amount of fluorescein that crossed the BRB into the vitreous. Because the amount of fluorescein leakage into the vitreous is related to the BRB permeability (Lobo, 1999), the excess of leakage indicates the breakdown of the BRB (Lobo, 2001, Lobo, 2004).

Although this and the previous version of this method are of interest in the follow-up of diabetic patients (Lobo, 1999), these are clearly invasive techniques requiring dedicated instrumentation and skilled personnel. The system is able to produce a map of fluorescein leakage, to compare this leakage map to a healthy reference leakage map and to compute an eye fundus reference. From this comparison, it is possible to indicate which areas present normal leakage values and which areas present an increased leakage, therefore indicating BRB break down locations.

2.2 Optical coherence tomography

The OCT is a noninvasive imaging device that provides cross-sectional tomograms of the structure of the retina. A low coherence near-infrared light beam from a Super Luminescent Diode (SLD) is emitted to the retina and to a moving reference mirror to produce high resolution profiles, A-scans, resorting to interferometry. Repeating this procedure in the lateral direction enables two dimensional high resolution data sets referred as B-scans (Fig. 1) (Fujimoto, 2003).

The new generation of spectral domain OCT devices, e.g. Cirrus HD-OCT (Carl Zeiss Meditec, Dublin, CA, USA), resorts to Fourier domain analysis of the reflected light signals making moving parts in the reference arm needless (Schuman, 2008). With these new approach manufacturers were able to increase data acquisition speed to 27000 A-scans per second on a $6 \times 6 \times 2$ mm³ volume of either $512 \times 128 \times 1024$ or $200 \times 200 \times 1024$ voxels (Fig. 2). Lateral resolution is 20 μm in tissue and axial resolution was increased to 5 μm in tissue by using a broader SLD when compared to the previous versions.

2.3 Healthy and patient comparison

To assess differences between healthy and diseased retinas, a set of 6 eyes from healthy volunteers were examined by the Cirrus HD-OCT using the $512 \times 128 \times 1024$ voxels Macular Cube Protocol. Similar scans were performed on Diabetic

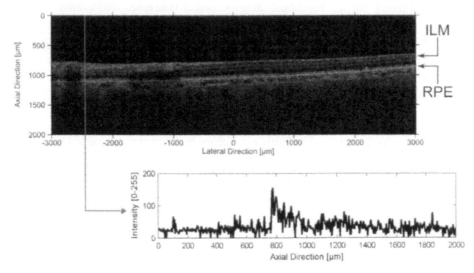

Figure 1. Optical coherence tomograph B-scan image (top) and intensity plot of the 30th A-scan (bottom). Top: the upper dark region of the image represents the vitreous, immediately followed by the retina (delimited by the Inner Limiting Membrane—ILM and by the Retinal Pigment Epithelium—RPE), the RPE, the choroid and a shadow area bellow the RPE/choroiod.

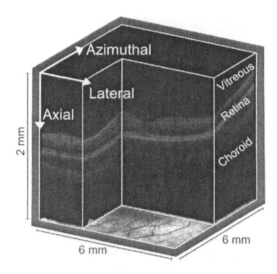

Figure 2. Optical coherence tomography volumetric data display. The fundus image reference underneath the volume is automatically computed from the volume and corresponds to the line integral along the axial direction (depth-wise data).

Retinopathy (DR), Age related Macular Degeneration (AMD), Diabetic Macular Edema (DME) and Cystoid Macular Edema (CME) patients.

Using the segmentation algorithm on the Cirrus HD-OCT device, the Inner Limiting Membrane (ILM) and RPE were identified to compute the histograms of B-scans intensity values of the whole retina, from the ILM to the RPE. These histograms were scaled to correct for differences in acquisition and brought into alignment by their respective maximum values to compute the average and standard deviation for the healthy control population.

This same procedure was used to compare healthy to diseased eyes.

2.4 *OCT versus leakage*

In this work patients performed the RLA in order to map sites of BRB disruption (areas of increased leakage) and areas of intact BRB (areas of normal leakage).

By co-registering images of fundus references from the RLA and HD-OCT, it becomes possible to correlate HD-OCT intensity distribution data according to the classification received from the RLA, that is, it becomes possible to compare HD-OCT intensity distribution data, from the ILM to the RPE, from areas of intact BRB to areas of disrupt BRB (Fig. 3).

These comparisons were performed using the intensity histograms normalized to the number of

voxels therefore resulting in a Probability Density Function (PDF).

Each PDF, one from an area of intact BRB and one from and area of disrupt BRB were brought into alignment by their respective maximum values and the Sum of the Squared Difference (SSD) was computed.

Additionally, SSD were computed from different areas with the same classification on the RLA, intact or disrupt, to assess the expected level of difference and to demonstrate the

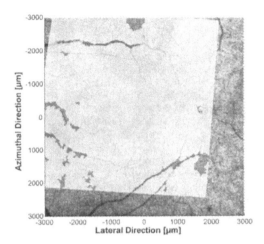

Figure 3. Perspective image co-registration result between HD-OCT and RLA fundus references. The overlaid gray square like area represents the projected RLA map with the identified disrupted BRB areas (leakage) as the darker areas. Beneath, the computed line integral image along the depth-wise direction, the HD-OCT eye fundus reference.

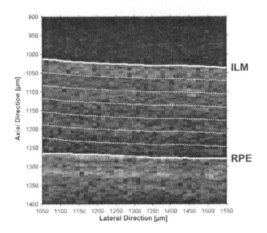

Figure 4. Detail of a HD-OCT B-scan showing the Cirrus device segmentation of the ILM and RPE in white and the evenly split of the retina into 7 layers (white dashed lines).

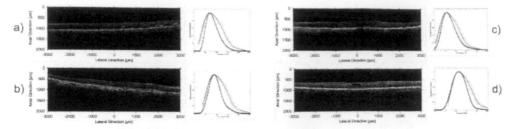

Figure 5. Four representatives HD-OCT B-scans from pathological eyes and the plot of average (solid line) one standard deviation (dashed lines) of the healthy reference and the patient's eyes normalized histograms (solid dotted line). Cases: a) diabetic retinopathy; b) age-related macular degeneration; c) diabetic macular edema; and d) cystoid macular edema. The normalized histograms of the reference population and of the patients were aligned by their maximum scaled to one for comparison purposes.

higher differences found when comparing areas receiving different classifications, i.e. intact-to-disrupt in comparison to intact-to-intact or disrupt-to-disrupt areas.

We went a step further in our analysis by considering seven different retinal layers (evenly split between the ILM to the RPE, Figure 4) and performed the above comparison considering each retinal layer independently, as opposed to the above approach where the entire retina, from the ILM to the RPE, was considered.

3 RESULTS

The comparison of normalized histograms between healthy and DR, AMD, DME and CME eyes can be seen in Figure 5. The differences between healthy and diseased eyes histograms demonstrate the associated changes from the retina optical properties viewpoint.

Two cases, one DR eye (male, 53 years) and one AMD eye (female, 68 years), were segmented in seven retinal layers and comparisons between areas of intact-to-intact, disrupt-to-disrupt and intact-to-disrupt were performed to compare the sum of squared differences as shown in Table 1. The differences found are of one to two orders of magnitude when comparing distinct BRB status to similar BRB status (Table 1).

Moreover, when analized by retinal layer (Table 2) these differences are notorious on the top layers (layers 1–3) therefore being in aggreement with the distribution of retinal vascular network. This suggests these changes are associated to changes in the optical properties of the retina closely related to changes in BRB status, i.e. instact or disrupted.

This hypothesis is supported by the statistical significant difference ($p < 0.0001$) between the ratio of the SSD values of layers 1 to 3 and 4 to 6 (Table 2).

Table 1. Summary of 50 runs for randomly selected A-scans sets (5000 A-scans per set) from each BRB function status. Please note the order of magnitude of the average of the sum of squared differences between probability density functions of the same and of distinct area types.

| | Sum of squared differences | |
Comparison (Status–Status)	DR case m(SD) $\times 10^{-9}$	AMD case m(SD) $\times 10^{-9}$
Intact–Intact	5.9(9.3)	2.8(3.6)
Disrupt–Disrupt	1.6(4.5)	2.2(1.6)
Intact–Disrupt	66.2(16.1)	176.3(26.1)

Table 2. Average (N = 10) ratio between different and same BRB function status SSD values of probability density functions of intensity values at each layer of the retina.

| | Ratio between SSD of different and same BRB function status | |
	DR case m(SD)	AMD case m(SD)
Layer 1	84.4(84.0)	16.1(8.7)
Layer 2	20.3(13.9)	80.1(88.6)
Layer 3	19.3(12.9)	17.3(10.8)
Layer 4	6.5(5.7)	8.4(8.4)
Layer 5	4.1(3.8)	4.4(4.4)
Layer 6	7.7(2.4)	2.8(1.6)
Layer 7	45.9(22.6)	4.0(2.4)

4 CONCLUSIONS

The quest for the in vivo assessment of BRB function has involved many groups over time. The difficulty of the techniques involved and the need for dedicated instrumentation, such as with the confocal scanning laser ophthalmoscope,

(Lobo, 1999, Bernardes, 2005) preclude the possibility of spreading the technique.

In this work we have demonstrated, based on quantitative techniques, the presence of indirect information of the blood-retinal barrier status on optical coherence tomography data.

As a starting point, we have demonstrated the global differences between healthy reference eyes and eyes with diabetic retinopathy, age-related macular degeneration, diabetic macular edema and cystoid macular edema. These two groups, healthy vs unhealthy eyes, present a clear difference in their plot of distribution of intensities within the retina as gathered by optical coherence tomography.

Because the OCT measures and quantifies the reflections/scattering of the infrared laser beam directed into the retina, and these reflections/scattering are due to changes in the refractive indexes along the light path, any change in distribution of reflection/scattering results in a change in the optical properties on the tissue under analysis.

We went a step further by identifying changes in the retina optical properties within the same eye and scan. We have resorted to a proprietary technique, the retinal leakage analyzer, to identify regions of intact and sites of disrupted blood-retinal barrier and analyzed the reflectance/scattering distribution in between these regions to find a clear dissimilarity.

The optical coherence tomography imaging modality is spreading very fast to the clinical practice relatively to human eye imaging due to two main reasons, because it is non-invasive and because it gives detailed information on the human eye fundus structure.

In addition to the original purpose, Wehbe et al. 2007 have achieved blood flow measurement, while Bizheva et al. 2006 have demonstrated the changes in optical properties of the retina due to light stimuli.

Furthermore, we demonstrate herewith a new functionality for the OCT which may lead to a large impact on the way patients, especially diabetic patients, are followed by their ophthalmologist.

The possibility of gathering information on the blood-retinal barrier from the OCT, a non-invasive imaging technique, offers the opportunity for dismissing the sodium fluorescein injection with all the associated advantages: no medical and nursing staff required, no adverse events due to dye injection (Yannuzzi et al. 1986) and the possibility of repeating the exam frequently, should the need arise.

ACKNOWLEDGEMENTS

This study is supported in part by the Fundação para a Ciência e a Tecnologia (FCT) under the research project PTDC/SAU-BEB/103151/2008 and program COMPETE (FCOMP-01-0124-FEDER-010930). The authors would like to thanks Dr. Melissa Horne and Carl Zeiss Meditec (Dublic, CA, USA) for their support on getting access to HD-OCT data through the Research Browser software. This study is registered at ClinicalTrials.org (ID: NCT00797524).

REFERENCES

Alfaro, V., Quiroz-Mercado, H., Gómez-Ulla, F., Figueroa, M. & Villalba, S. 2006. *Retinopatia Diabética—Tratado Médico Quirúrgico.* MAC LINE, S.L.

Bernardes, R., Dias, J., Cunha-Vaz, J. 2005. Mapping the Human Blood-Retinal Barrier Function. *IEEE Trans Biomed Eng* 52:106–116.

Bizheva, K., Pflug, R., Hermann, B., Povazay, B., Sattmann, H., Qiu, P., Anger, E., Reitsamer, H., Popov, S., Taylor, J., Unterhuber, A., Ahnelt, P. & Drexler, W. 2006. Optophysiology: Depth-resolved probing of retinal physiology with functional ultrahigh-resolution optical coherence tomography. *Proc. Natl. Acad. Sci. U.S.A.* 103:5066–5071.

Cunha-Vaz, J. 2006. *Retinopatia Diabética.* Sociedad Española de Oftalmologia, MAC LINE, S.L.

Fujimoto, J. 2003. Optical Coherence Tomography: Principles and Applications. *The Review of Laser Engineering* 31:635–642.

Lobo, C., Bernardes, R., Santos, F. & Cunha-Vaz, J. 1999. Mapping Retinal Fluorescein Leakage with Confocal Scanning Laser Fluorometry of the Human Vitreous. *Arch Ophthalmol* 117:631–637.

Lobo, C., Bernardes, R., Abreu, J. & Cunha-Vaz, J. 2001. One-year Follow-up of Blood-Retinal Barrier and Retinal Thickness Alterations in Patients with Type 2 Diabetes Mellitus and Mild Nonproliferative Retinopathy. *Arch Ophthalmol* 119:1469–1474.

Lobo, C., Bernardes, R., Figueira, J., Abreu, J. & Cunha-Vaz, J. 2004. Three-Year Follow-up Study of Blood-Retinal Barrier and Retinal Thickness Alterations in Patients With Type 2 Diabetes Mellitus and Mild Nonproliferative Diabetic Retinopathy. *Arch Ophthalmol* 122:211–217.

Schuman, J. 2008. Spectral domain optical coherence tomography for glaucoma (an AOS Thesis). *Trans Am Ophthalmol Soc* 106:426–458.

Wehbe, H., Ruggeri, M., Jiao, S., Gregori, G., Puliafito, C. & Zhao, W. 2007. Automatic retinal blood flow calculation using spectral domain optical coherence tomography. *Optics Express* 15:15193–15206.

Yannuzzi, L., Rohrer, K., Tindel, L., Sobel, R., Costanza, M., Shields, W. & Zang, E. 1986. Fluorescein angiography complication survey. *Ophthalmology* 93:611–617.

Technology and Medical Sciences – Natal Jorge et al. (eds)
© 2011 Taylor & Francis Group, London, ISBN 978-0-415-66822-4

OCT noise despeckling using a 3D nonlinear complex diffusion filter

C. Maduro

Association for Innovation and Biomedical Research on Light and Image (AIBILI), Coimbra, Portugal
Institute of Biomedical Research on Light and Image (IBILI), Portugal

R. Bernardes

Association for Innovation and Biomedical Research on Light and Image (AIBILI), Coimbra, Portugal
Institute of Biomedical Research on Light and Image (IBILI), Portugal
Faculty of Medicine, University of Coimbra, Coimbra, Portugal

P. Serranho

Institute of Biomedical Research on Light and Image (IBILI), Portugal
Faculty of Medicine, University of Coimbra, Coimbra, Portugal

T. Santos & J. Cunha-Vaz

Association for Innovation and Biomedical Research on Light and Image (AIBILI), Coimbra, Portugal
Institute of Biomedical Research on Light and Image (IBILI), Portugal

ABSTRACT: An improved despeckling method, based on complex diffusion filtering, is herein presented to enhance structure segmentation in high-definition spectral domain optical coherence tomography data. We propose to extend the filter concept from 2- to 3-dimensions, taking into account the consistency of noise along the entire 3D data volume.

This method compares favorably to existing methods reducing speckle noise and preserving edges and features.

Keywords: Speckle denoising, complex diffusion, optical coherence tomography, spatial filtering

1 INTRODUCTION

The Optical Coherence Tomography (OCT) is a non-invasive imaging modality with several applications. It provides in vivo high-resolution cross-sectional imaging of the retinal tissue through light scattering. However, as any imaging technique that has his image formation based on coherent waves, OCT images suffer from speckle noise which reduce its quality (Drexler, Morgner, Ghanta, Kärtner, Schuman & Fujimoto 2001).

Speckle noise is a random phenomenon generated by interference of waves with random phases (Fercher 2008), being a common problem to other imaging modalities as ultrasound, Synthetic-Aperture Radar (SAR) or laser imaging, leading to research and resulting on many speckling reduction techniques (Fercher 2008).

It creates a grainy appearance that can mask diagnostically significant image features and reduces the accuracy of segmentation and pattern recognition algorithms (Fercher 2008), (Puvanathasan & Bizheva 2007), Please refer to (Fercher 2008), (Schmitt, Xiang & Yung 1999) for a further description of the speckle in OCT characteristics.

The statistical mechanism of laser speckle formation was first presented by Goodman (Goodman 1976). Besides the theoretical results, this study also supports the idea that speckle noise could be rejected by linear filtering. On the other hand, Wagner et al. (Wagner, Smith, Sandrik & Lopez 1983), Burckhardt et al. (Burckhardt 1978) and Abbott et al. (Abbott & Thurstone 1979) conclude that linear filtering, the way it was presented in (Goodman 1976), suppresses the noise at the cost of smoothing out image details.

Some speckle reducing methods were proposed based on modifications to the OCT system design, such as the angular compounding (Schmitt 1997),

(Bashkansky & Reintjes 2000), (Iftimia, Bouma & Tearney 2003), the frequency compounding (Shankar & Newhouse 1985), (Pircher, Gotzinger, Leitgeb, Fercher & Hitzenberger 2003) and the spatial compounding (Kilm, Miller, Kim, Oh, Oh & Milner 2005).

The requirements on modifying the hardware led to the development of post-processing methods, being the CLEAN algorithm one of the first image processing techniques for OCT despeckling (Schmitt 1998). Among these are the median filtering (Bernstein 1987), homomorphic Wiener filtering (Franceschetti, Pascazio & Schirinzi 1995), enhanced Lee filter (ELEE) (Lee 1981), Symmetric Nearest Neighbor (SNN) filter, adaptive smoothing (Kuan, Sawchuk, Strand & Chavel 1985), multiresolution wavelet analysis (Xiang, Zhou & Schmitt 1998), filtering techniques based on rotating kernel transformations (Rogowska & Brezinski 2000), Kuwahara filter (Kuwahara, Hachimura, Eiho & Kinoshita 1976) and anisotropic diffusion filtering (Perona & Malik 1990), (Salinas & Fernádez 2007).

Fernández et al. (Fernández, Salinas & Puliafito 2005) and Salinas et al. (Salinas & Fernández 2007) have shown that a nonlinear complex diffusion filter can be successfully applied to remove OCT speckle noise while preserving image features.

Current despeckling methods applied to process noisy optical coherence tomography data take into consideration each B-scan individually, therefore looking to the 3D data as a set of individual 2D images (Ozcan, Bilenca, Desjardins, Bouma & Tearney 2007), (Puvanathasan & Bizheva 2007), (Salinas & Fernández 2007). In this way, the consistency of noise along the entire 3D data volume is not taken into account.

In the work herewith presented, we have extended the application of complex diffusion filters from 2- (Salinas & Fernández 2007) to 3-dimensions therefore considering the entire volume as a single entity and not as a set of aggregated 2D entities.

As a proof-of-concept, the proposed method will be compared resorting to quantitative measures with filtering methods from the literature.

2 MATERIAL AND METHODS

2.1 Optical coherence tomography

The OCT working principle is similar to ultrasound and adopted some of its terminology from that field.

The volumetric OCT information is composed of a set of A-scans (depth-wise information on refractive index changes) (Fig. 1). The scanning is performed along a series of parallel lines covering the 20° field-of-view of the eye fundus.

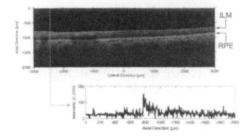

Figure 1. Optical coherence tomography example of a B-scan (top) and an A-scan profile (bottom).

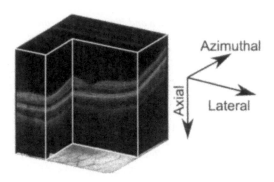

Figure 2. Volumetric OCT data shown over an eye fundus reference.

In this work the high-definition spectral domain Cirrus OCT (Carl Zeiss Meditec, Dublin, CA, USA) was used.

This retinal imaging system allows for an acquisition scan of $200 \times 200 \times 1024$ or $512 \times 128 \times 1024$ voxels for the lateral, azimuthal and axial directions, respectively, with a depth resolution of $5\,\mu m$ in tissue. This volumetric data is obtained from a $6000 \times 6000 \times 2000\,\mu m^3$ volume of the human macula (Fig. 2).

2.2 3D-nonlinear complex diffusion filter

The application of diffusion filters to image processing is based on the analogy to physical diffusion processes, the rational being to balance different concentrations without creation or destruction of mass/energy (Weickert 1997).

Here, the concentration becomes the image and the diffusion equation becomes:

$$\frac{\partial I}{\partial t} = \nabla \cdot \left(D \nabla I \right), \tag{1}$$

where the initial condition is given by the original image ($I_{t=0} = I_0$), D is the diffusion coefficient, ∇ is the gradient operator and $\nabla \cdot$ is the divergence operator.

Commonly, the diffusion coefficient is chosen to be dependent on the image gradient (Perona & Malik 1990), hence

$$D = d(|\nabla I|), \qquad (2)$$

where $|\cdot|$ denotes the magnitude.

Fernández et al. (Fernández, Salinas & Puliafito 2005) and Salinas et al. (Salinas & Fernández 2007) shown that a nonlinear complex diffusion filter can be successfully applied to remove the OCT speckle noise while preserving image features. Both defined the diffusion coefficient as

$$d(\mathrm{Im}(I)) = \frac{e^{i\theta}}{1 + \left(\dfrac{\mathrm{Im}(I)}{k\theta}\right)^2}, \qquad (3)$$

where Im $(\cdot)$ is the imaginary value, $i = \sqrt{-1}$, k a threshold parameter and θ a phase angle (Salinas & Fernández 2007).

This choice relies on the fact that for small θ the imaginary part can be considered as a smoothed second derivative of the initial signal factored by θ and time (t) (Gilboa, Sochen & Zeevi 2004) (4).

$$\lim_{\theta \to 0} \frac{Im(I)}{\theta} = t \Delta g * I_0, \qquad (4)$$

where g is a gaussian and $*$ the convolution operator.

This formulation does not require to compute derivatives of the image, avoiding the numerical instabilities at early stages and is a good choice for edge preservation.

In the work herewith presented we extended this application from 2- to 3-dimensions taking advantage of the volumetric information provided by the Cirrus OCT.

The extension to 3D is proposed by implementing a Forward in Time and Centered in Space (FTCS) finite difference scheme, being the iterative update given by:

$$I_{i,j,m}^{(n+1)} = I_{i,j,m}^{(n)} + \Delta t \left(\bar{D}_{i,j,m}^{(n)} \Delta_h I_{i,j,m}^{(n)} + \nabla_h D_{i,j,m}^{(n)} \cdot \nabla_h I_{i,j,m}^{(n)} \right), \qquad (5)$$

where Δ_h and ∇_h are, respectively, the discrete second order laplacian and gradient operators, Δt is the step in time, i, j and m are the indexes for the voxels of I and $\bar{D}$ is given by

$$\bar{D}_{i,j,m}^{(n)} = \frac{6D_{i,j,m}^{(n)} + D_{i\pm 1,j,m}^{(n)} + D_{i,j\pm 1,m}^{(n)} + D_{i,j,m\pm 1}^{(n)}}{12}. \qquad (6)$$

As shown in (Araújo, Barbeiro & Serranho 2010) this explicit method is stable if

$$\Delta t \le \frac{1}{\alpha \max_{i,j,m} \left[\mathrm{Re}\left(D_{i,j,m}^{(n)} \right) + \left| \mathrm{Im}\left(D_{i,j,m}^{(n)} \right) \right| \right]}, \qquad (7)$$

where $\Delta x = \Delta y = \Delta z = 1$ and $\alpha = 8$. So, the maximum step in time is of 0.25 s or 0.125 s for the 2D or 3D case, respectively (Araújo, Barbeiro, Serranho 2010).

2.3 Quality metrics

For the quantitative evaluation of filters' performance, two quality metrics used in (Ozcan, Bilenca, Desjardins, Bouma & Tearney 2007), (Puvanathasan & Bizheva 2007) and (Salinas & Fernández 2007) were applied. The metrics used are the Mean Squared Error (MSE) and the edge preservation parameter (χ).

The MSE is given by:

$$\mathrm{MSE} = \frac{1}{MN} \sum_{m=1}^{M} \sum_{n=1}^{N} (I(m,n) - I_f(m,n))^2, \qquad (8)$$

where $I(m, n)$ denotes the original image, $I_f(m, n)$ denotes the filtered image, M and N are the number of pixels in row and column directions, respectively.

To evaluate the edge preservation we use the correlation coefficient χ (9) as in (Salinas & Fernández 2007), (Puvanathasan & Bizheva 2007), where ΔI and ΔI_f are the laplacian of the original and filtered image, respectively, and the $\Delta \bar{I}$ and $\Delta \bar{I}_f$ the respective mean values.

In order to quantify the smoothness of Homogeneous regions (H) the Equivalent Number of Looks (ENL) is computed according to equation 10.

$$ENL = \frac{1}{H} \sum_{h=1}^{H} \frac{\mu_h^2}{\sigma_h^2}, \qquad (10)$$

where μ_h and σ_h^2 are the mean and variance, respectively, of the regions H.

3 RESULTS

In order to evaluate the performance of the filter herewith presented, eyes of 30 healthy volunteers and eyes of patients with age-related macular degeneration (20), diabetic retinopathy (23), cystoid macular edema (2) and choroidal neo-vascularization (13) underwent the high-definition spectral domain Cirrus OCT using both the $200 \times 200 \times 1024$ and the $512 \times 128 \times 1024$ Macular Cube protocols.

The volumetric scans were filtered using the here proposed 3D-NCDF, as well as using its 2D version (Salinas & Fernández 2007), the Perona-Malik (PM) with the diffusion coefficient $d(|\nabla I|) = \exp(-(|\nabla I|/k)^2)$, where $k = 50$ (Perona & Malik 1990), and the adaptive Lee filter with a window of 3×3 pixels (Lee 1981).

Table 1. Filter performance metrics (m ± SD). MSE—mean square error; χ—edge preservation metric; PM—Perona-Malik; NCDF–nonlinear complex diffusion filter; AMD—age-related macular degeneration; DR—diabetic retinopathy; CME—cystoid macular edema; CNV—choroidal neo-vascularization.

Metric	Filter	Healthy (N = 30)	Diseased eyes AMD (N = 20)	DR (N = 23)	CNV (N = 13)	CME (N = 2)
MSE	Lee	129.38 ± 11.51	124.69 ± 9.65	125.15 ± 7.99	120.55 ± 4.64	129.53 ± 14.36
	PM	162.16 ± 13.12	156.23 ± 12.04	158.11 ± 12.04	153.08 ± 5.78	162.58 ± 16.16
	2D-NCDF	119.34 ± 7.35	116.71 ± 6.10	117.95 ± 5.05	115.23 ± 2.91	120.10 ± 8.64
	3D-NCDF	135.62 ± 8.00	132.59 ± 6.96	134.26 ± 5.72	136.40 ± 9.47	131.89 ± 3.69
χ	Lee	0.27 ± 0.00	0.26 ± 0.01	0.27 ± 0.01	0.28 ± 0.01	0.27 ± 0.01
	PM	0.24 ± 0.04	0.19 ± 0.03	0.19 ± 0.03	0.20 ± 0.02	0.20 ± 0.03
	2D-NCDF	0.61 ± 0.03	0.58 ± 0.04	0.57 ± 0.04	0.55 ± 0.01	0.59 ± 0.04
	3D-NCDF	0.70 ± 0.03	0.68 ± 0.03	0.67 ± 0.03	0.69 ± 0.03	0.66 ± 0.02

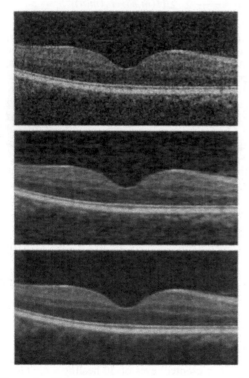

Figure 3. Original B-scan (top) and the respective 2D-NCDF (middle) and 3D-NCDF (bottom) filtered versions of an healthy volunteer's retina.

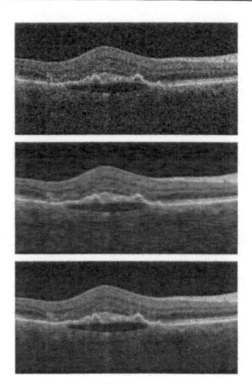

Figure 4. Original B-scan (top) and the respective 2D-NCDF (middle) and 3D-NCDF (bottom) filtered versions of a CNV diseased eye.

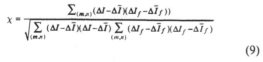

$$\chi = \frac{\sum_{(m,n)}(\Delta I - \Delta \bar{I})(\Delta I_f - \Delta \bar{I}_f))}{\sqrt{\sum_{(m,n)}(\Delta I - \Delta \bar{I})(\Delta I - \Delta \bar{I})\sum_{(m,n)}(\Delta I_f - \Delta \bar{I}_f)(\Delta I_f - \Delta \bar{I}_f)}}$$

(9)

The exact same diffusion time (2.4 s) was used which correspond to 10 and 20 iterations with a step in time of 0.24 and 0.124 s to the 2D and 3D cases, respectively. The 2D and 3D-NCDF were applied using $k = 10$ and $\theta = \pi/30$, as in (Salinas & Fernández 2007).

To perform the quantitative measurement of the filter performance the MSE and the χ metrics were computed for each of the 88 volumetric scans. The results from the quantitative analysis are shown in Table 1.

The average computing time for each volume of $200 \times 200 \times 1024$ voxels OCT data is of 97 minutes

Table 2. ENL comparison for the original B-scans and the corresponding filters' results.

Metric	Filter	Healthy (N = 10)	Diseased eyes AMD (N = 10)	DR (N = 10)	CNV (N = 10)	CME (N = 2)
ENL	Original	5.84 ± 0.77	5.57 ± 0.69	5.53 ± 0.83	5.60 ± 0.99	6.17 ± 0.41
	Lee	18.39 ± 2.39	17.13 ± 1.53	16.70 ± 2.60	16.83 ± 4.69	19.25 ± 2.56
	PM	71.28 ± 11.45	66.90 ± 10.41	61.45 ± 15.87	69.46 ± 25.73	75.33 ± 9.66
	2D-NCDF	39.50 ± 5.79	37.57 ± 03.85	34.73 ± 7.58	37.06 ± 12.23	41.47 ± 5.69
	3D-NCDF	111.03 ± 11.99	107.58 ± 8.91	102.74 ± 29.42	99.85 ± 33.54	112.67 ± 2.10

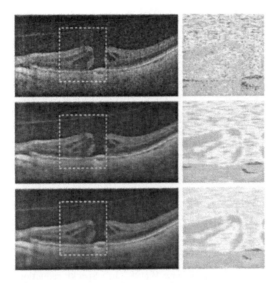

Figure 5. An original B-scan (top-left). Color-coded inset from the dashed area on the left (top-right). Filter results for the 2D-NCDF (middle) and the 3D-NCDF (bottom), with the corresponding color-coded insets on the right. All color-coded figures use the same color map and color limits for ease of comparison. Note the well-defined membrane in the vitreous region.

for the Lee filter, 2 minutes for the Perona-Malik (PM) (2D) filter, 3 minutes for the 2D-NCDF (Salinas & Fernández 2007) filter and 11 minutes for the 3D-NCDF here proposed. The total diffusion time for PM, 2D-NCDF and the 3D filter is of 2.4 s.

These tests were performed using a 2.4 GHz Intel Core 2 Quad Q6600 CPU, 3 GB of RAM to run Matlab on the Ubuntu operating system.

Figures 3 to 5 show the result of the application of the 2D-NCDF to a particular B-scan and the same B-scan after the respective 3D-NCDF filtered data. In figure 3 it is shown an healthy volunteer's retina example where is possible to note the good performance of the 3D-NCDF filter in reducing speckle while preserving retinal layers. Figures 4 and 5 show results from a CNV and an

AMD cases, respectively. For easy of comparison a region is zoomed in and shown in insets using a pseudo-color (Fig. 5). Please note the good preservation and better visualization of a retinal membrane after the 3D-NCDF application and the increased homogeneity of the vitreous.

To quantify the filters performance in homogeneous areas, one B-scan of each volumetric data was selected and the ENL was computed on a vitreous region. The results are presented in Table 2.

4 CONCLUSIONS

In the work herewith presented we propose to extend the application of a nonlinear complex diffusion filters from 2- to 3-dimensions and quantitatively and qualitatively demonstrate its advantages.

The natural drawback is the required computing time. On the other hand, we should note the increased edge preservation while simultaneously achieving much smoother areas as demonstrated by the χ and ENL parameters, respectively.

Additionally, the visual inspection allows to see the increased definition of the several retinal layers.

Then facts allow us to speculate that the 3D filtering presented may represent an important preprocessing towards a better image segmentation process.

FUNDING

This study is supported in part by the *Fundação para a Ciência e a Tecnologia* (FCT) under the research project PTDC/SAU-BEB/103151/2008 and program COMPETE (FCOMP-01-0124-FEDER-010930). The authors would like to thanks Dr. Melissa Horne and Carl Zeiss Meditec (Dublic, CA, USA) for their support on getting access to OCT data and AIBILI Clinical Trial Center technicians for their support in managing data, working with patients and performing scans. This study is registered at ClinicalTrials.org (ID: NCT00797524).

REFERENCES

Abbott, J. & Thurstone, F. (1979). Acoustic speckle: Theory and experimental analysis. *Ultrasonic Imaging 1*, 303–324.

Araújo, A., Barbeiro, S. & Serranho, P. (2010). Stability of finite difference schemes for complex diffusion processes. *DMUC report*, 10–23.

Bashkansky, M. & Reintjes, J. (2000). Statistics and reduction of speckle in optical coherence tomography. *Opt. Lett. 25*(8), 545–547.

Bernstein, R. (1987, Nov). Adaptive nonlinear filters for simultaneous removal of different kinds of noise in images. *IEEE Trans. Circuits Syst. 34*(11), 1275–1291.

Burckhardt, C. (1978). Speckle in ultrasound b-mode scans. *IEEE Trans. on Sonics and Ultrasonics 25*(1), 1–6.

Drexler, W., Morgner, U., Ghanta, R., Kärtner, F., Schuman, J. & Fujimoto, J. (2001, April). Ultrahigh-resolution ophthalmic optical coherence tomography. *Nat. Med. 7*(4), 502–507.

Fercher, A. (2008). *Optical Coherence Tomography: Technology and Applications* (illustrated ed.)., Chapter 4, pp. 119–146. New York: Springer.

Fernández, D., Salinas, H. & Puliafito, C. (2005). Automated detection of retinal layer structures on optical coherence tomography images. *Opt. Express 13*(25), 10200–10216.

Franceschetti, G., Pascazio, V. & Schirinzi, G. (1995). Iterative homomorphic technique for speckle reduction in synthetic-aperture radar imaging. *J. Opt. Soc. Am. A 12*(4), 686–694.

Gilboa, G., Sochen, N. & Zeevi, Y. (2004, August). Image enhancement and denoising by complex diffusion processes. *IEEE Trans. Pattern Anal. Mach. Intell. 26*(8), 1020–1036.

Goodman, J. (1976). Some fundamental properties of speckle. *J. Opt. Soc. Am. 66*(11), 1145–1150.

Iftimia, N., Bouma, B. & Tearney, G. (2003). Speckle reduction in optical coherence tomography by "path length encoded" angular compounding. *J. Biomed. Opt. 8*(2), 260–263.

Kim, J., Miller, D., Kim, E., Oh, S., Oh, J. & Milner, T. (2005). Optical coherence tomography speckle reduction by a partially spatially coherent source. *J. Biomed. Opt. 10*(6), 064034.

Kuan, D., Sawchuk, A., Strand, T. & Chavel, P. (1985, March). Adaptive noise smoothing filter for images with signal-dependent noise. *IEEE Trans. Pattern Anal. Mach. Intell. 7*(2), 165–177.

Kuwahara, M., Hachimura, K., Eiho, S. & Kinoshita, M. (1976). Processing of riangiocardiographic images. *Digital Processing of Biomedical Images*, 187–203.

Lee, J. (1981, September). Speckle analysis and smoothing of synthetic aperture radar images. *Comp. Graph. and Image Process. 17*(1), 24–32.

Ozcan, A., Bilenca, A., Desjardins, A., Bouma, B. & Tearney, G. (2007). Speckle reduction in optical coherence tomography images using digital filtering. *J. Opt. Soc. Am. A 24*(7), 1901–1910.

Perona, P. & Malik, J. (1990). Scale-space and edge detection using anisotropic diffusion. *IEEE Trans. Pattern Anal. Mach. Intell. 12*(7), 629–639.

Pircher, M., Gotzinger, E., Leitgeb, R., Fercher, A. & Hitzenberger, C. (2003). Speckle reduction in optical coherence tomography by frequency compounding. *J. Biomed. Opt. 8*(3), 565–569.

Puvanathasan, P. & Bizheva, K. (2007). Speckle noise reduction algorithm for optical coherence tomography based on interval type ii fuzzy set. *Opt. Express 15*(24), 15747–15758.

Rogowska, J. & Brezinski, M. (2000). Evaluation of the adaptive speckle suppression filter for coronary optical coherence tomography imaging. *IEEE Trans. Med. Imaging 19*(12), 1261–1266.

Salinas, H. & Fernández, D. (2007, June). Comparison of pde-based nonlinear diffusion approaches for image enhancement and denoising in optical coherence tomography. *IEEE Trans. Med. Imaging 26*(6), 761–771.

Schmitt, J. (1997). Array detection for speckle reduction in optical coherence microscopy. *Phys. Med. Biol. 42*(7), 1427–1439.

Schmitt, J. (1998). Restoration of optical coherence images of living tissue using the clean algorithm. *J. Biomed. Opt. 3*(1), 66–75.

Schmitt, J., Xiang, S. & Yung, K. (1999). Speckle in optical coherence tomography. *J. Biomed. Opt. 4*(1), 95–105.

Shankar, P. & Newhouse, V. (1985, Jul). Speckle reduction with improved resolution in ultrasound images. *IEEE Trans. on Sonics and Ultrasonics 32*(4), 537–543.

Wagner, R., Smith, S., Sandrik, J. & Lopez, H. (1983). Statistics of speckle in ultrasound b-scans. *IEEE Trans. on Sonics and Ultrasonics 30*(3), 156–163.

Weickert, J. (1997). A review of nonlinear diffusion filtering. In *Proceedings of the First International Conference on Scale-Space Theory in Computer Vision*, London, UK, pp. 3–28. Springer-Verlag.

Xiang, S., Zhou, L. & Schmitt, J. (1998). Speckle noise reduction for optical coherence tomography. *Optical and Imaging Techniques for Biomonitoring III in Proc. SPIE 3196*(1), 79–88.

Technology and Medical Sciences – Natal Jorge et al. (eds)
© *2011 Taylor & Francis Group, London, ISBN 978-0-415-66822-4*

Possible relations between female pelvic pathologies and soft tissue properties

P.A.L.S. Martins & R.M. Natal Jorge
IDMDEC—Polo FEUP
Faculty of Engineering, University of Porto, Porto, Portugal

A.L. Silva-Filho
Department of Gynecology and Obstetrics
Faculty of Medicine, Federal University of Minas Gerais, Belo Horizonte, Brazil

A. Santos & L. Santos
Forensic Sciences Centre of the Sciences and Technologies Foundation (FCT), Porto, Portugal
National Institute of Legal Medicine, North Branch Porto, Portugal
Faculty of Medicine, University of Porto, Porto, Portugal

T. Mascarenhas
Department of Gynecology and Obstetrics
Faculty of Medicine, University of Porto, Porto, Portugal

A.J.M. Ferreira
Faculty of Engineering, University of Porto, Porto, Portugal

ABSTRACT: The female pelvic pathologies constitute a significant public health problem. The lack of fundamental knowledge on the pelvic cavity, led recently to significant research efforts. In particular, some studies have been addressed to evaluate the biomechanical properties of pelvic ligaments and vaginal tissue. These studies present themselves to the clinicians as potential diagnostic complementary techniques. This could be achieved either by using accurate simulations based on the finite element method or by the direct use of biomechanical parameters. This information is also relevant for the improvement of prostheses used in prolapse correction and/or incontinence surgeries. Despite these investigations, the biomechanical repercussions of the overloaded vaginal tissues caused by POP remain unclear.

The mechanical tests performed in this work belong to the category of destructive tests. This means that the specimens tested are completely (at least irreversibly) damaged. There are alternative techniques to infer/estimate the biomechanical properties of soft biological tissues without damage. However, the information acquired is not adequate for an accurate estimation of these properties, specially in loading conditions outside the physiologic range. Extreme biological functions such as birth, or even a violent cough, may stress pelvic tissues to their physiologic limit.

The aim of this study is to search possible relations between female pelvic pathologies and soft tissue properties. This will be achieved through the analysis of the Biomechanical properties extracted from uniaxial tension tests, following the techniques and processes outlined by.

1 INTRODUCTION

Female pelvic pathologies, in particular Urinary Incontinence (UI) and Pelvic Organ Prolapse (POP), have heavy social, psychological and financial impacts (Jelovsek *et al.*, 2007, Kenton and Mueller 2006, Birnbaum *et al.*, 2003). These pathologies are multi-factorial (Liu *et al.*, 2006, Dietz 2007, Lowenstein *et al.*, 2009, Turner *et al.*, 2009), an obstacle to the understanding of their mechanisms. Acquiring fundamental knowledge on the pelvic cavity is of paramount importance for a better understanding of these pathologies. Although much remains to be done on the medical field, engineering techniques, in particular the study of Biomechanical properties and Biomechanical simulation (FEM models), are regarded by some of the most renowned specialists as important tools (Petros, 2007, Ch. 7). As a direct response to this situation, on the last few years there was a significant increase of mixed collaborations between medical doctors (mainly urogynecologists and obstetricians) and engineers. Several studies were focused on the Biomechanical properties of pelvic ligaments and vaginal tissue (Cosson et al., 2003, Cosson et al., 2004, Goh, 2002, Lei et al., 2007, Rubod et al., 2008, Calvo et al., 2009, Martins et al., 2010, Peña et al., 2010), while others presented simulations of the pelvic tissues and structures (Haridas et al., 2006, Janda, 2006, Martins et al., 2006, Parente et al., 2008, Chen et al., 2009, Zhang et al., 2009).

These studies present themselves to the clinicians as potential diagnostic complementary techniques. This could be achieved either by using accurate simulations based on the finite element method or by the direct use of biomechanical parameters. This information is also relevant for the improvement of prostheses used in prolapse correction and/or incontinence surgeries (Goh, 2003). Despite these investigations, the biomechanical repercussions of the overloaded vaginal tissues caused by POP remain unclear. The mechanical tests performed in this work belong to the category of destructive tests. This means that the specimens tested are completely (at least irreversibly) damaged. There are alternative techniques to infer/estimate the Biomechanical properties of soft biological tissues without damage (Kauer, 2001, Kauer et al., 2002, Epstein et al., 2007, Cox et al., 2008). However, the information acquired is not adequate for an accurate estimation of these properties, specially in loading conditions outside the physiologic range. Extreme biological functions such as birth, or even a violent cough, may stress pelvic tissues to their physiologic limit.

The aim of this study is to search possible relations between female pelvic pathologies and soft tissue properties. This will be achieved through the analysis of the Biomechanical properties extracted from uniaxial tension tests, following the techniques and processes outlined by Martins et al. (2006).

2 MATERIALS AND METHODS

POP patients were submitted to pelvic surgeries for prolapse correction. During surgery, as a consequence of the anatomical reconstructive procedures, there were portions of vaginal tissue excised. As a standard practice these tissues are incinerated, in compliance with waste disposable procedures of Health institutions. The Ethical Research Ethics Committee guidelines of *Hospital de So Joo* (Porto, Portugal) were followed throughout the study. There was also the informed consent provided by all patients involved in the investigation.

This study includes 25 patients suffering from POP. The vaginal tissue analyzed was from the anterior vagina. The patients were preoperatively evaluated in terms of history, physical examination and a urodynamic study was performed when

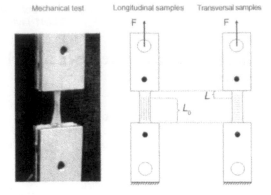

Figure 1. Vaginal tissue fibers.

indicated. The Pelvic Organ Prolapse Quantification (POP-Q) system (Bump et al., 1996) was used to quantify the pelvic organ prolapse severity on all the patients. Patients were excluded when: the tissue sample was too small or too damaged to be tested; there was not enough data (on the patient) to support its inclusion in the study.

The tissue was excised in the longitudinal axis of the middle third vagina in the anterior and posterior vaginal walls. The samples were preserved in a saline bath and kept at 5° Celsius until 15 minutes before the mechanical tests were performed. The storage time of the soft tissues (until testing) did not exceed 6 hours, and for most of the samples it was inferior to 4 hours.

Prior to the mechanical test, the individual specimens were prepared from the original sample. The samples presented a diversity of shapes and sizes. In addition, it was also established a preferential cutting direction in reference to the dominant fiber direction (Figure 1) and a tissue defect exclusion policy. Tissue defects (like scars or deep forceps marks) were excluded because they could affect the local stiffness (ex. stress concentration effect) altering the mechanical test outcome. These factors were accounted while cutting the specimens in strips (approximately rectangular) using scalpel and tweezers.

Geometrical properties were acquired through digital image analysis using the techniques detailed in (Martins et al., 2010).

2.1 The uniaxial tensile test

The uniaxial tensile test, also called simple tension test requires an experimental setup. There are commercial solutions available from companies like Bose (ElectroForce Systems Group), INSTRON or MTS however, the budget constraints of the research project led to an alternative solution. The scheme in Figure 2 represents each component of

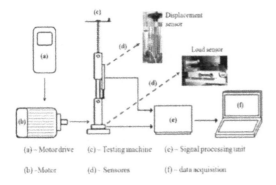

(a) – Motor drive   (c) – Testing machine   (e) – Signal processing unit

(b) – Motor   (d) – Sensores   (f) – data acquisition

Figure 2.   Diagram of the experimental setup.

the uniaxial tensile test setup. The video/image setup was left out of the scheme because it is an add-on to the basic system, despite its importance to the testing solution. The experimental approach used was validated for hyperelastic, rubber-like materials (silicon rubber) (Martins *et al.*, 2006), and later successfully applied to the testing of biomaterials (polypropylene meshes) (Afonso *et al.*, 2008) and human soft tissues (Calvo *et al.*, 2009, Martins *et al.*, 2010). The mechanical testing of soft tissues requires particular care in every step of the process. The sample was mounted on the testing machine, using a set of light aluminum grips. Due to the fragile nature of the tissues, it was required a grip support system to mount the samples on the testing machine. This procedure minimizes sample damage prior to the test beginning. It also provides for an easier adjustment of the sample in the test rig.

2.2 *Biomechanical properties assessment*

The Biomechanical properties were evaluated by means of uniaxial tensile tests. The load (N) and displacement (mm) data were acquired using a load cell; ($F_{max} = 200\ N$) and a displacement sensor. A constant displacement rate of 5 mm·min^{-1} was maintained throughout the test and for all tests. Both load and displacement data were recorded till complete specimen rupture. One of the video cameras previously employed for geometry measurement was used to record each mechanical test on video. This procedure enabled the quality control of each test, by a posteriori elimination of tests where an inadequate alignment or slippage was detected. There is a variety of Biomechanical properties that can be obtained directly from the experimental data, Figure 3. The properties considered on the scope of the present study are the tangent modulus (E_t) defined as

$$E_t = \frac{\Delta\sigma_1}{\Delta\lambda_1} \tag{1}$$

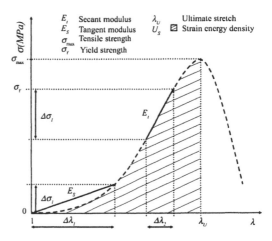

Figure 3.   Typical mechanical behavior of biological soft tissues. *Classical* mechanical properties of soft tissues.

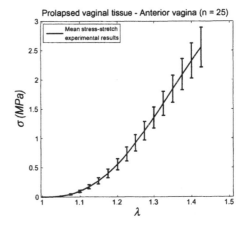

Figure 4.   Typical mechanical behavior for the anterior vaginal wall. Prolapsed vaginal tissue, POP group. Longitudinal (fiber oriented) direction.

and tensile strength (σ_{max}) obtained directly from the experimental curves as shown in Figure 3.

3   RESULTS

Nonlinear theories like hyperelasticity (Calvo *et al.*, 2009, Martins *et al.*, 2010, Peña *et al.*, 2010) or viscoelasticity (Peña *et al.*, 2010) are able to describe the complex mechanical behavior of vaginal tissue with great accuracy. However, a common criticism of such models is their inherent complexity, because they rely on the optimization of a set of interdependent variables. The solution of this multi-variable optimization problem is not unique, there is a set of possible solutions with a given error. It is also fair to state that in such models, it is quite difficult to have a sense of the underlying physics associated to each of the variables. The Biomechanical properties considered (E_t, σ_{max}) are extracted directly from the experimental data. Figure 4 shows the typical mechanical behavior for the anterior vaginal wall (longitudinal direction). The mean stress-stretch curve was truncated to $\lambda = 1.425$. This limit corresponds to the maximum common stretch for the tested samples. The error bars represent the variability of the results, and were calculated using the Standard Error of the Mean (SEM).

The numerical values of the Biomechanical properties were 13.1 ± 0.8 MPa for E_t and 5.3 ± 0.5 MPa for σ_{max}.

4 CONCLUSIONS

The anatomical changes associated with female POP are very well documented (Silva-Filho et al., 2010, Wallner et al., 2009, Ashton-Miller and Delancey 2009, Ashton-Miller and DeLancey 2007). Recently Salman et al., (2010) demontrated that "Uterine prolapse is associated with connective tissue alterations including total amount of connective tissue components and diameter and distribution of collagen fibers". An active remodeling of the vagina and its supportive tissues in response to different environmental stimuli is to be expected (Alperin and Moalli 2006). Therefore, the abnormal morphology of the pelvic cavity in women suffering with POP (Salman et al., 2010, Badiou et al., 2008) may have it's source on the tissue alterations reported.

These observations hint that Biomechanical properties of prolapsed pelvic tissues, and in particular prolapsed vaginal tissues, may differ from those of normal pelvic tissue. Comparing the results obtained, 13.1 ± 0.8 MPa for E_t and 5.3 ± 0.5 MPa for σ_{max}, with those reported by Martins et al., (2010a) for women without prolapse (anterior vagina), 6.9 ± 1.1 MPa for E_t and 2.6 ± 0.4 MPa for σ_{max}, it is observed a clear and significant difference of the Biomechanical properties.

The evidence presented supports the thesis that associated with POP there are changes on the Biomechanical properties of prolapsed pelvic tissues, in this case on the anterior vagina.

ACKNOWLEDGEMENTS

The funding by Ministrio da Cincia, Tecnologia e Ensino Superior FCT, Portugal, under grants PTDC/SAU-BEB/71459/2006 and SFRH/BD/41841/2007, and Euro-Brazilian Windows (Working Programme for Staff/Post-Doctoral Mobility) is gratefully acknowledged.

REFERENCES

Afonso, J., Martins, P., Girao, M., Natal Jorge, R., Ferreira, A., Mascarenhas, T., Fernandes, A., Bernardes, J., Baracat, E., Rodrigues de Lima, G. & Patricio, B. (2008, March). Mechanical properties of polypropylene mesh used in pelvic floor repair. International Urogynecology Journal 19(3), 375–380.

Alperin, M. & Moalli, P. (2006). Remodeling of vaginal connective tissue in patients with prolapse. Current Opinion in Obstetrics and Gynecology 18(5), 544–550.

Ashton-Miller, J.A. & DeLancey, J.O.L. (2007, Apr). Functional anatomy of the female pelvic floor. Ann N Y Acad Sci, 1101, 266–296.

Ashton-Miller, J.A. & Delancey, J.O.L. (2009). On the biomechanics of vaginal birth and common sequelae. Annu Rev Biomed Eng, 11, 163–176.

Badiou, W., Granier, G., Bousquet, P.-J., Monrozies, X., Mares, P. & de Tayrac, R. (2008, May). Comparative histological analysis of anterior vaginal wall in women with pelvic organ prolapse or control subjects. a pilot study. Int Urogynecol J Pelvic Floor Dysfunct 19(5), 723–729.

Birnbaum, H., Leong, S. & Kabra, A. (2003). Lifetime medical costs for women: cardiovascular disease, diabetes, and stress urinary incontinence. Women's Health Issues 13(6), 204–213.

Bump, R., Mattiasson, A., Bo, K., Brubaker, L., DeLancey, J., Klarskov, P., Shull, B. & Smith, A. (1996). The standardization of terminology of female pelvic organ prolapse and pelvic floor dysfunction. American Journal of Obstetrics and Gynecology 175(1), 10–17.

Calvo, B., Peña, E., Martins, P., Mascarenhas, T., Doblaré, M., Natal Jorge, R. & Ferreira, A. (2009, March). On modelling damage process in vaginal tissue. Journal of Biomechanics 42(5), 642–651.

Chen, L., Ashton-Miller, J.A. & DeLancey, J.O. (2009). A 3d finite element model of anterior vaginal wall support to evaluate mechanisms underlying cystocele formation. Journal of Biomechanics 42(10), 1371–1377.

Cosson, M., Boukerrou, M., Lacaze, S., Lambaudie, E., Fasel, J., Mesdagh, H., Lobry, P. & Ego, A. (2003). A study of pelvic ligament strength. European Journal of Obstetrics Gynecology and Reproductive Biology 109(1), 80–87.

Cosson, M., Lambaudie, E., Boukerrou, M., Lobry, P., Crépin, G. & Ego, A. (2004). A biomechanical study of the strength of vaginal tissues: Results on 16 postmenopausal patients presenting with genital prolapse. European Journal of Obstetrics Gynecology and Reproductive Biology 112(2), 201–205.

Cox, M.A.J., Gawlitta, D., Driessen, N.J.B., Oomens, C.W.J. & Baaijens, F.P.T. (2008). The non-linear mechanical properties of soft engineered biological tissues determined by finite spherical indentation. Computer Methods in Biomechanics and Biomedical Engineering 11(5), 585–592.

Dietz, H.P. (2007, April). Levator trauma in labor: a challenge for obstetricians, surgeons and sonologists. Ultrasound in Obstetrics and Gynecology 29, 368–371(4).

Epstein, L., Graham, C. & Heit, M. (2007). Systemic and vaginal biomechanical properties of women with normal vaginal support and pelvic organ prolapse. American Journal of Obstetrics and Gynecology 197(2), 165.e1–165.e6.

Goh, J. (2002). Biomechanical properties of prolapsed vaginal tissue in pre- and postmenopausal women. *International Urogynecology Journal and Pelvic Floor Dysfunction 13*(2), 76–79.

Goh, J. (2003). Biomechanical and biochemical assessments for pelvic organ prolapse. *Current Opinion in Obstetrics and Gynecology 15*(5), 391–394.

Haridas, B., Hong, H., Minoguchi, R., Owens, S. & Osborn, T. (2006). Pelvicsim–A computational-experimental system for biomechanical evaluation of female pelvic floor organ disorders and associated minimally invasive interventions. *Stud Health Technol Inform 119*, 182–187.

Janda, S. (2006, January). *Biomechanics of the pelvic floor musculature*. Ph.D. thesis, TUD Technische Universiteit Delft.

Jelovsek, J., Maher, C. & Barber, M. (2007). Pelvic organ prolapse. *Lancet 369*(9566), 1027–1038.

Kauer, M. (2001). *Inverse Finite Element Characterization of Soft Tissues With Aspiration Experiments*. Ph.D. thesis, Swiss Federal Institute Of Technology, Switzerland.

Kauer, M., Vuskovic, V., Dual, J., Szekely, G. & Bajka, M. (2002). Inverse finite element characterization of soft tissues. *Medical Image Analysis 6*(3), 275–287.

Kenton, K. & Mueller, E. (2006). The global burden of female pelvic floor disorders. *BJU International 98*(SUPPL. 1), 1–5.

Lei, L., Song, Y. & Chen, R. (2007). Biomechanical properties of prolapsed vaginal tissue in pre- and postmenopausal women. *International Urogynecology Journal 18*, 603–607.

Liu, X., Zhao, Y., Pawlyk, B., Damaser, M. & Li, T. (2006). Failure of elastic fiber homeostasis leads to pelvic floor disorders. *Am J Pathol 168*(2), 519–528.

Lowenstein, L., Gamble, T., Deniseiko Sanses, T., Van Raalte, H., Carberry, C., Jakus, S., Kambiss, S., Mcachran, S., Pham, T., Aschkenazi, S., Hoskey, K. & Kenton, K. (2009). Sexual function is related to body image perception in women with pelvic organ prolapse. *Journal of Sexual Medicine 6*(8), 2286–2291.

Martins, J., Pato, M.P., Pires, E., Jorge, R., Parente, M. & Mascarenhas, T. (2006). Finite element studies of the deformation of the pelvic floor. *Journal of Biomechanics 39*(Supplement 1), S347–S347. Abstracts of the 5th World Congress of Biomechanics, Munich, Germany, 29 July-04 August 2006.

Martins, P., Natal Jorge, R., Salema, C., Roza, T., Ferreira, A., Parente, M., Pinotti, M., Mascarenhas, T., Santos, A., Santos, L. & Silva-Filho, A. (2010). Vaginal tissue properties versus increased intra-abdominal pressure: a biomechanical study. *Gynecologic and Obstetric Investigation (DOI: 10.1159/000315160)*.

Martins, P., Peña, E., Calvo, B., Mascarenhas, T., Doblaré, M., Natal Jorge, R. & Ferreira, A. (2010, June). Prediction of nonlinear elastic behaviour of vaginal tissue: experimental results and model formulation. *Computer Methods in Biomechanics and Biomedical Engineering 13*(3), 327–337.

Martins, P.A.L.S., Jorge, R.M.N. & Ferreira, A.J.M. (2006). A comparative study of several material models for prediction of hyperelastic properties: Application to silicone-rubber and soft tissues. *Strain 42*(3), 135–147.

Parente, M., Jorge, R., Mascarenhas, T., Fernandes, A. & Martins, J. (2008, January). Deformation of the pelvic floor muscles during a vaginal delivery. *International Urogynecology Journal 19*(1), 65–71.

Peña, E., Calvo, B., Martínez, M., Martins, P., Mascarenhas, T., Jorge, R., Ferreira, A. & Doblaré, M. (2010, February). Experimental study and constitutive modeling of the viscoelastic mechanical properties of the human prolapsed vaginal tissue. *Biomechanics and Modeling in Mechanobiology 9*(1), 35–44.

Peña, E., Martins, P., Mascarenhas, T., Natal Jorge, R.M., Ferreira, A., Doblaré, M. & Calvo, B. (2010). Mechanical characterization of the softening behavior of human vaginal tissue. *J. Mech. Behav. Biomed. Mater. (submitted)*.

Petros, P.P. (2007). *The Female Pelvic Floor: Function, Dysfunction and Management According to the Integral Theory, 2nd ed.* Springer.

Rubod, C., Boukerrou, M., Brieu, M., Jean-Charles, C., Dubois, P. & Cosson, M. (2008). Biomechanical properties of vaginal tissue: preliminary results. *International Urogynecology Journal, 19*, 811–816.

Salman, M., Ozyuncu, O., Sargon, M., Kucukali, T. & Durukan, T. (2010, February). Light and electron microscopic evaluation of cardinal ligaments in women with or without uterine prolapse. *International Urogynecology Journal 21*(2), 235–239.

Silva-Filho, A.L., Saleme, C.S., Roza, T., Martins, P.A., Parente, M.M., Pinotti, M., Mascarenhas, T., Ferreira, A.J.M. & Jorge, R.M.N. (2010). Evaluation of pelvic floor muscle cross-sectional area using a 3d computer model based on mri in women with and without prolapse. *Eur J Obstet Gynecol in press (doi:10.1016/j.ejogrb.2010.07.005)*.

Turner, C.E., Young, J.M., Solomon, M.J., Ludlow, J. & Benness, C. (2009, Jun). Incidence and etiology of pelvic floor dysfunction and mode of delivery: an overview. *Dis Colon Rectum 52*(6), 1186–1195.

Wallner, C., Dabhoiwala, N.F., DeRuiter, M.C. & Lamers W.H. (2009, Apr). The anatomical components of urinary continence. *Eur Urol 55*(4), 932–943.

Zhang, Y., Kim, S., Erdman, A.G., Roberts, K.P. & Timm, G.W. (2009, Jul). Feasibility of using a computer modeling approach to study sui induced by landing a jump. *Ann Biomed Eng 37*(7), 1425–1433.

Technology and Medical Sciences – Natal Jorge et al. (eds)
© *2011 Taylor & Francis Group, London, ISBN 978-0-415-66822-4*

Processing and classification of biological images: Application to histology

Bruno Nunes & Luís Miguel Rato
Departamento de Informática, CITI—Centro de Investigação em Tecnologias de Informação da, Universidade de Évora, Universidade de Évora, Évora, Portugal

Fernando Capela Silva
Departamento de Biologia, Instituto de Ciências Agrárias e Ambientais Mediterrânicas (ICAAM), Universidade de Évora, Évora, Portugal

Ana Rafael & António Silvério Cabrita
Instituto de Patologia Experimental, Faculdade de Medicina da Universidade de Coimbra, Coimbra, Portugal

ABSTRACT: This article deals with a histological problem by using image processing and feature extraction in images of renal tissues of rats and their classification through various methods such as: Bayesian inference, decision trees and support vector machines.

Keywords: Image Processing, Segmentation, Classification, Kidney, Renal Glomeruli, Histology, Feature Extraction, Xenobiotics

1 INTRODUCTION

The observation in photonic microscopy of histological sections allows us to evaluate the structural changes of an individual's exposure to xenobiotics.

This evaluation can be made through quantitative criteria by using computational tools and algorithms to make the process faster and more accurate.

2 OBJECTIVES

This work intends to evaluate the morphological changes in the kidney of rats, caused by exposure to xenobiotics, through computer-assisted histomorphometric analysis.

3 IMAGE PROCESSING

In this work, we used 210 kidney photomicrographs of 21 Wistar rats belonging to three groups: Group I [Control, n = 7], Group II [Pesticide Thiram, n = 6) and Group III [Corn Oil, n = 8] (Fialho, Capela e Silva, Rafael & Cabrita, 2001).

Samples were collected after 35 days of testing and processed by histological routine techniques, in Instituto de Patologia Experimental, Faculdade de Medicina da Universidade de Coimbra.

The final preparations were observed with a Nikon Eclipse 600 microscope, using a magnification of 200X, and the images were acquired using a Nikon DN100 digital camera.

For each animal of each group was selected a section and, for each of them, there were randomly observed 10 renal corpuscles (Figure 1).

The images were then processed using several tools from the program *ImageJ* (Rasband 2009)

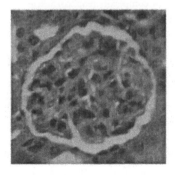

Figure 1. Example of a renal corpuscle.

together with an existing plugin called *MultiCell Outliner* (MCO) (Latxiondo 2006), in order to highlight the renal corpuscles.

3.1 *Methodology*

The methodology we used was divided in two different steps: the delimitation and the extraction of the renal corpuscle.

3.1.1 *Delimitation*

In this first step, the objective was to define the contour of the renal corpuscle and fill it's interior.

Depending on the three complexity degrees of the images: low, medium and high, there were different types of approach.

Low complexity images

We say that an image has a low complexity degree when the Bowman's capsule is clearly visible and without any breaks, as we can see in Figure 2.

In these cases, we were able to fully trace the outline of the renal structure using only the MCO plugin, as left image from Figure 3 shows.

Once the outline is highlighted, we've painted it's interior with the black color, using the *Fill* tool, as shown in the right image from Figure 3.

The result from a low complexity image delimitation is shown in Figure 4.

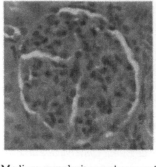

Figure 5.   Medium complexity renal corpuscle.

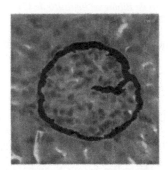

Figure 4.   Final result from a delimitation in a low complexity image.

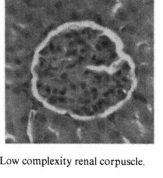

Figure 2.   Low complexity renal corpuscle.

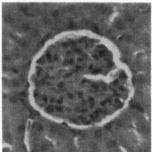

Figure 3.   Delimitation and filling of a low complexity renal corpuscle.

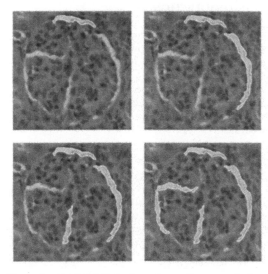

Figure 6.   Partial delimitation of a medium complexity renal corpuscle.

Medium complexity images

In images with a medium complexity degree, despite it contains some breaks, the Bowman's capsule shape is perfectly recognizable.

In these cases, we only managed to outline the renal corpuscle partially using MCO plugin. The following figure shows the partial delimitation step by step.

After the partial delimitation was completed, the inside of each highlighted part was painted with the black color using the *Fill* tool.

The following figure shows the result after the partial delimitation of the renal corpuscle.

To complete the process, it was necessary to manually finish the Bowman's capsule's contour, using the brush tool with 3 pixels size.

High complexity images
Images with high complexity degree are the worst case scenario. In these images, the Bowman's capsule's shape is difficult to identify or barely can be seen.

We didn't obtained satisfactory results using the MCO plugin in these cases, so the renal corpuscle had to be entirely delimited by hand, using the brush tool with 3 pixels size. The delimitation steps and the final result can be seen in figure below.

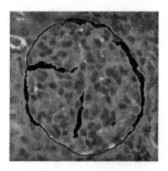

Figure 9. Final result from the complete delimitation of a medium complexity renal corpuscle.

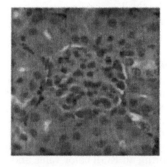

Figure 10. High complexity renal corpuscle.

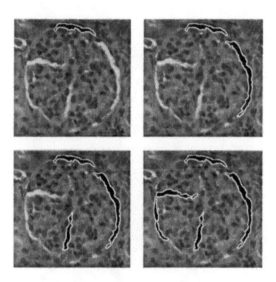

Figure 7. Filling the partial delimitation of a medium complexity renal corpuscle.

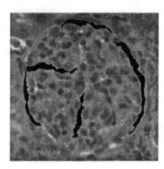

Figure 8. Partial delimitation in a medium complexity case.

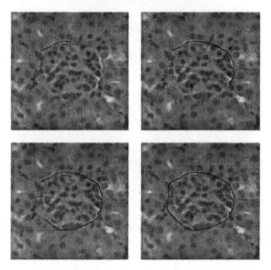

Figure 11. Delimitation of a high complexity renal corpuscle.

235

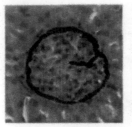
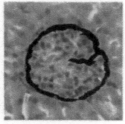

Figure 12.   RGB to Grayscale conversion.

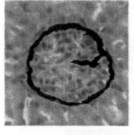
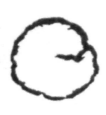

Figure 13.   Highlight of renal structure through threshold technique.

3.1.2 *Extraction*

In the second step, the objective was to isolate the regions painted in black previously, under the form of binary images.

To do this, we've made a RGB to Grayscale conversion, as can be seen in Figure 12.

After this conversion, each of the image's pixels stops storing an RGB color value and starts to store a gray intensity, being the strongest intensity the black color and the weakest intensity the white color.

Then we've applied the threshold technique on top of the grayscale image, in order to highlight the renal corpuscle silhouette, as shown in Figure 13.

4   FEATURE EXTRACTION

After isolating the renal corpuscles, and based on the resulting images from processing and segmentation, we used *ImageJ* again to measure several morphological features that served to identify and distinguish the renal corpuscles.

The following features were considered:

In addition to these features, we've also considered the fractal dimensions of the renal corpuscle.

Finally, after measuring all these features for the complete set of images, the resulting data was stored in the form of a vector of features for each image.

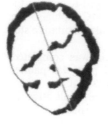

Figure 14.   Diameter and Perimeter of Bowman's capsule.

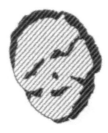
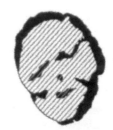

Figure 15.   Bowman's capsule's and glomeruli's total area.

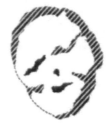
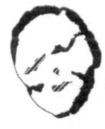

Figure 16.   Exterior and interior Bowman's space.

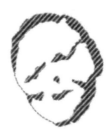
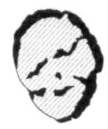

Figure 17.   Total Bowman's space and glomerular capillaries area.

5   CLASSIFICATION

Once the entire data set was obtained, we applied several algorithms for classifying data using *WEKA* (Witten & Frank, 2005). The used classifiers were:

- Zero rule
- One rule

- Naive Bayes
- J48 Tree
- Support Vector Machines

The classification results, with and without feature selection, may be seen in Table 1.

In order to reduce uncertainty in the final results we made some transformations on the data, namely the aggregation of image data concerning to the same animal.

The classification results after aggregation of instances, with and without feature selection, may be seen in Table 2.

Comparing the results there have been some improvements on some classifiers, however, a high accuracy rate not always means a good classification. This can be observed through the example of Tables 3 and 4, corresponding to Naive Bayes and Zero Rule confusion matrices, both with feature selection and instance aggregation.

Naive Bayes has 85,7143% of accuracy rate and correctly classifies all the pesticide instances and the most of the healthy instances.

Table 1. Percentage of accuracy rate of the different classifiers.

Classifier	No. selection	Selection
Zero Rule	71,3636	71,3636
One Rule	70,4545	72,7273
Naive Bayes	64,5455	73,6364
J48 Tree	70,4545	73,1818
SVM	69,0909	78,1818

Table 2. Percentage of accuracy rate of the different classifiers with instance aggregation.

Classifier	No. selection	Selection
Zero Rule	71,4286	71,4286
One Rule	66,6667	66,6667
Naive Bayes	85,7143	85,7143
J48 Tree	71,4286	66,6667
SVM	76,1905	80,9524

Table 3. Naive Bayes confusion matrix.

Classified as →	Healthy	Pesticide
Healthy	12	3
Pesticide	0	6

Table 4. Zero Rule confusion matrix.

Classified as →	Healthy	Pesticide
Healthy	15	0
Pesticide	6	0

Table 5. FP Rate and Precision of the different classifiers with instance aggregation for pesticide class.

Classifier	FP Rate	Precision
Zero Rule	0	0
One Rule	0,267	0,429
Naive Bayes	0,200	0,667
J48 Tree	0,333	0,500
SVM	0,200	0,571

On the other hand, Zero Rule classifies well all the healthy instances but fails completely when classifying the pesticide instances. On this case, the high accuracy rate (71,4286%) is purely justified with the existence of more healthy instances then pesticide instances.

One way to avoid these type of misunderstandings, it's to consider other variables such as false positive rate and precision of the class of interest. The table below shows values from both variables for each classifier.

Given these facts, when choosing one of the classifiers we should always consider not only it's accuracy rate but also the the lowest false positive rate an the highest precision on the class of interest. Therefore, based on the previous tables, we can conclude that the best classifier options would be Naive Bayes followed by SVM.

6 CONCLUSION

The results of this work may be considered positive since, by analyzing the information obtained through all the process, it was possible to say with an acceptable degree of certainty, whether or not histological changes occured at the level of renal corpuscles. However, given that there remains an uncertainty in the results of some classifiers, improvements can be made by including other image features.

REFERENCES

Fialho, I., Capela e Silva, F., Rafael, A. & Cabrita, A. (2001). Effects of tetramethylthiuram disulfide (thiram) on kidney metallothionein expression in rats. In *Biomarkers of Environmental Contamination*, 24–26 September 2001, Póvoa de Varzim, Portugal, p. 191.

Latxiondo, K. (2006). Multicell outliner. http://rsbweb. nih.gov/ij/plugins/multi-cell-outliner.html [accessed July-2010].

Rasband, W.S. (1997–2009). *ImageJ*. Bethesda, Maryland, USA: U.S. National Institutes of Health. http://rsb.info.nih.gov/ij/ [accessed July-2010].

Witten, I.H. & Frank, E. (2005). *Data Mining: Practical Machine Learning Tools and Techniques* (2nd ed.). Morgan Kaufmann.

Technology and Medical Sciences – Natal Jorge et al. (eds)
© *2011 Taylor & Francis Group, London, ISBN 978-0-415-66822-4*

Reducing and preventing drug interactions–An approach

R. Barros
Faculdade de Ciências e Tecnologia da, Universidade Nova de Lisboa, Caparica, Portugal
Siemens S.A, Sector Healthcare, Matosinhos, Portugal

F. Janela
Siemens S.A, Sector Healthcare, Matosinhos, Portugal

ABSTRACT: Polypharmacy is commonly used in clinical practice and it is related with adverse drug reactions. These are one of the leading causes of morbidity and can result in hospitalization or even death. In the United States, two millions serious adverse drug reactions, and one hundred thousand deaths occur yearly. The aim of this study is to contribute to decrease the number of adverse drug reactions, especially drug interactions, in Portugal. It is necessary to investigate different nonproprietary names of drugs and the pharmacotherapeutic classifications used in the different places of world. Drug interactions databases need to identify which diseases and related health problems are caused by a given drug; thus it is necessary to identify the diseases classifications and terminologies. The main features considered in this analysis are the drugs identification systems, the diseases' classification and the types of drug interactions.

1 INTRODUCTION

In the last century, scientific progress, especially in pharmacology, led physicians to prescribe drugs more frequently. The increment of polytherapy situations (simultaneous treatment of more than one disease) led to an increasing number of drugs prescribed simultaneously, or polypharmacy.

Nowadays, polypharmacy is common in clinical practice and is associated with the risk of drug interactions, which is a frequent cause of morbidity. It can lead to hospitalization and even death. It is also estimated that the incidence of clinical drug interactions vary from 3 to 5% in patients who have up to six prescription drugs, increasing to 20% or more in patients who use more than 10 drugs (Goodman Gilman et al. 1996).

In the United States, two millions serious adverse drug reactions, and one hundred thousand deaths occur yearly (Lazarou et al. 1998).

In order to reduce potential risks associated with polypharmacy, it was developed the present study with the aim of establishing the basis for supervision of the electronic prescription of drugs. This study will allow alerting the physician whenever one or more drug interactions are detected in a prescription.

In order to achieve this goal, it is necessary to identify the type of interactions, the various types of classifications, the existing databases and, then, choosing the one that presents the greatest potential.

2 APPROACH

The aim of this study is the identification of database (s) capable of indicating the different types of interactions that best suits the Portuguese health system.

2.1 Types of drug interactions

This section identifies and describes the different existing types of interactions:

Drug/drug—this type of drug interaction occurs when one drug alters the behavior of others. Polypharmacy increases the likelihood of this type of interaction.

The drugs can interact with other medication, but there are other forms of drug interaction, such as:

Drug/Allergy—this is the interaction of drug with an allergy that patient may have. If the patient is allergic to lactose, the drug can not contain lactose to prevent the allergy manifestation. With the knowledge of the patient's allergies, we can obtain the drug interaction between prescription drugs and allergies. To be efficient this process requires an electronic health record.

Drug/Food and Beverage—this type of IM occurs when the behavior of the drug in the body is altered by the intake of one or more kinds of food or beverages. To be efficient this process requires an electronic health record.

Drug/Alternative Therapies—in recent years there has been an increasing demand for alternative therapies such as herbal, dietary supplements and homeopathic remedies to treat severe medical conditions. Unfortunately, when these products are taken in wrong doses or in combination with medications they can cause drug interactions.

Drug/Laboratory Interference—are changes that can occur in laboratory tests due to the consumption of drugs. It can be misleading to read the analysis.

Contraindications, the predisposing factors such as age (extremes of life) and sex, genetic factors such as polymorphism and physiological factors like pregnancy and concomitant diseases may also influence the effectiveness of the prescribed medication.

2.2 Methods

The first step in the study of drug interactions is to understand the identification of the drug. There are different classifications in this area. The first one is the identification of the drug by the name. The second is the pharmacotherapeutic classification that identifies the organ or system in which the active substance will act.

The second step in the study of drug interactions is the identification of diseases', which aims to identify and codify the diseases, hence the disease or reaction resulting from a given drug interaction, to be able to develop an unequivocal system, reducing medical errors.

The third step is to identify the databases that summarise interactions. This type of database can be used into electronic prescribing software, in electronic health record or in an isolated way. These databases may indicate more than one type of IM.

3 RESULTS

3.1 Drug name

Regarding the drug name, we identified three possibilities: the chemical name, the brand name and the nonproprietary name. The chemical name is an unambiguous description of the chemical structure of a drug, which usually uses guidelines by international organizations, as International Union of Pure and Applied Chemistry (IUPAC), but frequently is a difficult designation and it is not commonly used in the prescription act. The brand name is the name chosen by the manufacturer, which is simple, attractive to the public and protected by patent. The brand name of the same drug can change depending on the manufacturer or the country, leading to unnecessary misunderstandings. The nonproprietary name

identifies the active substance, being simple, concise, distinguished in spelling and sound and is not susceptible to be confused with other names in common use. The nonproprietary name is public property and is chosen by the entities responsible for each country or by the WHO (Kopp-Kubel 1995), (Aronson 2000), (World Health Organization–Division of Drug Management Policies 1997).

This kind of name is divided in national nonproprietary name, such as, the British Approved Name (BAN), the Japanese Accepted Name (JAN) and the United States Adopted Name (USAN),

The entities responsible for national nonproprietary names in collaboration with WHO develops International Nonproprietary Name (INN), aiming to standardize the name of an active substance, reducing the errors in the identification of drug.

3.2 Pharmacotherapeutic classification

This classification system follows encodings with hierarchical structure, which divide drugs by different groups, according to the organ or system in which they will operate, for its therapeutic, pharmacological and chemical properties.

This study identifies some pharmacotherapeutic classifications, with different structural levels and nonproprietary names.

One example of pharmacotherapeutic classification is American Hospital Formulary Service (AHFS), developed in the USA, uses 4 levels to identify the active substance and uses USAN as nonproprietary name (American Society of Health-System Pharmacists 2010). Another example is the Anatomical Therapeutic Chemical Classification (ATC), developed by WHO, uses 5 levels to identify the active substance and uses INN as nonproprietary name (WHO Collaborating Centre for Drug Statistics Methodology Norwegian Institute of Public Health 2010). The *Classificação Farmacoterapêutica* (CFT) developed in Portugal, uses 4 levels to identify the chemical group of drug is other example. Finally, the Hierarchical Ingredient Code (HIC3), developed in the USA, uses 4 levels to identify the active substance and uses USAN as nonproprietary name.

The pharmacotherapeutic classifications are define by the site of action of the drug. Since the same drug can be used for more than one therapy, each drug may have more than one code, which can increase the errors in the identifications of drug.

3.3 Classification of diseases

To decrease costs and errors made by the health professionals, several classifications to standardize diseases' identification were developed. This study identifies some classifications of diseases, such as:

The International Classification of Diseases (ICD), developed by WHO, is used worldwide for morbidity and mortality stats. It's been used on the management in healthcare providers, through the identification of diseases and the wide variety of signs, symptoms, abnormal aspects, complaints, social circumstances and external causes for injury or illness. The ICD-10th used alone it's an incomplete classification. In order to adapt to healthcare evolution, the WHO created modules for specialties, such as, Oncology (ICD-O-3) and modules of interventions and procedures, such as, ICD-10th-Clinical Modification (ICD-10th-CM) and ICD-10th-Procedure Classifications System (ICD-10th-PCS). Therefore it is the most complete classification of diseases (Colorado Department of Public Health and Enviroment 2001), (Administração Central do Sistema de Saúde (ACSS) 2009).

The International Classification of Primary Care (ICPC-2) is used in diagnostics of diseases. Its biaxial structure makes it a simple and logical classification. However it's only focused on primary care, which makes it the a less detailed classification than ICD. Since the creation of ICPC, it has been developed a relationship table between ICPC and ICD, which shows the collaboration between entities responsible for both classifications (Administração Central do Sistema de Saúde (ACSS) 2009), (WONCA International Classification Commitee (WICC) 2010).

The SNOMED-CT is one extensive and dynamic clinical terminology for health care provision. It uses a hierarchical structure to identify clinical concepts and description associated with the concepts. That structure allows the indexation, archive, gathering and storing of clinical information for the several specialties. It is a complex terminology, mapped with several versions of ICD, and used by some international organizations (Administração Central do Sistema de Saúde (ACSS) 2009), (U.S. National Library of Medicine 2003).

The WHO-Adverse Reaction Terminology (WHO-ART) and the Medical Dictionary for Regulatory Activities (MedDRA) are terminologies that classify and encode adverse drug reactions and allow the reporting of adverse events that occur with drugs, to the responsible entities (Bousquet et al. 2008). The WHO-ART is a simple and robust terminology, while MedDRA is detailed and complex. The collaboration between the agencies responsible for these terminologies resulted in the mapping of all WHO-ART terms in MedDRA (the Uppsala Monitoring Centre 2010). The use of MedDRA is recommended by the responsible entities for medicines in Europe, the European Medicines Agency (EMEA), and in the U.S., the Food and Drug Administration (FDA) (MedDRA Maintenance and Support Services Organization 2010).

The use of classifications has different purposes. For example the ICD-10th-CM, SNOMED-CT and ICPC-2 are used in diagnostics of disease; the ICD-10th-CM, ICD-10th-PCS and SNOMED-CT are used at interventions and procedures made by health care providers.

3.4 Drug interaction databases

The databases capable of detecting drug interactions have been developed in order to increase patient safety and to reduce the possibility of errors in prescribing drugs and the costs associated with these. During this study were identified different databases of drug interaction that has as many features and it are shown below:

The ABDATA-Datenbank is a drug database, developed in Germany. It is divided in several modules, which contain detailed information about 50.000 drugs used in Germany. One of the modules in this database is the *Interaktionen* (*Drug interactions*), which allows analysis of drug interactions of type drug/drug and drug/food and beverages, only for two drugs at the same time. This database identifies the drug through the INN, the brand name used at Germany and the ATC (ABDATA Pharma-Daten-Service 2005).

The Danish Drug Interaction Database (Lægemiddelstyrelsens) is available online. The drug is identified in database through the INN, the brand name used at Denmark and the ATC. This database describes, in Danish, about 2.500 drug interactions, in majority drug/drug interaction and some drug/alternative therapies. It also has the capacity to identify drug interactions between two or more drugs at the same time (Lægemiddelstyrelsen 2010).

The DrugBank is a database developed in Canada, available online. This database contains more than 100 research fields with detailed chemical, pharmaceutical, medical and biological information about the 4.900 approved drugs in Asia, Europe and North America. The DrugBank has the ability to detect drug interactions of the drug/drug and drug/foodtypes. However this database doesnot evidence the interaction between two or more drugs, it just gives information about one drug. The drug is identified in database through the INN, the brand name, the chemical name—IUPAC and the pharmacotherapeutic classification ATC and AHFS (Wishart et al. 2008).

The Drug Information Database (DRUID) is a drug interactions database developed in Norway and available online. This database has the capability to identify drug interactions between two or more drugs of the drug/drug and drug/food and beverages types. However it only identifies foods and beverages that most often interact with medicines, such as foods rich in vitamin K and alcohol. The drug is identified in database through the INN, the brand name and the ATC (Spigset & Rekda 2010).

The MedicineOne software is an electronic health record developed in Portugal, which manages all clinical and administrative information of users. It is structured in modules representing different types of health care. The MedicineOne has the ability to identify drug interactions between two or more drugs. The physician has access to the comprehensive monographs of drugs from INFARMED and *Simposium Terapêutico* and to an alert system for drug interactions such as: drug/drug, drug/allergy, drug/food and beverages, drug/alternative therapies, drug/lab interferences types and indicating also the contraindications of the drug to the predisposing factors. The drug is identified in database through the INN, the brand name and the ATC. For the identification of diseases, the MedicineOne uses the **ICD-10th e ICPC-2** (Tomé et al. 2008).

The National Drug Data File (NDDF) is a drug database developed in U.S.A. with the aim of improving safety in drug prescribing, dispensing and administration. This database has access to all the information about drugs from the book "AHFS Drug Information". Therefore, this database is very useful when connected to a health record, helping the physician to choose the drug and dosesproperly. This connection allows the emission of drug interaction alerts such as: drug/drug, drug/allergy, drug/food and beverages, drug/alternative therapies, drug/lab interferences types, indicating also the contraindications of the drug to the predisposing factors. It can detect and prevent duplicate drug therapies. The drug is identified in database through the USAN, the U.S.A. brand name and the pharmacotherapeutic classification AHFS and HIC3. In the identification of diseases, the NDDF has connection with ICD-9th-CM (First Data Bank, Inc 2010).

The Qscan is a security platform developed in the USA, which assesses drug interactions, drug/drug type, using a statistical analysis, especially logistic regression. It has the ability to correlate drugs with reactions, age and sex of the patient and allows the analysis of more than two drugs at the same time (DrugLogic, Inc 2008).

The VantageRx is a drug database developed in U.S.A., with the aim of reducing adverse drug reactions and, consequently, costs. This database is useful when connected to a health record, helping the physician to choose the drug and doses properly. This connection allows the emission of drug interaction alerts such as: drug/

drug, drug/allergy, drug/food and beverages types, indicating also the contraindications of the drug to the predisposing factors. It can detect and prevent duplicate drug therapies. The drug is identified in the database through the USAN, the U.S.A. brand name (Cerner® Multum 2009).

4 DISCUSSION

After the identification and study of each database for drug interactions, a comparison between them and the nonproprietary names used was made.It can be seen in Table 1, that the databases developed in Europe use the nonproprietary name INN, while the database developed in North America uses as reference the USAN. This is due to the choice of nonproprietary name for the entity responsible for the drugs in each country. In Portugal, INFARMED uses Denominação Comum Internacional (DCI), which is the Portuguese translation into of INN. Thus the European databases are the most suited to this study.

It was also made a comparison between the databases and the pharmacotherapeutic classifications used, as indicated in Table 2. After reviewing the table, it can be seen that the European databases usethe ATC, the NDDF uses the AHFS, the QScan

Table 1. Comparison of nonproprietary name in the drug interaction databases.

Databases	INN	USAN
ABDA	✓	
Danish Drug Interaction	✓	
DrugBank		✓
DRUID	✓	
MediceOne	✓	
NDDF		✓
Qscan		✓
VantageRx		✓

Table 2. Comparison of pharmacotherapeutic classifications in the drug interaction databases.

Databases	ATC	AHFS
ABDATA	✓	
Danish Drug Interaction	✓	
DrugBank	✓	✓
DRUID	✓	
MediceOne	✓	
NDDF		✓
Qscan		
VantageRx database		

Table 3. Comparison of types of drug interaction in the databases of drug interaction.

Database	Drug / Drug	Drug / Allergy	Drug / Food & Beverages	Drug / Alternative Therapy	Drug / Lab Interference	Dosage	ContraIndication	Duplicate Therapy	2 or + Drugs
ABDATA	✓		✓				✓		
Danish Drug Interaction	✓			✓					✓
DrugBank	✓		✓						
DRUID	✓		✓						✓
Medice One	✓	✓	✓	✓	✓		✓		✓
NDDF	✓	✓	✓	✓	✓	✓	✓	✓	✓
Qscan	✓								
VantageRx	✓	✓	✓			✓	✓	✓	✓

and VantageRx donot use any classification and DrugBank provides the two classifications. In Portugal, INFARMED uses the pharmacotherapeutic classification ATC and CFT. The European databases are the best suited to this study.

In Table 3 are listed the types of drug interaction that each database identifies. It can be seen that most databases have more than one type of drug interactions. The QScan is the only database that identifies just one type of interactions: Drug/Drug.

The ABDATA, DrugBank and DRUID identify the following type of interactions: Drug/Drug and Drug/Food and Beverage. The ABDATA still has the ability to indicate the contraindications of the drug to the predisposing factors.

The Danish Drug Interaction Database identifies the following type of interactions: Drug/Drug and Drug/Alternative Therapies.

The database MedicineOne and NDDF have identical abilities, both identify all the interactions documented in this study. However the MedicineOne does not indicate the dose levels and does not prevent possible duplication. VantageRx has similar capabilities to NDDF however it does not identify Drug/Alternative Therapies and Drug/Lab Interferences types of drug interactions. These databases function is maximized using the electronic health record.

One important aspect of Table 3 is the databases' ability to make interactions with two or more drugs. The DrugBank only shows the list of interaction for each drug, while the ABDATA and QScan show the interactions between two drugs. All other databases in this study have shown the ability to identify and display interactions with more than two drugs. These databases are ideal for the prevention of drug interactions in the polypharmacy used today.

The NDDF and MedicineOne are, of the databases studied, the ones with the greatest potential for establishing the basis for a supervision tool in the electronic prescription of drugs, because they have the ability to detect most of the requisites applications, as evidenced in Table 3. What differentiates them is the surrounding reality, causing differences in language, and in the used classifications, influenced by the responsible entities in each country.

Since MedicineOne is developed in Portugal, it respects and uses the common name pharmacotherapeutic classifications and disease classifications recommended by INFARMED. The NDDF uses the common name pharmacotherapeutic classifications and classifications of diseases developed in the U.S., with exception of the classification of diseases ICD. The North American databases require adjustments in order to be applicable in Portugal.

5 CONCLUSION

The aim of this project is the reduction of adverse drug reactions, by issuing warnings at the time of the drug prescription by a physician. The determination of the most appropriate database(s) is dependent on several factors, such as language or the classifications recommended by the national health systems.

The MedicineOne uses the International Nonproprietary Name to identify the drugs' name. It uses the Anatomical Therapeutic Chemical Classification to identify the pharmacotherapeutic classification and recognizes the disease by the International Classification of Diseases, and others international classifications reference.

The National Drug Data File is original from the United States and uses the United States Adopted Name to identify the drugs' name. It uses the American Hospital Formulary Service and the Hierarchical Ingredient Code to identify the

243

pharmacotherapeutic classification and recognizes the disease by linkage with ICD-9th. This database requires adjustments in order to be applicable in Portugal.

The National Drug Data File and the MedicineOne are the drug interactions databases with the greatest potential, because they have the capability to identify all the different drug interactions related in this study, such as, drug-drug, drug-allergy, drug-food and drinks, drug-laboratory interference, drug-alternative therapy and contraindications. The detection of most types of drug interactions is only possible if you can access information stored in electronic health record.

Thus, according to those factors, the National Drug Data File and MedicineOne are the databases that have the most potential to develop prescription tools and to decrease the number of adverse drug reactions in Portugal.

REFERENCES

ABDATA Pharma-Daten-Service, 2005. ABDA-Datenbank—Drug Information Database. Available at: http://data.getafreelancer.com/project/76196/DB_Kurzinfo_englisch_0905.pdf [Acedido Janeiro 21, 2010].

Administração Central do Sistema de Saúde (ACSS), 2009. RSE–Registo de Saúde Electrónico–R1: Documento de Estado da Arte. Available at: http://www.portugal.gov.pt/pt/Documentos/Governo/MS/RSE_R1_Estado_da_Arte_V2_0.pdf [Acedido Abril 27, 2010].

American Society of Health-System Pharmacists, 2010. AHFS Pharmacologic-Therapeutic Classification System. Available at: http://www.ahfsdruginformation.com/class/index.aspx [Acedido Abril 23, 2010].

Aronson, J.K., 2000. Where name and image meet—the argument for "adrenaline". *BMJ: British Medical Journal*, 320(7233), 506–509.

Bousquet, C. et al., 2008. Semantic categories and relations for modelling adverse drug reactions towards a categorial structure for pharmacovigilance. *AMIA ... Annual Symposium Proceedings / AMIA Symposium. AMIA Symposium*, 61–65.

Cerner® Multum, 2009. VantageRx Database. Available at: http://www.multum.com/VantageRxDB.htm [Acedido Junho 16, 2010].

Colorado Department of Public Health and Enviroment, 2001. New International Classification of Diseases (ICD-10): The History and Impact. *Brief Health Statistics Section*, (41). Available at: http://www.cdphe.state.co.us/hs/briefs/icd10brief.pdf

DrugLogic, Inc, 2008. Qscan® from DrugLogic®: The Multi-Database Safety Platform for Risk Evaluation and Mitigation Strategies. Available at: http://www.druglogic.com/sites/default/files/105894_DrugLogic_Market.pdf [Acedido Junho 14, 2010].

First DataBank, Inc, 2010. NATIONAL DRUG DATA FILE (NDDF) PLUS. Available at: http://www.firstdatabank.com/Products/national-drug-data-file-NDDF.aspx [Acedido Junho 15, 2010].

Goodman Gilman, A. et al., eds., 1996. *Goodman & Gilman's The Pharmacological Basis of Therapeutics* Ninth., McGraw-Hill.

Kopp-Kubel, S., 1995. International Nonproprietary Names (INN) for pharmaceutical substances. *Bulletin of the World Health Organization*, 73(3), 275–279.

Lægemiddelstyrelsen, 2010. Lægemiddelstyrelsen–Interaktionsdatabasen.dk. Available at: http://www.interaktionsdatabasen.dk/Default.aspx [Acedido Junho 7, 2010].

Lazarou, J., Pomeranz, B.H. & Corey, P.N., 1998. Incidence of Adverse Drug Reactions in Hospitalized Patients: A Meta-analysis of Prospective Studies. *JAMA*, 279(15), 1200–1205.

MedDRA Maintenance and Support Services Organization, 2010. Regulatory Information. *MedDRA MSSO–Medical Dictionary for Regulatory Activities*. Available at: http://www.meddramsso.com/public_aboutMedDRA_regulatory.asp [Acedido Junho 25, 2010].

Spigset, O. & Rekda, M., 2010. DRUID–Drug information database–Legemiddelinformasjon for norske klinikere. Available at: http://www.interaksjoner.no/default.asp [Acedido Junho 7, 2010].

Tomé, A., Broeiro, P. & Faria-Vaz, A. 2008. Os sistemas de prescrição electrónica. *Rev Port Clin Geral*, 24(5), 632–640.

The Uppsala Monitoring Centre, 2010. Mapping tool to MedDRA. *Adverse Reaction Terminology WHO-ART*. Available at: http://www.umc-products.com/DynPage.aspx?id=73560&mn1=1107&mn2=1664&mn3=6045 [Acedido Maio 12, 2010].

U.S. National Library of Medicine, 2003. FAQs: Inclusion of SNOMED CT in the UMLS. Available at: http://www.nlm.nih.gov/research/umls/Snomed/snomed_faq.html [Acedido Abril 29, 2010].

WHO Collaborating Centre for Drug Statistics Methodology Norwegian Institute of Public Health, 2010. The Anatomical Therapeutic Chemical (ATC). Available at:http://www.whocc.no/atc/structure_and_principles/ [Acedido Abril 23, 2010].

Wishart, D.S. et al., 2008. DrugBank: a knowledgebase for drugs, drug actions and drug targets. *Nucleic Acids Research*, 36 (Database issue), D901-D906.

WONCA International Classification Commitee (WICC), 2010. The International Classification of Primary Care. Available at: http://www.globalfamilydoctor.com/wicc/icpcstory.html [Acedido Abril 29, 2010].

World Health Organization - Division of Drug Management Policies, 1997. Guidelines On The Use Of International Nonproprietary Names (INNs) For Pharmaceutical Substances. Available at: http://whqlibdoc.who.int/hq/1997/WHO_PHARM_S_NOM_1570.pdf [Acedido Abril 5, 2010].

Technology and Medical Sciences – Natal Jorge et al. (eds)
© *2011 Taylor & Francis Group, London, ISBN 978-0-415-66822-4*

Registration of bone ultrasound images to CT based 3D bone models

Paulo J.S. Gonçalves
Polytechnic Institute of Castelo Branco, Castelo Branco, Portugal
IDMEC / IST, Technical University of Lisbon, Lisboa, Portugal

Pedro M.B. Torres
Polytechnic Institute of Castelo Branco, Castelo Branco, Portugal

ABSTRACT: This paper presents a study on state-of-the-art algorithms to register ultrasound images (US) to 3D bone models. An experimental apparatus developed to evaluate the algorithms is also presented. This experimental apparatus was developed under the framework of a previously developed 3D medical visualization software and a robotic system to support orthopedic surgery. The study is based in a 3D bone model obtained from Computer Tomography (CT) images, in the pre-operative scenario. In the intra-operative scenario, the 2D US images of the bone are acquired and then registered to the 3D bone model. The experimental results obtained from a cow femur bone, real CT and US images were acquired, demonstrate the validity of the approaches and the comparative study.

1 INTRODUCTION

In orthopedic surgery, physicians and engineers pursuit the exact bone position and orientation during surgery. This is very important because the surgery outcome largely depends on precise bone machining, for example to place the implants or to perform resurfacing. Moreover, with the increasing deployment of robots in the operating room (Taylor and Stoianovici 2003, Casals et al. 2009), this point is even more critical.

Nowadays surgeons obtain the position and orientation of the bone using invasive approaches. This approaches place directly in the bone screws to attach metallic structures, in which are attached infrared emitters that allow a stereo system to obtain the relative position and orientation of the bone to the stereo system. Other approach, often used in the operating room, is by x-ray imaging that due to its biological effects to the patient and health professionals should be less used in the future. Using ultrasound images overcomes the two previous stated drawbacks, invasiveness and x-ray emission, used in the actual approaches. However the precision of the US imaging can be a drawback. This in the near future can be overcome due the increasing precision of US systems.

In this paper is performed a survey on state-of-the-art US to CT image registration, and used Open-Source software to obtain the 3D bone model, e.g. MeVisLab, Invesalius and MedInria.

The comparison between US to CT image registration, based on 3D data points obtained from the acquired images is performed in Matlab. The methods applied were the Iterative Closest Point and the Coherent Point Drift. The output of the compared methods is a transformation matrix, containing the rotation and translation, between the CT and US 3D points. The results were validated in an experimental setup to obtain images form a femur of a cow.

This paper is organized as follows. Section 2 describes briefly how the femur 3D bone model. Section 3 presents very briefly the state-of-the-art in US to 3D bone model registration, and also the Iterative Closest Point and the Coherent Power Drift algorithms. Section 4 describes the experimental setup and presents the obtained results, where the transformation matrix was obtained. Finally, Section 5 presents the conclusions and the future work.

2 3D BONE MODEL FROM CT IMAGES

Medical image processing comprises a set of techniques used to extract information for use by health professionals, for medical diagnostics. The medical imaging comprises a set of methods of data collection ranging from the best-known conventional radiology, ultrasound, Computed Tomography (CT), Magnetic Resonance Imaging (MRI), among others.

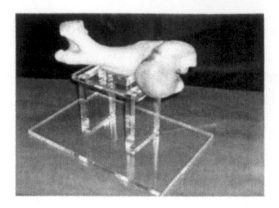

Figure 1. Cow femur bone.

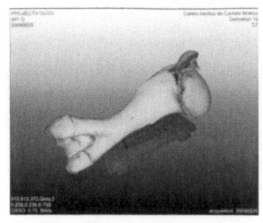

Figure 2. MeVisLab 3D bone model.

Traditionally, these images are presented in the form of two-dimensional images from devices that generate them using the international standard DICOM (Digital Image Communications in Medicine). Software platforms have been increasingly developed to handle these two-dimensional medical images and obtain a 3D model of the structure under analysis. The 3D reconstruction of anatomical structures has revolutionized medicine by allowing the viewing of more detailed anatomical human structures in a non-invasiveway.

In recent decades, there has been remarkable progress in reconstruction, both regarding quality and the speed of reconstruction. Nowadays, it is routine in operating rooms the use of medical images from computed tomography, magnetic resonance imaging or even ultrasound in pre-surgery. With this, medical doctors get a fairly accurate picture of the situation inside the human body before beginning surgery.

With the increasing processing power of computers, these, from the images captured get a three-dimensional representation of the anatomical (s) structure (s) of interest. Using software developed for this purpose, it is possible to analyze from different angles and depths three-dimensional images. In the following are presented three freeware programs used to obtain the 3D model of the femur bone of cow, depicted in Figure 1.

2.1 3D model reconstruction

The 3D bone model from the femur cow was obtained directly from the Open Source Software packages: MeVisLab, Invesalius, MedInria.

2.1.1 MeVisLab

(MeVisLab 2010), is a software consisting of several modules dedicated to processing and visualization of medical images. Has been developed by Mevis Research, GmbH, Germany, and use the

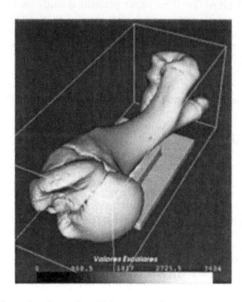

Figure 3. Invesalius 3D bone model.

libraries VTK—Visualization Toolkit (Schroeder et al. 2010) for the model. Figure 2 presentes the result of applying the software to the femur bone in the study.

2.1.2 Invesalius

(Martins et al. 2007), is a software consisting of several modules dedicated to processing and visualization of medical images. It is developed by the Center for Information Technology Renato Archer, Brazil, and use the libraries VTK—Visualization Toolkit (Schroeder et al. 2010). Figure 3 presents the result of applying the software to the femur bone under study.

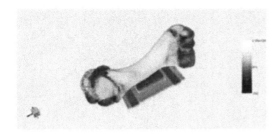

Figure 4. MedInria 3D bone model.

2.1.3 *MedInria*

(MedInria 2010), is a software consisting of several modules dedicated to processing and visualization of medical images. These were developed within a research group of INRIA, France and use the libraries VTK—Visualisation Toolkit (Schroeder et al. 2010). Figure 4 presents the result of applying the software to the femur bone under study.

Using the three programs, a valid 3D bone model is obtained. The three models are similar when comparing the Figures 2, 3, 4 because its base framework is the VTK library. For the three free software packages, the MedINRIA proved to be a little more sensitive to the threshold value for segmentation of bone in CT images, making the 3D model with more errors. The simplest program to use is the InVesalius.

3 US IMAGES TO 3D BONE MODEL REGISTRATION

Several methods have been developed in recent years to perform the registration of bone ultrasound images, obtained in the intra-operative scenario, to the 3D bone model, obtained from CT images.

The approaches presented by the research community are nowadays a active field of research, due to the need of a high precision system. In fact, the following approaches can perform US images to 3D bone model registration on several parts of the human body but still need to improve its overall accuracy. The approaches tackle the Spine (Brendel et al. 2002), the shoulder (Tyryshkin et al. 2007) and the nose (Descoteaux et al. 2006). None of them tackled the femur.

The method proposed by (Brendel et al. 2002) estimates the translation and rotation parameters between images and is based in the mean value of the pixel grey values. The nearest neighbor, k-NN, approach estimates the location of the correspondent grey area between images. Finally the Levenberg-Marquart optimization method is used to estimate the rotation and translation parameters.

The sum of the pixel bright grey values of the US image, i.e. the surface of the bone, are used by (Brendel et al. 2008) to calculate the correspondences between images.

(Beek et al. 2008) uses 3D points, obtained from an 3D US machine and from the classical TC, to apply the Iterative Closest Point (ICP) algorithm (Besl and McKay 1992), to obtain the translation and rotation parameters of the transformation. The mutual information approach is used by (Chen and Abolmaesumi 2005) to register intraoperative US images to preoperative US images. The preoperative images are also used to construct the 3D volume of the bone. When the 2D intraoperative US image is registered to the preoperative US image, the 3D position od the bone in the operating room can be easily known.

The above presented methods, apart from digital image processing to obtain the bone contours, all rely on the registration of the 3D contour points obtained from US to the ones obtained from CT images (preoperative 3D bone model). The most commonly method used is the ICP. Recently (Myronenko and Song 2010) have proposed a new method, that relies on a probabilistic framework to perform the registration.

3.1 *Iterative Closest Point method*

The Iterative Closest Point (ICP) method is the standard method used to perform registration between two set of 3D points. It transforms two sets of points to a common coordinate frame. If the exact correspondences of the two data set could be known, then the exact translation t and rotation R can be found. The main issue of the method is then to find the corresponding points between the two data sets, $Y = (y_1, ..., y_M)^T$ and $X = (x_1, ..., x_M)^T$.

The assumption in the ICP method is that the closest points between the data sets correspond to each other, and are used to compute the best transformation, rotation and translation, between them. The original method have been extended to line segment sets, implicit curves, parametric curves, triangle sets, implicit surface and parametric surfaces. In this paper point sets are considered for comparison to the CPD method.

To obtain the closest point of Y to a point in X, the Euclidean distance is applied. When all points of the data set Y are associated to the point in X the transformation is estimated by minimizing a mean square cost function:

$$E_{ICP} = \sum_i \| R \cdot x_i + t - y_i \|^2 \qquad (1)$$

From the obtained parameters, the points in the X data set are transformed and the error between them and the ones in Y calculated. If the error is above a pre-defined threshold then the points must be re-associated and the previous steps again performed until the error is below the threshold.

3.2 Coherent Point Drift method

Coherent Point Drift (CPD) is a probabilistic method for point set registration, described in (Myronenko and Song 2010). Given two n-dimensional point sets and fit a GMM (Gaussian Mixture Models) to the first point set, whose Gaussian centroids are initialized from the points in the second set.

The second point set is expressed as $Y = (y_1, ..., y_M)^T$ and should be aligned with the reference point set $X = (x_1, ..., x_N)^T$. Points in Y are considered the centroids of the GMM, and fit it to the data points X by maximizing the likelihood function. Y_0 has the initial centroid positions and define a continuous velocity function υ for the template point set such that the current position of centroids is defined as

$$Y = \upsilon(Y_0) + Y_0 \tag{2}$$

Bayes theorem is used to find the parameters Y by maximizing the posteriori probability, or minimizing the energy function:

$$E_{CPD}(Y) = -\sum_{n=1}^{N} log \sum_{m=1}^{M} e^{-\frac{1}{2}\left\|\frac{x_n - y_m}{\sigma}\right\|^2} + \frac{\lambda}{2}\phi(Y) \tag{3}$$

where $\phi(Y)$ is a function that is related to the smoothness of the motion.

4 EXPERIMENTAL RESULTS

4.1 Experimental setup

For obtaining the CT images, a Siemens commercial machine (special thanks to Centro Médico de Castelo Branco) was used with 0.75 [mm] between slices. The ultrasound images were acquired through the experimental apparatus shown in Figure 5, which consists of a tub with water (to place the femur of cow and its support), a echograph Sonoline Siemens Versa Pro, a PC equipped with a standard video capture (not shown Figure 5) and a stereo vision system (Morgado et al. 2009) to determine the 3D coordinates of the markers in the ultrasound probe, depicted in Figure 6. The pixel value of the US image is $[1.5120 \times 1.7166]$ (mm).

An ultrasound image representative of all those obtained from the femur of the cow is shown in Figure 7. The probe of 3.5 MHz was placed on

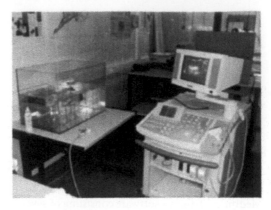

Figure 5. Ultrasound acquisition system.

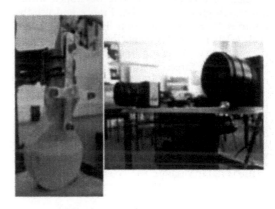

Figure 6. Ultrasound probe with markers (left). Stereo Vision System (right).

the water surface. The image corresponds to the central section of the bone, where can be observed the upper surface of the bone, with brighter gray levels and the absence of other bone surfaces, since all the ultrasound is reflected by the upper surface.

4.2 Registration results

In this section are presented the registration results obtained using the experimental setup developed for this work, and also using the ICP and CPD algorithms. This algorithms allow the registration of the 3D data points obtained from US images to the 3D bone model obtained from the CT images. The 3D data points are depicted in Figure 8, where are presented the femur contour points from ten slices of CT images in red. In blue are presented femur contour points from the slice obtained from the US image. The US slice was acquired to correspond to the 5th slice of the CT, from bottom to top. The first slice of CT was

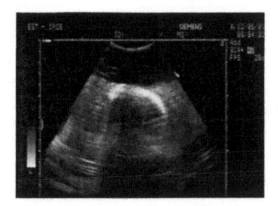

Figure 7. Ultrasound image of the femur.

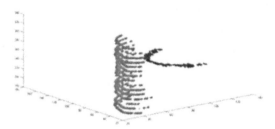

Figure 8. 3D data points. 10 slices of CT data points (red) and 1 slice of US data points (blue).

acquired 183 [mm] from the right extreme od the femur, see Figure 1.

$$RMSE = \sqrt{\frac{1}{n}\sum(\hat{y}_i - y_i)^2} \qquad (4)$$

From the US image of the femur bone, depicted in Figure 7, the root mean square errors, RMSE, (4) were obtained using the ICP and CPD algorithms. The errors obtained are presented in Table 1. The ICP algorithm obtained the best result of the two methods. To further investigate this difference the registered 3D points must be presented.

In Figure 9 and in Figure 10 are presented the results obtained from the ICP and CPD algorithms respectively. It can be observed that the CPD algorithm fails to match to the 5th slice. This fact helps to explain the error obtained. The ICP error is due to several factors, first is the speckle present in US images, second is the error of the stereo visual system $(2 \times 2 \times 2)$ [mm²].

The final transformation matrix, containing the rotation and translation, between the CT and US 3D points obtained with the ICP algorithm, follows.

Table 1. Registration errors.

Method	RMSE [mm]
ICP—Iterative Closest Point	14.3218
CPD—Coherent Point Drift	22.4808

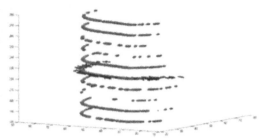

Figure 9. ICP algorithm. 10 slices of CT data points (red) and 1 slice of registered US data points (blue).

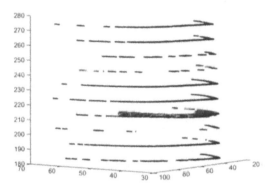

Figure 10. CPD algorithm. 10 slices of CT data points (red) and 1 slice of registered US data points (blue).

$$^{CT}T_{US} = \begin{pmatrix} 0.2642 & 0.2642 & -6.7980 & 45.1166 \\ 0.2183 & 0.4038 & 6.8311 & 0.3790 \\ 0.0001 & 0.0002 & 0.1452 & 103.1364 \\ 0 & 0 & 0 & 1 \end{pmatrix}$$

5 CONCLUSIONS

This paper presents a study on the registration of femur bone US images to its 3D model, obtained from CT images. The US image obtained in the intraoperative scenario is then registered to the preoperative scenario. The methods presented by the research community need to register the 3D data obtained from the US image to the 3D bone model. The ICP method is the must used in common practice, but recently the CPD method have been proposed. This work compares the two algorithms for the femur application.

To perform the comparison, an experimental setup was developed and dozens of tests were performed. The results obtained validate both approaches for the femur application and showed that the ICP method performs better.

To obtain more accurate results, the stereo vision system must be replaced by the well known Polaris Spectra state-of-the-art system. The bone contours should be better described in order to speed up the system and reduce the errors. Further research will also be focused in the application of this US based registration approaches to robotic assisted surgery.

ACKNOWLEDGEMENTS

The authors would like to thank: the Centro Médico de Castelo Branco; the Portuguese Science Foundation, FCT, for the funding to IDMEC through the Associated Laboratory in Energy, Transports, Aeronautics and Space (LAETA); the FCT project: PTDC/EME-CRO/099333/2008.

REFERENCES

Brendel, B., Winter, S., Rick, A., Stockheim, M. & Ermert, H. (2002). Registration of 3d ct and ultrasound datasets of the spine using bone structures. *Computer Aided Surgery 7(3)*, 146–155.

Brendel, B., Winter, S., Pechlivanis, I., Schmieder, K. & I.C. (2008). Registration of ct and intraoperative 3-d ultrasound images of the spine using evolutionary and gradient-based methods. *IEEE Transactions on Evolutionary Computation 12(3)*, 284–296.

Beek, M., Abolmaesumi, P., Luenam, S., Ellis, R., Sellens, R. & Pichora, D. (2008). Validation of a new surgical procedure for percutaneous scaphoid fixation using intra-operative ultrasound. *Medical Image Analysis 12(2)*, 152–162.

Besl, P.J. & McKay, N.D. (1992). A method for registration of 3-d shapes. *IEEE Transactions on Pattern Analysis and Machine Intelligence 14(2)*, 239–250.

Casals, A., Frigola, M. & Amat, J. (2009). La robtica una valiosa herramienta cirugia. *Revista Iberoamericana de de Automtica e Informtica Industrial 6(1)*, 5–19.

Chen, T. & Abolmaesumi, P. (2005). A mutual information based registration algorithm for ultrasound-guided computer-assisted orthopaedic surgery. *Medical Imaging 2005: Visualization, Image-Guided Procedures 5744*, 111–122.

Descoteaux, M., Audette, M., Chinzei, K. & Siddiqi, K. (2006). Bone enhancement filtering: application to sinus bone segmentation and simulation of pituitary surgery. *Computer aided surgery: official journal of the International Society for Computer Aided Surgery 11*, 247–255.

Martins, T.A.C.P., Barbara, A.S., Silva, G.B.C., Faria, T.V., Cassaro, B. & Silva, J.V.L. (2007). Invesalius: Three-dimensional medical reconstruction software. In *3rd International Conference on Advanced Research in Virtual and Rapid Prototyping, Leiria—Portugal. Virtual and Rapid Manufacturing, Taylor and Francis*, pp. 135–142.

MedInria (consulted in 15/07/2010). http://www.sop.inria.fr/asclepios/software/medinria/

MeVisLab (consulted in 15/07/2010). http://www.mevislab.de

Morgado, P., Caldas Pinto, J., Martins, J.M.M. & Gonçalves, P. (2009). Cooperative eye-in-hand/stereo eye-to-hand visual servoing. In *Proc. of RecPad 2009—15th Portuguese Conference in Pattern Recognition*, Aveiro, Portugal.

Myronenko, A. & Song, X. (2010). Point set registration: Coherent point drift. *IEEE Transactions on Pattern Analysis and Machine Intelligence 99* (PrePrints).

Schroeder, W.J., Geveci, B. & Malaterre, M. (consulted in 15/07/2010). Compatible triangulations of spatial decompositions. *http://www.vtk.org/VTK/img/Ordered Triangulator.pdf*

Taylor, R. & Stoianovici, D. (2003). Medical robotics in computer-integrated surgery. *IEEE Transactions on Robotics and Automation 19(5)*, 765–781.

Tyryshkin, K., Mousavi, P., Beek, M., Ellis, R., Pichora, D. & Abolmaesumi, P. (2007). A navigation system for shoulder arthroscopic surgery. *Proceedings of the Institut of Mechanical Engineers. Part H, Journal of engineering in medicine 221 (7)*, 801–812.

Technology and Medical Sciences – Natal Jorge et al. (eds)
© *2011 Taylor & Francis Group, London, ISBN 978-0-415-66822-4*

Segmentation and 3D reconstruction of the vocal tract from MR images—A comparative study

S.R. Ventura
School of Allied Health Science—Porto Polytechnic Institute, V.N. Gaia, Portugal

D.R. Freitas
Faculty of Engineering, University of Porto, Porto, Portugal

I.M. Ramos
Faculty of Medicine, University of Porto, São João Hospital Porto, Porto, Portugal

João Manuel R.S. Tavares
Faculty of Engineering, Institute of Mechanical Engineering and Industrial Management,
University of Porto, Porto, Portugal

ABSTRACT: Speech production is an important human function involving a set of organs with specific morphological and dynamic aspects. The inter-speaker variability, the coarticulation or the nasality are some interesting aspects to improve a realistic 3D modeling of the vocal tract. For this, the understanding of the mechanism of speech production is crucial, as the current image data is not sufficient to reproduce truthfully the speaker's anatomy and articulation. Hence, the goal of 3D modeling is to generate the complete geometrical and dynamical information concerning the vocal tract from medical images, such as from Magnetic Resonance Imaging (MRI). This work aims to describe and compare two different segmentation techniques to attain the 3D shape of the vocal tract during speech production from MR images: the former based on manual tracing of the vocal tract contours and the latter based on image thresholding. Thus, the segmented cross-sectional areas were measured, and 3D models were built from the sagittal data by blending the contours obtained from the two segmentation techniques. The mean error of the measures computed were low for both segmentation techniques, which let us conclude that the techniques are useful to evaluate the vocal tract geometry accurately. Additionally, the 3D models built using both segmentation techniques were also very similar and truthful. However, when the coronal data was used, various difficulties occurred.

1 INTRODUCTION

Magnetic Resonance Imaging (MRI) is a promising technique in all clinical research fields; the multiplanar imaging acquisition, high soft-tissue resolution and safety of MRI are some of the most important advantages for its use (Shadle et al. 1999; Narayanan et al. 2004). Vocal tract morphology is one of the main aspects to be considered during speech articulation that confers potential inter-speaker differences (Fuchs, Winkler, and Perrier 2008).

Until now, the knowledge concerning the morphology and articulation measurements of the vocal tract, based on MRI, is not sufficient to reproduce accurately the speaker's anatomy (Birkholz and Kroger 2006). However, this knowledge is demanded by different areas, such as bioengineering, medicine or speech therapy (Ventura, Freitas, and Tavares 2009).

Three-dimensional (3D) imaging based on magnetic resonance is essential to acquire the full geometry of the vocal tract, and thus to provide better knowledge concerning vocal tract shape and to obtain more data its realistic 3D modeling (Bresch et al. 2008; Apostol et al. 1999; Badin and Serrurier 2006; Kim, Narayanan and Nayak 2009).

In order to study the vocal tract from MRI data, the acquired images must be processed considering the following main steps: image segmentation and 3D shape reconstruction. The former is the most important and difficult; mainly, because there are common problems related with the determination of the air-tissue boundaries, as previously reported by (Demolin, Metens and Soquet 1996) and (Soquet et al. 1998), and is decisive to obtain suitable 3D models in the second step. For example, to achieve the completion of these tasks, (Serrurier and Badin 2005; Badin et al. 1998) extracted the vocal tract shape manually and the 3D mesh reconstruction was realized by intersecting these contours along a semipolar grid. However, manual edition, besides of being very arduous and time consuming, is extremely user-dependent (increasing the uncertainty of results). On the other hand, (Behrends and Wismuller 2001) introduced a simple algorithm based on 3D region growing; and (Narayanan et al. 2004) focuses on methods to automatically segment and track the real-time MRI data using Kalman snakes and optical flow.

Despite the level of automation in performing the image processing tasks, the analysis of vocal tract from images remains complex, given the various problems that persist. Some of these problems are related with the MR image acquisition technique and with the morphology of the vocal tract (i.e. the non-identification of teeth and the similarity of signal intensity between the vocal tract and of some of the surrounding structures).

According to (Soquet et al. 1998), that presents a comparative study to assess the accuracy of three different segmentation techniques, the image thresholding method revealed an inferior dispersion, but the overall results presented small average error and large error distribution.

In this work, we describe and compare two different segmentation techniques to extract the contours to be used in 3D reconstruction of the vocal tract during speech production from MR images: one based on the manual tracing of the segmentation contours, and another based on image threshold.

The remaining of this paper is organized as follows. In the next section, the description of the MRI protocol, the speech corpus and the image analysis and assessment are described. Then, in section three, the area measurements obtained by using the two segmentation techniques under comparison are presented and discussed, and the 3D models built for the vocal tract are shown and examined. Finally, the conclusions are pointed out in the last section.

2 METHODS

According to the usual regulated safety procedures for MRI, the subject was previously informed about the undergoing imaging exam and subsequently instructed about the procedures to be adopted, whereupon the subject signed a consent form.

2.1 MRI protocol and speech corpus

This study was performed using a 1.5T Siemens Magneton Symphony system and a head array coil, involving one healthy young male, with speech

therapy skills. Using a fast image acquisition mode, we collected an overall of seven slices in two different image orientations, considering the following acquisition parameters: field of view 150 mm, image matrix 128 × 128 and image resolution 0.853 px/mm.

The subject sustained the articulation during 9 s for the acquisition of three sagittal slices (slice thickness of 5 mm) and 9.9 s for the four coronal slices (slice thickness of 6 mm and with 10 mm of gap between slices) for each speech sound. The acquisition time was defined adopting a compromise between image resolution and the duration of the sustained articulation allowed by the subject.

The speech corpus consisted in four European Portuguese sounds: the vowels [i] and [u] and the lateral consonants.

Due to the MR acoustic noise produced during the acquisition process, the speech recording had not enough quality, and therefore, it was discarded.

2.2 Image analysis and assessment

The analysis of the 2D images was performed using ImageJ–Image Processing and Analysis in Java (from NIH, USA–http://rsb.info.nih.gov/ij/). Subsequently, the 3D models of the vocal tract were built using Blender (from Blender Foundation, Amsterdam, The Netherlands-http://www.blender. org/cms/Home.2.0.html).

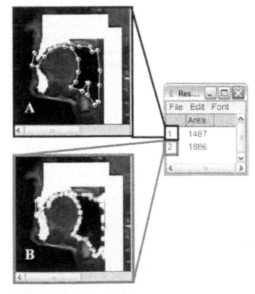

Figure 1. Measurement of the cross-sectional areas of the vocal tract obtained using manual tracing of the segmentation contours (A) and manual imaging threshold (B).

The vocal tract region was extracted from each image slice using two segmentation techniques:

1. Manual tracing of the segmentation contours-based on Bézier curves;
2. Manual imaging threshold.

The contour segmentation process resulted in a total of 28 2D contours, i.e. seven contours for each sound. Then, the resultant contours from all cross-sectional images were measured, Figure 1.

The contours obtained by the two segmentation techniques were then used to build the 3D skin models, after importing the contours in *.shapes* format, into the *Blender* software.

3 RESULTS AND DISCUSSION

3.1 *Cross-sectional area measurements*

The measurements on the cross-sectional areas, attained using manual tracing of the segmentation contours and manual imaging threshold in each image slice (Si), are indicated in Tables 1–3.

The manual tracing segmentation was taken as reference, mainly because the user can take into account its knowledge about the vocal tract anatomy in an easier way.

Tables 1 and 2 indicate the areas measured using the segmentation techniques based on manual tracing and imaging threshold, respectively. The sagittal slice 2 was situated at the midsagittal anatomic plane (a plane passing vertically through the

Table 1. Measurements (mm^2) on the cross-sectional areas obtained by manual tracing of the segmentation contours.

Speech corpus	Sagittal			Coronal			
	S1	S2	S3	S1	S2	S3	S4
[i]	1487	1540	1568	185	53	43	856
[u]	1686	1826	1911	379	973	134	43
[L]	1358	1650	1662	368	678	186	83
[lh]	1603	1812	1811	337	368	100	1294

Table 2. Measurements (mm^2) on the cross-sectional areas obtained by manual imaging threshold.

Speech corpus	Sagittal			Coronal			
	S1	S2	S3	S1	S2	S3	S4
[i]	1886	2022	1649	370	84	99	733
[u]	1480	1748	1906	404	969	114	57
[L]	1202	1612	1651	520	738	121	161
[lh]	1343	1577	1694	424	236	196	1395

Table 3. Mean cross-sectional areas and relative errors of the measurements (mm^2).

Speech corpus	Average sagittal area		Average coronal area	
	Relative error	SD	Relative error	SD
[i]	0.2094	147.63	0.1310	82.429
[u]	0.0533	101.74	0.0098	1.3066
[L]	0.0439	76.582	0.1711	34.969
[lh]	0.1171	58.342	0.0724	37.050

SD—Standard Deviation.

midline, dividing the body into left and right parts). The slice 1 and 3 were situated at right and left from slice 2, respectively.

The coronal (or frontal) plane was a vertical section that divides the body into anterior and posterior; sections 1, 2, 3 and 4 were situated in the oral cavity, from front to back, showing areas for the lips (S1), tongue apex (S2), tongue body (S3) and oropharynx (S4). The unrounded vowel [i] area at the lips plane (S1) is inferior to the area of rounded vowel [u] for both segmentation techniques. Similarly, these two vowels have different areas in slice 4: front vowel [i] area is superior to the back vowel [u] area.

In lateral consonants, an occlusion was observed some where along the tongue, while air was escaping at one or both sides of the tongue. As it can be realized from Tables 1 and 2, the coronal sections 2 and 3 of the palatal lateral approximant [lh] are inferior than slice areas 1 and 4 for both segmentation techniques. The consonant [L] is pronounced by the tongue's approximation to the velar region, as a result, the sections 3 and 4 areas are inferior when compared with sections 1 and 2 areas.

The average areas and standard deviation of the measurement errors between the two segmentation techniques under comparison are depicted in Table 3.

For both segmentation techniques, the results indicate in Table 3 allow to conclude that the mean error is relatively small and the distribution of the errors is highly dispersed.

3.2 *3D vocal tract models*

From the contours extracted it is possible to reconstruct the 3D vocal tract shape. Figure 2 depicts the 3D vocal tract models built from the cross-sectional sagittal data segmented by the two segmentation techniques.

The 3D vocal tract meshes created using the two segmentation techniques are very similar; i.e. the articulatory organs shape and position for these two vowels are identical. However, the non-rigid geometry of the vocal tract model generated

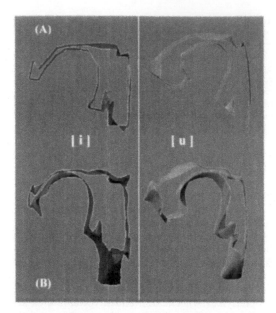

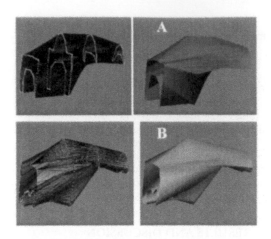

Figure 4. 3D vocal tract models built for consonant [L] from manual tracing of the segmentation contours (A) and manual imaging threshold (B).

Figure 2. 3D vocal tract models built for vowels [i] and [u] from manual tracing of the segmentation contours (A) and manual imaging threshold (B).

The coronal data is particularly important to realize the lateral dimension of the oral cavity and the tongue's position. The 3D vocal tract models generated by the interpolation of cross-sectional contours of lateral consonants are shown in Figures 3 and 4.

Contrasting with the 3D models built from sagittal data, the vocal tract shapes built applying the two segmentation techniques (Figures 3 and 4) on the coronal data are reasonably different. Despite the more likely anatomic shape provided by 3D models built from the segmentations done by manual imaging threshold, the lateral dimensions of the vocal tract are overestimated, probably because the non-identification of the teeth and the similarity of signal intensity between the vocal tract and of some of the surrounding structures (e.g. nasal cavity). Consequently, the 3D model of the vocal tract built from coronal data must be carefully analyzed in order to avoid inaccurate measures.

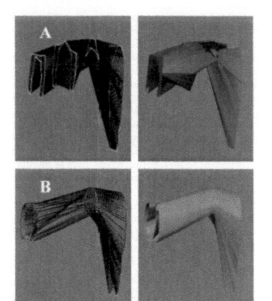

Figure 3. 3D vocal tract models built for consonant [lh] from manual tracing of the segmentation contours (A) and manual imaging threshold (B).

using the segmentation technique based on manual imaging threshold provides a more likely anatomic shape.

4 CONCLUSIONS

In this work, we compared the measurements attained on cross-sectional areas obtained by two different image segmentation techniques, one based on manual contours tracing and another one based on imaging thresholding, in MR images acquired during speech production. Additionally, 3D models were built by blending the segmented contours.

For both segmentation techniques under comparison, the measurement of the segmented cross-sectional regions allowed to attain accurate data concerning the vocal tract geometry during speech production. In fact, low mean errors and errors in a very dispersed manner were verified.

The success of the 3D modelling is conditioned by the segmentation technique used. By one hand, the technique based on the manual tracing of the segmentation contours gives results more accurate, while in the other hand, is more dependent on the user's skill and is more time consuming. The inferior dependency in the user's skill and the higher level of automation are advantages of the segmentation technique based on imaging threshold, but the vocal tract geometry reconstructed from this technique must be carefully analyzed as it can be inaccurate, particularly when applied on coronal data.

MRI data interpretation is difficult and some problems remain to be solved in order to obtainmore realistic and accurate 3D models, as the correct identification of the teeth and of the vocal tract limits. On the other hand, the low number of MR slices that are always acquired has a negative impact in the resultant 3D models.

ACKNOWLEDGMENTS

The images considered in this work were acquired at the Radiology Department of the S. João Hospital, in Portugal, and we would like to express to our gratitude to the technical staff.

The first author would like to thank the support and contribution of the PhD grant from IPP—Instituto Politécnico do Porto and ESTSP—Escola Superior de Tecnologia da Saúde, in Portugal.

REFERENCES

Apostol, Lian, Pascal Perrier, Monica Raybaudi and Christoph Segebarth. 1999. "3D Geometry of the Vocal Tract and Inter-speaker Variability. "pp. 443–446 in *14th International Congress of Phonetic Sciences (ICPhS 99)*. San Francisco, USA.

Badin, P., Bailly, G., Raybaudi, M. and Segebarth, C. 1998. "A Three-dimensional Linear Articulatry Model Based on MRI Data. "pp. 417–420 in *5th International Conference on Spoken Language Processing*, Eds Mannell, R.H. & Robert-Ribes, J. Sydney, Australia.

Badin, Pierre, and Antoine Serrurier. 2006. "Three-dimensional modeling of speech organs: Articulatory data and models." *Transactions on Technical Committee of Psychological and Physiological Acoustics* 36:421–426.

Behrends, Johannes and Axel Wismuller. 2001. "A Segmentation and Analysis Method for MRI Data of the Human Vocal Tract." *Forschungsberichte des Instituts fur Phonetik und Sprachliche Kommunikation der Universitat Phonetik und at Munchen (FIPKM)* 37:179–189.

Birkholz, Peter and Bernd J Kroger. 2006. "Vocal Tract Model Adaptation Using Magnetic Resonance Imaging." pp. 493–500 in *7th International Seminar on Speech Production*. Ubatuba, Sao Paolo, Brazil.

Bresch, Erik, Yoon-chul Kim, Krishna Nayak, Dani Byrd and Shrikanth Narayanan. 2008. "Seeing Speech: Capturing Vocal Tract Shaping and Real-time Magnetic Resonance Imaging." *IEEE Signal Processing Magazine* 123–129.

Demolin, D., Metens, T. and Soquet, A. 1996. "Three-dimensional measurement of the vocal tract by MRI." pp. 272–275 in *4th Internat. Conf. on Spoken Language Processing (ICSLP 96)*, Vol. 1p. Philadelphia, USA.

Fuchs, Susanne, Ralf Winkler and Pascal Perrier. 2008. "Do Speakers' Vocal Tract Geometries Shape their Articulatory Vowel Space?." pp. 333–336 in *8th International Seminar on Speech Production (ISSP)*. Strasbourg, France http://halshs.archives-ouvertes.fr/hal-00370715/.

Kim, Yoon-chul, Shrikanth S Narayanan and Krishna S Nayak. 2009. "Accelerated Three-Dimensional Upper Airway MRI Using Compressed Sensing." *Magnetic Resonance in Medicine* 61:1434–1440.

Narayanan, S., Nayak, K., Lee, S., Sethy, A. and Byrd, D. 2004. "An Approach to Real-time Magnetic Resonance Imaging for Speech Production." *Journal Acoustical Society of America* 115:1771–1776.

Serrurier, A. and Badin, P. 2005. "Towards a 3D articulatory model of the velum based on MRI and CT images." *ZAS Papers Linguistics* 40:195–211.

Shadle, C.H., Mohammad, M., Carter, J.N. and Jackson, P.J.B. 1999. "Multi-planar Dynamic Magnetic Resonance Imaging: New Tools for Speech Research." pp. 623–626 in *International Congress of Phonetics Sciences (ICPhS99)*. San Francisco.

Soquet, A., Lecuit, V., Metens, T., Nazarian, B. and Demolin, D. 1998. "Segmentation of the Airway from the Surrounding Tissues on Magnetic Resonance Images: A Comparative Study." pp. 3083–3086 in *5th International Conference on Spoken Language Processing (ICSLP 98)*. Sydney, Australia.

Ventura, Sandra Rua, Diamantino Freitas and João Manuel R S Tavares. 2009. "Application of MRI and biomedical engineering in speech production study Application of MRI and biomedical engineering in speech production study." *Computer Methods in Biomechanics and Biomedical Engineering* 12:671–681.

Technology and Medical Sciences – Natal Jorge et al. (eds)
© 2011 Taylor & Francis Group, London, ISBN 978-0-415-66822-4

Significance of fast and simple determination of catecholamines and their metabolites in patients with Down syndrome

L.I.B. Silva, M.E. Pereira & A.C. Duarte
CESAM & Department of Chemistry, University of Aveiro, Campus Universitário de Santiago, Aveiro, Portugal

A.M. Gomes & M.M. Pintado
Escola Superior de Biotecnologia, Catholic University, Porto, Portugal

H. Pinheiro & D. Moura
Faculty of Medicine, University of Porto, Porto, Portugal

A.C. Freitas
ISEIT/Viseu—Instituto Piaget, Galifonge, Lordosa, Viseu, Portugal

T.A.P. Rocha-Santos
CESAM & Department of Chemistry, University of Aveiro, Campus Universitário de Santiago, Aveiro, Portugal
ISEIT/Viseu—Instituto Piaget, Galifonge, Lordosa, Viseu, Portugal

ABSTRACT: The excretion of catecholamines and their precursor and the major dopamine metabolite in urine was studied in 3 to 18 year old Down Syndrome (DS) subjects. Adrenaline and noradrenaline concentrations were used as indicators of physiological stress and dopamine, L-3,4-dihydroxyphenylalanine (L-DOPA), and 3,4-dihydroxyphenylacetic acid (DOPAC) concentrations were used as indicators of the contribution of the dopaminergic system to the kidney function. An optical fiber biosensor was used with a view to assess the significance of such of fast and simple determination of catecholamines and their precursor and metabolite in DS patients.

1 INTRODUCTION

Down Syndrome (DS) or trisomy 21 is associated with physical and physiological perturbation which includes thyroid dysfunction, cardiovascular disorders, obesity, musculoskeletal disorders and autonomic nervous system dysfunction (Battarai et al., 2008, Barnhart & Connolly 2007). Down syndrome has also been found to be associated with improper regulation of catecholamine neurotransmitters. Catecholamines are biogenic amines and act either as neurotransmitters or hormones (Kumar et al., 2003, Ferry & Lecch 2005, Lisdat et al., 2007). They play an important role in the control and regulation of a number of brain functions and are implicated in several physiological conditions such as stress, sleep, vigilance, kidney function, food intake, temperature regulation, memory and learning (Whiting 2009). This work aims at the use of an optical fiber biosensor as a fast and simple methodology for analysis of adrenaline, noradrenaline, dopamine, L-3,4-dihydroxyphenylalanine (L-DOPA), and 3,4-dihydroxyphenylacetic acid (DOPAC) on urine from subjects with Down syndrome.

2 EXPERIMENTAL

2.1 Samples

Urine samples from patients with Down syndrom and healthy controls (age 3–18 years old) were collected for 24 h in plastic containers with 6 mol/L HCl to prevent spontaneous catecholamine oxidation and kept frozen until assay. Aliquots of 0.5 mL of acidified urine were placed in 5 mL conical vials with 50 mg alumina and adjusted to pH 8.6 by the addition of Tris buffer. The adsorbed catecholamines were then eluted from the alumina with 200 µL of 0.2 mol/L perchloric acid on Millipore microfilters (MFI). After preparation, the urine aliquots were analyzed by both Optical Fiber biosensor.

2.2 Analysis by optical fiber biosensor

This fast and simple methodology is basically constituted by two major components a) chromatographic column for separation of catecholamines and metabolites; b) optical fiber coated with laccase for detection. The experimental apparatus was described elsewhere by Silva *et al.*, (2010) andwas improved from a biosensor and a detector for developed for screening catecholamine and also described elsewhere by Silva *et al.*, (2009) and Ferreira *et al.*, (2009).

The standard mixtures of catecholamines (adrenaline (AD), Noradrenaline (NA), Dopamine (DA) and their precursor (L-DOPA) and the major dopamine metabolite (DOPAC)) or samples were injected with a micro-syringe (Hamilton) at the injection cell and carried by a constant flow (0.8 mL/min) of mobile phase (0.1 M sodium acetate, 0.5 M sodium octylsulphate and 8–10% methanol (v/v), pH 3.7) to the chromatographic column. The analytes after being separated in the chromatographic column reached the optical fiber coated with laccase (detection component) generating and analytical signal.

The principle of detection is based on changes in the refractive index of the optical fiber coating (laccase), due to the linkage of the catecholamines or its metabolites to laccase which results on a quinone. These changes in the refractive index are independent of the generated quinone and leads to changes in the reflected optical power, measured as the analytical signal. The optical power (analytical signal) returns to its initial value after the catecholamine or metabolite oxidation. The linkage of the catecholamine or its metabolite to the enzyme is the most relevant factor for the analytical signal generation, and the highest analytical signal and sensitivity obtained for dopamine when compared to the other catecholamine under study could be attributed to the high affinity of the enzyme to this catecholamine, with consequent increase of the optical power change amplitude.

3 RESULTS AND DISCUSSION

Figure 1 shows the decrease in optical power obtained with the optical fiber biosensor for a standard mixture of L-DOPA (53 pmol/mL), noradrenaline (62 pmol/mL), adrenaline (57 pmol/mL), DOPAC (53 pmol/mL), and dopamine (69 pmol/mL).

The chromatogram displayed in Figure 1 showed a good separation of the five analytes in retention times of 0.85, 1.5, 1.7, 2.2, and 2.6 min for L-DOPA, noradrenaline, adrenaline, DOPAC and dopamine, respectively, of a total analytical time of around 3 min. The detection limits based on three times the residual standard deviation (Miller & Miller 2005) were 4.10, 5.30, 5.50, 4.20 and 3.70 pmol/L for dopamine, noradrenaline, adrenaline, L-DOPA and DOPAC, respectively.

The performance of the optical fiber biosensor was previously evaluated by comparison with

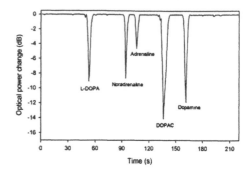

Figure 1. Chromatogram obtained with the optical fiber biosensor (analytical signals obtained for a standard mixture solution of L-DOPA (53 pmol/mL), noradrenaline (62 pmol/mL), adrenaline (57 pmol/mL), DOPAC (53 pmol/mL), and dopamine (69 pmol/mL).

HPLC-ED method of different amounts of the three catecholamines and two metabolites (Silva *et al.*, 2010).

The results obtained for the analysis of catecholamines and their metabolites (Tables 1–2) showed that: a) DA concentration in urine was above the pathological (2618 pmol/L) and normal (1280 pmol/L) levels (Pussard *et al.*, 2009) in 4 and 9 (out of 40) patients, respectively; b) adrenaline concentration was above pathological levels (262 pmol/L) and normal levels (71 pmol/L) in 9 and 15 patients, respectively; c) noradrenaline concentration was almost below the normal levels (390 pmol/L); and d) L-DOPA concentrations ranged between <4.20 and 6000 pmol/L while DOPAC ranged between <3.70 and 30000 pmol/L; e) the urinary concentration ratio DA/L-DOPA was 7.8 ± 1.2 (mean ± SEM, n = 34) and the ratio DOPAC/DA was 4.1 ± 1.7 (n = 33).

As the human adrenal medulla content of adrenaline is 3-fold higher than that of noradrenaline, increased secretion in response to stress follows the same pattern in blood and urine. Thus adrenaline is preferentially increased during response to stress. These results suggest that patients with DS may have a general increase on the level of stress. DA urinary concentrations as well as the urinary concentration ratios DA/L-DOPA and DOPAC/DA were high. As healthy tubular cells decarboxylate large amounts of L-DOPA to form dopamine and deaminate large amounts of DA to form DOPAC, those values indicate that the contribution of the dopaminergic system to the kidney function in our subjects is intact (Pestana *et al.*, 1997).

An optical fiber biosensor has been successfully used for monitoring the concentration of adrenaline, noradrenaline, dopamine, L-DOPA and DOPAC. The optical fiber biosensor showed

Table 1. Catecholamine Dopamine (DA), Noradrenaline (NA) and Adrenaline (AD)) concentrations on urine from 40 subjects with Down syndrome.

Patient	Catecholamine (pmol/L)		
	DA	NA	A
1	261.69 ± 0.07	305.04 ± 0.06	536.27 ± 0.04
2	2278.14 ± 0.09	312.49 ± 0.04	531.79 ± 0.06
3	112.10 ± 0.05	<5.30	14.81 ± 0.03
4	2316.26 ± 0.07	165.42 ± 0.04	808.93 ± 0.05
5	627.27 ± 0.03	222.85 ± 0.04	8.17 ± 0.03
6	193.52 ± 0.02	4.527 ± 0.03	<5.50
7	42.81 ± 0.05	6.63 ± 0.06	<5.50
8	1163.59 ± 0.07	155.39 ± 0.09	227.02 ± 0.06
9	2252.09 ± 0.09	181.22 ± 0.04	<5.50
10	32.64 ± 0.05	<5.30	<5.50
11	1038.54 ± 0.04	<5.30	7.93 ± 0.01
12	41.65 ± 0.04	6.27 ± 0.07	12.54 ± 0.07
13	719.15 ± 0.09	56.24 ± 0.07	86.33 ± 0.04
14	474.85 ± 0.06	171.32 ± 0.05	11.77 ± 0.06
15	1121.92 ± 0.09	103.87 ± 0.08	251.50 ± 0.05
16	2988.70 ± 0.03	335.17 ± 0.03	557.17 ± 0.05
17	4554.03 ± 0.04	192.37 ± 0.04	545.17 ± 0.05
18	376.79 ± 0.01	43.62 ± 0.05	56.94 ± 0.04
19	23.07 ± 0.04	<5.30	6.78 ± 0.03
20	54.49 ± 0.07	<5.30	< 5.50
21	62.21 ± 0.05	39.47 ± 0.03	175.88 ± 0.06
22	2174.28 ± 0.02	125.31 ± 0.06	344.10 ± 0.05
23	1978.15 ± 0.05	236.70 ± 0.07	322.60 ± 0.02
24	31.13 ± 0.07	<5.30	<5.50
25	37.90 ± 0.04	<5.30	<5.50
26	52.74 ± 0.01	12.97 ± 0.03	140.96 ± 0.02
27	3932.91 ± 0.08	150.22 ± 0.04	2279.84 ± 0.02
28	145.24 ± 0.01	<5.30	13.79 ± 0.05
29	44.46 ± 0.01	<5.30	<5.50
30	1058.85 ± 0.04	81.79 ± 0.03	97.48 ± 0.02
31	41.25 ± 0.05	8.74 ± 0.08	<5.50
32	46.54 ± 0.02	< 5.30	<5.50
33	129.48 ± 0.05	45.66 ± 0.07	<5.50
34	433.12 ± 0.07	45.38 ± 0.07	<5.50
35	24.29 ± 0.04	<5.30	<5.50
36	4550.91 ± 0.01	425.10 ± 0.07	603.24 ± 0.07
37	31.74 ± 0.08	11.51 ± 0.04	16.37 ± 0.04
38	34.06 ± 0.01	< 5.30	<5.50
39	17.49 ± 0.01	< 5.30	<5.50
40	60.67 ± 0.04	2.12 ± 0.06	<5.50

Table 2. Catecholamine metabolites (L-DOPA and DOPAC) concentrations on urine from 40 subjects with Down syndrome.

Patient	Catecholamine metabolite (pmol/L)	
	L-DOPA	DOPAC
1	334.03 ± 0.07	14887.9 ± 0.2
2	302.51 ± 0.03	7113.5 ± 0.1
3	<4.20	43.67 ± 0.02
4	178.32 ± 0.06	6403.1 ± 0.3
5	283.14 ± 0.09	2230.8 ± 0.1
6	<4.20	<3.70
7	17.76 ± 0.02	13.46 ± 0.02
8	172.93 ± 0.08	3426.5 ± 0.3
9	176.05 ± 0.07	5909.2 ± 0.2
10	24.65 ± 0.02	24.59 ± 0.03
11	37.28 ± 0.03	52.80 ± 0.07
12	<4.20	28.34 ± 0.02
13	155.22 ± 0.05	1688.2 ± 0.1
14	75.07 ± 0.03	606.87 ± 0.09
15	117.38 ± 0.07	2695.04 ± 0.08
16	370.17 ± 0.09	9054.0 ± 0.3
17	272.61 ± 0.09	8265.8 ± 0.4
18	21.52 ± 0.04	1553.9 ± 0.1
19	19.88 ± 0.02	38.06 ± 0.01
20	4.57 ± 0.02	<3.70
21	<4.20	46.96 ± 0.05
22	233.54 ± 0.09	5787.3 + 0.3
23	257.07 ± 0.08	6899.2 ± 0.4
24	22.61 ± 0.03	36.12 ± 0.02
25	24.87 ± 0.02	<3.70
26	7.61 ± 0.01	<3.70
27	252.80 ± 0.09	9397.8 ± 0.1
28	938.00 ± 0.09	44.83 ± 0.03
29	8.49 ± 0.01	13.12 ± 0.02
30	130.49 ± 0.08	2443.95 ± 0.09
31	5.46 ± 0.02	21.81 ± 0.01
32	22.31 ± 0.04	28.20 ± 0.03
33	7.17 ± 0.02	366.27 ± 0.08
34	18.41 ± 0.03	1555.22 ± 0.09
35	23.20 ± 0.01	<3.70
36	5906.7 ± 0.1	28471.3 ± 0.5
37	<4.20	504.13 ± 0.09
38	<4.20	<3.70
39	17.13 ± 0.07	<3.70
40	20.35 ± 0.04	9.73 ± 0.02

a high analytical signal and a linear response, allowing the determination of catecholamines with detection limit lower than 5.50 pmol/L and catecholamine metabolites lower than 4.20 pmol/L. In addition, this optical fiber biosensor was able of rapid, single and inexpensive detection of catecholamines, its precursor and metabolites, constituting an excellent alternative to the more classical methods such as HPLC-ED for catecholamines detection.

AKNOWLEDGEMENTS

This work has been developed under the scope of the FCT (Portugal) funded research project

PTDC/QUI/70970/2006 and FCOMP-01-0124-FEDER-010896: "Development of a new Optical Fiber Biosensor for Determination of Catecholamines (CATSENSOR)", and research grants ref. SFRH/BPD/48028/2008 and ref. SFRH/BPD/65410/2009.

REFERENCES

Barnhart, R.C. & Connolly, B. (2007). Aging and Down syndrome: implications for physical therapy. *Phys-Ther.* 87, 1399–1406.

Bhattarai, B., Kulkarni, A.H., Rao, S.T. & Mairpadi, A. (2008). Anesthetic consideration in Down syndrome-a review. *Nepal Med Coll J.* 10, 199–203.

Ferreira, F.D.P., Silva, L.I.B., Freitas, A.C., Rocha-Santos, T.A.P. & Duarte, A.C. (2009). High performance liquid chromatography coupled to an optical fiber detector coated with laccase for screening catecholamines in plasma and urine. *J. Chromatogr A.* 1216, 7049–7054.

Ferry, Y. & Leech, D. (2005). Amperometric Detection of Catecholamine Neurotransmitters Using Electro-catalytic Substrate Recycling at a Laccase Electrode. *Electroanalysis.* 17, 113–119.

Kumar, A.M., Fernandez, B., Antoni, M.H., Eisdorfer, S. & Kumar, M. (2003). Catecholamine quantification in body fluids using isocratic, reverse phase HPLC-CoulArray multielectrode chemical detector system: investigation of sensitivity, stability, and reproducibility. *J. Liq Chrom Rel Technol.* 26, 3433–3451.

Lisdat, F., Wollenberger, U., Makower, A., Hörtnagl, H., Pfeiffer, D. & Scheller, F.W. (1997). Catecholamine detection using enzymatic amplification. *Biosens. Bioelectron.* 12, 1199–1211.

Miller, J.N. & Miller, J.C. (2005). Statistic and chemometrics for analytical chemistry. Pearson Prentice Hall, New York.

Pestana, M., Faria, M.S., Oliveira, J.G., Baldaia, J. Santos, A., Guerra, L.E. & Soares-da-Silva, P. (1997) Assessment of renal dopaminergic system activity during the recovery of renal function in human kidney transplant recipients. *Nephrol Dial Transplant.* 12, 2667–2672.

Pussard, E., Neveux, M. & Guigueno, N. (2009). Reference intervals for urinary catecholamines and metabolites from birth to adulthood. *Clin Biochem.* 42, 536–539.

Silva, L.I.B., Gomes, A., Pintado, M., Pinheiro, H., Moura, D., Freitas, A.C., Rocha-Santos, T.A.P. & Duarte, A.C. (2010). Optical fiber-based biosensor for measurement of catecholamines and their metabolites in urine samples from patients with Down syndrome. *Anal Bioanal Chem.* Submitted.

Silva, L.I.B., Ferreira, F.D.P., Freitas, A.C., Rocha-Santos, T.A.P. & Duarte, A.C. (2009). Optical fiber biosensor coupled to chromatographic separation for screening of dopamine, norepinephrine and epinephrine in human urine and plasma. *Talanta.* 80, 853–857.

Whiting, M.J. & Doogue, M.P. (2009). Advances in biochemical screening for phaeochromocytoma using biogenic amines. *Clin Biochem Rev.* 30, 3–17.

Technology and Medical Sciences – Natal Jorge et al. (eds)
© 2011 Taylor & Francis Group, London, ISBN 978-0-415-66822-4

Study of pressure sensors placement using an Abdominal Aortic Aneurysm (AAA) model

L.A. Rocha, A. Sepulveda, A.J. Pontes & J.C. Viana
Institute for Polymers and Composites/I3N, University of Minho, Guimarães, Portugal

Isa C.T. Santos & João Manuel R.S. Tavares
Instituto de Engenharia Mecânica e Gestão Industrial/Faculdade de Engenharia, Universidade do Porto, Porto, Portugal

ABSTRACT: An Abdominal Aortic Aneurysm (AAA) model for post-EVAR (endovascular aneurysm repair) analysis, including the blood flow, the bifurcated stent-graft, the aorta aneurysm wall motion and the stagnant blood inside the aneurysm sac, was built and solved using a Fluid Structure Interaction (FSI) code. The post-EVAR analysis aims to check the feasibility of EVAR surveillance using a remote pressure sensor, and the study of the pressure variations inside the aneurysm sac to determine the best placement position for the pressure sensor(s). First results suggest that aneurysm sac pressure measurement is feasible and can be a good indicator of aneurysms post-EVAR evolution.

Keywords: AAA Model, CFD, Aneurysm pressure sensing

1 INTRODUCTION

1.1 *Abdominal Aortic Aneurysms (AAA)*

An aneurysm can be defined as a permanent and irreversible localized dilatation of an artery, having at least a 50% increase in diameter compared with the healthy one. It can appear anywhere, but it occurs most commonly in the aorta, as well as in arteries located at the base of the brain and in the legs.

Two treatments are currently available for the treatment of aneurysms: conventional surgical repair (open surgery) (Myers et al. 2001) and endovascular aneurysm repair (EVAR) (Parodi et al. 1991). The first involves the replacement of the damaged section of the aorta with a prosthetic graft through a surgical procedure (a large incision in the abdomen). EVAR is a minimally invasive procedure in which a stent-graft is guided from the femoral artery to the affected artery segment in order to prevent wall rupture shielding the aneurysm from the blood pressure. The latter is usually associated with less physiological derangement, lower morbidity and mortality, and more rapid recovery than open surgery (Chuter et al. 2004) but, after the procedure, regular surveillance to detect and prevent complications such as graft migration, stent fracture, endoleaks, enlargement of the aneurysm sac, and AAA rupture is required.

Comparing both treatments, EVAR is preferable due to the fact of being less stressful and reducing significantly systemic complications (Rutherford & Krupski, 2004), as well as having lower costs of inpatient stay and less or no need for intensive care facilities during recovery. The durability of open surgery, established with long-term follow-up studies, is excellent (Rutherford & Krupski, 2004), so good that there is little or no requirement for long-term surveillance, in contrast with EVAR whose current results suggest that there is a need for increased surveillance and re-intervention (Hayter et al. 2005). Considering the longer life expectancies and the rising public expectations for quality of life, the costs associated to the follow-up can jeopardize EVAR's effectiveness.

1.2 *EVAR surveillance*

The current surveillance protocol involves imaging at 1, 6, and 12 months after the procedure, and thereafter, on an annual basis. In order to reduce and even eliminate these exams, new surveillance technologies are being investigated and the most promising technique identified so far is remote pressure sensing (Springer et al. 2007). Up to now, existing sensors are randomly placed on the aneurysm sac and only provide information, namely the pressure, regarding a single point.

Several studies using full AAA models (stent-graft, aorta and aneurysm sac) have been presented in the literature (Li & Kleinstreuer, 2006, Frauenfelder et al. 2006, Scotti & Finol, 2007), but they mainly studied the drag forces on the stent-graft, or the stresses on the vessel that can lead to rupture.

This paper introduces a Computational Fluidic Model (CFD) with Fluid Structure Interaction (FSI) of an AAA to study the pressure variations inside the aneurysm sac after stent-graft placement. The goal is to determine if there is a best location for placement of pressure sensors and to check if more information (besides the aneurysm sac pressure) can be retrieved. Additionally, the influence of AAA geometry on the sac pressure is also analyzed.

2 AAA MODEL

2.1 Geometry

A full parametric script was implemented in a CAD software for the 3D modeling of the AAA geometry (Fig. 1). The geometry of the AAA is based on typical fusiform aneurysms geometries, including models built from CT-scan available in literature (Li & Kleinstreuer, 2006, Vorp, 2007).

For the study presented here, aorta radius and aorta wall thicknesses of 2.5 cm and 2.5 mm respectively, were used. The aneurysm has a length of 10.5 cm and a main radius of 6.7 cm.

2.2 Material properties

The transient simulation used considers the pulsate nature of blood flow. The model includes the blood flow, the bifurcated stent-graft, the aorta wall motion (including the aneurysm wall) and the stagnant blood inside the aneurysm sac (essential for the pressure simulation inside the sac).

The ANSYS multiple code coupling (MFX) with FSI coupling between Ansys and CFX was used to solve the model. Newtonian, laminar and incompressible blood flow was assumed with a density of $\rho = 1.05$ g/cm^3 and a viscosity of $v = 0.0035$ Pa·s.

The diseased AAA wall was modeled as a non-linear, isotropic, elastic material with a density $\rho = 1.2$ g/cm^3, a Young's Modulus E = 4.6 MPa and a Poisson's ratio of 0.49 (Li & Kleinstreuer, 2006). The healthy part of the aorta (AAA neck) and iliac were also assumed to be a non-linear, isotropic, elastic material with a density $\rho = 1.2$ g/cm^3, a Young's Modulus E = 2 MPa and a Poisson's ratio of 0.45. The stent graft-graft was modeled with SHELL elements, and was assumed to be a non-linear, isotropic material

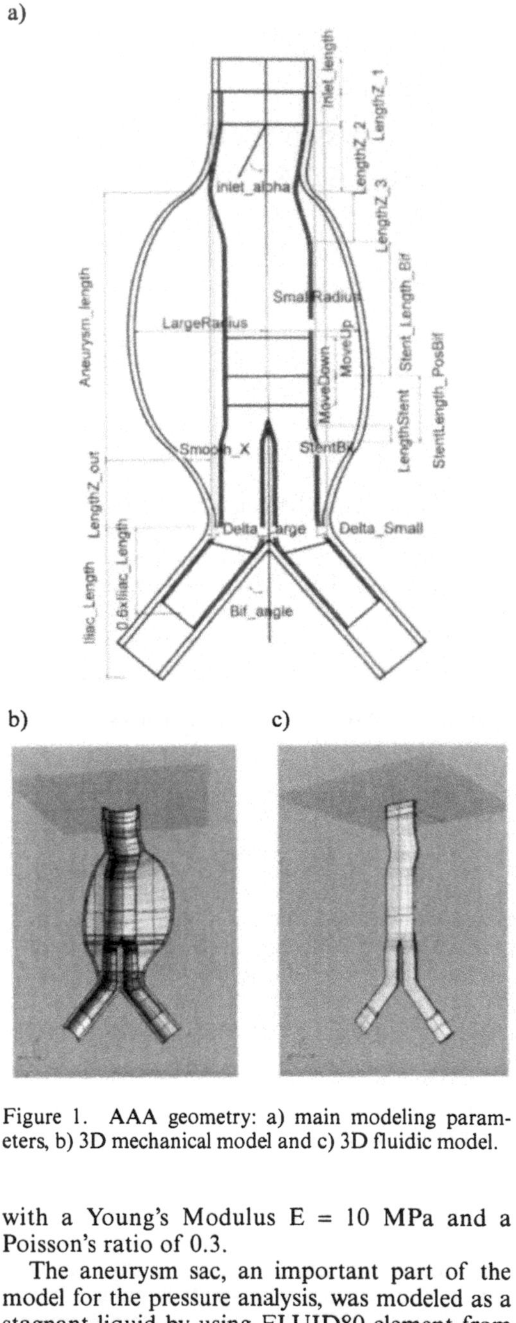

Figure 1. AAA geometry: a) main modeling parameters, b) 3D mechanical model and c) 3D fluidic model.

with a Young's Modulus E = 10 MPa and a Poisson's ratio of 0.3.

The aneurysm sac, an important part of the model for the pressure analysis, was modeled as a stagnant liquid by using FLUID80 element from the ANSYS element library. This element allows the simulation of stagnant fluids in containers with no flow.

2.3 Boundary conditions

The mechanical domain of the simulation was assumed to have zero displacement at the top of

a)

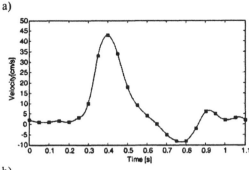

b)

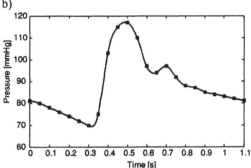

Figure 2. Fluidic boundary conditions: a) inlet velocity and b) outlet pressure.

the AAA neck and at the bottom of the iliacs, while a time dependent uniform velocity was applied at the inlet of the fluidic domain (Fig. 2a) and a time dependent normal traction (due to luminal pressure) on the outlet (Fig. 2b). A full cardiac cycle (1.1 s) was simulated.

3 RESULTS AND DISCUSSION

3.1 *Simulation results*

Initially, a simpler AAA model without stent-graft was used to validate the FSI solver. These initial simulation results showed a maximum aorta displacement of 1.9 mm and a maximum stress (von Mises) around 0.4 MPa in good agreement with the data from Li & Kleinstreuer, 2006 (using a similar geometry size).

Next, the full AAA model with stent-graft was simulated and Figure 3 shows the pressure inside the aneurysm sac at systolic pressure (t = 0.5 s). Clearly, some pressure variations along the aneurysm sac are visible with the minimum pressure occurring close to the stent-graft bifurcation. A closer look to the stent-graft displacement at the same simulation time (Fig. 3) suggests that the minimum pressures are related to the maximum stent-graft displacements.

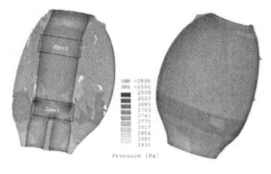

Figure 3. Results of the aneurysm sac pressure during systolic pressure (t = 0.5 s).

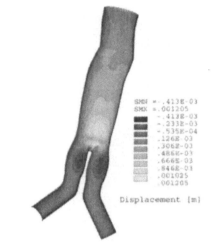

Figure 4. Stent-graft displacement during systolic pressure (t = 0.5 s).

In order to assess the pressure variations inside the aneurysm sac during one cardiac cycle, two zones were defined (zone 1 and 2 in Fig. 3) and the mean pressures within those regions were plotted along with the pressure boundary condition at the outlet. The results are depicted in Figure 4.

3.2 *Discussion*

These initial simulations imply that the pressure variations within the aneurysm sac are related to the displacement of the stent-graft caused by the luminal pressure. If this is the case, the placement of one sensor on the region with less structural stability (higher displacement) might be a good indicator, when compared to other sensor placed elsewhere within the aneurysm sac, of the structural integrity of the stent-graft.

Since the pressure variations inside the aneurysm sac seem to be related to the stent-graft material (structural behavior), a second set of simulations were performed using a higher Young's Modulus for the stent-graft material, E = 60 MPa.

The second set of simulations (Fig. 6) clearly shows that the pressure within the aneurysm sac depends on the structural behavior of the stent-graft material. In fact, simulations reveal that a

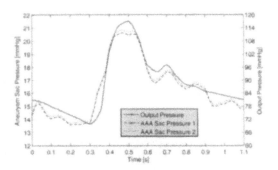

Figure 5. Pressures inside aneurysm sac (zone 1 and 2 in Fig. 3) and pressure boundary condition at the outlet.

a)

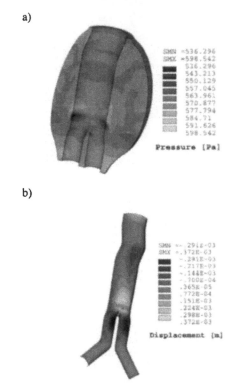

b)

Figure 6. AAA simulations using a Young's Modulus of 60 MPa for the stent-graft material: a) aneurysm sac pressure and b) stent-graft displacement during systole (t = 0.5 s).

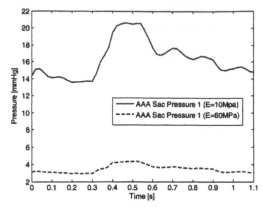

Figure 7. Pressures inside aneurysm sac on zone 1 (Fig. 3) for different stent-graft material properties.

large drop on the pressure within the aneurysm (>10 mmHg) sac occurs when the Young's Modulus is increased from 10 MPa to 60 MPa. As in the previous simulation, the minimum pressures within the aneurysm sac occur around the area where the stent-graft displacement is higher (Fig. 6b).

Figure 7 compares the aneurysm sac pressure on zone 1 (Fig. 3) during the total cardiac cycle for the two simulated models. In both cases, the aneurysm sac transient pressure changes are related to the luminal pressure.

4 CONCLUSIONS

An abdominal aortic aneurysm CFD model with FSI was developed to study the suitability of using pressure sensors to detect post-EVAR complications. The results demonstrate that pressure sensing in the aneurysm sac can be used both for leakage detection and to measure systolic and diastole blood pressures and indicate that the pressure within the aneurysm sac depends on the stent-graft material structural behavior.

Although more simulations are required to evaluate the best location for the placement of a cluster of pressure sensors, the results obtained suggest that the differences in pressure within the aneurysm sac can be an indicator of the stent-graft material integrity.

ACKNOWLEDGEMENTS

This work is supported by FCT under the project MIT-Pt/EDAM-EMD/0007/2008.

REFERENCES

Chuter, T., Parodi, J.C. & Lawrence-Brown, M. 2004. Management of abdominal aortic aneurysm: a decade of progress. *Journal of Endovascular Therapy*, 11(Sup. II): S82-S95.

Frauenfelder, T., Lotfey, M., Boehm, T. & Wildermuth, S. 2006. Computational fluid dynamics: hemodynamic changes in abdominal aortic aneurysm after stent-graft implantation. *Cardiovascular and interventional radiology*, 29(4), 613–623.

Hayter, C.L., Bradshaw, S.R., Allen, R.J., Guduguntla, M. & Hardman, D.T. 2005. Follow-up costs increase the cost disparity between endovascular and open abdominal aortic aneurysm repair. *Journal of Vascular Surgery*, 42(5), 912–918.

Li, Z. & Kleinstreuer, C. 2006. Analysis of biomechanical factors affecting stent-graft migration in an abdominal aortic aneurysm model. *J.Biomechanics*, 39(12), 2264–2273.

Myers, K., Devine, T., Barras, C. & Self, G. 2001. Endoluminal Versus Open repair for abdominal aortic aneurysms. *2nd Virtual Congress of Cardiology*.

Parodi, J.C., Palmaz, J.C. & Barone, H.D. 1991. Transfemoral intraluminal graft implantation for abdominal aortic aneurysms. *Annals of Vascular Surgery*, 5(6), 491–499.

Rutherford, R.B. & Krupski, W.C. 2004. Current status of open versus endovascular stent-graft repair of abdominal aortic aneurysm. *Journal of Vascular Surgery*, 39(5), 1129–1139.

Scotti, C. & Finol, E. 2007. Compliant biomechanics of abdominal aortic aneurysms: A fluid–structure interaction study. *Computers & Structures*, 85(11–14), 1097–1113.

Springer, F., Günther, R.W. & Schmitz-Rode, T. 2007, Aneurysm sac pressure measurement with minimally invasive implantable pressure sensors: An alternative to current surveillance regimes after EVAR?. *CardioVascular and Interventional Radiology*. 31(3): pp. 460–467.

Vorp, D.A. 2007. Biomechanics of abdominal aortic aneurysm. *J. Biomechanics*, 40(9), 1887–1902.

Technology and Medical Sciences – Natal Jorge et al. (eds)
© 2011 Taylor & Francis Group, London, ISBN 978-0-415-66822-4

Termographic assement of internal derangement of the temporomandibular joint

M. Clemente
Assistant of Occlusion, TMJ and Orofacial Pain in the Faculty of Dentistry, University of Porto, Porto, Portugal

A. Sousa
Monitor of Occlusion, TMJ and Orofacial Pain in the Faculty of Dentistry, University of Porto, Porto, Portugal

A. Silva & J. Gabriel
IDMEC—Polo FEUP, Faculty of Engineering, University of Porto, Porto, Portugal

J.C. Pinho
Chairman of Occlusion, TMJ and Orofacial Pain in the Faculty of Dentistry, University of Porto, Porto, Portugal

ABSTRACT: This article presents a clinical study where an infrared thermal camera was included in the protocol, as a complementary diagnostic method for TMD disorders.

This patient showed the presence of signs and symptoms characteristic of TMD, such as pain in the TMJ during mandibular function and palpation of the TMJ, noises in the TMJ and deviation of mandibular movements. Facial thermography was made using right and left lateral projections during clench and when eating. Results showed an increase of 1.2°C between the left TMJ and the right TMJ. The spot temperature over the region of the involved TMJ demonstrated an increase temperature compared to the normal TMJ.

This clinical research study appears to be consistent to indicate that there is a presence of thermal asymmetry in a patient with a TMJ disorder. However, further studies should be made to validate this non-invasive diagnostic technique.

1 INTRODUCTION

The clinical assessment of temporomandibular disorders (TMDs) should involve a patient evaluation that integrates the clinical findings, after performing a through physical examination, including the patient history and other diagnostic data that the clinician finds important to achieve a correct diagnosis. Magnetic Resonance Imaging (MRI) is the preferred imaging used to obtain a more accurate diagnosis of an internal derangement, Emshoff et al. (2002), nevertheless there are some inconvenient in this kind of examination, especially the economic aspect, once it is very expensive.

Thermography has been used in the assessment of craniomandibular disorders, Gratt et al. (1994), once he demonstrated that thermal symmetry, regarding the right and left sides of the body, would represent a normal thermal image, for symptom free patients. While, on the other hand, the presence of a significant temperature difference between corresponding areas of opposite sides of the body could be used as an indicator of medical dysfunction, Gratt et al. (1993a).

TMD can share common characteristics of orofacial pain, masticatory dysfunction, chronic musculoskeletal pain, Suvinen et al. (1995), such as back pain, involving the cervical zone, were the trapezius area could be affected or originating headaches that can include frontal, temple and occipital headache sites. The clinical condition of the TMD can also involve sounds during mandibular movements and limited mandibular movement, Okeson (1996). In dental research, parafunctional activities and dental occlusion are the two factors that have received most attention, although it is important to recognize that the cause of TMD is multifactorial involvingbehavioral, environmental and psychological factors, Turner et al. (2004).

Likewise, patients believed to have TMD generally present to the dentist with pain and confounding disorders of the contiguous and noncontiguous structures of the head and neck, upper quadrant and systemic musculoskeletal disease.

Our study aimed to assess the relationship of the thermal data collected in a patient with TMD symptoms and correlate them with previous clinical findings. This project has the intent of analyzing the correlation between temperature measurements of certain structures of the cranio-cervical-mandibular complex and distinguishes between normal and abnormal individuals, regarding TMDs. In previous studies, temporomandibular joints (TMJ) with temperature differences ranging 0.4°C to 0.5°C indicate the presence of TMD, Gratt et al. (1993b). While a difference of 0.5°C or greater, left versus right side is indicative of potentially clinically significant pathology, once it is possible to correlate with the anatomical distribution of pain in actual patients, Weinstein et al. (1991).

2 MATERIALS AND METHODS

The patient gave written informed consent to participate in this study; she had pain in the temporomandibular joint during jaw function, upon palpation and limited jaw excursion movements, which fulfilled the inclusion criteria, of a patient with TMD.

The procedure involved the patient sitting on a common bench, with their feet resting on the floor, and her head looking straight forward (Figure 1A).

The thermography was conducted using an infrared Flir A325 camera, and the software Therma CAM Researcher Pro, (Figure 1B).

The facial thermal images were made using frontal, right and left projections (Figure 2A). It was allowed ten minutes for facial temperature equilibration, in between the series of evaluation of the mastication. Three different kinds of food consistency were offered to the subject (Figure 2B), in order to evaluate if any type of difference in the body temperature of the TMJ and the masticatory muscles, occurred (Figure 2C).

The patient presented during the extra-oral muscle examination tenderness of the posterior cervical muscles, especially on the trapezius muscle. In this case, the postural apparatus and related neuromusculatures were taken into account during the thermographic examination, with individual mapping areas to identify thermal points and their respective temperature measurement (Figure 3A).

It is important to mention, as a general guideline that when using thermography as an aid tool for examination, certain parameters have to be taken into account to achieve a correct diagnosis. These are temperature room control, with no windows, closed doors, and also the bra strap of the patient, which can induce a body temperature difference because of the pressure that is applied on the trapezius. On the other hand, having pimples on your skin, in this particular case on the back of the patient can mislead the diagnosis when analyzing the digitized color images. This can lead to a failure in the diagnostic accuracy

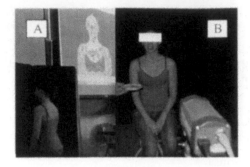

Figure 1. Patient sitting on bench with her back straight and her head in an upright position (A).The thermography was conducted using a Flir A325 thermovision camera (B).

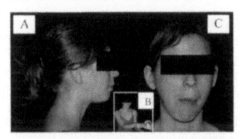

Figure 2. Lateral facial thermal image of a 21-year-old female patient having internal derangement of the TMJ. Lateral view (A) and front view (C), evaluated when masticatory function was active (eating a cake, B).

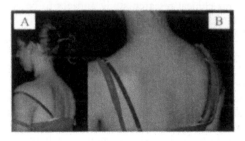

Figure 3. Temperature measurements were made on the occipital and trapezius muscles of the patient (A). To provide objective classification of the measurements, special attention should be taken to the bras strap and any kind of dermatological inflammations (B).

of the examiner having the wrong perception of a presence of a thermal point corresponding to a possible pain zone (Figure 3B).

3 RESULTS

The results of the clinical examination which included the thermographic assesment of detrimental anatomic regions in a patient with TMD, included findings on: (1) temporomandibular joint, (2) deep masseter muscle, (3) anterior temporalis muscle, (4) posterior cervical muscle—trapezius and (5) sternocleidomastoid muscle. The (6) orbicular oris muscle was also associated in this study, as a relevant anatomic region, due to significant changes in temperature observed when comparing the rest position and when eating food with different kinds of consistency. Therefore the main clinical parameters that have changed in this study were muscles and joint.

The symptom prevalence data obtained in the questionnaire filled by our patient where she reported pain symptoms in the left temporomandibular joint (TMJ), is in consistency with the thermal image obtained at a rest position (Figure 4).

The measurements of thermal asymmetry of the TMJ regions indicate pathology among these structures, since it is possible to observe differences of 1.2°C.

The subject presented also pain symptoms that consisted in headaches and pain associated with the left TMJ, back and neck. After clinical examination it was possible to confirm joint sounds (clicking) at the left TMJ, and at our extra-oral muscle examination, (4) posterior cervical muscles—trapezius, left side, were tender to palpation.

It is important to examine very carefully the relationship of thermal findings and clinical palpation examination. In this particular case,the imagesshowed an area, were we could believe the there was a tender point in the trapezius region, and actually, it corresponded to a dermatological inflammation of the patient, were the temperature score values were higher (Figure 5).

The images should be obtained with a correct protocol and small details analyzed carefully. Otherwise it can actually mislead the clinician to an inaccurate diagnosis.

Another particular aspect is the management of the hair, so that infrared thermography can be reliable when performing the study of the occipital muscles. These images were not included in our examination due to the fact they were asymptomatic in our patient, and because of the presence of images artifacts (Figure 5). Thus in this case, it was not possible to correlate the cervical temperature measurements to the patient's symptoms.

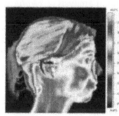
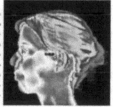

Figure 4. Right and left TMJ thermal measurements, 37.5 and 38.7°C respectively.

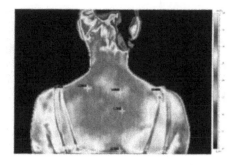

Figure 5. The palpation of the symptomatic trapezius muscle were performed on the patient's back and apparentlyit was coincident with artifact image.

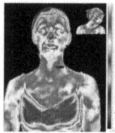
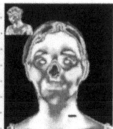

Figure 6. Thermography spot of the left sternocleidomastoid muscle before and after head and neck rotation.

When comparing the (5) sternocleidomastoid muscle group as mentioned previously, we can notice that the temperature scores raises, after repeated rotation of the head and neck, corresponding to the minimal tenderness the patient initially referred (Figure 6). The spot temperature of the left and right sternocleidomatoid was 37.7°C and 37.8°C respectively, compared with the 38.7°C and 38.8°C after the head and neck rotation. Theseinterpretations of the cranio-cervical-mandibular complex thermal images correspond with the detailed history obtained from the patient and can conduct to an appropriate physical assessment.

The subject of our study was a ballerina for the past 12 years and is also a dental medical student; this frequently causes an abnormal posture which involves an extended head-neck position, with a forward head position.

Comparisons of the facial temperature points, demonstrated significant differences from the left symptomatic side to the right asymptomatic side. These findings could be expected in a patient that experiences head and orofacial pain and since one of the most important functions that the TMJ is under load, is mastication, we can observe the differences of the (1) TMJ, (2) deep masseter muscle, (3) anterior temporalis muscle when the subject was eating cheese (Figure 7), eating a cake and chewing a gum, Table 1.

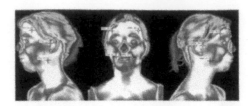

Figure 7. Lateral (left and right) and frontal facial thermal image where it is possible to notice the different thermal patterns.

Table 1. Comparison of thermal spot measurement of orofacial anatomic zones measured in this study on a TMD patient.

Temperature°C	TMJ left	TMJ right	Deep masseter muscle left	Deep masseter muscle right	Anterior temporalis left	Anterior temporalis right	Orbicular oris left	Orbicular oris right
Rest position	38.7	37.5	37.9	37.6	38.8	37.4	38.1	38.4
Eating chease	37.9	38.2	37.8	37.4	38.9	38.0	37.8	38.3
Eating cake	38.4	38.0	38.3	38.2	39.0	38.2	38.2	38.8
Chewing gum	38.8	38.4	38.5	38.2	39.2	38.2	38.8	38.2

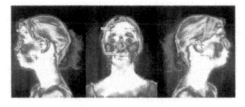

Figure 8. Lateral (left and right) and frontal facial thermal images. The thermal patterns do not changed when compared to the patterns of Figure 7 (soft food consistency). It is possible to observe that the thermal spot of the left TMJ is always higher.

The TMJ can adapt to biomechanical stresses allowing the tissues of the joint to maintain a normal function, when loading changes occur. Nevertheless it was possible to observe the functional movements of the jaw of the patient when eating, which demonstrates excessive mechanical stress in the left TMJ, possibly because of unique structural or functional characteristics of the masticatory system, for example when chewing a gum, corresponding to a hard food consistency (Figure 8).

4 CONCLUSIONS

In this study, it was comparedthe thermal images of a normal TMJ from an abnormal TMJ. It was also possible torelate the thermal images with painful clicking joints, clinical palpation findings, especially in the orofacial region. Therefore this study suggests that the assessment of an internal derangement of the TMJ can take advantage of the aid of a thermal camera. This patient was previously examined by a TMJ specialist, and submitted to an Arcus Digma test, which confirmed an internal derangement of the left TMJ.

Future studies should be made with a larger sample, observing also non-pain symptoms patients, because they exist and appear to be far less prevalent as an incentive for searching professional treatment for TMD. With this imaging technique, which is easy and quick to perform, it may be possible to detect signs before they proceed to symptoms and may create discomfort to the patient.

This imaging technique is not painful neither invasive, and can be repeated without any inconvenience to the physician or patient, allowing a physiological-anatomic evaluation of the desired structures during function.

ACKNOWLEDGEMENTS

The authors would like to thank to Fundação para a Ciência e Tecnologia (FCT), for the support of the project PTDC/EEA-ACR/75454/2006.

REFERENCES

Emshoff, R., Brandlmaier, I., Bosch, R. et al. 2002. Validation of the clinical diagnostic criteria for temporomandibular disorders for the diagnostic subgroup—disc derangement with reduction. *J Oral Rehabil*; 29:1139–1145.

Gratt, B.M. & Sickles, E.A. 1993. Thermographic characterization of the asymptomatic (normal) TMD. *J. Orofacial Pain*; 7:7–14.

Gratt, B.M., Sickles, E.A. & Wexler, C.E. 1993. Thermographic characterization of oseoarthrosis of the TMD. *J. Orofacial Pain*; 7(4):345–353.

Gratt, B.M., Sickles, E.A., Ross, J.B., Wexler, C.E. & Gorbein, J.A. 1994. Thermographic assessment of craniomandibular disorders: diagnostic interpretation versus temperature measurement analysis. *J. Orofacial Pain*; 8:278–288.

Suvinen, T.I. & Reade, P.C. 1995. Temporomandibular disorders: a critical review of the nature of pain and its assessment. *J. Orofacial Pain*; 9:317–339.

Okeson, J.P. (ed). 1996. Orofacial Pain. Guidelines for assessment, diagnosis, and management. Carol Stream, IL: Quintessence Publ. Co. Inc.

Turner, J.A. & Dworkin, S.F. 2004. Screening for psychosocial risk factors in patients with chronic orofacial pain. *J. American Dental Association*; 135:1119–1125.

Weinstein, S.A., Weinstein, G., Weinstein, E.L. & Gelb, M. 1991. Facial Thermography, Basis, Protocol, and Clinical Value. *J. Craniomandibular Practice*; 9:201–211.

Technology and Medical Sciences – Natal Jorge et al. (eds)
© 2011 Taylor & Francis Group, London, ISBN 978-0-415-66822-4

The action of middle ear muscles using the finite element method

F. Gentil
IDMEC, ESTSP, Clínica ORL—Dr. Eurico Almeida, Widex, Portugal

C. Garbe, M. Parente, P. Martins & R.M. Natal Jorge
IDMEC, Faculdade de Engenharia da, Universidade do Porto, Portugal

ABSTRACT: The human middle ear is composed by three ossicles, ligaments and muscles tendons. These muscles (tensor tympani and stapedius) have a protection action of the inner ear, avoiding that loud sounds can be harmful. The behavior of these muscles is studied in this work, looking for the correct influence on the biomechanics of the middle ear. A model of the eardrum and the ossicles, based in images of Computerized Tomography (CT), was made (Gentil et al. 2009). The discretization of this 3D solid model was done using the ABAQUS program. Using the Hill model, the simulation of these muscles was made and the results are compared considering passive and active behavior.

1 INTRODUCTION

The ear is the hearing organ. It is divided in external, middle and inner ear. The middle ear is a cavity that contains a chain of 3 little bones (ossicles: malleus, incus and stapes) that connect the eardrum to the inner ear.

The middle ear also contains two tiny muscles. The tendon of the tensor tympani muscle, innervated by the trigeminal nerve, is attached to the upper part of the handle of the malleus; it helps to tune and protect the ear. The stapedius muscle, innervated by the facial nerve, is attached to the stapes; it contracts in response to a loud noise, making the chain of ossicles more rigid so that less sound is transmitted. Contraction of the tensor tympani pulls the handle of the malleus inward and, as the name of the muscle suggests, tenses the tympanic membrane. Contraction of the stapedius pulls the stapes footplate outward from the oval window. This response, called the acoustic reflex, helps protect the delicate inner ear from sound damage.

In this work, the behavior of these muscles is studied, looking for the correct influence on the biomechanics of the middle ear.

Using a finite element method, a model of the eardrum and the ossicles, based in images of Computerized Tomography (CT), was made (Gentil 2009). The mechanical properties used in this work are available in the literature (Prendergast 1999, Sun 2002). The respective boundary conditions are considered.

2 MATERIALS AND METHODS

2.1 Geometric and finite element mesh

The geometry of the ossicles and eardrum is constructed from CT images. The obtained slices had 0.5 mm of thickness. The discretization of this 3D solid model was done using the ABAQUS program (ABAQUS 2007) and the related finite element meshes were obtained, Figure 1. Therefore, the finite element meshing of the middle ear is then carried out, including the ligaments (superior, lateral and anterior of malleus, superior and posterior

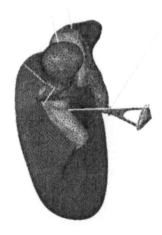

Figure 1. Middle ear model.

of the incus and annular ligament of the stapes), two muscle tendons, tensor tympani (Figure 2) and the stapedius (Figure 3) and the simulation of the cochlear fluid.

The boundary conditions applied to the finite element model include the tympanic annulus (around pars tensa of eardrum), the connection between the stapes footplate and the cochlea (stapes annular ligament) and the connection of the suspensory ligaments and muscle tendons to the temporal bone. The five suspensory ligaments are all fixed in their free extremities. The tensor tympanic muscle is fixed in the handle of the malleus, in a lateral direction and the stapedius muscle in the posterior crus of stapes.

2.2 Material properties

In the present work, the eardrum and the ossicles were assumed to have viscoelastic behavior, with their elastic properties summarized in Table 1, assuming an isotropic behavior. The Poisson's ration is assumed equal to 0.3 for all viscoelastic materials. The connection between ossicles, malleus/incus and incus/stapes, is done using contact formulation (Gentil 2007).

Considering the Yeoh model (Yeoh 1990), this work also uses hyperelastic non-linear behavior for the ligaments and muscle tendons. The density for all components is $1.0E + 3$ kg/m³.

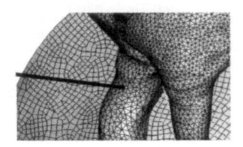

Figure 2.   Tensor tympani muscle.

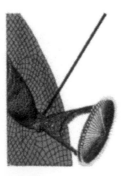

Figure 3.   Stapedius muscle.

Table 1.   Material properties for the eardrum and ossicles.

Material properties		Young's modulus (N/m²)	Density (kg/m³)
Eardrum:			1.20E + 3
Pars flaccida		10.0E + 6	
Pars tensa	Layer 1	10.0E + 6	
	Layer 2	$E_\theta = 20.0E + 6$	
		$E_r = 32.0E + 6$	
	Layer 3	10.0E + 6	
Ossicles:		1.41E + 10	
Malleus:			
- head			2.55E + 3
- neck			4.53E + 3
- handle			3.70E + 3
Incus:			
- body			2.36E + 3
- short process			2.26E + 3
- long process			5.08E + 3
Stapes			2.20E + 3

Assuming the Yeoh constitutive model, the strain-energy function can be written in the following form, where I_1 is the first right Cauchy-Green tensor invariant (Holzapfel 2000) and c_1, c_2 and c_3 are the material constants, for all ligaments and muscle tendons (Martins 2006).

$$\psi = c_1 (I_1 - 3) + c_2 (I_1 - 3)^2 + c_3 (I_1 - 3)^3 \qquad (1)$$

3   RESULTS

Considering a Sound Pressure Level (SPL) of 120 dB (20 Pa), applied on the eardrum, stapes footplate pressure was obtained for different activation values applied on two muscles.

Using the Hill model (Martins 1998), the simulation of two middle ear muscles was made and the results are compared considering passive and active behavior.

In order to determine the most appropriate activation, we considered, initially, the two muscles with equal activation to a sound pressure level of 120 dB SPL (20 Pa), applied to the eardrum.

The pressure obtained at the stapes footplate, when the muscles are passive (zero activation) was 741 Pa (Figure 4).

It can be concluded that by assigning an activation between 0 and 8.0E-02, the pressure obtained in the stapes footplate does not undergo significant change, but from this value, the pressure decreases, reaching a value of 430 Pa, for an activation level of 1.4E-01.

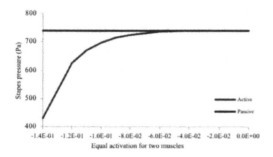

Figure 4. Variation of the pressure obtained at the stapes footplate

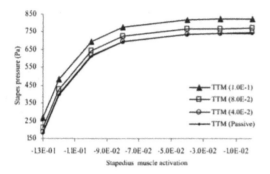

Figure 5. Pressure variation obtained in the stapes footplate with the activation of tensor tympani muscle for a sound pressure level of 120 dB SPL on the eardrum.

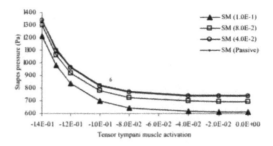

Figure 6. Pressure variation obtained in the stapes footplate with the activation of stapedius muscle for a sound pressure level of 120 dB SPL on the eardrum.

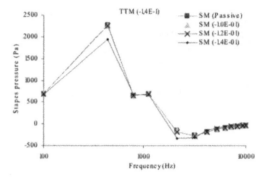

Figure 7. Pressures obtained in the stapes footplate to 120 dB SPL, for a frequency range between 100 Hz and 10 kHz.

The activation of the Tensor Tympani Muscle (TTM) was fixed by varying the activation of the Stapedius Muscle (SM) (Figure 5).

Keeping tensor tympani muscle activation and activating the stapedius muscle to 8.0E-02 there is no great variation, assuming a similar behavior to the state of the two muscles are passive. Increasing the activation of the stapedius muscle, there will one drop of this pressure, even to the value of 183 Pa, at a level of activation of 1.3E-01. If we increase the activation of tensor tympani muscle, the pressure in the stapes is not as pronounced.

Then, the procedure was done contrary, i.e., activation of stapedius muscle was fixed by varying the activation of tensor tympani muscle (Figure 6).

Keeping passive stapedius muscle, it appears that activation of tensor tympani muscle greater than 8.0E-02 cause an increase of the pressure on the stapes footplate.

Then a dynamic study was done for a frequency range between 100 and 10 kHz, for different levels of activation.

In Figure 7 we can see that for any level of activation, the most significant differences are found in low frequencies. The greatest pressure on the stapes footplate is to a greater activation of the tensor tympani muscle.

These results are in agreement with clinical records that tell us that the muscles of the middle ear have a greater influence on the bass frequencies.

4 CONCLUSIONS

The muscles of the middle ear, the tensor tympani and the stapedius, can influence the transmission of sound by the ossicular chain. These muscles contract in response to loud sounds, thereby reducing the transmission of sound to the inner ear. This is called the acoustic reflex.

If we keep activation of the tensor tympani muscle fixed with the increasing of the activation of the stapedius muscle there will be a decrease of pressure on stapes footplate. These results are consistent with clinical data that indicate that the stapedius muscle tends to decrease the pressure at the stapes footplate.

Doing the opposite procedure, the activation of stapedius muscle was fixed by varying the activation

273

of tensor tympani muscle. Keeping stapedius muscle passive it appears that activation of tensor tympani muscle greater than 8.0E-02 there is a tendency to increase the pressure on the stapes footplate, which is also in agreement with clinical records that indicate than the function of tensor tympani muscle is to increase the fluid pressure labyrinth. When we activate the stapedius muscle, it offers a resistance to the pressure increase.

ACKNOWLEDGEMENTS

The authors truly acknowledge the funding provided by Ministério da Ciência, Tecnologia e Ensino Superior—Fundação para a Ciência e a Tecnologia (Portugal) and by FEDER, under grants PTDC/EME-PME/81229/2006 and PTDC/SAU-BEB/104992/2008.

REFERENCES

ABAQUS 2007. Analyses User´s Manual, Version 6.5.

Gentil, F., Jorge, R.N., Parente, M.P.L., Martins, P.A.L.S. & Ferreira, A.J.M. 2009. Estudo biomecânico do ouvido médio, Clínica e Investigação em Otorrinolaringologia, 3 (1), 24–30.

Gentil, F., Natal, R.M., Ferreira, A.J.M., Parente, M.P.L., Moreira, M. & Almeida, E. 2007. Estudo do efeito do atrito no contacto entre os ossículos do ouvido médio, Revista Internacional de Métodos Numéricos para Cálculo y Diseño en Ingeniería, 23 (2), 177–187.

Holzapfel, G.A. 2000. Nonlinear solid mechanics, John Wiley & sons, Ltd., New York.

Martins, J.A.C., Pires, E.B., Salvado, R. & Dinis, P.B. 1998. A Numerical model of passive and active behavior of skeletal muscles, Computer methods in applied mechanics and engineering, 151, 419–433.

Martins, P.A.L.S., Jorge, R.M.N. & Ferreira, A.J.M. 2006. A Comparative Study of Several Material Models for Prediction of Hyperelastic Properties: Application to Silicone-Rubber and Soft Tissues. Strain, 42, 135–147.

Prendergast, P.J., Ferris, P., Rice, H.J. & Blayney, A.W. 1999. Vibro-acoustic modelling of the outer and middle ear using the finite element method, Audiol Neurootol, 4, 185–191.

Sun, Q., Gan, R.Z., Chang, K.H. & Dormer, K.J. 2002. Computer-integrated finite element modeling of human middle ear, Biomechanics and Modeling in Mechanobiology, 1, 109–122.

Yeoh, O.H. 1990. Characterization of elastic properties of carbon-black-filled rubber vulcanizates, Rubber Chemistry and Technology, 63, 792–805.

Technology and Medical Sciences – Natal Jorge et al. (eds)
© *2011 Taylor & Francis Group, London, ISBN 978-0-415-66822-4*

The contribution of the scapular patterns to the amplitude of shoulder external rotation on thrower athletes

A.M. Ribeiro & A.G. Pascoal
Faculty of Human Kinetics, Technical University of Lisbon, Lisbon, Portugal
CIPER, Neuromechanics Group

ABSTRACT: Despite the recognized importance of the scapular patterns to the amplitude of shoulder External Rotation (ER) on throwers, the clinical assessment does not take enough care with the traditional exams. Twenty-four healthy males were equally divided into athletes and non-athletes and their throwing arm was tested during active fast arm movements. The humeral and scapular 3D position were recorded at the shoulder end-range and compared across groups using a mixed-model two-way ANOVA. At the end-range of humeral ER the throwers showed a scapula more in retraction, also showed less humeral external rotation. Glenohumeral amplitude was reduced at the end-range of ER. On both groups when axial rotation velocity increases the peaks of external HRs decreases. No significant interaction was found between speed motions. Correlation analysis between spinal tilt and TH and GH position at the end-range of ER reveal a positive correlation on the control group, a negative correlation on volleyball players and absence of correlation on handball players. Clinical Relevance: Current study provides clinicians with an understanding of the types of adaptations that may be observed in normal, healthy throwing athletes, while using kinematic resources at the clinical trials.

1 INTRODUCTION

The shoulder joint is a complex of great mobility, and its static and dynamic stability depends on the synchronized action of rotator cuff muscles and capsuloligamentous structures. The demands on these structures are even higher during the practice of sports such as tennis, volleyball, handball, baseball and swimming.

Repetitive throwing at high velocities over time leads to chronic adaptations to soft and osseous tissues in the glenohumeral joint. These anatomic adaptations likely lead to differences in Range Of Motion (ROM) when shoulders are compared bilaterally and when overhead-throwing is compared to non-overhead throwing athletes. Although ROM changes may be adaptive, some changes in ROM are associated with pain, decreased performance and shoulder disorders.

Optimal scapular positioning is believed to be necessary for ideal muscles lengths, force production, and assisting with glenohumeral joint stability. In general, the scapula demonstrates a pattern of progressive upward rotation, external rotation and posterior tilting as the humerus is elevated. (Tsai, McClure et al., 2003).

Physical examination of overhead-throwing athletes consistently demonstrates adaptive glenohumeral internal and external rotation range if motion of the dominant shoulder when compared with the non-dominant limb. Based on the results of several studies (Osbahr, Cannon et al., 2002; Myers, Laudner et al., 2005; Oyama 2006; Gomes 2009), it can be concluded that throwers demonstrate significantly increased glenohumeral external rotation (external rotation gain) and significantly decreased glenohumeral internal rotation (glenohumeral internal rotation deficit) in the throwing arm.

During clinical range of motion testing in patients, it is common practice to measure maximal external rotation in one or two arm positions only. This provides insufficient information to describe patterns of external rotation during humeral motion. These patterns may be essential for insight in the shoulder movement and several shoulder disorders. Deviating patterns of external rotation or the inability to externally rotate the humerus sufficiently may change the scapula-humeral rhythm leading to several impairments (Stokdijk, Eilers et al., 2003).

An assessment of internal and external rotation is a standard part of a clinical examination of the shoulder. It is important for clinicians to understand that these measurements are dependent on the plane tested and how end range is determined. In addition, the scapula must be considered in evaluation specially its relationship to the humerus.

Thus the purpose of this study was to understand the contribution of the scapular patterns to the amplitude of shoulder external rotation on thrower athletes.

2 METHODS

Twenty-four subjects divided in two groups were studied: the throwers group with 6 volleyball players (height = 181 ± 4,7 cm; age = 22 ± 4,0 years; body mass: 75 ± 7,6 kg) and 6 handball players (height = 184 ± 3,7 cm; age = 22 ± 0,9 years; body mass = 81 ± 5,6 kg); and the non-thrower group with 12 non-thrower athletes (height = 176 ± 4,7 cm; age = 26 ± 2,9 years; body mass = 73 ± 7,5 kg). Humeral and scapular 3D positions were recorded by means of an 6DOF electromagnetic tracking device (100 Hz) with a four sensors setup:thorax sensor attach over T1; the arm sensor, placed just below the deltoid attachment, by mean of a cuff; and the scapular sensor, attached to the superior flat surface of the acromion process. A 4th sensor mounted on a hand-held stylus (± 6,5 cm) was used on bony landmarks digitalization in order to link sensors to Local anatomical Coordinate Systems (LCS) and subsequently calculated segments and joint rotations by combining the LCSs with the sensor motions. Segments LCSs and joint rotations definition, expressed in Euler angles, were made according to the shoulder ISB standardization protocol (Wu, van der Helm et al. 2005). Humeral axial rotation (internal and external) and scapular 3D position were recorded at the end-range of active fast and slow (subject self-selected end of range) glenohumeral external rotation ER), with subjects in a seated position and the dominant arm supported by there searcher at 90° of humeral elevation on the scapular plane. Humeral axial rotation was described with respect to the scapula, the glenohumeral (HRs) angles, and with respect to thorax, the thoracohumeral (HRt). Scapular position was described with respect to the thorax as protraction (Syt), lateral rotation (Sxt) and spinal tilt (Szt). A mixed-model two-way ANOVA was used to test the main effect of group (between-group factor) on 3 scapular (Syt, Sxt and Szt) and 2 humeral (HRt and HRs) dependent variables, as well as test for an interaction of group and speed motion (slow vs. fast; within-subjects factor). A bivariate correlation test was running in order to describe the relationships between scapular spinal tilt (Szt) and shoulder thoracohumeral and scapulohumeral rotation.

3 RESULTS

No significant interaction between group and speed motion was found for any of the 3 scapular and the 2 humeral dependent variables. The throwers group had significantly (p <.05) less scapular protraction (15° difference; P = 0.00) and less HRs amplitude (23° difference; P = 0.04) at the peak of ER. On the fast arm condition amplitude of HRs was lower at the end-range of external rotation (13,6° difference; P = 0.04). On both groups when axial rotation velocity increases the peaks of ER decrease. On throwers, scapula was also kept more in retraction at the end-range of ER (Table 1).

Between Szt and TH and GH a positive correlation was found on the control group, a negative correlation on volleyball players and no correlation on handball players. The scapula shows a position more in posterior tilt. In the control group we found a linear relation, so, with higher external rotation, less scapular tilt is shown.

Table 1. Mean ± SD (degrees) of humerus and scapula 3D position at the end-range of external rotation on both groups (throwers and non-throwers) and on fast condition. Humerus position with-respect-to (wrt) to the thorax (HRt) and wrt scapula. Scapular protraction (Syt), lateral rotation (Sxt) and spinal tilt (Szt), wrt thorax.

	Non-Throwers group	Throwers group
	Fast	Fast
HRt	−96,3 ± 26,8	−77,5 ± 19,2
HRs	−90,4 ± 29,2	−65,6 ± 19,5
Syt	32,5 ± 14,0	17,4 ± 5,6
Sxt	42,1 ± 9,8	39,4 ± 12,1
Szt	8,3 ± 7,1	9,9 ± 6,5

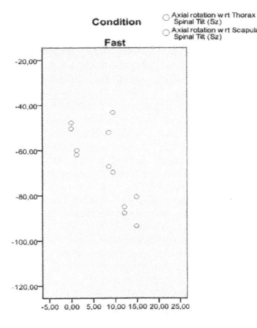

Figure 1. Correlation between spinal tilt (degrees) (Szt) and shoulder axial rotation (degrees) wrt thorax (TH) and wrt scapula (degrees) (GH) in the fast condition.

276

At the non-throwers group movement occurs more in the GH while in volleyball we have movement in GH and scapula. At fast condition a negative correlation was shown (Figure 1). This means that, on volleyball players, scapula assumes a position on posterior spinal tilt (acromion backward) when humerus is positioned more in external rotation. No correlation was found between volleyball and the slow condition.

4 DISCUSSION

During throwing motion athletes should keep their scapula stable, even while moving the arm too fast. This means that, scapular position is crucial on throwers namely when arm speed increased.

Our primary purpose was to identified, in throwers, the effect of arm speed on the extreme amplitude of shoulder external rotation. Additionally, the patterns of relative contribution of scapular motion were described in order to understand the contribution of the scapular patterns to the amplitude of shoulder external rotation in throwers.

The results showed no interaction between arm speed, groups and scapular and humeral variables. Although, the throwers demonstrated a scapula more in retraction (acromion backwards) when compared with non-throwers. This seems to be protective for the glenohumeral joint. In fact, the inability to retract the scapula, appears to impart several negative biomechanical effects on the shoulder, including a narrow subacromial space, increased strain on the anterior-inferior glenohumeral ligament, reduced impingement-free arc of upper limb elevation, reduced isometric elevation strength tested in the sagital plane. Concerning this, throwers on our study seem to have developed an adaptation towards stability.

While in clinical trial these kinds of patterns are important to evaluate, to allow a better rehabilitation, but with the traditional methods this does not seem possible. Using 3D kinematic analysis, scapular positioning could be recorded and morpho functional adaptations could be identified, and also the specific movement of throwers. While using traditional goniometry this cannot be possible.

Concerning axial shoulder rotation, scapular contribution is crucial. Although it is recognized that not all of the external rotation needed to perform the throwing motion occurs at the glenohumeral joint (Werner, Guido et al., 2006).

Excessive motion is required at the shoulder joint during throwing, yet the glenohumeral joint must remain stable to resist injury. We found that volleyball players show a more posterior tilted scapula when arm is positioned more in external rotation, while the control group showed an anterior

tilted scapula tilt. This seems to demonstrate that shoulder adaptation on volleyball players, while throwing, does not occur only at the glenohumeral joint, as it is evaluated in clinical trial, but supported by the trunk, where a scapula in retraction and posterior tilt, gives the necessary stability to achieve best performance.

This is why proper 3D position of the scapula relative to the humerus and trunk is important for muscle function, because scapula acts as the common point of attachment of the rotator cuff and primary humeral movers such as the biceps, deltoid and triceps, as well as several scapular stabilizers. Poor position of the scapula can lead to alterations to the relationship between length and tension of each muscle, thus adversely affecting muscle force generation (Myers, Laudner et al., 2005).

An imbalance in external rotators will lead to alterations in scapular tilt (McCully, Kumar et al., 2005). Concerning the movement, clinical trials use passive and active motion. But the active motion used is usually a slow motion, and not simulating the sports practice. In our study we looked for active motion. Besides using an elevated position as testing position, the calibration one, was following the protocol (Wu, van der Helm et al., 2005) as mentioned in methods, with the arm at a side. While testing we hoped that when raising the arm to the elevated position (arm at 90° flexion and abduction) the zero stayed the same, we didn't expect to have any complementary rotation (Codman's paradox), and it happened that way. So the main reason to find more external rotation at non-throwers is possibly the fact that we were evaluating active motion and not passive one.

Knowledge of joint ranges of motion and speeds of movement along with joint forces and moments will provide a scientific basis for improved and rehabilitative protocols for throwers.

As a limitation of this study we would include possible skin artifacts, especially at the arm sensor. To avoid this situation we used a sensor mounted on a cuff tiny adjusted to the arm just below the deltoid attachment, trying to ensure the position of the sensor towards the skin.

5 CONCLUSIONS

Speed was not an interaction factor between groups. The throwers group showed a scapula more in retractionin maximal external rotation of the humerus, they also showed less external rotation in active motion. Scapula on throwers group was also more in posterior tilt. This means that, on volleyball players, scapula assumes a position on posterior spinal tilt (acromion backward) when humerus is positioned more in external rotation.

No such correlation was found in the control group or the handball players, possibly due to sports adaptation.

REFERENCES

Gomes, R.R.T. a. J.L.E. (2009). "Measurement of Glenohumeral Internal Rotation in Asymptomatic Tennis Players and Swimmers." American Journal of Sports Medicine 37, 1017–1023.

McCully, S.P. Kumar, N, et al. (2005). "Internal and external rotation of the shoulder: Effects of plane, end-range determination, and scapular motion." J Shoulder Elbow Surg 14(6), 602–610.

Myers, J.B, Laudner, K.G, et al. (2005). "Scapular position and orientation in throwing athletes." Am J Sports Med 33(2), 263–271.

Osbahr, D.C, Cannon, D.L, et al. (2002). "Retroversion of the humerus in the throwing shoulder of college baseball pitchers." Am J Sports Med 30(3), 347–353.

Oyama, S. (2006). Profiling Physical Characteristics of the Swimmer's Shoulder: Comparison to Basebol Pitchers and Non-Overhead Atheletes., University of Pittsburg.

Stokdijk, M, Eilers, P.H, et al. (2003). "External rotation in the glenohumeral joint during elevation of the arm." Clin Biomech (Bristol, Avon) 18(4), 296–302.

Tsai, N.T, McClure, P.W, et al. (2003). "Effects of muscle fatigue on 3-dimensional scapular kinematics." Arch Phys Med Rehabil 84(7), 1000–1005.

Werner, S.L, J.A, Guido, Jr., et al. (2006). "Relationships between throwing mechanics and shoulder distraction in collegiate baseball pitchers." J Shoulder Elbow Surg.

Wu, G, van der Helm, F.C. et al. (2005). "ISB recommendation on definitions of joint coordinate systems of various joints for the reporting of human joint motion—Part II: shoulder, elbow, wrist and hand." J Biomech 38(5), 981–992.

Technology and Medical Sciences – Natal Jorge et al. (eds)
© *2011 Taylor & Francis Group, London, ISBN 978-0-415-66822-4*

Influence of an unstable shoe on compensatory postural adjustments

Andreia S.P. Sousa, Rui Macedo & Rubim Santos
Centro de Estudos de Movimento de Actividade Humana, Escola Superior de Tecnologias da Saúde do Instituto Politécnico do Porto, Portugal

João Manuel R.S. Tavares
Faculdade de Engenharia da Universidade do Porto, Departamento de Engenharia Mecânica e Gestão Industrial; Instituto de Engenharia Mecânica e Gestão Industrial, Portugal

ABSTRACT: This study attempted to evaluate the influence of using an unstable shoe in muscle recruitment strategies and Center of Pressure (CoP) displacement after the application of an external perturbation.

Fourteen healthy female subjects participated in this study. The electromyographic activity of medial gastrocnemius, tibialis anterior, rectus femoris, biceps femoris, rectusabdominis and erector spinaemuscles and the kinetic values to calculate the CoP were collected and analyzed after the application of an external perturbation with the subject in standing position, with no shoes and using unstable footwear.

The results showed increased in medial gastrocnemius activity during the first compensatory postural adjustments and late compensatory postural adjustments when using an unstable shoe. There were no differences in standard deviation and maximum peak of anteroposterior displacement of CoP between measurements.

From the experimental findings, one can conclude that the use of an unstable shoe leads to an increase in gastrocnemius activity with no increase in CoP displacement following an unexpected external perturbation.

Keywords: postural control strategies, electromyography, center of pressure, Masai Barefoot Technology

1   INTRODUCTION

The postural control system manages body position in space in order to promote balance and orientation, based on the central integration of proprioceptive, visual and vestibular information and an internal representation of body orientation in space. The internal model of body position is continually updated based on this multi-sensorial feedback that is used to create motor commands to control body position in space, taking into account environmental constraints [Massion, 1994; Mergner, 1998].

Any perturbation, either external, such as a sudden change in the base of support, or internal, such as a rapid movement of the upper and lower extremities, changes the projection of the Center of Mass (CM) closer to the limits of the base of support and the alignment between the CM and the Center of Pressure (CoP), which can result in postural imbalances. To minimize the danger

of loss of balance, the central nervous system uses Anticipatory Postural Adjustments (APA) in the form of feedforward mechanisms prior to the imbalance [Aruin, 1995b; Belenkiy, 1967; Li, 2007; Massion, 1992] and Compensatory Postural Adjustments (CPA) that are initiated by sensory feedback signals [Alexandrov, 2005; Park, 2004].

There are different balance strategies. The most common strategy of movement in response to aforward imbalance is the ankle strategy, which involves shifting the CM by rotating the body about the ankle joints with minimal movement of hip and knee joints. The hip strategy changes the CM position through flexion or extension of the hip. A stepping strategy realigns the base of support under the center of body mass with rapid steps towards the external source of perturbation [Horak, 1987]. The use of each strategy depends on the configuration of the base of support and on the intensity of the perturbation. Postural adjustments occur not only as a result of sensory feedback in response to unexpected external perturbations but also as a result of feed forward in anticipation of expected disruptions [Horak, 1987]. Maintaining posture on unstable bases of support requires higher levels of the control system and a fundamental change in the mode of using proprioceptive information [Ivanenko, 1997].

Maintaining balance in the standing position has been described as an effective method for the rehabilitation [Wester, 1996] and prevention of musculoskeletal injuries [Bahr, 1997; Caraffa, 1996; Wedderkopp, 1999]. The Masai Barefoot Technology (MBT), an unstable shoe, aims to promote continuous stability training. This study aims to evaluate the influence of using an unstable shoe, MBT Sport Black model, USA, on kinetic and electromyographic parameters during CPA following an external perturbation.

2 METHODOLOGY

2.1 Subjects

Fourteen healthy female individuals were tested (age = 34.6 ± 7.7 years, body weight = 65.3 ± 9.6 kg, height = 1.59 ± 0.06 m and Q angle = 15.14 ± 0.79 degrees; mean ± S.D.), being excluded subjects presenting one or more of the following conditions: 1) history of recent musculoskeletal injury in the lower limbs [Lord, 1994], 2) history or signs of neurological dysfunction which could affect motor performance, balance and sensory afferents [Lord, 1994; Ramstrand, 2010], 3) history of surgery of the lower limbs, 4) presence of pain in the legs and lower trunk in the 12 months preceding the study [Ramstrand, 2010; Tinetti, 1988], 5) cognitive changes [Lord, 1994], 6) individuals under the influence of medication, 7) balance disorders and visual deficits, 8) individuals with experience of using unstable footwear prior to the study [Ramstrand, 2010], 9) individuals with abdominal skinfold thickness exceeding 0.2 cm.

All trials were performed using the dominant limb, which was identified by asking subjects to kick a ball [Keating, 1996]. In all individuals the right lower extremity was the dominant member.

The study was conducted according to the involved institutions'ethical norms and conformed to the Declaration of Helsinki, dated 1964, being informed consent obtained from all participants.

2.2 Instrumentation

A Biopac Systems, Inc.—MP 100 Workstation™ (Biopac Systems, Inc. 42 Aero Camino Goleta, CA 93117) was used to collect all electromyographic (EMG) data, which were sampled at 2000 Hz

with a bandpass filter between 10 and 500 Hz, amplified (Common Mode Rejection Ratio (CMRR) >110 dB, gain = 1000) and analogical-to-digital converted (12 bit). Data were collected on Tibialis Anterior (TA), Medial Gastrocnemius (MG), Rectus Femoris (RF), Biceps Femoris (BF), rectusabdominis (RA) and Erector Spinae (ES) muscles using steel surface electrodes (TSD150, from BIOPAC Systems, Inc. (USA)), with bipolar configuration, a 11.4 mm contact area and an inter-electrode distance of 20 mm, and a ground electrode. This equipment presents good reliability and validity [Soderberg, 2000].

CoP values were obtained from a force plate, model FP4060-10 from Bertec Corporation (USA), connected to an amplifier with default gains and a 1000 Hz sampling rate. The amplifier was connected to a Biopac 16-bit analogical-digital converter from BIOPAC Systems, Inc. (USA). The Intraclass Correlation Coefficient (ICC) reliability of the instrument is 0.88 [Hanke, 1992].

The magnitude of the destabilizing force induced to subjects was monitored using an isometric dynamometer (Globus Italia, Italy). (Reliability: ICC = 0.97–0.98 [Bohanon, 1986]).

We used a caliper to measure the abdominal skinfold thickness (Harpenden Skinfold Caliper HSB-BI model, Victoria Road Burguess Hill, UK).

2.3 Assessment

Each individual was exposed to a postural stress, whose protocol was adapted from [Wolfson, 1986], being applied a forward destabilizing force at the lower trunk level with a magnitude of 4.5% of body weight.

All individuals were asked to remain upright, comfortably standing, with the base of support aligned across the width of the shoulders, upper limbs along the body, and not to take any step or elevate the heels, keeping the balance [Fiedler, 2005]. They were also given a target two meters away at eye level on which to focus [Fiedler, 2005].

No advance warning of the impending perturbation was provided; instead the subjects wore earphones and listened to music delivered via a mini audio player. A forward destabilizing force was applied, maintained for at least three seconds and subsequently eliminated instantaneously. Each subject performed three repetitions of the procedure.

We evaluated the electromyographic activity (EMGa) of TA, MG, RF, BF, RA and ES muscles at predetermined intervals. The integral of the EMGa during the procedure was analyzed in two epochs, each of 150 ms duration in relation to the time of application of the destabilizing force, herein designated by "time zero" (T0). The time windows for the two epochs were the following: 1) from −100 ms to +50 ms (Compensatory Postural Adjustments 1 (CPA1)) and 2) from +200 ms to 350 ms (late Compensatory Postural Adjustments (CPA2)). The window of CPA was chosen based on the literature data regarding the time of corrective responses observed in the trunk and leg muscles following external perturbations, see, for example, [Henry, 1998], and following the protocol described in [Santos, 2009]. This interval was divided in two epochs to differentiate reflex responses (CPA1) from voluntary reactions (CPA2) [Latash, 2008].

The EMGa integral, Int_{EMGi} for each epoch was subsequently corrected by the EMG integral of the baseline activity from −500 ms and −450 ms in relation to T0:

$$Int_{EMGi} = \int_{twi} EMG - \int_{-500}^{-450} EMG \quad (1)$$

The Int_{EMGi} within each 150 ms epoch twi, i = 1, 2, and $\int_{-500}^{-450} EMG$ is the 50 ms of the EMG baseline activity defined as the integral of EMG signal from −500 ms to −450 ms in relation to T0 [Aruin, 1995a; Santos, 2009].

The Standard Deviation (SD) and maximum peak-to-peak amplitude (CoPmax) of displacement of the CoP for each interval of 150 ms was calculated and corrected for baseline values between −500 ms and −450 ms. The time durations for each interval for the CoP were similar to those used to calculate the Int_{EMGi}. However, they were shifted 50 ms forward for each epoch to account for the electromechanical delay [Cavanagh, 1979; Howatson, 2008]. This resulted in the following intervals: (1) +100 a 250 ms (CPA1); (2) +250 a 400 ms (CPA2).

2.4 Statistics

The data were processed using the Statistic Package Social Science (SPSS Inc., an IBM Company Headquarters, 233 USA) version 13.0. The sample characterization was performed using descriptive statistics.

The Wilcoxon test was used to examine the influence of using an unstable shoe on the degree of muscle activity recruited after the application of an external perturbation, and the T-test for paired samples was used to analyze the same influence on the parameters for the CoP. For inferential analysis, a statistical significance of 0.05 was adopted.

3 RESULTS

Tables 1 and 2 show mean values, SD, maximum and minimum EMGa integral of TA, MG, RF, BF, RA

Table 1. Mean values, SD, maximum (Max.) and minimum (Min.) EMGa integral of TA, MG, RF, BF, RA and ES muscles, measured with and without MBT shoes during CPA1.

Muscles	Series	Mean	SD	Max.	Min.
TA	Barefoot	0.00005	0.000039	0.00015	0.000001
	MBT	0.00008	0.00009	0.00038	0.000019
MG	Barefoot	0.00011	0.000063	0.00015	0.000001
	MBT	0.00049	0.000080	0.00300	0.000087
RF	Barefoot	0.00001	0.000008	0.00003	0.000006
	MBT	0.000003	0.000004	0.00017	0.000007
BF	Barefoot	0.00002	0.000037	0.00015	0.000007
	MBT	0.00003	0.000040	0.00017	0.000007
RA	Barefoot	0.00001	0.000007	0.00003	0.000005
	MBT	0.00002	0.000023	0.00008	0.000005
ES	Barefoot	0.00001	0.000005	0.00002	0.000006
	MBT	0.00003	0.000044	0.00018	0.000006

Table 2. Mean values, SD, maximum (Max.) and minimum (Min). EMGa integral of TA, MG, RF, BF, RA and ES muscles, measured with and without MBT shoes during CPA2.

Muscles	Series	Mean	SD	Max.	Min.
TA	Barefoot	0.00004	0.000047	0.00019	0.000009
	MBT	0.00006	0.000077	0.00032	0.000014
MG	Barefoot	0.00010	0.000070	0.00004	0.000007
	MBT	0.00040	0.000680	0.00257	0.000085
RF	Barefoot	0.00001	0.000008	0.00004	0.000007
	MBT	0.00003	0.000038	0.00015	0.000007
BF	Barefoot	0.00002	0.000025	0.00010	0.000006
	MBT	0.00003	0.000038	0.00014	0.000008
RA	Barefoot	0.00001	0.000001	0.00001	0.000005
	MBT	0.00001	0.000020	0.00008	0.000005
ES	Barefoot	0.00001	0.000006	0.00003	0.000007
	MBT	0.00003	0.000039	0.00015	0.000007

and ES muscles, obtained in the standing position after the application of an external perturbation, with and without MBT shoes. Both for CPA1 and CPA2, the Wilcoxon test has shown statistically significant differences between measurements obtained with and without the shoes in MG muscle activity, Table 3.

When analyzing the displacement of the CoP (SD and CoPmax) following the application of an external perturbation, it can be seen that, both in terms of SD and CoPmax, there was an increase in the CoP displacement in the series performed with MBT shoes, Figures 1 and 2. However, the results obtained after applying the T-test for paired samples showed no evidence of statistically

Table 3. P values obtained using the Wilcoxon test to compare muscle activity between measurements taken with and without MBT shoes, during CPA1 and CPA2.

Muscles		Time window	P value	Time window	P value
TA	Barefoot MBT		0.221		0.245
MG	Barefoot MBT		0.001		0.008
RF	Barefoot MBT	CPA1	0.551	CPA2	0.572
BF	Barefoot MBT		0.331		0.064
RA	Barefoot MBT		0.660		0.346
ES	Barefoot MBT		0.245		0.173

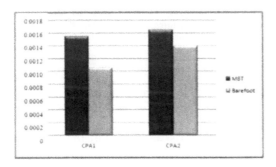

Figure 1. SD of CoP displacement after the application of an external perturbation with unstable shoes (MBT) and without shoes (Barefoot).

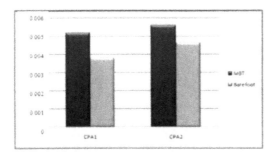

Figure 2. CoPmax displacement after the application of an external perturbation with unstable shoes (MBT) and without shoes (Barefoot).

significant differences in these two variables, with and without MBT shoes (PCA1, p = 0.315 (SD), p = 0.331 (CoPmax); PCA2, p = 0.712 (SD), p = 0.650 (CoPmax)).

4 DISCUSSION

The results of this study show that when using MBT shoes there is higher muscle activity during CPA (CPA1, CPA2). According to [Santos, 2009], there is a relationship between APA and CPA in the control of posture and the possibility of optimal use of CPA in postural control. These findings are supported by several previous observations. Firstly, the EMGa of the trunk and leg muscles during CPA may be associated with a failure in APA, as was observed in children [Hadders-Algra, 2005; van der Fits, 1998] and in individuals with neurological damage [Bazalgette, 1987]. Moreover, as already mentioned, APA are mitigated in situations of postural instability [Arruin, 1998]. Thus, in this case, compensatory muscle activity becomes necessary to maintain body equilibrium.

In terms of CPA, this study has shown an increase in activity only in the MG muscle when using unstable shoes. According to [Ivanenko, 1997], when standing on an unstable support base, the CM deviation is accompanied by changes in ankle and plantar pressure distribution, which is compensated by tricepssurae muscle activation. When standing on a movable platform, the postural pattern regulation is slightly different: usually humans do not move the CM, shifting instead the point of contact of the rocking platform with the ground under the CM, which leads to an increased need for MG activation.

While analyzing the anteroposterior Cop displacement, no differences were found in SD and CoPmax during CPA, with and without the use of unstable footwear. The values of the CoP anteroposterior displacement did not correlate with changes in MG.

According to [Shumway-Cook, 2003], the time needed to stabilize the CoP is a variable to take into account during postural adjustments. Thus, although there were no changes in terms of SD and CoPmax displacement, there might have been differences in the time needed to stabilize the CoP. Thus, it is suggested as future work to monitor this variable in order to ascertain whether it may relate to changes in MG activity during CPA.

5 CONCLUSION

The use of unstable footwear leads to an increase in muscle activity recruited by the medial gastrocnemius muscle during compensatory postural adjustments. Additionally, no differences were observed in the tibialis anterior, rectus femoris, biceps femoris, rectus abdominis and erector spinae muscles after the application of an external perturbation. Finally, the use of unstable footwear did not imply an increase in anteroposterior center of pressure displacement, both in terms of standard deviation and peak-to-peak amplitude in compensatory postural adjustments after the application of an external perturbation.

ACKNOWLEDGEMENTS

This work was supported in part by PROTEC, SFRH/BD/50050/2009.

REFERENCES

Alexandrov, A.V., Frolov, A.A., Horak, F.B., Carlson-Kuhta, P. & Park, S. 2005. Feedback equilibrium control during human standing. *Biological Cybernetics* 93: 309–322.

Arruin, A.S., Forrest, W.R. & Latash, M.L. 1998. Anticipatory postural adjustments in conditions of postural instability. *Electroencephalography and Clinical Neurophysiology* 109(4): 350–359.

Aruin, A.S. & Larash, M.L. 1995a. The role of motor action in anticipatory postural adjustments studied with self-induced and externally triggered perturbations. *Experimental Brain Research* 106: 291–300.

Aruin, A.S. & Latash, M.L. 1995b. Directional specificity of postural muscles in feed-forward postural reactions during fast voluntary arm movements. *Experimental Brain Research* 103: 323–332.

Bahr, R., Lian, O. & Bahr, L.A. 1997. A twofold reduction in the incidence of acute ankle sprains in volleyball after the introduction of an injury prevention program: a prospective cohort study. *Scandinavian Journal of Medicine and Science in Sports* 7: 172–177.

Bazalgette, D., Zattara, M., Bathien, N., Bouisset, S. & Rondot, P. 1987. Postural adjustments associated with rapid voluntary arm movements in patients with Parkinson's disease. *Advanced Neurology* 45: 371–374.

Belenkiy, V., Gurfinkel, V. & Pal'tsev, Y. 1967. Elements of control of voluntary movements. *Biofizika* 10: 135–141.

Bohanon, RW. 1986. Test–retest reliability of hand-held dynamometry during a single session of strength assessment. *Physical Therapy* 66(2): 206–209.

Caraffa, A., Cerulli, G., Projetti, M., Aisa, G. & Rizzo, A. 1996. Prevention of anterior cruciate ligament injuries in soccer. A prospective controlled study of proprioceptive training. *Knee surgery, Sports Traumatology, Arthroscopy* 4: 19–21.

Cavanagh, P.R. & Komi, P.V. 1979. Electromechanical delay in human skeletal muscle under concentric and eccentric contractions. *European Journal of Applied Physiology* 24(3): 159–163.

Fiedler, A., Haddad, J.M., Gagnon J.L., Van Emmerik, R.V. & Hamill, J. (2005). *Postural control strategies in dancers and non dancers.* Paper presented at the International Society of Biomechanics in Sports.

Hadders-Algra, M. 2005. Development of postural control during the first 18 months of life. *Neural Plasticity* 12(2–3): 99–108.

Hanke, A. & Rogers, W. 1992. Reliability of ground reaction force measurements during dynamic transitions from bipedal to single-limb stance in healthy adults *Physical Therapy* 72(11): 810–816.

Henry, S.M., Fung, J. & Horak, F.B. 1998. EMG responses to maintain stance during multidirectional surface translations. *Journal of Neurophysiology* 80(4): 1939–1950.

Horak, F.B. 1987. Clinical measurement of postural control in adults. *Physical Therapy* 67(12): 1881–1885.

Howatson, G., Glaister, M., Brouner, J. & van Someren, K.A. 2008. The reliability of electromechanical delay and torque during isometric and concentric isokinetic contractions. *Journal of Electromyography and Kinesiology*.

Ivanenko, Y.P., Levik, Y.S., Talis, V.L. & Gurfinkel, V.S. 1997. Human equilibrium on unstable support: the importance of feet-support interaction. *Neuroscience Letters* 235: 109–112.

Keating, J.L. & Matyas, T.A. 1996. The influence of subjsct and test design on dynamometry measurements of extremity muscles. *Physical Therapy* 76(8): 866–889.

Latash, M.L. (2008). *Neurophysiological basis of movement* (second ed.). Champaign: Human Kinetics.

Li, X. & Aruin, A.S. 2007. The effect of short-term changes in the body mass on anticipatory postural adjustments. *Experimental Brain Research* 181: 333–346.

Lord, SR., Ward, J.A., Williams, P. & Anstey, J. 1994. Physiological factors associated with falls in older community-dwelling women. *Journal of American Geriatric Association* 42: 1110–1117.

Massion, J. 1992. Movement, posture and equilibrium: interaction and coordination. *Progress in Neurobiology* 38: 35–56.

Massion, J. 1994. Postural Control System. *Current Opinion in Neurophysiology* 4: 877–887.

Mergner, T. & Rosemeier, T. 1998. Interaction of vestibular, somatosensory and visual signals for postural control under terrestrial and microgravity conditions: a conceptual model. *Brain Research Review*: 118–135.

Park, S., Horak, F.B. & Kuo, A.D. 2004. Postural feedback responses scle with biomechanical constraints in human standing. *Experimental Brain Research* 154: 417–427.

Ramstrand, N., Thuesen, A.H., Nielsen, D.B. & Rusaw, D. 2010. Effects of an unstable shoe construction on balance in women aged over 50 years. *Clinical Biomechanics*.

Santos, M.J., Aruin, A., Kanekar, N. & Aruin, A.S. 2009. The role of anticipatory postural adjustments in compensatory control of posture: 1. Electromyographic analysis. *Journal of Electromyography and Kinesiology*.

Shumway-Cook, A., Hutchinson, S., Kartin, D., Price, M. & Woolacott, M. 2003. Effect of balance training on recovery of stability in children with cerebral palsy. *Developmental Medicine and Child Neurology* 45: 591–602.

Soderberg, G. & Knutson, L. 2000. A Guide for Use and Interpretation of Kinesiologic Electromyographic Data. *Physical Therapy* 80(5): 485–498.

Tinetti, M.E., Speddchlev, M. & Ginter, S.F. 1988. Risk factors for falls among eldery persons living in the community. *New England Journal of Medicine* 319: 1701–1707.

van der Fits, I.B., Klip, A.W., van Eykern, L.A. & Hadders-Algra, M. 1998. Postural adjustments accompanying fast pointing movements in standing, sitting and lying adults. *Experimental Brain Research* 120(2): 202–216.

Wedderkopp, N., Kaltoft, M., Lundgaard, B., Rosendahl, M. & Froberg, K. 1999. Prevention of injuries in young female players in European team handball. A prospective intervention study. *Scandinavian Journal of Medicine and Science in Sports* 9: 41–47.

Wester, J.U., Jesperson, S.M., Nielsen, K.D. & Neumann, L. 1996. Wobble board training after partial sprains of the lateral ligaments of the ankle: a prospective randomized study. *Journal of Orthopaedics and Physical Therapy* 23: 332–336.

Wolfson, L.I. Whipple, R. Amerman, P. et al. 1986. Stressing the postural response: a quantitative method for testing balance. *Journal of American Geriatric Society* 34: 845–850.

Technology and Medical Sciences – Natal Jorge et al. (eds)
© *2011 Taylor & Francis Group, London, ISBN 978-0-415-66822-4*

The use of muscle recruitment algorithms to better assess problems for children with gait deficiency

M. Voinescu
Politehnica University of Timisoara, Timisoara, Romania

D.P. Soares & M.P. Castro
Faculty of Sports, University of Porto, Porto, Portugal

A.T. Marques & R.M. Natal Jorge
Faculdade de Engenharia da, Universidade do Porto, Porto, Portugal

ABSTRACT: Gait deficiencies are usually determined based on simpler mathematical models that are meant to virtually reconstruct the experiment that the data was taken from. This assessment is usually faster to make, but has the disadvantage of being somewhat lacking in depth and usually the muscles on the body are either not present in the model or they are highly simplified. This work proposes the use of the advanced musculoskeletal modeling software AnyBody® to further understand the mechanical elements in human gait. A 2.5 year old girl with birth malformation and a healthy child of the same age were investigated. The analysis provided detailed data regarding the angles of the different body elements during the motion together with information related to the forces and moments that act on the joints in order to perform the movement. Further conclusions can be reached upon analyzing the extracted data.

1 INTRODUCTION

The determination of forces and moments in lower limb has been the purpose of many studies. The inverse dynamics approach is one of the most used methods for this goal, considering that is not invasive and allows the analysis of different skills like gait and running. Even though, it has the disadvantage of being somewhat lacking in depth and usually the muscles on the body are either not present in the model or they are highly simplified.

Prosthetics and Orthotics are devices that are used to substitute or help parts of the body to improve their lack of movement. The prosthetics still present a pattern of movement further from a normal gait, with high asymmetry (Nolan et al., 2001) and a higher metabolic cost (Schmalz et al., 2002).

The study of the parameters that influence the gait with deficiencies, namely the mechanisms that are associated with the pattern and the muscle efforts involved, could help in the building of prosthesis and orthotics that allows an improvement in the quality of life of this population. Of the works presented on the literature only a few analyze the deficient gait in a tridimensional approach, reinforcing the importance of this kind of studies.

Considering this, the purpose of this study is to use musculoskeletal modeling software AnyBody® to further understand the mechanical elements in human abnormal gait, and apply the results in a case study of a child with deficiencies in gait pattern.

When conducting such a study, care must be taken regarding the fact that children under the age of 3 have still to achievemature gait and will tend to have more ankle dorsiflexion during stance and greater knee flexion (Sutherland et al., 1988).

2 METHODS

The children used for this case study were a 2.5 year old girl that had birth malformations in both legs. Namely she had missing ligaments in the right knee and the knee was subsequently rigidized using an orthotics specifically developed, in a way that did not allow the hyperextension during gait. In the left leg, she had a malformation similar to a below knee amputation. The left leg was also very rigid since the child had a prosthetic device that allowed no flexion of the knee and a rigid foot. The second subject was a young boy of similar age that had no deformities and no limitation in gait pattern.

Both children were asked to walk on an 8 m walkway and pass over a Kistler® force plate (1000 Hz) while wearing their own shoes at a self selected speed. The markers used to collect the motion data were 15 in number and based on the protocol described by Vaughan *et al.*, (2002) and the data was registered using 3 synchronized high speed cameras (50 Hz).

The synchronization of the kinematic and kinetic variables was achieved using a MATLAB® routine that was developed to facilitate the exporting of experimental data into the AnyBody® modeling system. The application can be used to interpolate additional values in the coordinate strings for each of the markers and allow a much smoother motion for the 3d reconstruction. The MATLAB® routine is also used to obtain the COP displacement during gait. This determination is based on a Kistler® force plate formula found in literature and also takes into account the depth of the force platform sensors (Vaughan, 1999).

Another feature of the routine is the capacity to export the synchronized data directly into Any-Body® modeling software format, what faster the overall process. The starting point for this particular application was the GaitUniMiamiTD® model that is provided with the version 1.0 of the repository from Aalborg technology (Horsman, 2007). The application was altered to suit the experimental data, namely one force plate, different marker configuration and a different file for applying the ground reaction forces.

The virtual child model was based on the anthropometric data taken from the two subjects and was scaled down to suit the needs.

The variables analyzed were the ankle, knee and hip moments and range of motion in the major three planes of movement. As it is a comparison between two subjects, only descriptive analysis was made, not using any statistical procedure.

3 RESULTS

3.1 *Ground reaction forces*

The reaction forces show a similar stance on both legs in the case of the child with malformations, this is due to the fact that the bilateral rigidization of the knees severely limits the motion and the body has to cope with this by extending the motion of the hip and not flexing the ankle so much.

3.2 *Joint moments*

Figure 2 shows the moments in the ankle (A) in the knee (B) and in the hip joint (C) in the sagital plane for the normal gait, sound limb and amputee limb.

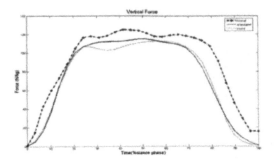

Figure 1. Resultant ground reaction forces from the force platform in the three conditions analyzed.

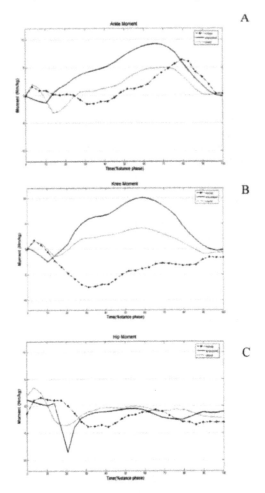

Figure 2. A, B, C: MA, MK, MH in sagital plane. Positive values are clockwise internal moments.

The MA in normal gait and sound limb show a dorsiflexion moment in the beginning of stance phase due to the control in placing the foot in the ground. As expected, the moment charts were

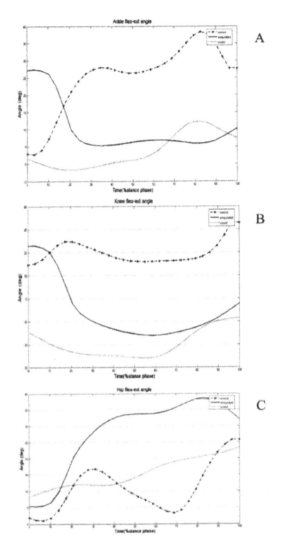

Figure 3. A, B, C: Angle values for the motion in the ankle, knee and hip joint. Positive is clockwise movement.

similar in shape due to the fact that the knees had little mobility if any and the child had to adapt to using the hip for locomotion and help from the ankle where the ankle was present.

The ankle moment pattern was different from that of an adult for both children, but this can be explained by the fact that children this young are still learning to properly balance themselves during walking, so in the first phase of the movement the child tries to get extra equilibrium and only after achieving this, does the second phase of the motion, the roll and toe off, begin (Fig. 2A). Similar shapes of this curve are present in both

the case of the normal child and in the child with disabilities, for the leg with intact ankle.

The larger values of the moment in ankle for the case of the amputee can be explained by the fact that she needs to displace as much force as possible in order to keep the balance and be able to completely swing the body forward. The motion recorded being very energetic on this part.

The knee moment charts for the child with birth malformation were similar in shape for each leg but completely opposite to those of the normal child. This is due to the hyperextension of the knee, since in one knee there are ligaments missing and the body has to rely on an external device to achieve stability. The situation is similar for the second leg with the transtibial amputation, and the body has to perform a flexor moment in the joint in order for any kind of motion to be possible in this situation.

The hip joint is responsible for most of the motion in the case of the child with malformation but the forward motion is similar to that of the normal child, suggesting that a partial recovery of a more correct posture would be possible with a device that can limit the knee joint motion to a more natural one.

ACKNOWLEDGEMENT

This work was partially supported by the strategic grant POSDRU 6/1.5/S/13, Project ID6998 (2008), co-financed by the European Social Fund—Investing in People, within the Sectoral Operational Programme Human Resources Development 2007–2013.

REFERENCES

Horsman, K. (2007). The Twente Lower Extremity Model, http://doc.utwente.nl/58231/1/thesis_Klein_Horsman.pdf

Nolan, L., Wit, A., Dudzinski, K., Lees, A., Lake, M. & Wychowanski, M. Adjustments in gait symmetry with walking speed in trans-femoral and transtibial amputees, 2002.

Schmalz, T., Blumentritt, S. & Jarasch, R. Energy expenditure and biomechanical characteristics of lower limb amputee gait: The influence of prosthetic alignment and different prosthetic components, 2002.

Sutherland, DH., Olshen, RA., Biden, EN. & Wyatt, MP. The development of mature walking. London: Mac Keith Press, 1988.

Vaughan, C., Davis, B. & O'Connor, J. (1999). Dynamics of human gait, Kiboho Publishers, 0-620-23558-6, Cape Town, South Africa.

Vaughan, K. (1999). Extracting force plate information from C3D, http://isbweb.org/software/movanal/vaughan/kistler.pdf

Technology and Medical Sciences – Natal Jorge et al. (eds)
© *2011 Taylor & Francis Group, London, ISBN 978-0-415-66822-4*

Using an Infra-red sensor to measure the dynamic behaviour of N_2O gas escaping through different sized holes

A.P. Slade, D. Convales & J. Vorstius
Medical Engineering Research Institute, University of Dundee, Dundee, Scotland

G. Thomson
Engineering and Applied Science, Aston University, Aston Triangle, Birmingham, UK

ABSTRACT: An anastomosis is a surgical procedure that consists of the connection of two parts of an organ and is commonly required in cases of colorectal cancer. About 80% of the patients diagnosed with this problem require surgery. The malignant tissue located on the gastrointestinal track must be resected and the most common procedure adopted is the anastomosis. Therefore, an anastomotic leak represents a significant problem and increases the duration of hospital stay, which is associated with remedial treatment and recovery, causing, as a result, a negative financial impact.

A number of techniques to treat, prevent and even detect an anastomotic leakage are under investigation. However, studies show that these techniques are not always able to prevent an anastomotic leak from occurring.

This paper discusses the monitoring of leakage through differently sized and differently positioned leak holes in phantom colons, using physical experiments and a Computational Fluid Dynamics package called FloWorks.

1 INTRODUCTION

An anastomosis is a surgical procedure that consists of the connection of two parts of an organ, and is commonly required in cases of colorectal cancer where 80% of the patients diagnosed with this condition require surgery (Scholefield & Steele 2002). The malignant tissue located on the gastrointestinal track must be resected and the most common procedure adopted is the anastomosis (Fernadez et al., 2008). Unfortunately, this procedure is not 100% effective. Studies made with 2980 patients receiving this kind of operation, showed that the leakage through the anastomosis was 5.1% (Thomson 2007). A gastroesophageal anastomotic leak after cancer resection, for example, has a mortality rate of up to 60% and significant morbidity, no matter what type of treatment is applied after it (Walker et al., 2004). A perfect anastomosis depends to a high degree on the surgeon's performance (Roy-Choudhury et al., 2001), though there is some evidence that robot-assisted may be more accurate (Fielding et al., 1980). Therefore, an anastomotic leak represents a big problem for many surgeons (Frye et al., in press). In addition to the clinical complications of leakage there are significant financial costs associated with remedial treatment and recovery (Tsereteli et al., 2008).

A number of techniques to treat, prevent and even detect an anastomotic leakage are under investigation. However, studies show that these techniques are not always able to prevent an anastomotic leak from occurring (Fernadez et al., 2008). Ways of detecting leakage have also been explored, such as applying air (Tcileppi et al., 2005; Hochberger et al., 1995) or saline (Beard et al., 1990; Royle 1993; Gilbert & Trapnell 1988) through the rectum. These methods however, faced some problems as they need to apply relatively large volumes of pressurized air or liquid via the rectum to be able to assess the integrity of the anastomosis (Fernadez et al., 2008). An alternative approach, presented in this paper uses a gas sensor and a small volume of trace gas to evaluate leakage through the anastomosis.

The selection of the trace gas and associated sensor required careful study as most gas sensors are usually made to detect dangerous gases and this project requires the use of safe gases. Several sensors for poisonous or flammable gases, such as hydrogen sulphide, ammonia, hydrogen and hydrocarbons, are easily found in the market. However, only a few are built for gases such as, helium and nitrous oxide. A problem with helium is that as a noble gas, it is hard to detect, as noble gases react to very little. Gases such as carbon dioxide and nitrous oxide are already used in surgery. Carbon Dioxide is used to inflate the abdominal cavity during laparoscopic surgery, which would make detecting any leakage of trace CO_2 difficult if the technique was applied in this type of work. Nitrous oxide by contrast is used in anesthesia, making this gas more suitable for this study.

There are two types of sensor available to detect Nitrous oxide, electrochemical or optical. As a quick and accurate answer from the sensor is necessary, optical sensors would be better suited to this application than electrochemical sensors.

This paper discusses the dynamic behavior of N_2O gas through different sized leakages as detected by an Infra-Red gas sensor and how the sensors response time changes depending on the leakage size. Tests were made experimentally and also using a Computational Fluid Dynamics (CFD) package called FloWorks which is part of the Solid Works suite of programmes. The results will be compared and discussed in this paper.

2 MATERIALS AND METHODS

2.1 Experimental

The experimental arrangement is shown in Figure 1. A box with dimensions of $115 \times 115 \times 57$ mm was used to simulate the interior part of the abdomen. The colon was represented by a sealed rigid pipe placed inside the box. A flexible pipe from the box goes to the inlet of the N_2O infra-red sensor and gas is pulled through the sensor by a pump with a flow rate of 1 L/min. An injection pipe goes through the box into the rigid tube to allow gas to be injected into the rigid pipe.

The anastomic leak was simulated by drilling small holes of 1, 2 & 3 mm diameter into the rigid tubes used to represent the colon. A 0.68 ml gelatine capsule filled with N_2O gas at a pressure of 2 bar would be placed into a syringe that was used to break the capsule and inject the gas into the pipe. After the gas was released, the sensor would detect the N_2O gas that would leak from the hole in the pipe.

The aim of these experiments was to measure the parts per million (ppm) increase of N_2O over time with the different sized holes in the pipe, and to see if there was any noticeable difference that would allow the change in gas concentration to be used to quantify the size of leak in the pipe.

3 COMPUTATIONAL

For the computational analysis, Solid Works was used to generate a model of the actual physical experiment. FloWorks (included in Solid Works) was used to simulate the gas flow in the model and to calculate the ppm increase. FloWorks uses conservation laws (Navier-Stokes equations) to calculate the air flows.

To replicate the same conditions used in the experimental tests, it was necessary to use a fan with a flow rate of 1 l/mim because pumps are not included in the software toolbox. The box was filled with air at atmospheric pressure, 101325 Pa, at a temperature of 293.2 K. The CAD model used for the computational simulations is shown in Figure 2.

4 RESULTS AND DISCUSSIONS

For both the physical and computational experiments the analyses were performed for three different sized holes (1, 2 & 3 mm) in the pipe. In all the experiments the outlet hole was placed at the top of the pipe and the sensor to the lower right as shown in Figure 2 above. An average of the results from the physical experiments for each size of hole was compared to the computational experiment and is shown in the figures below.

To enable the software to simulate the experiment it was necessary to include a run the simulation

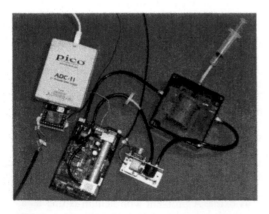

Figure 1. The experimental apparatus.

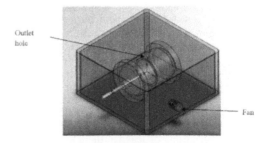

Figure 2. The CFD model.

for 5 seconds before the N_2O gas was injected into the model. Due to the length of time the simulations took to run, the experiments were limited to a period of 180 seconds.

4.1 Case 1; 1 mm hole

While at the beginning of the experiment the values of the curves differ by around 12%, after 180 seconds the values for the concentration of N_2O are only differing by around 4%. A strong similarity between the curves is shown in the first 55 seconds, but between 55 seconds and 140 seconds the computational curve varies considerably from the curve obtained by the actual experiment. Simulations with different meshes and step times were performed in an attempt to identify the reason for this unexpected result, but in all of them a similar result was observed during this time interval.

One of the possible explanations for this result is that FloWorks does not appear to break up the period of simulation into evenly spaced iterations (Dray et al., 2009). If this is true, then during the first 55 seconds the software used one number of iterations and during the next 55 seconds it would use a different number of iterations, leading to the inaccuracies shown in the graphs.

4.2 Case 2; 2 mm hole

The response time for the physical experiment in this case is faster than in the first case due to the fact that the area of the hole now is bigger allowing more gas to exit from the hole in the same time.

As in the previous case both curves present a similar behaviour with a difference of 7% up to 55 seconds, when the curves vary widely again for the interval between 55 seconds and 145 seconds with a difference of 50%, after which the curves are broadly corresponding.

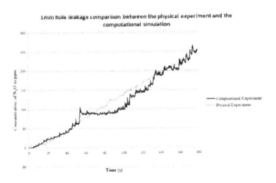

Figure 3. Comparison of results for a leakage through a 1 mm hole.

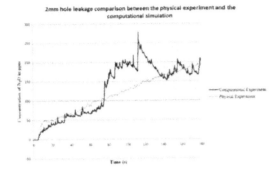

Figure 4. Comparison of results for a leakage through a 2 mm hole.

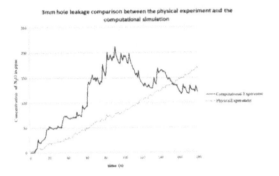

Figure 5. Comparison of results for a leakage through a 3 mm hole.

4.3 Case 3; 3 mm hole

Both curves in Figure 5 show an instantaneous response time but a big discrepancy between them over the whole period of the experiment. Again the interval between 55 seconds and 160 seconds shows the same trend in the simulation curve of measuring a high concentration than the physical experiment.

The curve for the physical experiment demonstrates a normal behaviour. Its angle and the final concentration of N_2O are smaller than the ones in Figures 3 and 4 as expected.

5 CONCLUSIONS

The consequences of a failure in the Anastomosis of the colon are serious and any steps that can be taken to reduce the likelihood of such failure must be welcomed. These tests have shown that it is possible to develop a system to detect the presence and location of a small hole in a colon analogue. The use of small quantities of a trace gas coupled to sensing technology could offer more dignified and safer methods to intra operatively test the integrity of Anastomosis than are available at present.

In all three physical experiments the curve is essentially linear over the whole time period investigated (0–180 seconds) but showing a different final value of gas concentration in the box. The FloWorks simulations do not exhibit any such correspondence between the graphs, and although the end point for the 1 and 2 mm simulations are similar to the physical experiment the end point for the 3 mm hole is 20% lower for the simulation.

It would appear that FloWorks does not break up the period of simulation into evenly spaced iterations, therefore it is difficult to make any meaningful comparison between the two methods. On balance it would appear that the results from the physical experiments are in line with what was expected.

From the results of the physical experiments it would appear that this technique is a viable one for detecting an anastomostic leakage after a surgical procedure. Further experiments are required to develop a system that could be suitable for use in a surgical situation.

In summary, this paper describes a system in which an N_2O infra-red sensor could be used to detect an anastomtic leakage immediately post surgery before final closure. Therefore avoiding the problem of further infection caused by bacteria growth at the leakage site.

ACKNOWLEDGEMENTS

The authors wish to acknowledge the support given by the Engineering & Physical Sciences Research Council to this work, under Grant ref. EP/D003040/1.

REFERENCES

Beard, J.D., Nicholson, M.L., Sayers, R.D., Lloyd, D. & Everson, N.W. Intraoperative air testing of colorectal anastomoses: a prospective, randomized trial. Brit J Surg, 77, (1990), 1095–1097.

Dray, X., Redding, S.K., Shin, E.J., Buscaglia, J.M., Giday, S.A., Wroblewski, R.J., Assumpcao, L., Krishnamurty, D.M., Magno, P. Pipitone, L.J., Marohn, M.R., Kalloo, A.N. & Kantsevoy, S.V. Hydrogen leak test is minimally invasive and highly specific for assessment of the integrity of the luminal closure after natural orifice transluminal next term endoscopic surgery procedures, Gastrointest Endosc, 69, (2009), 554–560.

Fernandez, V., Thomson, G. & Slade, A. Integrity of Colorectal Anastomosis: A Review of Technological Assets, BioMed 2008, Innsbruck, Austria, Feb 2008, 283–287.

Fielding, L.P., Stewart-Brown, S., Blesovsky, L. & Kearney, G. Anastomotic integrity after operations for large bowel cancer: A multi-centre study, Brit Med J, 281(6237), (1980), 411–414.

Frye, J., Bokey, E.L., Chapuis, P.H., Sinclair, G. & Dent, O.F. Anastomotic leakage after resection of colorectal cancer generates prodigious use of hospital resources, Colorectal Disease, Accepted for publication, DOI: 10.1111/j.1463-1318.2008.01728.x.

Gilbert, J.M. & Trapnell, J.E. "Intraoperative testing of the integrity of left-sided colorectal anastomoses: a technique of value to the surgeon in training". Ann Roy Coll Surg, 70, (1988), 158–160.

Hochberger, J., Kusch, B., Franke, F., Ell, C. & Hahn, E.G. Successful endoscopic occlusion of a postoperative anastomotic leakage using collagen fleece and fibrin glue over a variceal ligation overtube: A case report, Gastrointest Endosc, 41(4), (1995), 305.

Roy-Choudhury, S.H., Nicholson, A.A., Wedgwood, K.R., Mannion, R.A.J., Sedman, P.C., Royston, C.M.S. & Breen, D.J. Symptomatic Malignant Gastroesophageal Anastomotic Leak: Management with Covered Metallic Esophageal Stents. Am. J. Roentgenol, 176(1), (2001), 161–165.

Royle, C.A.J.P. "An inexpensive method of quality assessment in anastomosis workshops". J Royal Army Medical Corps, 139, (1993), 105–108.

Scholefield, J.H. & Steele, R.J. Guidelines for follow up after resection of colorectal cancer, Gut, 51, (2002) Supplement V; v3–5.

Scileppi, T., Li, J.J., Iswara, K. & Tenner, S. The use of a Polyflex coated esophageal stent to assist in the closure of a colonic anastomotic leak, Gastrointest Endosc, 62(4), (2005), 643–645.

Thomson, G.A. An investigation of leakage tracts along stressed suture lines in phantom tissue, Med Eng Phys 29, (2007), 1030–1034.

Tsereteli, Z., Sporn, E., Geiger, T.M., Cleveland, D., Frazier, S., Rawlings, A.S., Bachman, L. Miedema, B.W. & Thaler, K. Placement of a covered polyester stent prevents complications from a colorectal anastomotic leak and supports healing: Randomized controlled trial in a large animal model. Surgery, 144(5), (2008), 786–792.

Walker, S.W., Bell, M.J.F.X., Rickard, D., Mehanna, O.F., Dent, P.H. & Chapuis, E.L. Bokey, Anastomotic leakage is Predictive of diminished survival after potentially curative resection for colorectal cancer. Ann Surg, 240(2), (2004), 255–259.

Visual tracking of surgical instruments, application to laparoscopy

Paulo J.S. Gonçalves
Polytechnic Institute of Castelo Branco, Castelo Branco, Portugal
IDMEC/IST, Technical University of Lisbon, Lisboa, Portugal

A.M.D. Gonçalves
Polytechnic Institute of Castelo Branco, Castelo Branco, Portugal

ABSTRACT: This paper presents a study on the performance of classical visual tracking algorithms when applied to track surgical instruments in images. Successful deployment of robots in the operating room depends on its perception of the environment and the surgical instruments that the robot holds in its hand. In this study an laparoscopic training system was built and the Lucas-Kanade, Kanade-Lucas-Tomasi, and homography based, were implemented in C++ and its results compared for tracking laparoscopic instruments, e.g. a grasper. The results obtained showed that the best method is Kanade-Lucas-Tomasi, since it have showed best robustness to differences between consecutive images and consequentially less tracking points lost.

1 INTRODUCTION

In laparoscopic surgery, the instruments, e.g. graspers, scissors, cameras are operated by the surgeons in the operating room. These instruments enter the human body via a trocar. Usually there are used three trocars, two as the extension of the surgeon hand, operated by him, and another one for the camera (operated by a fellow worker). The last one is the extension of the surgeons hand. This setup have a long history of success in the Operation Room (OR).

In recent years, robots are been increasingly applied in the OR to help the surgeons in surgical tasks (Casals, et al. 2009). The main goal with robot usage is to improve the accuracy of the tasks and in some times, to perform the surgery in a remote location by tele-operation. Since the robot is performing surgical tasks, the overall system must have visual sensors in order to the robot have feedback of the work environment.

In laparoscopic surgery, the work environment is the human body with the introduction os the laparoscopic instruments. So the robot must be able to identify the instruments and the region to operate, in order to perform the task. This is the main goal of the paper, to identify and track the laparoscopic instruments. For that an experimental setup was developed, an acrylic box, with a camera, two trocars and two laparoscopic graspers. The camera can capture images of the work environment and a laptop was used to implement the tracking algorithms, to track the two instruments.

In this paper is presented a study on three tracking algorithms: Lucas-Kanade, Kanade-Lucas-Tomasi, and a homography based method (ESM). These methods are applied to track the laparoscopic graspers. The output of this study is to obtain some insight on the methods and to define which is best for the application at hand, laparoscopic surgery.

This paper is organized as follows. Section 2 describes briefly the three visual tracking methods. Section 3 describes the experimental setup and presents the obtained results, where arc also discussed. Finally, Section 4 presents the conclusions and the future work.

2 VISUAL TRACKING

This section presents three tracking algorithms: Lucas-Kanade, Kanade-Lucas-Tomasi, and a homography based method (ESM).

2.1 Lucas-Kanade

The goal of the original paper of the algorithm (Lucas and Kanade 1981), (Baker and Matthews 2004) is to align a template image $T(x,y)$ with an input image $I(x,y)$, where x and y are the image pixel coordinates. When $I(x,y)$ is a subimage of the initial image, the tracking can be faster.

Considering a set of allowable warps $W(X;P)$, where $X = [x,y]^T$ and $P = [p_x,p_y]^T$. The later is a set of parameters used for translations:

$$W(X;P) = \begin{pmatrix} x + p_x \\ y + p_y \end{pmatrix} \tag{1}$$

The best alignment is obtained by the minimization of the dissimilarity measure:

$$D = \sum_x \left[I(W(X;P)) - T(X) \right]^2 \tag{2}$$

This measure is non-linear because the pixels relations for both images (T and I) are generally non-linear.

It is assumed that some P is known and best increment ΔP is sought. Then the modified problem arises:

$$D = \sum_x \left[I(W(X;P + \Delta P)) - T(X) \right]^2 \tag{3}$$

and is solved regarding to ΔP. When it is found, then P is updated by:

$$P \leftarrow P + \Delta P \tag{4}$$

Equation 2 can be linearized using the first order Taylor series expansion:

$$D \approx \sum_X \left[I(W(X;P)) + \nabla I \frac{\partial W}{\partial P} \Delta P - T(X) \right]^2 \tag{5}$$

where ∇I is the gradient of the image and $\partial W/\partial P$ is the jacobian of the warp. Since the unknown is ΔP, equation 5 must be derived to obtain its minimum. Setting the obtained equality to zero the unknown is obtained by:

$$\Delta P = H^{-1} \sum_x \left[\nabla I \frac{\partial W}{\partial P} \right]^T \left[T(x) - I(W(X;P)) \right] \tag{6}$$

where H is the Hessian matrix:

$$H = \sum_x \left[\nabla I \frac{\partial W}{\partial P} \right]^T \left[\nabla I \frac{\partial W}{\partial P} \right] \tag{7}$$

The Lucas-Kanade algorithm have the following steps:

1. warp $I(X)$ with $W(X; P)$
2. warp the gradient ∇I with $W(X; P)$
3. evaluate the jacobian $\partial W/\partial P$ at $(X;P)$ and the compute the steepest descent image $\nabla I \, \partial W/\partial P$

4. compute the hessian matrix H
5. compute ΔP
6. update the parameters $P \leftarrow P + \Delta P$

The algorithm ends when the following condition is satisfied:

$$\| \Delta P \| \leq \varepsilon \tag{8}$$

where ε is a user predefined threshold.

Assuming n warping parameters and N pixels in the template image $T(x, y)$, the computational effort of the Lucas-Kanade algorithm is $O(n^2 N + n^3)$.

2.2 Kanade-Lucas-Tomasi

(Shi and Tomasi 1994), have proposed a new definition of the dissimilarity measure defined in equation 2, between the images T and I.

$$D = \iint \left[I\left(X + \frac{P}{2}\right) - T\left(X - \frac{P}{2}\right) \right]^2 \omega(X) dX \tag{9}$$

where usually $\omega(X)$ is set to 1. The difference between equation 2 and equation is that the term $\left[I(X + P/2) - T(X - P/2) \right]$ makes the previous term $[I(W(X; P + \Delta P)) - T(X)]$ now symmetric to both images.

When applying the same methodology used in the Lucas-Kanade pioneer work, described previously, to find the new displacement ΔP is used the following expression:

$$\Delta P = \iint [I(X) - T(X)] g(X) \omega(X) dX \tag{10}$$

where $g(X) = \left[\frac{\partial}{\partial x}\left(\frac{I+T}{2}\right) \frac{\partial}{\partial y}\left(\frac{I+T}{2}\right) \right]^T$

2.3 Homography based

The method proposed in (Benhimane and Malis 2007) is based in an efficient real-time homography estimation and template based tracking. This approach is suitable for high inter-frame displacements. The algorithm is named Efficient Second-order Minimization, ESM, and is suited for tracking planar targets in the environment.

An overview of the method is depicted in Figure 1, that was designed to track a pattern in a sequence of images containing it. The output of the method is the homography that relates the reference pattern to the reprojected current pattern, using the actual homography. The ESM method starts with an initial prediction of the homography, if none is available then the identity matrix is used. The method then minimizes the Sum of Squared Differences (SSD) between the reference pattern T and the actual pattern W reprojected

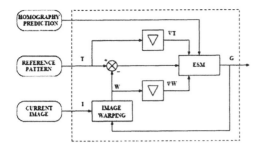

Figure 1. ESM method overview.

using the captured current homography. Both its derivates, ∇T and ∇W are calculated to obtain a second order update. A detailed description of the tracking method can be found in (Benhimane and Malis 2007).

3 EXPERIMENTAL RESULTS

3.1 *Experimental setup*

The experimental setup for simulating/training laparoscopic surgery was built on the lab and is depicted in Figure 2. It is an acrilic box with two trocars that are placed in a light brown leather. On the top is placed a laptop for the operator (surgeon) to see inside the box. The webcam that captures the images is below the laptop, not seen in the picture. The laparoscopic instruments used are two graspers, that the three methods must track. The methods were implemented in C++ on the laptop, using the OpenCV library, in Microsoft Visual Studio for Windows. The two graspers have a yellow marker to increase the contrast on the part of the image to be tracked. This fact decreases the probability of each method to lose tracking points, and is also a common procedure during surgery.

3.2. *Tracking results*

For both the Lucas-Kanade and Kanade-Lucas-Tomasi methods, the initial points were set manually by the operator close to the yellow marker.

The Lucas-Kanade method was tested in dozens of image sequences and the points were not lost during the tracking if the image differences were not very large. An example of the points (in red) tracked in one grasper is depicted in Figure 3.

The Kanade-Lucas-Tomasi method can track the points with larger image differences than lucas-kanade. The points tracked are shown in red in Figure 4. The four images presented show that the laparoscopic grasper have a large number of red points attached, stating that the instrument is

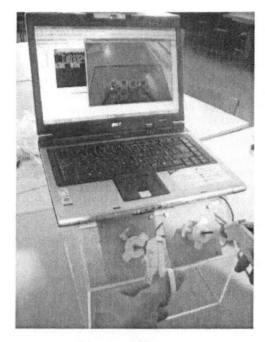

Figure 2. Laparoscopic training system.

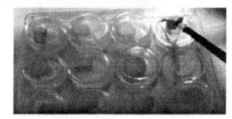

Figure 3. Tracking results for the Lucas-Kanade method. Example image.

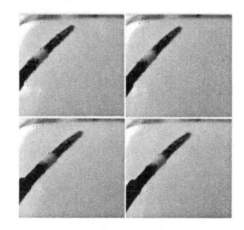

Figure 4. Tracking results for the Kanade-Lucas-Tomasi method. Top left image, the first frame. Bottom right, the last frame.

correctly tracked. This experiment was replicated a dozen of times with the same good results, including quick movements.

The ESM method was applied with no initialization of the homography matrix, so the identity matrix was used as described in the original paper. Although the method is suitable to planar targets, the results obtained in the laparoscopic graspers were very good. Only in few experiments the tracking of the pattern, depicted in Figure 5, was lost. In Figure 6 the six images show the tracking of the pattern that is no longer a square, as expected for a planar object, although the method can track the grasper. The method should be extended to the case where the object is not planar for more precise results, and without losing the grasper. In this setup the object is cylindrical.

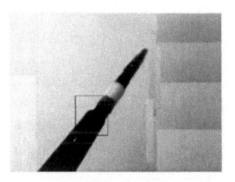

Figure 5. Pattern to track by the ESM method, inside the square in the image center.

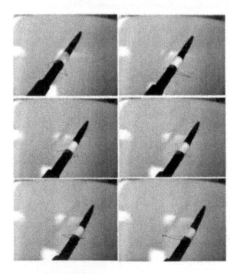

Figure 6. Tracking results for the ESM method. Top left image, the first frame. Bottom right, the last frame.

4 CONCLUSIONS

This paper presents a study on three tracking algorithms: Lucas-Kanade, Kanade-Lucas-Tomasi, and a homography based method (ESM). These methods were applied to track a laparoscopic grasper in a specially developed experimental setup. The strengths and weaknesses of each method, when applied to track a laparoscopic grasper were discussed in the paper. The output of this study was to obtain some insight on the methods and to define which is best for the application at hand, laparoscopic surgery.

From the three methods studied, the Kanade-Lucas-Tomasi is the best suited for tracking the grasper, a cylindrical object. Its superior robustness to abrupt changes between consecutive images of the object lead to this conclusion, when compared with the classical Lucas-Kanade. The ESM method can track the grasper but with less accuracy and often loses the object, which is not planar. This method has excellent results with planar objects and with considerable changes between consecutive images.

To improve the tracking of the laparoscopic grasper, the ESM tracker can be developed in the future to deal with other types of objects, not only planar, like the cylindrical type of the grasper.

ACKNOWLEDGEMENTS

The authors would like to thank: the Portuguese Science Foundation, FCT, for the funding to IDMEC through the Associated Laboratory in Energy, Transports, Aeronautics and Space (LAETA); the FCT project: PTDC/EME-CRO/099333/2008.

REFERENCES

Baker, S. & Matthews, I. (2004). Lucas-Kanade 20 years on: A unifying framework. *International Journal of Computer Vision 56(3)*, 221–255.

Benhimane, S. & Malis, E. (2007). Homography-based 2d, visual tracking and servoing. *International Journal of Robotics Research 26(7)*, 661–676.

Casals, A., Frigola, M. & Amat, J. (2009). La robótica una valiosa herramienta cirugia. *Revista Iberoamericana de de Automática e Informática Industrial 6(1)*, 5–19.

Lucas, B.D. & Kanade, T. (1981). An iterative image registration technique with an application to stereo vision. In *Proceedings of the 7th International Conference on Artificial Intelligence*, pp. 674–679.

Shi, J. & Tomasi, C. (1994). Good features to track. In *IEEE Conference on Computer Vision and Pattern Recognition*, pp. 593–600.

Technology and Medical Sciences – Natal Jorge et al. (eds)
© 2011 Taylor & Francis Group, London, ISBN 978-0-415-66822-4

Wavelet analysis of the pupil's autonomic flow

G. Leal & P. Vieira
IBEB—Institute of Biophysics and Biomedical Engineering, Lisbon, Portugal
FCT/UNL—Faculty of Science and Technology, New University of Lisbon, Portugal

C. Neves
IMM—Institute of Molecular Medicine, Lisbon, Portugal

ABSTRACT: This project presents the preliminary results of the Pupillometer project, developed last year in the Institute of Molecular Medicine, in Lisbon. The Pupillometer is a stable and robust optical equipment for detecting, with high resolution, the area of the pupil and its variation on a temporal scale. It allows us to detect the pupil's oscillations, which represent the autonomic nervous system behavior, that is, the parasympathetic and sympathetic equilibrium. The Pupillometer has an algorithm developed in Matlab, which detects the pupil's properties at the output of the acquisition system (Leal *et al.*, 2009). We can thus register the variation of the pupil's area, perimeter, centroids and diameter during the period of the acquisition of data. Using the Matlab Wavelet toolbox some time-frequency analysis was made of the first results. These were obtained giving the subjects a stimulus such as a flash of light or putting their hand in a bucket of cold water. A Pupillogram, an ECG and a Pneumogram were simultaneously acquired of the subject and, during that time, the stimulus was applied. By examining the time-frequency analysis, we can see the same frequency components behavior in the subjects, but it is still too soon to be certain. Although we have not reached many results yet, we believe that in a couple of months we will have gathered more significant and interesting results.

1 INTRODUCTION

The pupil moves in response to the variation in light intensity in the retina, with a view to assisting the optimizing of visual perception. In dim light, pupil dilation (midriasis) is an effective way to maximize the number of photons reaching the retina, which in turn activates adaptive to low light intensity. When exposed to bright light, miosis causes an adequate reduction in the intensity of light in the retina, acting asimmediate response to the mechanisms of adapting to intense light (Kardon, 2003). The study of the enlarging of the pupil is of relevant clinical interest, for it acts as an objective result of the optical nerve. The permanent oscillations of the pupil are due to the balance between two opposite neural flows: the sympathetic and parasympathetic. The state of a person's pupil allows for several diseases to be diagnosed, among which sleep disturbances (narcolepsy), Alzheimer's, Adie's Syndrome, narcotic addiction, among others (Smith and Smith, 2001).

The autonomic nervous system behaves like a two oscillators model. We have the parasympathetic oscillator and the sympathetic one. These oscillators are competing with each other for predominance. This equilibrium is altered when one of these oscillators is inhibited. This phenomenon allows the other oscillator to take over. The inhibition of the sympathetic system is faster compared to the inhibition of the parasympathetic one. We can see this balance disturbed in the pupil. If we apply a light stimulus to the eye, the pupil contracts given to a superimposed central sympathetic inhibition (Heller *et al.*, 1990). Then the dilation follows, due both to the parasympathetic relaxation and also the increase of sympathetic activity.

By understanding the high frequency structure of these signals we can correlate them to other physiological activity and investigate neurological disorders.

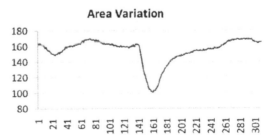

Figure 1. Example of the pupil's area variation in time. Note that the area is given in pixels². The study could be made using metric units like millimeters, but since we are measuring variation it does not really make a difference.

2 METHODS

2.1 Experimental procedure

This experiment was made with a group of subjects with no known physiological pathologies. An ECG and a Pneumogram were acquired of each subject during ten minutes in a dark room using a Powerlab equipment from AD Instruments company. After this we applied an eye anesthetic to the subject, in order to give him the ability to withstand his eye open for a long period (60 s). We then acquired a pupillogram during 60 s. The video files were acquired at the camera's maximum resolution and maximum acquisition rate, 1392 × 1040 pixels and 30.3 fps respectively. Afterwards we gave the subject an artificial tear to lubricate the eye and then we acquired a 30 s pupillogram in which we applied 2 light flashes unknown to the subject to avoid adaptability.

2.2 PCD*—Pupil Contour Detection

The pupil contour was calculated with an algorithm that preallocates all the frames of an '.avi' file and, given a threshold value, measures the pupil's area, perimeter, horizontal and vertical diameters and the coordinates of the pupil's centroid in each frame.

The algorithm removes the LED ring in a user inferface and then uses Threshold fundamentals and egde filters to measure de pupil boundaries. By acquiring the portion of interest it binarizes the image, creates a region and then calculates the dimensional values. After that it uses the wavelet toolbox functions to plot the original signal along with its frequency components. We then can correlate the acquired pupil signal with the signals acquired using the Powerlab equipment. The Powerlab application allows us to export the output ECG and Pneumogram signals to Matlab.

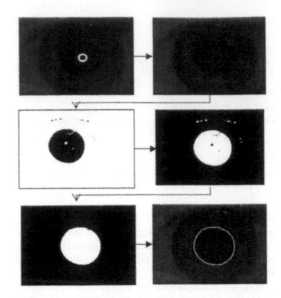

Figure 3. Detecting the pupil region. First we remove the LED ring illuminator and then we process the image to measure pupil dimensions.

For this study we present 5 examples of acquired signals below.

Table 1. Properties of the video files. Note that all video files have 60 s duration, but we only processed the region of interest. We can see four examples of signals acquired during stimulation and a signal of the basal sympathetic activity (with no stimulation applied).

Video file	Frame rate	Duration	Threshold value
Flash 1	30.3 fps	10.23 s	0,150
Flash 2	30.3 fps	8.45 s	0,300
Flash 3	30.3 fps	16.63 s	0,255
Flash 4	30.3 fps	17.98 s	0,320
Basal 1	30.3 fps	30.00 s	0,135

2.3 Wavelet analysis

Many physiological signals may be described either as isolated pulses or as quasi-periodic sequences of isolated pulses. Wavelets are a powerful tool for the representation and analysis of such physiologic waveforms because a wavelet has finite duration (compact support), as contrasted with Fourier methods based on sinusoids of infinite duration (Strang, 1994).

The frequencies of the sympathetic and parasympathetic neural flows in the pupil are unknown because this is a poorly studied topic. So, we made the time-frequency analysis using Wavelets, since we do not have to worry about which frequency windows to choose.

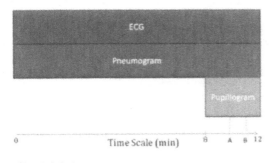

A- Direct light flash
B- Indirect light flash

Figure 2. Experimental procedure's time scale.

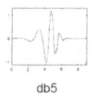

db5

Figure 4. Daubechies wavelet family of order 5 (Misiti *et al.*).

The Wavelet analysis was made using the Matlab Wavelet Toolbox. The Daubechies Wavelet family of order 5 (Figure 4 was chosen, since this family is very much used in discrete analysis studies).

The Daubechies wavelets are a family of orthogonal wavelets defining a discrete wavelet transform and characterized by a maximal number of vanishing moments for some given support. With each wavelet type of this class, there is a scaling function (also called father wavelet) which generates an orthogonal multi resolution analysis (Wikipedia, accessed 20-07-2010).

3 RESULTS

Below we can see an example of a signal acquired in which we applied a flash of light as a stimulus and an example of a signal acquired where no stimulus was applied.

The Figure 5 shows us the original signal and Figures 6 and 7 the time-frequency analysis of the video file *'flash 2.avi'*.

The Figure 8 shows us the original signal of the *'basal 1.avi'* video file and Figures 9 and 10 the time frequency analysis.

We used the Wavelet toolbox to apply a discrete Wavelet transform db5 to the original signal.

3.1 *Stimulated subjet's results*

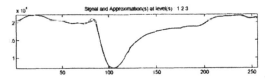

Figure 5. Original signal with the approximations 1, 2 and 3.

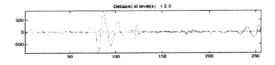

Figure 6. Details 1, 2, 3 of the three approximations.

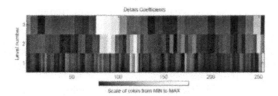

Figure 7. Coefficients of the analysis.

3.2 *Non-stimulated subjet's results*

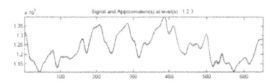

Figure 8. Original basal signal.

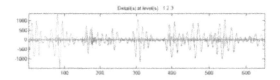

Figure 9. Details 1, 2, 3 of the three approximations.

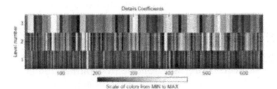

Figure 10. Coefficients of the analysis.

4 DISCUSSION

The original signals (Figures 5 and 8) shows us the area of the pupil in pixels^2 per frame. Since we are studying the pupil's variation, a conversion to millimeters is not needed.

By analyzing first the data from the subject to whom stimuli were applied (Figure 5) we see, in the beginning of the pupil contraction, that the detail 3 (d3) has maximum value (white) of scale in its frequency analysis (Figures 6 and 7). This means that this component has higher activity in this area. At the same time the detail 1 (d1) has minimum value (black). When the pupil starts to dilate, d1 takes a lower value and d3 takes max value. This behavior occurs in all the processed data, but it is better seen in Flash 1 and Flash 2. These antagonist components can be related to the autonomic activity.

Since the pupil contraction, given a light stimulus, is a response of an over imposed Sympathetic activity, we can better see the different frequency components during the application of a stimulus.

If we apply for example other stimuli, like putting the subject's hand in cold water, we can better see the parasympathetic activity since the pupil dilates.

When we analyze the basal original signal (Figure 8) we see, in detail, that the pupil oscillates even when we do not have any applied stimuli. By looking at the frequency analysis results (Figures 9 and 10) we see activation and inhibition of some frequency components.

More subjects must be tested in order to strengthen the objective that we are trying to accomplish. A better wavelet must be found and the algorithm must be enhanced in order to be more accurate and fast (like using parallel computing).

5 CONCLUSIONS

This is still a preliminary study, in order to find the frequency components of the sympathetic and parasympathetic activity in the pupil.

Possibly we will see two distinct frequency components, one faster than the other, corresponding to the Sympathetic and Parasympathetic Autonomic Nervous Systems, respectively.

We still do not know what kind of frequencies we are looking for. We are now acquiring more data and, by the time of the conference, we intend to present more accurate results and conclusions.

In the future we will apply the Pupillometer to subjects suffering from neuro-ophthalmologic disorders, so that we can infer conclusions and hopefully make the Pupillometer a diagnosis tool. That will make it possible to determine the ratio between the sympathetic and parasympathetic control systems.

We are already working in a more accurate acquisition method using "OpenCV" instead of the combination of the Camera's SDK + Matlab. In the future all the acquisition will be made in a single application designed specifically for this purpose and the aim is that it will give us results in real-time acquisition.

REFERENCES

Heller, Philip H., *et al.* "Autonomic Components of the Human Pupillary Light Reflex". *Investigative Ophthalmology & Visual Science*. Vol. 31, No.1, January 1990. 156–162.

Hohlfeld, R.G., Rajagopalan, C. and Neff, G.W. "Wavelet Signal Processing of Physiologic Waveforms". *Wavelet Technologies*, Inc., 2004.

http://en.wikipedia.org/wiki/Daubechies_wavelet. Accessed in 20-07-2010

Iacoviello, Daniela, Matteo Lucchetti. "Parametric characterization of the form of the human pupil from blurred noisy images". *Computer Methods and Programs in Biomedicine* (2005) 77, 39–48.

Iacoviello, Daniela, A. de Santis. "Optimal segmentation of pupillometric images for estimating pupil shape parameters". Computer methods and programs in biomedicine 84 (2006) 174–187.

Kardon, Randy. "Pupil". *Adler's Physiology of the Eye*. Edited by Paul L. Kaufman and Albert Alm. 10th Edition. St Louis: Mosby, 2003. 713–743.

Kaiser, Gerald. *A Friendly Guide to Wavelets*. Boston, Basel, Berlin:Birkhauser. 1994.

Klingler, Jeff, Rakshit Kumar. and Pat Hanrahan. Measuring the Task-Evoked Pupillary Response with a Remote Eye Tracker.

Leal, Gonçalo, Vieira, Pedro, Neves, Carlos. "Development of an instrument to measure pupil dynamics in subjects suffering from neuro-ophtalmological disorders". *Proceedings of the Medical Physics and Biomedical Engineering World Congress 2009*. 7–12 September 2009. Munich.

Mallat, Stéphane. *A Wavelet Tour of Signal Processing: The Sparse Way*. Third edition. Burlington: Academic Press, 2009.

Misiti, Michel, Yves Misiti, Georges Oppenheim, Jean-Michel Poggi "Wavelet Toolbox™ 4User's Guide". *The Mathworks*.

Smith, Shirley A. and Smith, S.E. "Pupil function: tests and disorders". Christopher J. Mathias and Sir Roger Bannister. *Autonomic Failure: A Textbook of Clinical Disorders of the Autonomic Nervous System*. 4th Edition Oxford: Oxford University Press, 2001.

Strang, Gilbert. "Wavelets". *American Scientist* 82. April 1994. 250–255.

Technology and Medical Sciences – Natal Jorge et al. (eds)
© 2011 Taylor & Francis Group, London, ISBN 978-0-415-66822-4

White matter segmentation in simulated MRI images using the Channeler Ant Model

E. Fiorina

Dipartimento di Fisica Sperimentale, Universita' degli Studi di Torino, Torino, Italy
Istituto Nazionale di Fisica Nucleare, Sezione di Torino, Torino, Italy

ABSTRACT: The Channeler Ant Model (CAM) is an algorithm that makes use of virtual ant colonies and exploits their natural capabilities to modify the environment by pheromone deposition and communicate with each other. The CAM is able to segment 3D structures with different shapes, intensity and background. Its performance has been validated with 3D artificial objects segmentation and its use has already started for the detection of lung nodules in CT scans. The incidence increase of Alzheimers Disease (AD) and other neurodegenerative diseases, related to the life expectancy increasing, demands more and more efforts for its early diagnosis. Therefore, it is required to analyze increasing amounts of neuroimages obtained by Magnetic Resonance (MRI) or Positron Emission Tomography (PET). The evaluation of the atrophy degree of some interesting anatomical structures and the study of the connections between different brain regions can provide lots of useful information. The CAM is a good candidate to segment the different tissues present in the brain and could help researchers, for example, to determine the degree of atrophy in the hyppocampal region, an acknowledged index of AD presence and progression.

1 INTRODUCTION

1.1 *The Simulated Brain Database*

The Simulated Brain Database is provided by the Brain Imaging Centre, Montreal Neurological Institute, McGill University and is available on-line (http://www.bic.mni.mcgillca/brainweb/). It contains a large number of brain MRI images with different noise levels (from 0% to 9%) and different bias-field levels (from 0% to 40%). The database also includes the images of the phantom used to obtain the simulated ones, in which, for each voxel the intensity is proportional to the percentage of white matter. The phantom represents a standard segmentation and can be used as a gold standard to evaluate the CAM segmentation result. In Fig. 1 one slice of a T1 images stack is compared to its gold standard, whose white voxels, at intensity 255, correspond to 100% of white matter.

1.2. *The Channeler Ant Model*

The Channeler Ant Model (CAM), described in Cerello et al. (2010), has already been successfully applied to the detection of nodules in lung CTs.

For this new application the model has been upgraded by removing the limit to the number of visits to a voxel: in this way, voxels are considered as fully reconstructed (i.e., containing 100% of white matter) when their pheromone content

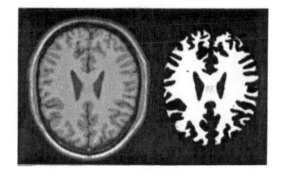

Figure 1. T1 weighted MRI image with 0% of noise and 0% of RF-bias-field and its white matter gold standard.

reaches a preset saturation threshold. After that, they become forbidden destinations.

It's important to remark the role of the pheromone deposition rule that is defined (Cerello et al. (2010)) by:

$$T = H_{Jac} \cdot \Delta_{ph} \tag{1}$$

where H_{Jac} is a constant and, together with the fixed pheromone threshold, is related to algorithm speed.

Δ_{ph} plays a crucial role in image segmentation: it represents the connection between the image intensity and the ant perception of it, it's the link between the real and the virtual world.

In Cerello et al. (2010), Δ_{ph} is given by:

$$\Delta_{ph} = I(v_j) - I_{min} \qquad (2)$$

where $I(v_j)$ is the image intensity of the voxel v_j and I_{min} is the minimum intensity of the image.

If Δ_{ph} is calculated with Eq. (2) the ant colonies segment voxels with a high intensity value: by changing the Δ_{ph} definition it's possible to segment volumes with different intensity features.

As a result of analysing the intensity distribution of the simulated brain image and of the real MRI images shown in Fig. 2, a new gaussian pheromone rule is implemented using the following Δ_{ph} definition:

$$\Delta_{ph} = I(v_j) \cdot e^{-\frac{(I(v_j)-<I>)^2}{2\sigma^2}} \qquad (3)$$

where $<I>$ and σ are the parameters calculated from the gaussian fit of the peak of the structure to segment (i.e. white matter) in the intensity distribution.

This Δ_{ph} definition makes the CAM able to segment structures with any intermediate value of intensity and not only with the highest or lowest ones.

2 METHOD

2.1 The CAM parameters

The CAM parameters and their values are the same used for the artificial objects and lung CT analysis: this is a proof of the CAM adaptability to images with different range of intensity and noise levels.

The pheromone saturation threshold is set to the value that corresponds, for both the pheromone deposition rule, to an average of about 40 visits to saturate the voxels that fully belong the white matter volume.

2.2 Data set

A portion of 15 slices in the middle of the stack of T1 weighted images with $1 \times 1 \times 1$ mm voxel dimension was considered, as in Huang et al. (2008).

3 RESULTS

3.1 Performance indicators

The sensitivity S and contamination C are defined as follows:

$$S = \frac{N_R}{N_T} \qquad (4)$$

$$C = \frac{N_{TR} - N_R}{N_T} \qquad (5)$$

N_R is the number of voxels correctly segmented by the CAM, N_{TR} the total number of segmented voxels and N_T the number of voxels that belong to the gold standard structure. Also, like in Huang et al. (2008), the Jaccard Similarity Index SI is defined:

$$SI = \frac{N_{TR} \cap N_T}{N_{TR} \cup N_T} = \frac{1+C}{S} \qquad (6)$$

3.2 Analysis

In Fig. 3 the pheromone maps obtained by CAM segmentation with both of pheromone deposition rules compared to gold standard are shown. Voxels with pheromone saturated to the fixed value are represented in black. The results obtained with different Δ_{ph} definition are comparable and also the graphs of the number of ants per cycle show the same (Fig. 4).

To obtain the white matter segmentation, the pheromone map must be analysed.

a.
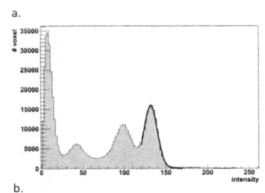
b.
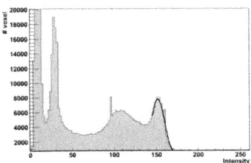

Figure 2. a. The intensity distribution of simulated brain images with 5% of noise and 0% of RF-bias with the gaussian fit of white matter peak; b. The intensity distribution of real MRI images with the gaussian fit of white matter peak.

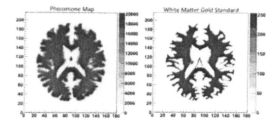

Figure 3. Pheromone map for an image with 0% of noise and 0% of RF-bias-field and the related gold standard (high intensity pheromone deposition rule).

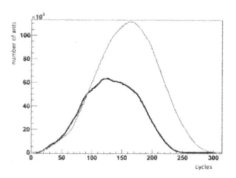

Figure 4. The number of ant per cycle: in black the result with the high intensity pheromone deposition rule, in gray the result with the gaussian rule.

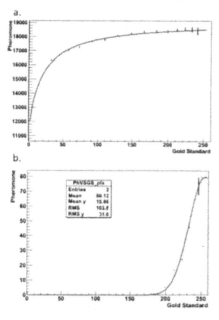

Figure 5. The correlation between the pheromone deposition and the percentage of white matter for the images with 0% of noise and 0% of RF-bias-field (a. high intensity pheromone deposition rule; b. gaussian pheromone deposition rule).

First of all, the calibration curve that gives the percentage of white matter as a function of the released pheromone quantity must be calculated.

To obtain the calibration curve it's necessary to study the relationship between the average of pheromone value (*ph*) and the known Gold Standard (*GS*).

The calibration curve changes with the Δ_{ph} definition. For the deposition rule used to segment the voxels with a high intensity, the calibration curve is hyperbolic:

$$Ph = p_0 + \frac{p_1}{GS + p_2} \qquad (7)$$

instead, for the gaussian deposition rule, it's obtained through a gaussian fit:

$$Ph = p_0 + e^{-\frac{(GS - p_1)^2}{2\,p_2^2}} \qquad (8)$$

In Figure 5, for the two different pheromone deposition rules, the average correlation between the released pheromone and the gold standard values is shown.

These graphs show that the high intensity deposition rule has much predictive power in the low gold standard value (i.e. in the voxels in which there is a low percentage of white matter); instead the gaussian pheromone deposition rule is much discriminating in the high gold standard zone and it isn't predictive at all for a gold standard of less then 180.

Such a different result in the quantitative segmentation is expected from the two different configurations.

After the calibration curve determination, the pheromone map is analysed and each voxel is associated to a percentage of white matter that represents the CAM segmentation result.

To check the CAM segmentation reliability, the result is compared to the known gold standard. The analysis is divided in two steps: first, only the voxels that the CAM segments as fully white matter (i.e. the voxels that reach the pheromone saturation value) are considered and, second, the quantitative analysis of the voxels that, for the CAM, do not contain only white matter is made.

Figure 6 shows the ROC curve obtained in the first step for the two algorithm configurations.

With the gaussian pheromone deposition rule the CAM reaches very high sensitivity values (i.e. $S = 0.985$) with a contamination equal to 0.03. The ROC curve obtained from the high intensity segmentation, on the other hand, shows a contamination higher then the gaussian one.

In order to evaluate the performance of the CAM is also important to analyze the exploration level: it's shown in Fig. 7 as the percentage of the voxels that are visited by ants as a function of the gold standard value. The high intensity segmentation rule is able to explore much more then the other one, so there's a sort of trade-off between the capability of an algorithm to have a low contamination and an high exploration level. For the gold standard values close to 100% of white matter both of the CAM configuration reach an exploration level of 90–100%.

In the second part of the result analysis, the CAM white matter fraction estimation power in the voxels that are not only formed by that is evaluated.

The difference between the CAM result and the gold standard value is considered and, as shown in Figure 8, it provides the resolution of the segmentation method for each CAM configuration. A normalization to the value corresponding to the 100% of white matter is made.

This analysis shows that for the high intensity segmentation CAM the difference $WM-GS$ could be very large: it's explained by the contamination and the higher exploration level.

The result obtained with the gaussian pheromone deposition rule is interesting and very important: it proves that the CAM could make a quantitative segmentation, in fact the 50% of

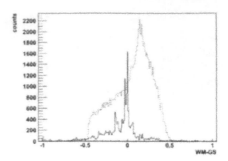

Figure 8. The normalized difference between the CAM result (WM) and the gold standard (solid: gaussian pheromone deposition rule; dashed: high intensity pheromone deposition rule).

voxels with a intermediate value of pheromone are classify with a $WM-GS$ less than 10%.

4 CONCLUSIONS

The results, although preliminary, confirm that there is room for improvements and confirm the adaptability of the CAM to segment complex structures in different kinds of images, regardless of their dynamic range.

The important role that the pheromone deposition rule plays is underlined: changing from the high intensity segmentation to the gaussian one the performance improves and the reliability of the quantitative segmentation using the CAM increases.

In the future, we will try to apply the method to real MRI images to segment not only the white matter but also the grey matter and the cerebrospinal fluid. The CAM will then used for the analysis of hippocampal boxes, the most relevant brain structures for the assessment of the development of the Alzheimers disease.

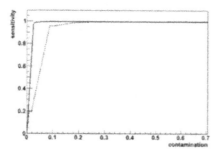

Figure 6. ROC curve for image with 0% of noise and 0% of RF-bias-field (solid: gaussian pheromone deposition rule; dashed: high intensity pheromone deposition rule).

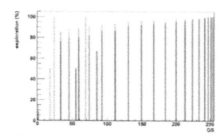

Figure 7. The percentage of the voxels that are visited by ants as a function of the gold standard values (solid: gaussian pheromone deposition rule; dashed: high intensity pheromone deposition rule).

ACKNOWLEDGMENTS

This work was carried out on behalf of the MAGIC-5 Collaboration.

REFERENCES

Cerello, P., Cheran, S.C., Bagnasco, S., Bellotti, R., Bolanos, L., Catanzariti, E., De Nunzio, G., Fantacci, M.E., Fiorina, E., Gargano, G., Gemme, G., Lopez Torres, E., Masala, G.L., Peroni, C. & Santoro, M. (2010). 3-d object segmentation using ant colonies. *Pattern Recognition.* 43, 1476–1490.

Huang, P., Cao, H. & Luo, S. (2008). An artificial ant colonies approach to medical image segmentation. *Computer Methods and Programs in Biomedicine.* 92, 267–273.

Abstracts

Technology and Medical Sciences – Natal Jorge et al. (eds)
© 2011 Taylor & Francis Group, London, ISBN 978-0-415-66822-4

In-silico models as a tool for the design of medical device technologies

J.M. García-Aznar, M.A. Pérez & M.J. Gómez-Benito
Aragón Institute of Engineering Research (I3A), Universidad de Zaragoza, Zaragoza, Spain

J.A. Sanz-Herrera & E. Reina-Romo
School of Engineering, University of Sevilla, Sevilla, Spain

ABSTRACT: As in other fields before, the use of mathematical and computer modeling is increasing in biomedical research. The design of new technologies in medicine and biology requires the development of in-vitro and in-vivo experiments needed to test different hypotheses that allow to understand observable phenomena. These experiments can be time-consuming, expensive and with a high difficulty to control all the parameters. Moreover, with a relevant socio-economic impact when animal experiments are required. In such cases, In-silico modeling can play a relevant role because computer simulations allow the possibility of considering and controlling factors that cannot be controlled or measured in experimental tests. In any case, we have to keep in mind that a computational model is a simplified and mathematical representation of a system to analyze the behaviour of this system under different conditions. Therefore, a model always requires validation. In fact, if a model is unable to reproduce some specific experiments, then the original hypotheses in which model is based should be revised and updated. Moreover, In-silico models can also improve experimental design by highlighting which measurements are needed to test a particular theory and whether additional information can be gained by collecting supplementary data. Therefore, modeling is an iterative process that is continually improved by means of comparison with experiments (Byrne, 2010).

Currently, this trend of using In-silico models in different fields of research in biology and medicine is being highly extended. Indeed, a considerable progress has been made, for example, in the mathematical modelling of cancer growth and its corresponding treatment (Byrne 2010). Another field where the development of models has been very important is in orthopaedic biomechanics, where Finite-Element-Analysis (FEA) has been applied to the design of medical devices (Prendergast, Lally & Lennon, 2009; Kluess, Mittelmeier & Bader, 2010). In fact, FEA has been also widely used to simulate mechanobiological problems (van der Meulen & Huiskes, 2002), where the main aim is to understand the way cells sense and respond to mechanical forces, modifying and updating the extracellular matrix of the involved tissues.

In this work, we present four examples of application of FEA to the design of different devices and/or protocols. Firstly, the design of cemented implants is mainly defined by the long-term failure of the cemented mantle, computer models have been used to determine the role of the cement in four different concepts of hip prostheses design: Exeter, Charnley, Elite Plus and ABG II stems (Pérez, García-Aznar, Doblaré, Seral & Seral, 2006). Secondly, an external fixator able to stimulate the fracture with high frequency low magnitude (LMHF) mechanical stimulus has been designed with FEA and implanted in sheep, improving successfully the healing course (Gómez-Benito, Grasa, Seral, González-Torres, Gómez-Arrue, Server & García-Aznar 2010). In a third example of application, we show how computer models allow to estimate the most adequate distraction rate to achieve a success bone healing in a clinical process of bone distraction (Reina-Romo, Gómez-Benito, García-Aznar, Domínguez & Doblaré, 2009). Finally, a fourth example, involved in bone tissue engineering is shown. Bone scaffolds can be designed through the use of FE models based on a mechanobiological approach (Sanz-Herrera, García-Aznar & Doblaré, 2009).

REFERENCES

Byrne, H. (2010). Dissecting cancer through mathematics: from the cell to the animal model. *Nat Rev Cancer 10(3)*: 221–230.

Gómez-Benito, M.J., Grasa, J., Seral, B., González-Torres, L., Gómez-Arrue, Server R. & García-Aznar, J. (2010). Mechanical stimulation of fracture healing by low-amplitude, high-frequency external loads in sheep. *Clinical Biomechanics*.

Kluess, D., Mittelmeier, W. & Bader, R. (2010). From theory to practice: Transfer of fea results into clinical applications. *Journal of Biomechanics 43S1*: S3–S14.

Pérez, M., García-Aznar, J., Doblaré, M., Seral, B. & Seral, F. (2006). A comparative fea of the debonding process in different concepts of cemented hip implants. *Med Eng Phys 28(6)*: 525–533.

Prendergast, P., Lally, C. & Lennon, A. (2009). Finite element modelling of medical devices. *Medical Engineering and Physics 31(4)*: 419.

Reina-Romo, E., Gómez-Benito, M. García-Aznar, J. Domínguez, J. & Doblaré, M. (2009). Modeling distraction osteogenesis: analysis of the distraction rate. *Biomech Model Mechanobiol 8(4)*: 323–335.

Sanz-Herrera, J., García-Aznar, J. & Doblaré, M. (2009). On scaffold designing for bone regeneration: A computational multiscale approach. *Acta Biomater 5(1)*, 219–229.

Van der Meulen, M. & Huiskes, R. (2002). Why mechanobiology? a survey article. *Journal of Biomechanics 35(4)*: 401–414.

Technology and Medical Sciences – Natal Jorge et al. (eds)
© 2011 Taylor & Francis Group, London, ISBN 978-0-415-66822-4

3D biomechanical model of the human hand using FEM

Daniel Neves Rocha
Universidade Federal de Minas Gerais, Belo Horizonte, Brazil

R.M. Natal Jorge
Faculdade de Engenharia da Universidade do Porto, Porto, Portugal

Marcos Pinotti
Universidade Federal de Minas Gerais, Belo Horizonte, Brazil

ABSTRACT: The human hand is responsible for a significant part of daily activities, becoming one of the most important tools of the human body. Hand injuries caused by different pathologies, by trauma or by the use of manual instruments with low ergonomics are pointed as the cause of social problems affecting individuals with limited capacity of using their hands. Designs of more ergonomic instruments are an important step to obtain comfortable and useful instruments to prevent hand injuries. Information about the pressure in the palm of the hand and the acting forces in the tendons of the fingers and wrist are useful to study. The discomfort, pain, muscle-skeletal and tendon injuries are consequences of using non-ergonomic instruments. The utilization of 3D models of the human hand has become a valuable tool, aiding the studies for the design of artificial members with more accurate controls and design of ergonomic instruments. The aim of this work is to create a 3D finite element model of the human hand, characterize the constitutive tissues (bones, skin and ligaments) and perform the simulation of the index finger's flexion. The devised numerical model was successfully implemented leading to stable and easily converged results, showing that the 3D biomechanical model of human hand is robust.

Keywords: Finite Elements Method, Human Hand, Biomechanical, 3D Model

Technology and Medical Sciences – Natal Jorge et al. (eds)
© 2011 Taylor & Francis Group, London, ISBN 978-0-415-66822-4

Using radiobiology simulators for evaluation of ^{99m}Tc Auger electrons for targeted tumor radiotherapy

Adriana Alexandre S. Tavares & João Manuel R.S. Tavares
Faculdade de Engenharia da Universidade do Porto (FEUP), Porto, Portugal

ABSTRACT: Technetium-99m (^{99m}Tc) has been widely used as an imaging agent; however, few studies evaluated its potential use as therapeutic agent. The present study aimed to analyze the potential use of ^{99m}Tc Auger electrons for targeted tumor radiotherapy by computational methods. Thus, three different computational simulators were used to estimate the yield of DNA damage, the probability of correct repair and cell kinetic effects after irradiation with ^{99m}Tc electrons, iodine-131 beta minus particles and astatine-211 alpha particles. Based on the obtained results, it is possible to conclude that ^{99m}Tc CKMMX (all M-shell Coster-Kroning—CK—and super CK transitions) electrons and Auger MXY (all M-shell Auger transitions) are valuable for targeted tumor radiotherapy.

1 INTRODUCTION

Targetedtumour radiotherapy with Auger electron emitters is an appealing, but challenging approach for systemic radiation therapy. Auger electrons are emitted by approximately half radioisotopes decaying by either electronic capture or internal conversion, including Technetium-99m (^{99m}Tc). Over the past decade, ^{99m}Tc has been widely used as an imaging agent, but few studies have evaluated its potential use as therapeutic agent. Results already obtained with ^{99m}Tc are encouraging; nonetheless, the definitive role of ^{99m}Tc as a therapeutic agent is far from conclusive. A short half-life, stable daughter nuclide, Auger electron energies suitable for target tumour radiotherapy and ability to do *in vivo* imaging are some potentially advantageous characteristics of ^{99m}Tc (Tavares et al. 2010a). The present study aimed to analyze the potential use of ^{99m}Tc Auger electrons for targeted tumour radiotherapy by computational simulation.

2 METHODS

Three different computational simulators were used to estimate the yield of DNA damage—fast Monte Carlo damage algorithm (MCDS), the probability of correct repair—Monte Carlo Excision Repair algorithm (MCER), and cell kinetic effects—virtual cell radiobiology algorithm (VC), after irradiation with ^{99m}Tc electrons, iodine-131 (^{131}I) beta minus particles and astatine-211 (^{211}At) alpha particles (Semenenko & Stewart 2004; Stewart 2004; Semenenko et al. 2005; Semenenko & Stewart 2005).

3 RESULTS

The percentage of simple- and double-strand breaks after irradiation, calculated using the MCDS simulator, was always higher for ^{99m}Tc CKMMX (all M-shell Coster-Kroning—CK—and super CK transitions) electrons and Auger MXY (all M-shell Auger transitions) than that for ^{131}I beta minus particles and was similar to ^{211}At alpha particles. Ananalogous trend was observed for the percentage of complex single- and double-strand breaks. Besides, the remaining ^{99m}Tc electrons obtained by internal conversion were less able to induce DNA damage, which may be explained by the higher tissue range of these ^{99m}Tc electrons, whose behaviour is similar to beta minus particles (low LET particles).

Results from MCER simulator showed that regardless the repair process used, the probability of correct repair of single-strand breaks is lower for ^{99m}Tc CKMMX electrons and Auger MXY than that for ^{131}I beta minus particles and is comparable to ^{211}At alpha particles. Furthermore, probability of conversion to DSBs was higher for ^{99m}Tc CKMMX electrons and Auger MXY than that for ^{131}I beta minus particles and is comparable to ^{211}At alpha particles.

VC simulator main findings showed that: 1) ^{99m}Tc CKMMX electron and Auger MXY had a higher probability of inducing mutagenesis and genetic instability than ^{131}I beta minus; 2) ^{131}I beta minus particles were the most likely of all the irradiating agents studied to induce neoplastic transformation; and 3) ^{99m}Tc CKMMX electron and Auger MXY had a higher ability to induce lethal damage, due to mutations, than the other particles studied. This suggests that the higher probability of induced mutagenesis and enhancement of genetic instability of ^{99m}Tc CKMMX electron and Auger MXY will potentially lead to cell death or benign mutations and not to neoplastic transformation (Tavares et al. 2010b).

4 CONCLUSIONS

[99m]Tc electrons CKMMX and Auger MXY present a therapeutic potential comparable to high linear energy transfer [211]At alpha particles and higher than beta minus particles of ^{131}I, while all remaining ^{99m}Tc electrons have a therapeutic potential similar to ^{131}I beta minus particles.

Additionally, apoptosis induction probability was found to be higher for ^{99m}Tc electrons CKMMX and Auger MXY than ^{131}I beta minus particles and similar to [211]At alpha particles. Based on the obtained results, one can conclude that ^{99m}Tc CKMMX electrons and Auger MXY are valuable electrons for targeted tumor radiotherapy.

REFERENCES

Semenenko, V. & Stewart, R. 2004. A fast Monte Carlo algorithm to simulate the spectrum of DNA damages formed by ionizing radiation. *Radiat. Res.* 161: 451–457.
Semenenko, V. & Stewart, R. 2005. Monte carlo simulation of base and nucleotide excision repair of clustered DNA damage sites. II. Comparisons of model predictions to measured data. *Radiat. Res.* 164: 194–201.
Semenenko, V., Stewart, R & Ackerman, E. 2005. Monte Carlo simulation of base and nucleotide excision repair of clustered DNA damage sites. I. Model properties and predicted trends. *Radiat. Res.* 164: 180–193.
Stewart, R. 2004. Computational Radiation Biology Purdue University, School of Health Sciences, West Lafayette.
Tavares, A. & Tavares, J. 2010a. [99m]Tc Auger electrons for targeted tumour therapy: A review. *Int. J. Radiat. Biol.* 86:261–270.
Tavares, A. & Tavares, J. 2010b. Evaluating [99m]Tc Auger electrons for targeted tumour radiotherapy by computational methods. *Med. Phys.* 37: 3551–3559.

Technology and Medical Sciences – Natal Jorge et al. (eds)
© 2011 Taylor & Francis Group, London, ISBN 978-0-415-66822-4

Therapeutic contact lenses obtained by SCF-assisted imprinting processes: Improved drug loading/release capacity

M.E.M. Braga, M.H. Gil & H.C. de Sousa
CIEPQPF, Chemical Engineering Department, FCTUC, University of Coimbra, Coimbra, Portugal

F. Yañez, C. Alvarez-Lorenzo & A. Concheiro
Departamento de Farmacia y Tecnología Farmacéutica, Facultad de Farmacia, Universidad de Santiago de Compostela, Spain

C.M.M. Duarte
Nutraceuticals and Delivery Laboratory, Instituto de Biologia Experimental e Tecnológica (IBET), Oeiras, Portugal
Instituto de Tecnologia Química e Biológica (ITQB), Universidade Nova de Lisboa, Oeiras, Portugal

ABSTRACT: Conventional methods to load drugs into commercial Soft Contact Lenses (SCLs) such as soaking and sorption in concentrated drug solutions are usually inefficient and mostly limited to highly water-soluble drugs. Molecular imprinting methods involve the synthesis of polymeric networks having high affinity and selectivity for specific drug template molecules and that can be used as efficient Drug Delivery Systems (DDSs). The main objective of this work is to improve the flurbiprofen load and release capacity of daily- and monthly-wear Hilafilcon B commercial SCLs by using an innovative Supercritical Fluid (SCF) assisted molecular imprinting method that comprises the use of consecutive SCF drug impregnation (SSI) and extraction (SFE) steps. Conventional flurbiprofen soaking and removal methods were also employed for comparison purpose. Supercritical carbon dioxide (scCO$_2$) impregnation assays were performed at 12.0 MPa and 313 K while scCO$_2$ extractions were performed at 20.0 MPa and at 313 K. In vitro drug release kinetics profiles were obtained and compared. A molecular imprinting proof-of-concept was performed by using equimolar flurbiprofen, ibuprofen and dexamethasone aqueous solutions in conventional sorption experiments and in order to verify if the employed processes were able to create drug-loaded SCLs having improved and specific affinity for flurbiprofen. Processed samples were also characterized by SEM, FTIR-ATR and contact angle determination. Finally, monthly-wear SCF drug-imprinted contact lenses were recharged overnight (14 hours) in aqueous flurbiprofen solutions and later released for 8 hours, in order to simulate a potential typical SCLs patient wearing. Obtained results demonstrate the viability of preparing more efficient flurbiprofen-loaded Hilafilcon B daily- and monthly-wear contact lenses by applying the proposed SCF technologies. In addition, SCF-processed SCLs showed recognition ability and a higher affinity for flurbiprofen in aqueous solution than for the other employed drugs which suggests the creation of molecularly imprinted SCLs by these SCF-based methods. Finally, these scCO$_2$ processes did not alter the critical functional properties of SCLs, enabled the control of drug loaded/released amounts and permitted the preparation of hydrophobic drug-based therapeutic SCLs in much shorter process times than those using conventional aqueous-based molecular imprinting methods.

Keywords: Therapeutic contact lenses, molecular imprinting, supercritical fluid technology, flurbiprofen, drug loading/release capacity

Technology and Medical Sciences – Natal Jorge et al. (eds)
© 2011 Taylor & Francis Group, London, ISBN 978-0-415-66822-4

Supercritical solvent impregnation of natural bioactive compounds in *N*-carboxybutyl chitosan membranes for the development of topical wound healing applications

A.M.A. Dias, I.J. Seabra, M.E.M. Braga, M.H. Gil & H.C. de Sousa
CIEPQPF, Chemical Engineering Department, FCTUC, University of Coimbra, Coimbra, Portugal

ABSTRACT: Wound dressings are usually applied with the objective of accelerating wound healing by preventing bacterial infection and accelerating tissue regeneration. The main goals of wound care are prevention of infection and/or inflammation, maintenance of a moist environment, protection of the wound with minimum scar formation, stimulating healthy healing responses. According to modern insights, a wound dressing should present flexibility, controlled adherence to the surrounding tissue, gas permeability, durability, capacity to absorb fluids exuded from the wounded area and the ability to control water loss. Delivery of pharmacologically active compounds like antibiotics/analgesics across the skin is also an attractive alternative to oral dosing. This work addresses the use of natural-based polymers and of "greener" processes to develop biocompatible drug release systems for biomedical applications. Healing of dermal wounds with such natural polymers are attractive primarily because they are biocompatible and present non-irritant and non-toxic properties, being its application on dermis easy and safe. Moreover, they are inexpensive, readily available, capable of multitude of chemical modifications and potentially degradable. Film and foam-like structures of *N*-carboxybutyl chitosan (CBC) and agarose (AGA) were prepared and characterized in order to evaluate their possible application as wound dressing materials mainly in what concerns their fluid handling properties and sustained drug release capacity. Polymeric biomaterials were loaded with two natural bioactive compounds namely, quercetin (known to present an anti-inflammatory action) and thymol (known to present an anaesthetic action) and using a Supercritical Solvent Impregnation (SSI) technique, in order to develop topical membrane-type natural-based wound dressings. Impregnation experiments were carried out with supercritical carbon dioxide (scCO$_2$) at 10.0 and 20.0 MPa, and at 303.0 and 323.0 K to study the influence of impregnation conditions on the loaded amounts of quercetin and thymol. For quercetin, ethanol was used as co-solvent in order to improve its solubility in the supercritical fluid phase. Drug release kinetics studies were also performed for all the impregnated systems using UV spectrophotometry. Similar release profiles were observed for the same bioactive compound but the total released amount (for each bioactive compound) is always higher when membranes were loaded at higher pressure/temperature conditions. Higher diffusion coefficients in water were obtained for thymol what may be justified by its smaller molecular volume and higher solubility in water, when compared to quercetin. A more sustained release was observed for quercetin which can be mainly due to its lower solubility in water, higher molar volume (which difficult the diffusion of the molecule through the polymeric network) and also due to the known specific favourable interactions between quercetin and CBC which were detected by Scanning Electron Microscopy (SEM) and FTIR-ATR analyses. These interactions can greatly enhance the sustained release of this natural drug from the polymeric matrix by slowing its release and making it dependent on the external induced degradation of the biopolymer. Obtained results demonstrate that, by the conjugation of different materials with a "tunable" impregnation process, it is possible to prepare different biomaterials, with a specific set of properties, which enable them to be used for wound healing purposes.

Keywords: Wound healing, quercetin, thymol, *N*-carboxybutyl chitosan, agarose, supercritical solvent impregnation, drug delivery

Technology and Medical Sciences – Natal Jorge et al. (eds)
© 2011 Taylor & Francis Group, London, ISBN 978-0-415-66822-4

Potential and suitability of Ion Mobility Spectrometry (IMS) for breath analysis

V. Vassilenko
Center of Physics and Technological Research—CEFITEC, Physics Department, Faculty of Sciences and Technology, Universidade Nova de Lisboa, Caparica, Portugal

A.M. Bragança
NMT—Tecnologia, Inovação e Consultoria Lda., Madan Parque—Parque de Ciência e Tecnologia de Almada, Caparica, Portugal

V. Ruzsanyi & S. Sielemann
G.A.S., Gesellschaft für Analytische Sensorsysteme mbH, Dortmund, Germany

ABSTRACT: The detection and monitoring of biomarkers for oxidative stress by measurement of endogenous compounds in exhaled breath has received increasing attention in the past decade. Numerous studies have been performed in order to establish the physiological and pathophysiological meaning of Volatile Organic Compounds (VOCs) emission in human breath. Among the various techniques used in exhaled air analysis, there is one that stands out due to its high sensitivity, low cost, portability and ease in-use: the ion mobility spectrometry. In this paper we describe the sampling procedure of human breath and present spectra of exhaled air using ion mobility spectrometers obtained without any pre-concentration. The detection of different volatiles in human breath are discussed with special attention on detection limits for some different analytes occurring in human breath.

1 INTRODUCTION

General metabolic conditions and developing diseases in human beings can very often be traced by evaluating chemical markers present in exhaled air. This is principally due to an almost instantaneous equilibrium between the pulmonary blood and the air in the alveoli of the lung (Di Francesco et al. 2005). The matrix of breath is a mixture of nitrogen, oxygen, carbon dioxide, water, inert gases, and trace Volatile Organic Compounds (VOCs). The matrix elements in breath vary widely from person to person, both qualitatively and quantitatively, particularly for VOCs. More than 3000 trace VOCs have been identified in human breath with concentrations from ppmv to pptv range. Among these, only a small number of VOCs are common to everyone (Amann et al. 2007; Cao & Duan 2007). These substances may be produced anywhere in the body and can reflect a normal physiological biochemical process or a pathological condition, such as lipid peroxidation, liver disease, renal failure, allograft rejection, cancer, or glucose or cholesterol metabolism (Miekisch & Schubert 2006). Some metabolites have already been established as biomarkers, such as acetone (diabetes), nitric

acid (asthma), ammonia (hepatitis), isoprene (cholesterol), ethane and pentane (oxidative stress), methylated hydrocarbons (lung and breast cancer), among others (Amann et al. 2007; Miekisch & Schubert 2006).

Breath analysis is thus an attractive procedure for biochemical monitoring in order to follow the evolution of diseases or malfunctions of the human body. It can even help to predict such diseases, particularly because it is not an invasive procedure and so can be applied to a wide range of compounds (Amann, 2007). The breath sampling is painless and does not require skilled medical staff. Other possible application is related to the monitorization of work-related exposure to hazardous substances (halogenated compounds, solvents and toxic gases).

During the last decade, GC and GC-MS techniques have improved significantly and new methods have been introduced into breath analysis like Proton Transfer Reaction (PTR-MS), Selected Ion-Flow Tube (SIFT-MS), Ion Mobility Spectroscopy (IMS) or sensors. GC and GC-MS have been applied to separate and to identify the majority of compounds in human breath such as aliphatics, aromatics, alcohols, aldehydes, ketones, carboxylic acids, amines, ether, thioether, thiols, amines and halogenated compounds. So, large-scale clinical use of breath analysis requires portable, on-site instruments that provide information on well-understood biomarkers, and preferably in real time. A good candidate to be a part of this new generation of instruments is Ion Mobility Spectrometry (IMS), which due to its high sensitivity (low ppb range), portability and low cost maintenance could be useful as a screening test for many different diseases.

Although the application of IMS in the medical field is recent, its efficiency in the diagnosis and detection of several pathologies has been proved in a small number of studies. Diseases like lung cancer, sarcoidosis, pneumonie and Chronic Obstructive Pulmonary Disease (COPD) (Ruzsanyi et al. 2005; Baumbach 2009; Westhoff et al. 2007) were successfully detected/diagnosed using ion mobility spectrometry, demonstrating that there are significant differences on the breath profiles of healthy and non-healthy people.

2 EXPERIMENTAL & RESULTS

The analysis with ion mobility spectrometers is based on characterizing chemical substances through their gas phaseion mobilities in weak electric fields at ambient pressure. The limited selectivity of the IMS, especially in the case of the detection of complex mixtures, can be avoided by pre-separationon Multi-Capillary Columns (MCC). Because of the high capacity, the gas flow conditions of MCC are comparable to IMS gas flows and retention times achieved at ambient temperature in the range of minutes (Ruzsanyi et al. 2005; Baumbach 2006).

The presented experimental measurements were done on MCC-IMS apparatus. A sampling procedure of human breath is show to be one of the principal parameters regarding the repeatability and stability of results. The spectra were obtained in positive polarity at room temperature and ambient pressure. Detection limits and reduced mobility were determined for selected analytes present in human breath. Special attention was done on differentiation between healthy persons and patients suffering from different pulmonary lung infections.

3 CONCLUSIONS

The MCC–IMS exhibits sufficient high sensitivity for detecting organic metabolites in exhaled air. The fact that is does not require vacuum or further sample preparation and the possibility of on-site and rapid analysis makes this technique suitable to be used in hospitals and healthcare centers. Using MCC–IMS directly in the clinical diagnostic will provide new additional information within some minutes and facilitate building databases for several illnesses. Further clinical trials will be implemented in the near future for the detection of different pathologieslike diabetes, cholesterol, tuberculosis, liver diseases, among others.

REFERENCES

Amann, A. et al. 2007. Applications of breath gas analysis in medicine. *International Journal of Mass Spectrometry*, 239(2–3): 227–233.

Baumbach, J.I. 2006. Process analysis using ion mobility spectrometry. *Analytical and Bioanalytical Chemistry*. 384(5): 1059–1070.

Baumbach, J.I. 2009. Ion mobility spectrometry coupled with multi-capillary columns for metabolic profiling of human breath. *Journal of Breath Research*. 3: 1–16.

Cao, W.Q. & Duan, Y.X. 2007. Current status of methods and techniques for breath analysis. *Critical Reviews in Analytical Chemistry*. 37(1): 3–13.

Di Francesco, F. et al. 2005. Breath analysis: trends in techniques and clinical applications. *Microchemical Journal*. 79(1–2): 405–410.

Miekisch, W. & Schubert, J.K. 2006. From highly sophisticated analytical techniques to life-saving diagnostics: Technical developments in breath analysis. *Trac-Trends in Analytical Chemistry*. 25(7): 665–673.

Ruzsanyi, V. et al. 2005. Detection of human metabolites using multi-capillary columns coupled to ion mobility spectrometers. *J. Chromatogr.* A 1084: 145–151.

Westhoff, M. et al. 2007. Ion mobility spectrometry in the diagnosis of sarcoidosis: results of a feasibility study. *J Physiol Pharmacol.* Suppl 5 (Pt 2): 739–51.

Technology and Medical Sciences – Natal Jorge et al. (eds)
© 2011 Taylor & Francis Group, London, ISBN 978-0-415-66822-4

Phosphonium-based ionic liquids as new *Greener* plasticizers for poly(vinyl chloride) biomedical applications

S. Marceneiro, A.M.A. Dias, J.F.J. Coelho, A.G.M. Ferreira, P.N. Simões, M.E.M. Braga & H.C. de Sousa
CIEPQPF, Chemical Engineering Department, FCTUC, University of Coimbra, Coimbra, Portugal

C.M.M. Duarte
Nutraceuticals and Delivery Laboratory, Instituto de Biologia Experimental e Tecnológica (IBET), Portugal
Instituto de Tecnologia Química e Biológica (ITQB), Universidade Nova de Lisboa, Portugal

I.M. Marrucho, J.M.S.S. Esperança & L.P.N. Rebelo
Instituto de Tecnologia Química e Biológica (ITQB), Universidade Nova de Lisboa, Portugal

ABSTRACT: Poly(vinyl chloride) (PVC) is one of the most widely used thermoplastic materials mostly due to its known advantages such as availability, low cost, processability and broad range of properties, that enable its large variety of applications ranging from building construction (tubes, pipes, flooring) to biomedical applications (blood bags, catheters). Depending on the envisaged processing method and on the intended application, different levels of viscosity and of material softness and flexibility may be needed and this can be controlled and achieved by the incorporation of external plasticizers into rigid PVC. Plasticizers are usually physically mixed with PVC and their migration and release when in contact with a certain surrounding medium may occur in different extents. The most commonly employed plasticizers for PVC are phthalate esters. However, these are now being banned or highly controlled by the European Union for several applications such as plastic children toys and medical devices due to their potential toxicity and low biodegradability. Therefore, both alternative plasticizers and substitute plastic materials have been assessed for the substitution of phthalate-plasticized PVC but, for many applications, no material has yet been found that can satisfactorily substitute soft PVC and no low molar mass plasticizer has been able of replacing phthalate esters without inducing migration.

Ionic Liquids (ILs) are readily modifiable materials with physical properties that make these compounds amenable to a wide range of applications. Due to some of these properties (negligible vapor pressures, high thermal stability and a large liquid-phase temperature range) together with the large number of different ILs (with different properties) that can be prepared by the conjugation of different cations and anions, recently ILs have been proposed as new solvent media for polymerization reactions and/or as polymer plasticizers.

In this work, the effects of PVC molecular weight and of IL plasticizer type and composition on the properties of plasticized PVC were studied. Two different molecular weight PVC materials (1200 and 2000 Da) were incorporated (by film casting) with increasing amounts of a phosphonium-based IL (0, 5, 10 and 20% w/w), comprised by similar cations but with different anions having different hydrophylicities (namely Cl^-, Br^-, $N(SO_2CF_3)_2^-$ and $N(CN)_2^-$). A conventional organic plasticizer (diisononyl phthalate, DINP) was also used for comparison purposes. Films were prepared by a solvent film casting method and using THF as the organic solvent. The migration/leaching (in water and in pH 7.0 HBSS buffer solutions) of employed plasticizers from prepared films was quantified at different temperature and stirring conditions. Because the migration of plasticizers can lead to changes in the thermal stability of PVC, obtained films (before and after leaching) were characterized by DMTA, TGA and DSC. Samples were also characterized by water and water-vapor sorption, SEM-EDX, FTIR-ATR and by contact angle determination. Considering one of the desired final biomedical applications (plasticized PVC materials for blood bags) blood biocompatibility tests were also carried out for pure ILs and for plasticized films, and in order to verify their toxicity against rabbit blood cells. Obtained results showed that all the studied ILs presented similar or even superior performances as biocompatible plasticizers to the employed conventional PVC plasticizer (DINP). Amongst all employed ILs, (trihexyl)tetradecylphosphonium bis(trifluoromethylsulfonyl)imide presented the most interesting and promising results regarding plasticized PVC thermal stability, blood biocompatibility and plasticizer leaching results.

Keywords: poly(vinyl chloride), plasticizers, ionic liquids, migration, thermal stability, blood biocompatibility, biomedical applications

Technology and Medical Sciences – Natal Jorge et al. (eds)
© 2011 Taylor & Francis Group, London, ISBN 978-0-415-66822-4

New approach to bone surface reconstruction from 2.5D sonographic dataset

P. Krowicki, K. Krysztoforski, E. Świątek-Najwer & R. Będziński
Wroclaw University of Technology, Institute of Machines Design and Operation, Biomedical Engineering and Experimental Mechanics Laboratory, Wroclaw, Poland

ABSTRACT: The main aim of this work was to invent algorithms for bone surface reconstruction. Basement on this concept was to use navigated ultrasound probe with developed system. Algorithms were introduced to the system which enables virtual osteotomy and measuring geometric parameters. Two algorithms for bone reconstruction were developed. Workflow of each algorithm was data collection, model resize, registration and bone model deforming. Differences between algorithms with experiment design approach and random measurements are described. Reconstructed bones are compared with CT/MRI reconstruction.

Keywords: Bone surface reconstruction; navigation; 3D ultrasound imaging; freehand scanning

1 INTRODUCTION

Bone deformities are typically recognized on standard long standing radiograms. Noninvasive techniques are not commonly applied for bone diagnostics, because X-ray examination is easily applicable, less time-consuming, high quality imaging. However, nonradiological techniques are required, since harmful influence of X-ray radiation is proved. Model morphing algorithms are commonly used in medical reconstruction. Reconstruction of femoral head was made by Rajamani (2007) and compared with gold standard. Also specimen reconstruction was made by Sigal (2008) who used wrapper algorithm. In this paper two new algorithms for bone surface reconstruction are described. Fast and accurate reconstructions give possibility to plan osteotomies instead planning on radiograms (Keppler 1997, Świątek-Najwer 2008). Proposed algorithm for comparison of surfaces reconstructed basing on ultrasound dataset and CT/MRI is described. Developed system consists of infrared tracking device combined with ultrasound probe. There exist several types of algorithms used to reconstruct objects from USG scans. Sample bone surface reconstruction algorithm is divided into three phases (Keppler 2007): pre-processing (filtration of images), segmentation (delineation of bone contour) and bone reconstruction (calculation of mesh built of triangles with vertices defined by the points of bone contours). The filtration of sonographic scans is a very demanding procedure, because of various artifacts introduced by reverberations. Standard methods of filtration like mean and median filters were applied. Additionally two images were registered in the same location and subtracted to eliminate noises. To delineate the bone contour gradient mask was applied and the bone interface was determined from downwards. To reconstruct the shape, the Delaunay 2D algorithm was applied to determine the scheme of vertices connection into a mesh of triangles. On obtained virtual model the surgeon designs bone correction and simultaneously controls resulting limb geometrical parameters. The osteotomy procedure can be performed using straight or dome osteotomy plane.

2 ALGORITHM, MATERIAL & METHODS

2.1 Deformable computer model

Following workflow describing two algorithms which at the beginning are similar: in first step computer model of bone consisting of 4344 points

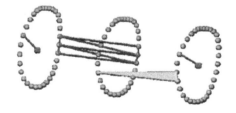

Figure 1. Points of computer model of shaft of femur bone.

connected by lines forming a network of triangles is scaled (Fig. 1). Using model allows to confine time consuming operations connected with meshing, contour determination and accelerate model tuning. Scale is determined from known and readily available points.

Next step was matching of resized computer model to real bone. Bone model is located in space. The main objective of the next steps is to reconstruct the central part of the bone reflecting the real shape. Therefore next calculations concerns mathematical model of reconstructed part.

2.2 Mathematical model

Let's consider femur shaft as cylinder which is build up from N smaller cylinders. Object consists of cone centers C_{N+1} and radii R_{N+1}. where radius $R_1 = R_2 = \ldots = R_N = R_{N+1}$ is constant. Each center has three-dimensional coordinates C_i (x_i, y_i, z_i). This assumption give very primitive mathematical model (Fig. 2).

Expanding it into the form consisting of N truncated cone's would better reflect reality. Equation 1 describes volumetric dependency of whole model.

$$V_C = \sum_{i=1}^{N} \frac{\pi}{3} h_i (R_i^2 + R_i R_{i+1} + R_{i+1}^2) \qquad (1)$$

where centers C_i of each cone are known and taken into account for height of cone calculations according to the formula:

$$h_i = \sqrt{(x_i - x_{i+1})^2 + (y_i - y_{i+1})^2 + (z_i - z_{i+1})^2} \qquad (2)$$

Therefore value of each radius could be different. Also cone centers could be placed at different positions. These facilities makes model more complicated and also more accurate. Connecting centers by straight line we obtain broken line. Individual parts are described by following linear equation:

$$\begin{cases} x = x_0 + ls \\ y = y_0 + ms \\ z = z_0 + ns \end{cases} \qquad (3)$$

where x_0, y_0, z_0 is the center of cone $C_i(x_i, y_i, z_i)$ and directional vector l, m, n is given by difference between corresponding centers C_i, C_{i+1}

$$\begin{cases} l = x_i - x_{i+1} \\ m = y_i - y_{i+1} \\ n = z_i - z_{i+1} \end{cases} \qquad (4)$$

Defined lines gives some lengths which could be measured and compared with other types of curves e.g. B-spline or polynomial. It could be criterion of accuracy. Another criterion could be the value of average distance between different line types, where distance is the closest point from curve to point on broken line. In this research we focus on volumetric comparison and local geometric accuracy which will be described in the next part of paper.

2.3 Design of experiment algorithm

When the mathematical model is obtained it is possible to tune it. At the beginning model and object having different locations (Fig. 3).

First step is connected with spatial placement of real object. It is to necessary to match the model to the object. Matching procedure provides the same spatial position of the object and model on the ends center (Fig. 4). Iterative Closest Points (ICP) algorithm was used to carry out matching procedure. Matching based on six anthropological points of the real object (femur bone). Matched model is ready to carry out tuning. Therefore algorithm designates regions of interest to be measured.

Considering the model measuring points are determined on the basis of D-optimal plan Rafajłowicz (1996). Reconstruction accuracy is fixed at a preset threshold $A_R = 3.0$ mm. First and last point of planning designate measurements borders as it is shown on (Fig. 5). Boundaries of measurements change

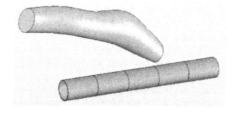

Figure 3. Mathematical model of cylinders (special case of cones) and real object.

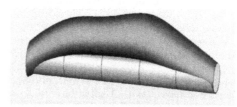

Figure 4. Matched mathematical model with real object.

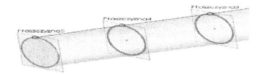

Figure 2. Sample model with constant radii R_{N+1} and indicated centers.

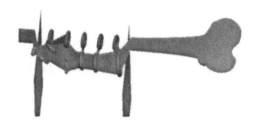

Figure 5. Reconstructed bone with planes demarcating the extent of correction by D-optimal planning.

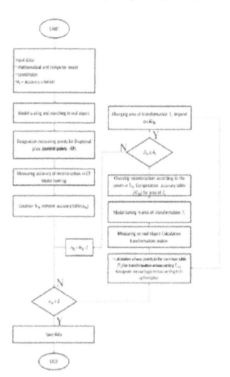

Scheme 1. Algorithm of reconstruction procedure.

during measurements. Changes depend on the accuracy obtained from measurement. For example if after first loop of accuracy condition is performed just for first and last points of plan, then the measurement table is changed. Also area of measurement is recalculated and new points of measuring are put in to the measuring array.

Scheme 1 presents workflow of all calculations which are performed during reconstruction.

2.4 Random reconstruction algorithm

Algorithm based on mathematical model was described above. For random reconstruction algorithm, the difference is that user performs any number of registration points on the real object. From randomized measurements centers and radii are taken into account. Computer model is adjusted on the basis of those parameters. Then, the accuracy is verified. Next the algorithm gives information about the repetition of measurements (depending on the accuracy value).

2.5 Calculating reconstruction accuracy

Model tuning reconstruction is locally tested by algorithm checking the distance to the nearest point of model and model surface. These two ways attempt allows to rate accuracy of model tuning. In case if one of two values meets accuracy condition, repetition of measurement is not required. Randomized algorithm works similar but measurement repetition allows to exercise survey in the whole measurement area.

2.6 Hardware specification

The computer system combines infrared optical tracking system (Polaris, NDI) and sonographic linear probe (with portable sonographic system EchoBlaster 128, Telemed). (Fig. 7).

Software developed in Microsoft Visual C++ 6.0 applies OpenGL standard specification to handle 3D computer graphics and DirectShow technology for any video stream controlling. Goal of this combined system is to create voxels from ultrasound scans registered with full description of position and rotation of scanning plane in space. The localization of scanning plane is tracked by the navigation system because of tracking of sensor mounted on ultrasound probe. To determine the coordinates a calibrating matrix is required. It describes the tilt of scanning plane in relation to the coordinate system of sensor mounted on probe. Mathematical apparatus of matrix transform between coordinate systems is implemented

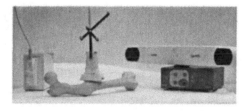

Figure 6. Bone reconstruction based on randomized measurements.

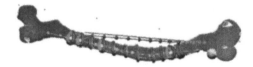

Figure 7. Navigated ultrasound head connected to Telemed control unit and Polaris navigation system.

Table 1. Volume accuracy test.

Method	Phantom	Patient
	Volume [cm³]	
Algorithm 1	412.5	511.2
Algorithm 2	432.0	520.6
CT/MRI*	500.6	633.9

* Depending on the bone.

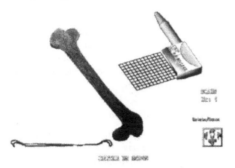

Figure 8. Checking the difference in the reconstruction of a scan.

Table 2. Area accuracy test.

Method	Phantom	Patient
	Difference in area [cm²]	
Algorithm 1	2.96 ± 0.39	3.22 ± 0.39
Algorithm 2	2.80 ± 0.33	3.15 ± 0.41

in the system. Points which are necessary to transformations and accuracy test were marked on the collected sonographical scans.

2.7 Accuracy tests

The accuracy tests were performed on deformed femur sawbone and in vivo on the bone of one proband. Sawbone was measured by computed tomography and the propositus was examined by MRI. The reconstruction based on data acquired by navigated ultrasound probe was performed using algorithms described above. Obtained value of reconstruction volumes using various techniques were compared (see Table 1).

Next test was to compare bone contours. For this purpose, an application was created (Fig. 8), which allows to move a virtual ultrasound probe, to indicate the locations where the contour plane is.

Two contours were obtained. Difference in field of CT/MRI reconstruction and applied algorithm were calculated. Results for three different positions are shown in Table 2.

Next test was to compare data obtained by palpation using navigated pointer to the points and surface of reconstructed bone based on US scans.

3 RECONSTRUCTION RESULTS

Algorithm using D-optimal path planning in the table is shown as Algorithm 1. Results from randomized measurement are presented as Algorithm 2.

The third test determined the accuracy of the reconstruction of the phantom, measured as average distance to the point equaling 2.75 mm and distance to the plane equaling 2.56 mm, for the reconstructed segment.

4 CONCLUSION

Model morphing algorithms are commonly used in medical reconstruction. Two algorithms of reconstruction using deforming of model were designed. Using the first algorithm assumed reconstruction accuracy was obtained. Number of loops and the time of calculations are satisfactory. The second algorithm due to lack of spatial constraints, finished calculations in a much shorter time. Obtaining such results for the whole bone would allow calculations of geometric parameters and planning osteotomies on the obtained model the measurements can be performed using the reconstructed model and virtual ultrasound probe.

ACKNOWLEDGEMENTS

This paper is supported by the Polish Ministry of Science and Higher Education in the framework of project with register number N R 13 0012 04.

REFERENCES

Keppler, P., Krysztoforski, K., Świątek-Najwer, E., Krowicki, P., Kozak, J., Gebhard, F. & Pinzuti, J.B. 2007. *A new experimental measurement and planning tool for sonographic-assisted navigation.* Orthopedics. Vol. 30, nr 10, suppl., pp. 144–147, 2007.

Keppler, P., Strecker, W., Anselment, K. & Kinzl, L. 1997. *Die sonographische Torsionwinkel und Langebestimmung der unteren Extremitaet*, Springer Verlag.

Rafajłowicz, E. 1996. *Algorytmy planowania eksperymentu z implementacjami w środowisku mathematica.* Warszawa.

Rajamani, K.T., Styner, M.A., Talib, H., Zheng, G., Nolte, L.P. & Gonzalez Ballester, M. 2007. *Statistical deformable bone models for rob ust 3D surface extrapolation from sparse data.* Medical image analysis nr 11, pp. 99–109, 2007.

Sigal, I.A., Hardisty, M.R. & Whyne, C.M. 2008. *Mesh-morphing algorithms for specimen-specific finite element modeling.* Jurnal of Biomechanics Vol. 41, pp. 1381–1389, 2008.

Świątek-Najwer, E., Będziński, R., Krowicki, P., Krysztoforski, K., Keppler, P. & Kozak, J. 2008. *Improving surgical precision – application of navigation system in orthopedic surgery*, Acta of Bioengineering and Biomechanics, Vol.10 (4), Wrocław.

Technology and Medical Sciences – Natal Jorge et al. (eds)
© 2011 Taylor & Francis Group, London, ISBN 978-0-415-66822-4

Metal-Organic Framework as potential drug carriers against inflammation

Iane Bezerra Vasconcelos Santos
Pós Graduate Materials Science, Federal University of Pernambuco, Recife, Brazil

Teresinha Gonçalves da Silva
Department of Antibiotics, Federal University of Pernambuco, Recife, Brazil

Severino Alves Júnior
Department of Chemistry, Federal University of Pernambuco, Recife, Brazil

Keywords: MOF, inflammation, drug delivery

1 INTRODUCTION

Inflammation is the reaction of tissue to an aggression, characterized by the reaction of blood vessels, leading to the accumulation of fluid and leukocytes in the site attacked. These characteristics have the following objectives: locate, isolate and destroy the harmful agents. But this answer does not always happen in a balanced manner, referring to disorders such as rheumatoid arthritis, rheumatoid fever, osteoarthritis, lupus erythematosus, among others, have been widely studied in order to develop new molecules or delivery systems able to reduce inflammation [1]. About this context, Metal-Organic Frameworks (MOFs) are networks of coordination, characterized as a class of porous material and consist of metal ions associated with organic ligands, which can certainly be used as drug delivery systems [2].

2 PURPOSE

To investigate the toxicity of MOF $(Zn(MeIM)_2)$ and the effect of MOF on the release of anti-inflammatory agents through study *in vitro*, by macrophage culture.

3 METHODS

The Ibuprofen loading (IBU-Zn) was performed by introducing, under stirring for 3 days, 100 mg of the dehydrated powder material (dried overnight at 150°C in an oven) in a 10 ml solution of hexane containing 300 mg of Ibuprofen. After the insertion of drug, remaining hexane was removed at 100°C. The adsorbed amount of Ibuprofen into the porous solids was estimated by Thermogravimetric Analysis (TGA), X-Ray Fluorescence (XRF) and elemental analysis. After this step, studies were performed *in vitro*. In this study the toxicity was performed using the MTT assay, colorimétrico 3-(4,5-dimethylthiazol-2-yl) 2,5-Diphenyl Bromide Tetrazoilium (MTT) Method described by Mosmann (1983) which is to indirectly measure cell viability by mitochondrial enzyme activity of living cells. Aiming to make the study more specific and to ascertain the feasibility of carrying out further steps forward in studies of inflammation, we performed the test culture of peritoneal macrophages of mice. The macrophages Were obtained from Swiss female mice 6–8 weeks old, weighing between 25 and 30 g from the vivarium of Department of Antibiotics, Federal University of Pernambuco. The peritoneal cavity of each animal were inoculated 3,0 mL of carrageenan three days before collection of cells. The sacrifice of animals was performed 72 h after separately by suffocation in a tank containing glass swab in ether. The animals were placed in support where they were detained by the legs with the abdomen upwards. Inside the laminar flow (Veco), after antisepsis of the abdomen with alcohol iodine 0,3% the peritoneum of mice was exposed with the aid of two clamps. Was then injected intraperitoneally 2.0 mL of solution of sodium chloride (0,9%). The abdomens were gently massaged and the cell suspension was collected with the aid of a disposable syringe and needle. The material was placed in plastic tubes and centrifuged at $225 \times g$ for 10 min and resuspended in the same solution, always kept at 4ºC. After this step, the macrophages were exposed substances under at different concentrations—1,25; 2,25; 5,0 and 10,0 µg.

4 RESULTS

The cytotoxicity of the MOF and IBU-Zn was not detected in the MTT assay. Still based on our results, the MOF and the system prepared did not affects macrophage viability at the concentrations tested.

5 CONCLUSIONS

The results showed it is possible to continue the studies in the area of inflammation, starting in vivo studies. This approach should allow the incorporation of new drugs in MOFs applications for future delivery of drugs.

REFERENCES

[1] Simmons, D.L. What makes a good anti-inflammatory drug target? *Inflammation Discovery Research* Vol. 11, Number 5/6. pp. 210–219, 2006.

[2] William J. Rieter, Kathryn M.L. Taylor and Wenbin Lin. Surface Modification and Functionalization of Nanoscale Metal-organic Frameworks for Controlled Realease and Luminescence Sensing. J Am Chem Soc. 2007 August 15;129 (32): 9852–9853. doi: 10.1021/ja073506r.

[3] Mosmann, T. Rapid colorimetric assay for cellular growth and survival: application to proliferation and cytotoxicity assays. J Immunol Methods. Vol. 65, n. 1–2, pp. 55–63, 1983.

Technology and Medical Sciences – Natal Jorge et al. (eds)
© 2011 Taylor & Francis Group, London, ISBN 978-0-415-66822-4

Knowledge based system for medical applications

C.S. Moura, P.J. Bártolo & H.A. Almeida
Centre for Rapid and Sustainable Product Development, Polytechnic Institute of Leiria, Leiria, Portugal

ABSTRACT: The development of computer-aided design and simulation tools to support tissue engineering is an important topic of research. This paper presents the initial stage of a project aiming at developing a knowledge based computer tool to support the selection of appropriate biomaterials for a certain medical application. The proposed tool is based on factual knowledge, case-based and rule-based reasoning algorithms, combining facts and heuristics and thus merging human knowledge with the computer power in solving problems. It is based on an extensive database of polymeric and ceramic biomaterials categorized by their nature, physical and biological characteristics.

Technology and Medical Sciences – Natal Jorge et al. (eds)
© *2011 Taylor & Francis Group, London, ISBN 978-0-415-66822-4*

In vitro method for test and measure the accuracy of implant impression

F.J. Caramelo
Institute of Biophysics and Biomathematics, Faculty of Medicine of Coimbra, IBILI, Coimbra, Portugal

P. Brito & J. Santos
Institute of Biophysics and Biomathematics and Faculty of Medicine of Coimbra, IBILI, Coimbra, Portugal
Superior Institute of Health Sciences—North, Portugal

A. Carvalho
Superior Institute of Health Sciences—North, Portugal

G. Veiga, B. Vasconcelos & J.N. Pires
Mechanical Engineering Department, Faculty of Sciences and Technology, University of Coimbra, Coimbra, Portugal

M.F. Botelho
Institute of Biophysics and Biomathematics and Faculty of Medicine of Coimbra, IBILI, Coimbra, Portugal

ABSTRACT: We developed a method for measuring the fitness of a prosthesis and implants. Since a robot arm is use for executing the impressions and part of the measuring procedure we gain high precision and reproducibility. We tested the measuring method regarding the operator dependence and tests confirm consistent results even with different users.

Keywords: Implant dentistry; implant impression; robot programming

1 INTRODUCTION

Single or multiple teeth faults are highly probable to occur in the lifetime of a person. If teeth are not replaced oclusal problems caused by migration, inclination or extrusion of the other teeth may arise. These problems cause defective mastication which in turn results in digestive problems. Although teeth replacement could be madevia removable or fixed prosthesis, implant surgery is generally accepted as the best technique and the most appropriatefor complete teeth replacement.

The long term success of the implant technique is multifactor dependent, being difficult to point out the major factor. Nevertheless, dental impression is the first step for transferring and recording the relationship between the pillars of the implants and reproduces their relationship as accurately as possible [3].

There is a plethora of work addressing the impression issue [1,2,4–8] using either "in vitro" techniques or "in vivo" data. "In vitro" studies,

generally use a simplify model with certain number of implants that could be angulated. Over this model different impression methods and materials are tested. The evaluation of the impression accuracy is only performed after the completion of the prosthesis by measuring the fitness between the prosthesis and the initial model. Various approaches have been proposed to determine the gap between the model (or the real implant for "in vivo" situations) and the dental prosthesis. The profile projector and thetraveling microscope are the most frequent methods employed for "in vitro" studies whereas visual inspection, tactile sensation and radiographs analysis are preferred for "in vivo" situations. Unfortunately, these methods are user dependent requiring well train staff to produce reliable results. Moreover the technique used for the impressionrelies also on the experience of the operator that unconsciously induces undetermined errors.

In this work we propose an "in vitro" method for evaluating impression (methods and materials) that avoids the operator for executing both the impression and the measuring. The proposed method is based on the use of a robot arm for performing the impression. For measuring the gap, between a realistic mandible made of a photoelastic polymer and the prosthesis obtain from the impression, we use a high quality photo camera and a specifically designed software.

2 METHODS

We constructed several realistic mandibles with a polymer material. We also devised an appropriate support for fixing tightly the mandibles by its condyles. We, then, programmed an ABB robot arm for collecting the impression material with a proper dental tray and executed the impression of the mandible that was previously prepared with 4 implants and the corresponding transfer posts. For the preparation of the mandible we also used the robot for positioning the implants with very high precision and reproducibility.

Directly from the polymer model we built a full-arch zirconia dental prosthesis that was fitted to plaster mandibles made from the impressions. The gap between the implant analog and the prosthesis was evaluated by taking 6 zoom photos of each of the implants. The camera was positioned by the robot arm. Figure 1 shows how photos were taken.

We implemented a Matlab routine for analyzing each of the photos. The developed routine is semi-automatic requiring the action of the user in some steps. Although a fully automatic routine would be faster, it is difficult to devise one successful enough since each photo is taken from different poses revealing different illuminations.

For measuring the gap we take advantage of two aspects. First, the edges of the implant and the corresponding support in the prosthesis are easily seen in each photo. Second, the head of the implant analog has a calibrate length (1.8 mm) that can be used as reference in each photo. Therefore the user is asked to define 5 points (with a mouse click) at the prosthesis edge (red line in Figure 2),

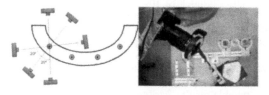

Figure 1. Left hand side: schematic representation of the photo arrangement for measuring the gap between the plaster mandibles and the zirconia dental prosthesis. Right hand side: photo of the actual arrangement.

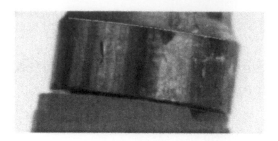

Figure 2. Photo of one implant analog and part of the prosthesis. The gap is well defined as the space between the red and the blues lines. The distance between the blue and the green line is used as reference.

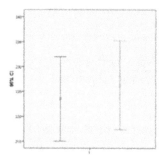

Figure 3. Error bar of the gap distance (μm) obtained for two users that tested three impressions each.

5 points at the superior edge of the implant head (blue line) and 5 points at the inferior edge of the head implant (green line).

The lines are defined based on the chosen points by fitting to them a parabolic curve. After the definition of the lines five points are evenly determine in the bottom line (red) and the distance to the middle line is calculated. The same procedure is applied to the middle line obtaining the distance of the reference measured in pixels. Finally, with 5 measures for the gap and five measures for the reference we do all the combinations of the quotients between the two distances writing in a file the 25 absolute measures of the gap (in mm). In fact, we construct a data base that can be easily accessed and analyzed with specific statistical software (e.g., SPSS).

To certify that the devise measure procedure is user independent we test for 3 mandibles the results obtained by two different operators. We applied to results a paired samples t-test ($\alpha = 5\%$).

3 RESULTS

In Figure 3, we show the error bar chart obtained for the gap in μm for three impressions when measure by two users. The overlap of the bars indicates that there are no differences statistically significant ($p > \alpha$).

4 DISCUSSION AND CONCLUSION

The developed method permits measuring with accuracy the fitness of prosthesis obtained using a certain impression technique. The use of a robot arm limits significantly random errors perform by an operator increasing as well the reproducibility of the complete procedure. Moreover, the measure process is consistent even with different operators.

REFERENCES

[1] Burns, J., Palmer, R., Howe, L. and Wilson, R. Accuracy of open tray implant impressions: an in vitro comparison of stock versus custom trays. *J Prosthet Dent*, 89(3):250–255, Mar 2003.

[2] Chee, W. and Jivraj, S. Impression techniques for implant dentistry. *Br Dent J*, 201(7):429–432, Oct 2006.

[3] Conrad, H.J., Pesun, I.J., DeLong, R. and Hodges, J.S. Accuracy of two impression techniques with angulated implants. *J Prosthet Dent*, 97(6):349–356, Jun 2007.

[4] Herbst, D. Nel, J.C. Driessen, C.H. and Becker, P.J. Evaluation of impression accuracy for osseointegrated implant supported superstructures. *J Prosthet Dent*, 83(5):555–561, May 2000.

[5] Lee, H., So, J.S., Hochstedler, J.L. and Ercoli, C. The accuracy of implant impressions: a systematic review. *J Prosthet Dent*, 100(4):285–291, Oct 2008.

[6] Lee, Y.-J., Heo, S.-J., Koak, J.Y. and Kim, S.-K. Accuracy of different impression techniques for internal-connection implants. *Int J Oral Maxillofac Implants*, 24(5):823–830, 2009.

[7] Vigolo, P., Majzoub, Z. and Cordioli, G. Evaluation of the accuracy of three techniques used for multiple implant abutment impressions. *J Prosthet Dent*, 89(2):186–192, Feb 2003.

[8] Wee, A.G. Comparison of impression materials for direct multi-implant impressions. *J Prosthet Dent*, 83(3):323–331, Mar 2000.

Technology and Medical Sciences – Natal Jorge et al. (eds)
© 2011 Taylor & Francis Group, London, ISBN 978-0-415-66822-4

Improving the resolution of scintigraphic images with super-resolution: Development of a dedicated device

R. Oliveira, F.J. Caramelo & N.C. Ferreira
Institute of Biophysics and Biomathematics, Faculty of Medicine of Coimbra, IBILI, Coimbra, Portugal

ABSTRACT: We developed a device for super-resolution imaging dedicated to scintigraphic images. Planar images obtained by a gamma camera usually present a poor resolution that can be improved at expenses of sensitivity. Other form of improving resolution is to acquire the object at different positions that are at distant from each other at subpixel level. The set of images can then be used to reconstruct an image with better resolution. Nevertheless, the success of the process is extremely dependent on the accuracy of the movements of the object. Therefore we devise and construct an inexpensive device for such movements. The device comprises two translational degrees of freedom and is easily controlled from a PC. The accuracy attained with the implemented solutions is less than 60 μm.

1 INTRODUCTION

Nuclear medicine images are obtained by detecting gamma photons with a specific collimated detector system that returns the radiotracer distribution. The detector is known as Gamma Camera (GC) and the general process of imaging is called planar scintigraphy, or simply scintigraphy. The GC can rotate around the patient, acquiring multiple views from different angular locations that are used to obtain tomographic images by appropriate reconstruction techniques. In this case the technique is denominate as SPECT (Single Photon Emission Computed Tomography). The design of the GC, original due to Hal Anger (1958) [1], has been subsequently improved and is currently close to the maximum of the efficiency to cost ratio. The main components of the gamma camera are the collimator, the scintillation crystal, the optical contact, the set of photomultiplier and electronics needed for signal discrimination. The collimator is a device, usually of lead, which is interposed between the crystal and the object and whose function is to stop the scattered rays that are not suitable for image formation. Because of the lack of refraction of the gamma-ray, collimators are essential in forming the image since it can establish a spatial correlation between the point of detection and the location of emission. However, the impact on sensitivity is enormous since only a fraction less than 1% of the photons reaching the collimator can pass through it and deposit their energy in the crystal [4]. Another aspect associated with collimators, is its direct influence on the spatial resolution (up to 8 mm) of the system. Besides the size of the holes, the distance between the object and the collimator affect the resolution of the GC. Hence, extremely careful is taken positioning the subject as close as possible to the GC in order to minimize the geometric effects of collimator in the resolution of the system. When high resolution is required (e.g. small animal imaging), specific collimators can be used—namely, high resolution collimators with parallel holes or pinhole collimators. High resolution collimator presents smaller holes, whereas the pinhole has just one hole. Both types have a tremendous impact on sensitivity, which therefore implies longer acquisition time or more dose of radiotracer. A better alternative is to use specific detectors that guarantee adequate spatial resolution for these applications. Super-resolution techniques may be an alternative to these dedicated GC. However, extremely accurate movements of the object must be performed in order to ensure the recovery of the resolution.

In this work, we implemented an affordable device that allows precise movements to use for super-resolution scintigraphic acquisitions.

2 THEORY

Super-resolution methods allow creating High-Resolution (HR) images from a set of images of Low Resolution (LR) of the same subject. If the LR images (samples) are acquired at distances that are smaller than the pixel size, then the new information contained in each sample can be exploited to obtain the HR image. If the offsets between images are known with excellent accuracy [3], the

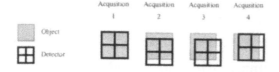

Figure 1. Principle of the super-resolution method. Four acquisitions at different positions are used to improve the resolution by a factor of 2. More acquisitions performed at closer positions may improve even more the resolution.

reconstruction of the HR image is possible [2]. The calculation of the HR image from the image samples can be understood as a reconstruction problem and, hence, typical algorithms of the field can be used (e.g. MLEM—Maximum Likelihood Expectation Maximization) [5]. Algebraically, the problem can be set as the solution of a linear equations system:

$$
\begin{bmatrix}
a_{11} & a_{12} & \cdots & a_{1N} \\
a_{21} & a_{22} & \cdots & a_{2N} \\
\vdots & & & \\
a_{M1} & a_{M2} & \cdots & a_{MN}
\end{bmatrix}
\begin{bmatrix}
s_1 \\
s_2 \\
\vdots \\
s_N
\end{bmatrix}
=
\begin{bmatrix}
L_1 \\
L_2 \\
\vdots \\
L_M
\end{bmatrix}
\quad (1)
$$

where s_i are the values of the pixels of the HR image, L_i the values of the pixels of the acquired LR images and the matrix with the elements a_{11} is the system matrix that links, through geometric relations, the HR image with the LR images. The s_i values can be obtained by calculating the pseudo-inverse matrix. However, due to noise this procedure is not always possible. Thus, as mentioned before, other methods are preferable.

In practice, the acquisition of the LR images is performed with the object (or the detector) at different positions. Fig. 1 shows, schematically, the acquisitions at 4 different positions which, theoretically, enable increasing the resolution by a factor of 2.

3 METHODS

We implemented a mechanism to carry out controlled simultaneous forward and backward movements in the horizontal xy coordinate axes. The dimensions of the developed system are 45×45 cm, with a base of 35×25 cm to allow the placement of a phantom or even a small animal.

The device is equipped with aluminum sliding guides that provide the linear displacement of the base platform, and this shift is caused by rotation of threaded shafts which are coupled to the ends of the platform. This movement is done by stepper motors, placed between them and the threaded

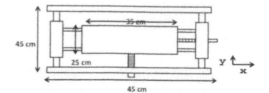

Figure 2. Scheme of the platform with two degrees of freedom. Both the linear movements in the xx and yy axis are achieved with threaded shafts that are coupled to suitable step motors.

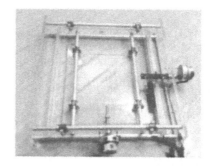

Figure 3. Final assembly of the platform.

shaft gearbox used to reduce the mechanical torque produced by the stepper motor, and increase the torque in the threaded shaft. The gearboxes present an output torque of 121×10^{-3} Nm.

We used lightweight materials to allow the system to be portable. Perspex (acrylic) was used in the external structure of the platform andin the basis. All other materials are made of light alloys.

For monitoring the absolute position we use a linear potentiometer since is an inexpensive device and also because when mounted properly the voltage signal is nearly linear. The position is paired to the resistance and, therefore to the voltage signal that can be easily and accurately measured. The analogue voltage signal is then transform into a digital signal by using a suitable ADC. To measure the spatial position and to control the stepper motors we used the data acquisition module UD128A8D (B & B), which has a 12 bits ADC and 8 digital inputs/outputs capable of interfacing with the PC. We also employ power drivers (ULN2003) with the purpose of supplying the correct power to the step motors.

After the final assembly of the platform we calibrate it by moving the motors 100 rotations and then measuring the position of the platform using a digital caliper. We then fit a line to the obtained pairs of values resulting in two calibration curves (one for each motion direction).

4 RESULTS

Results obtained so far (e.g. calibration curves) shows that the platform has an exactness less than 60 μm.

The PC control facilitates all the procedure since a user friendly GUI was implemented.

5 DISCUSSION AND CONCLUSION

The control procedure that we implemented (proportional control) shows some ripple behavior that we are correcting for. After the correction is accomplished we expect to improve the exactness of the system. Nevertheless, the results obtained until now are already satisfactory to improve the resolution (via super-resolution methods) in gamma cameras which is roughly 8 mm in normal conditions.

REFERENCES

[1] Anger, H.O. *J Nucl Med*, 5:515–531, Jul 1964.
[2] Caramelo, F.J. et al. In *IEEE NSS'07*, 6, 4452–4456, 2007.
[3] Caramelo, F.J. In *EANM'08, Munich, Germany*, 2008.
[4] Ricard, M. *NIMPRA*, 527(1–2):124–129, July 2004.
[5] Shepp, L.A. & Vardi, Y. *IEEE TMI*. 1(2):113–122, 1982.

Technology and Medical Sciences – Natal Jorge et al. (eds)
© 2011 Taylor & Francis Group, London, ISBN 978-0-415-66822-4

Hyperbolic surfaces for scaffold design

H.A. Almeida & P.J. Bártolo
Centre for Rapid and Sustainable Product Development—CDRsp, Polytechnic Institute of Leiria, Portugal

ABSTRACT: Tissue engineering represents a new, emerging interdisciplinary field involving combined efforts of biologists, engineers, material scientists and mathematicians towards the development of biological substitutes to restore, maintain, or improve tissue functions.

Most strategies in tissue engineering have focussed on using biomaterials as scaffolds to direct specific cell types to organise into three-dimensional structures and perform differentiated functions. Scaffolds provide a temporary mechanical and vascular support for tissue regeneration while shaping the in-growth tissues. These scaffolds must be biocompatible, biodegradable, with appropriate porosity, pore structure and pore distribution and optimal vascularisation, with both surface and structural compatibility. Surface compatibility means a chemical, biological and physical suitability to the host tissue. Structural compatibility corresponds to an optimal adaptation to the mechanical behaviour of the host tissue.

Recent advances in the tissue engineering field are increasingly relying on modelling and simulation. The design of optimised scaffolds based on the fundamental knowledge of its microstructure is a relevant topic of research. This paper proposes the use of novel geometric structures based on Schoen geometries, one of the Triple Periodic Minimal Surfaces. Geometries based on these surfaces enables the design of vary high surface-to-volume ratio structures with high porosity and mechanical/vascular properties.

Technology and Medical Sciences – Natal Jorge et al. (eds)
© *2011 Taylor & Francis Group, London, ISBN 978-0-415-66822-4*

Finite element analysis of a three layered cartilage

D.M. Freitas, P.J. Bártolo & H.A. Almeida
Centre for Rapid and Sustainable Product Development—CDRsp, Polytechnic Institute of Leiria, Portugal

ABSTRACT: Cartilage is a stiff and inflexible connective tissue found in many areas in living creatures located mainly in articular joints and intervertebral discs. Cartilage is composed of specialized cells called chondrocytes that produce a large amount of extracellular matrix composed of Type II collagen fibers, abundant ground substance rich in proteoglycan, and elastin fibers. Cartilage is classified in three types, elastic cartilage, hyaline cartilage and fibro cartilage, which differ in the relative amounts of these three main components. Unlike other connective tissues, cartilage does not contain blood vessels. The chondrocytes are supplied by diffusion, helped by the pumping action generated by compression of the articular cartilage or flexion of the elastic cartilage.

Many are the causes of damaged cartilage, such as diseases, trauma or genetic disorder. For instance, the failure of articular cartilage in the hip or knee may lead to hip or knee replacement. In order to overcome this issue, a new emerging interdisciplinary medical field, tissue engineering and regenerative medicine, have increased their importance due to the development of biological substitutes to restore, maintain, or improve tissue functions.

Most strategies in tissue engineering have focussed on using biomaterials as scaffolds to direct specific cell types to organise into three-dimensional structures and perform differentiated functions. Scaffolds provide a temporary mechanical and vascular support for tissue regeneration while shaping the in-growth tissues. These scaffolds must be biocompatible, biodegradable, with appropriate porosity, pore structure and pore distribution and optimal vascularisation, with both surface and structural compatibility.

Recent advances in the tissue engineering field are increasingly relying on modelling and simulation. This paper presents the undergoing research with the objective of defining a new mathematical formulation more adequate than the existing finite element models in order to simulate the cartilage behaviour and optimize the existing scaffold variables for cartilage applications. Firstly, swine cartilage was characterized and then a numerical model was defined and simulated using hiperelastic and viscoelastic models. after performing the simulations, the results were compared to the experimental results of the swine cartilage.

Technology and Medical Sciences – Natal Jorge et al. (eds)
© 2011 Taylor & Francis Group, London, ISBN 978-0-415-66822-4

External breast radiotherapy treatment planning verification using advanced anthropomorphic phantoms

J.A.M. Santos, J. Lencart, A.G. Dias & L.T. Cunha
Centro de Investigação do Instituto Português de Oncologia do Porto Francisco Gentil, EPE, Porto, Portugal

C. Relvas, A. Ramos & V.F. Neto
Departamento de Engenharia Mecânica, Universidade de Aveiro, Campus de Santiago, Aveiro, Portugal

ABSTRACT: Recent accidents in some countries involving incorrect radiation dose delivery to external radiotherapy patients revived an international discussion about the question of treatment plan verification and absolute dose accuracy delivered during the radiotherapy treatment course. The present work aims to develop a versatile and useful tool to verify the breast treatment planning by the Treatment Planning System (TPS) and, furthermore, that it will be delivered to the patient as expected. To achieve this goal, a female Alderson RANDO anthropomorphic phantom was used. A computationally designed polycarbonate (PC1000) breast simulating phantom was implanted on the RANDO surface after being designed following topographic laser scanning of the RANDO implantation interface for perfect fitting of both surfaces. The dose distribution inside the breast was measured at an inner plane with a radiochromic film and absolute dose near the thoracic wall was measured using a Farmer ionization chamber. The breast phantom was filled with water and silicone prosthesis was introduced to simulate tissue heterogeneity. The results proved to be of extreme importance especially during the acceptance testing of new or different algorithms of TPS and can be extended to other targets such as head and neck pathologies.

1 INTRODUCTION

1.1 Radiotherapy accidents

Patient safety in external radiotherapy treatment delivery has always been a concern (Shafiq, 2009) and can have several origins and consequences, such as dose variations of 5% (minor potential seriousness) to 25% dose variations (critical and lethal seriousness) leading to inefficiency of treatment, serious injury or even death. Reporting and studying such accidents (Derreumaux, 2008), through incident learning and prevention, double checking, *in-vivo* dosimetry, independent calculations (Sellakumar, 2010) and report management improvement, are tools usually used to decrease the probability of miscalculating or other errors that can influence the delivered dose to the patient (Clark, 2010). Also the reducing in the errors and uncertainties can have an important effect in the radiotherapy outcome (Van Dik, 1993).

1.2 TPS verification protocols

Several studies over the years have contributed to develop and upgrade protocols and guidelines for TPS verification (Mijnheer, 2005, AAPM, 1998, IAEA, 2005). The aim of these studies is focused on the verification of range of deviations between planned and delivered doses in situations as close as possible to a clinical procedure. Several methodologies can be used and the use of anthropomorphic phantoms is one of the most important choices, given the resemblance to the real clinical setting. In the present work, a special phantom simulating a breast treatment with two tangential beams was used. The specificity of the geometry, as well as the possibility of several dose measurement methodologies constitutes an important factor in the verification of the TPS.

2 MATERIALS AND METHODS

2.1 Phantom materials

A polycarbonate (PC1000; $1.2\,\mathrm{g\,cm^{-3}}$) material was chosen to make the breast replica to be positioned in a female Rando anthropomorphic phantom. This material was chosen after comparison with other polymeric materials in terms of fabrication possibilities, CT-number similarity to human tissue (positive CT-numbers), transparency to visible light, high radiation dose resistance and good mechanical properties.

Several materials were considered beside PC1000, such as polyethylene, polypropylene, ertacetal, PEEK carbon, Tectron and Teflon. Several CT scans were performed to determine the CT-number of all these materials and to determine if there was any significant change after irradiation until a maximum dose of a few hundred Gy. These values of absorbed dose are much higher than the dose absorbed by a complete fractionated treatment (typically, for breast irradiation, the value of absorbed dose at the volume of interest is around 50 Gy delivered in 25 daily fractions).

Beside the CT-number evaluation, a X-Ray Diffraction (XRD) analysis was performed before and after a megavoltage irradiation of 400 Gy by a radiotherapy *linac* (6 MV). The resultant experimental curves can be seen in Figure 2.

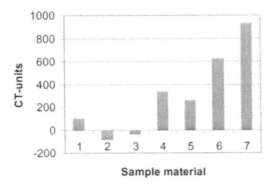

Figure 1. Results of CT-number determination by CT scanning of all the studied samples: PC1000 (1), polyethylene (2), polypropylene (3), ertacetal (4), PEEK carbon (5), Tectron (6) and Teflon (7).

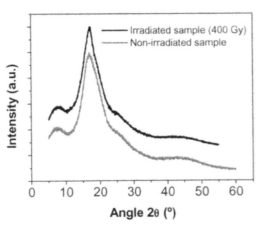

Figure 2. Results of X-Ray Diffraction (XRD) analysis of two PC1000 samples showing a clear insensibility to 400 Gy of radiation: the main peak occurs for the same angle and no extra peaks are observed either before or after irradiation.

2.2 *Phantom design and manufacturing*

To fabricate the breast phantom, one started by the acquisition of topographic data of the implantation surface on the Rando phantom using 3D laser scanning technology (Zscanner 700, Zcorporation, USA). The shape of contact area was accurately defined and a 3D CAD model was designed according to the specifications of the breast implant, allowing the housing of several radiation measuring devices (e.g. TLD dosimeters, radiochromic film and ionization chamber detectors). The breast phantom was fabricated by machining using computer numerical control technology. For breast heterogeneity simulation, before the phantom being filled with water, a prosthetic silicone implant could beoptionally placed inside.

2.3 *Treatment planning*

A 3D CT image volume was acquired and a treatment was planned for homogeneous breast irradiation using two *Varian Eclipse* TPS algorithms: *Pencil Beam Convolution* (PBC) and *Anisotropic Analytic Algorithm* (AAA). While PBC algorithms generates a dose distribution matrix by convolution of pencil beam kernels with a non-uniform field function, the AAA is a 3D pencil beam convolution superposition algorithm that has separate modeling for primary photons, scattered extra focal photons and electrons scattered from the beam limiting devices.

The treatment chosen was a conventional breast tangential two beam configuration. This treatment plan configuration consists usually in two tangential beams: one incident from the external side of the breast being treated (in our case we treated the left breast, so the external beam is positioned from the left side of the patient) and another from the internal side of the breast (incident from the right in the present case). Additionally, narrower beams (usually called segment beams) can be applied to achieve a better dose uniformity. The presented planned treatment to the phantom breast consisted in one tangential internal beam and two tangential external beams (the main beam plus a segment).

2.4 *Treatment delivery and dose measurements*

The phantom breast treatment irradiation was performed exactly as for a real patient (Figure 4), being irradiated 25 times (2 Gy per fraction at the volume of interest), with a few minutes interval between each fraction delivery instead of de daily daily fraction scheme used with patients.

During CT acquisition for treatment planning, an ionization chamber (Farmer type) was positioned in a specially designed inset space underneath the breast volume, close to the contact surface between the breast phantom and

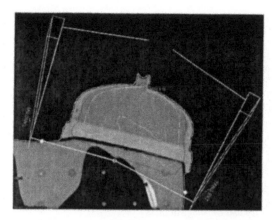

Figure 3. TPS view of the breast phantom during the treatment planning. The breast phantom is showed positioned in the RANDO anthropomorphic phantom. The isodose curves of 100% and 95% are showed.

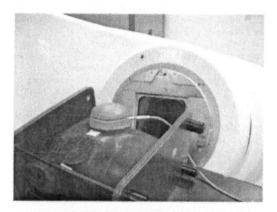

Figure 4. Anthropomorphic RANDO phantom placed for treatment delivery during an external tangential field irradiation.

the RANDO phantom. Also a circular shaped radiochromic film (Gafchromic EBT2) was positioned inside the phantom in a plane covering the whole breast base. The radiochromic film reading was performed with an *Epson Expression 10000XL* photo scanner with transparency adapter. A previous calibration curve was obtained for the film optical density from 0 to 7.5 Gy, with 0.2 Gy steps, for the same linear accelerator and energy used for the phantom irradiation. Only the red image channel was used due to its enhanced response to this wavelength (ISP, 2009).

The orientation of the scanning was the same for all the measurements to avoid anisotropic light scattering. The measurements were made 24 h after the irradiation to minimize the effects of post-exposure changes (ISP, 2009). The Gafchromic EBT2 red channel sensibility is high up to 8 Gy.

3 RESULTS

3.1 *Dose profiles*

After the irradiation, the radiochromic film was digitized for dose distribution verification and comparison with dose predicted by the TPS.

A previous irradiation with 6 Gy (the present gafchromic film is known to saturate at 8 Gy) was performed without the prosthesis and with the circular gafchromic film in place. In Figure 5, one shows the gafchromic dose profile measurement compared with the curves obtained by both TPS algorithms (PBC and AAA).

3.2 *Absolute dose measurements*

During the simulated treatment, the dose was measured using the Farmer ionization chamber associated with a PTW Unidos electrometer. The dose values measured with the ionization chamber were also evaluated and compared with the doses expected by the TPS using the PBC algorithm. The point of dose extracted from the TPS plan lied within the active region of the Farmer type ionization chamber, easily identified in the 3D CT scan. The doses from single beams and total dose delivered to this point are showed in Table 1.

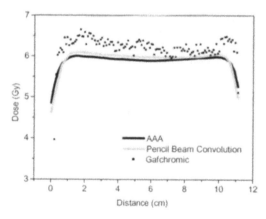

Figure 5. Comparison of the dose profiles obtained with the gafchromic film and the TPS algorithms (PBC and AAA).

Table 1. Comparison between the planned (PBC) and measured doses using the anthropomorphic phantom.

Field	Ext. tang.		Int. tang	
Measurement	Main	Segment	Main	Total
Meas. dose	0.889	0.091	1.035	2.016
Plann. dose	0.899	0.093	1.013	2.005
%	−1%	−2.5%	2.1%	0.5%

The table compares the measured dose for each of the individual beams with the planned dose for the same beam configuration. The total dose is calculated with PBC algorithm and also depicted in the table. For sake of analysis, the percent deviation of the measured dose relative to the planned dose is also showed.

4 CONCLUSIONS

One notices that the overall dose deviation of the absolute dose measurement is about 0.5%, which is clearly above the standard recommended limits (IAEA, 2005). However, the individual tangential fields present a deviation from the TPS value that exceeds the 2%, a fact not easily explainable but that can possibly be originated by a very small angular positioning error between the acquired CT and the position during treatment delivery. Nevertheless, a deviation in one field appears to compensate the deviation of the other field, canceling the overall dose variation.

The gafchromic results were also extremely satisfactory with a clear homogeneity and a relatively good agreement with the TPS profile for the same plane in the phantom. Although the dose measured with the gafchromic film presents a slightly higher value (around 4.7%), this is in accordance with the dose errors reported for gafchromic dosimetry (Butson, 2009; Hartmann, 2010). However, the shape of the gafchromic dose response closely resembles the predicted dose profiles as provided by the TPS algorithms (both PBC and AAA).

These results are a clear indication of the usefulness of this type of phantoms for TPS verification in a situation such as breast radiotherapy. The phantom can be also of extreme convenience during the acceptance and commissioning of new TPS and algorithm upgrade.

REFERENCES

AAPM, 1998. Quality assurance for clinical radiotherapy treatment planning. Report 53. *Med. Phys.* 25; 1773–1829.

Butson, M.J. *et al.* 2009. Dose and absorption spectra response of EBT2 Gafchromic film to high energy x-rays, Australasian Physical & Engineering Sciences in Medicine, Volume 32, Number 4.

Clark, B.G. *et al.* 2010. The management of radiation tretment error through incident learning. *Radiotherapy and Oncology* in press.

Derreumaux, S. *et al.* Lessons from recent accidents in radiation therapy in France. *Radiat Prot Dosimetry* (2008) 131(1): 130–135.

Hartmann, B. 2010. *Homogeneity of Gafchromic EBT2 film*, Medical Physics, 37(4): 1753–1756.

ISP, 2009. International Specialty Products, Gafchromic® EBT2 Self-Developing Film for Radiotherapy Dosimetry, Revision 1, February 19, 2009.

IAEA, 2005. Commissioning and quality assurance of computerized planning systems for radiation treatment of cancer. *Technical Report Series* 430.

Mijnheer, B. *et al.* 2005. Quality assurance of treatment planning systems. Practical examples for non-IMRT photon Beams. *ESTRO Booklet nº 7* (Brussels).

Sellakumar, P. *et al.* 2010. Comparison of monitor units calculated by radiotherapy treatment planning system and an independent monitor unit verification software. *Physica Medica* in press.

Shafiq, J., Barton, M., Noble, D., Lemer, C. & Donaldson, L.J. 2009. An international review of patient safety measures in radiotherapy practice. *Radiotherapy and Oncology* 92(1): 15–21.

Van Dik, J. *et al.* 1993. Commissioning and quality assurance of treatment planning computers. *Int. J. Radiat. Oncol. Biol. Phy.* 26 (1): 261–273.

Technology and Medical Sciences – Natal Jorge et al. (eds)
© 2011 Taylor & Francis Group, London, ISBN 978-0-415-66822-4

Blood Volume Pulse peak detector with a double adaptive threshold

J. Medeiros & R. Martins
Departamento de Física, Faculdade de Ciências e Tecnologia, Universidade de Coimbra, Coimbra, Portugal

S. Palma
PLUX—Wireless Biosignals, Lisboa, Portugal

H. Gamboa
PLUX—Wireless Biosignals, Lisboa, Portugal
CEFITEC—FCT—Universidade Nova de Lisboa, Lisboa, Portugal

M. Reis
Departamento de Engenharia Química, Faculdade de Ciências e Tecnologia, Universidade de Coimbra, Coimbra, Portugal

ABSTRACT: Blood Volume Pulse (BVP) signal processing is a method to access heart rate and other cardiovascular parameters. In this work we developed an algorithm that detects the cardiac systole from the BVP signal with high accuracy. The implemented algorithm consists of a Slope Sum Function (SSF), an adaptive threshold strategy and a backsearch routine which works as a double adaptive threshold to enhance the sensitivity of the systole detection. In order to evaluate the performance of our algorithm we synchronously acquired BVP and eletrocardiogram (ECG) signals from a group of nineteen volunteers. The QRS complexes were annotated in the ECG signals and used as reference to detect false positives and false negatives in BVP detected systoles. The algorithm detected 99.94% of the 20 210 BVP systoles evident.

Keywords: blood volume pulse sensor, pulse detector, adaptive threshold, backsearch routine, algorithm, signal processing

1 INTRODUCTION

The BVP signal is obtained with a photoplethysmography sensor. This sensor measures the changes in blood flow in arteries and capillaries during the cardiac cycle by shinning an infrared Light-Emission Diode (LED) through the tissues (Peper, et al. 2007 and Webster, 1997). The intensity of light that travels through the tissue and is detected in the photodetector changes proportionally to the amount of blood flowing in the tissues (Haahr, 2006).

Since the BVP signal reflects the blood changes that occur during a cardiac cycle it can be used as an alternative to ECG to assess instantaneous heart rate and the rr intervals. Some of the advantages of using a BVP sensor to extract the referred parameters are the fact that the sensor is non-invasive and is less obstrusive than an ECG sensor (Peper, et al. 2007). Additionally, it is possible to extract from this signal other parameters, such as pulse transit time and peripheral vasodilatation (Reisner, et al. 2008).

In the following sections we describe the development of an automated algorithm for detection of local maxima of the BVP pulses, which correspond to systoles in the cardiac cycle. An accurate detection of this parameter in the BVP signal is important for the computation of variables used to access the subject's health condition, such as heart rate variability (Haarh, 2006; Reisner, et al. 2008). Applications of this sensor and algorithm in health care range from internship and ambulatory healthcare to long-term patient monitoring. (Peper, et al. 2007).

2 METHODS

2.1 The algorithm

We implemented an algorithm that detects the local maxima of BVP pulses. The algorithm consists in three main steps: a Slope Sum Function (SSF), an adaptive threshold (Zong, 2003) and a backsearch routine.

When applied to the BVP signal, the SSF allows to keep pulses' information. The signal that results from the SSF is, then, checked for local maxima using an adaptive threshold and a decision criteria to determine whether or not a maximum occurs in each SSF pulse (Zong, 2003).

When a maximum is detected, the threshold (Th) is updated according to the value of that maximum. For each SSF pulse, the algorithm performs a local search for its maximum value between the two points where the threshold is crossed.

In order to avoid the loss of maxima due to big decays in the value of the maximum between consecutive BVP pulses, we implemented a backsearch routine. When (1) is verified the backsearch is activated and a lower threshold ($Th_{3.1}$) is set (Figure 1).

$$\Delta t_i > 110\% \times \Delta t_{i-1} \tag{1}$$

2.2 *Database and acquisition scenario*

To test the developed algorithm we collected a set of data composed of BVP and ECG from nineteen healthy volunteers with ages between 17 and 53 years old. Each volunteer was instrumented with a finger BVP sensor placed on the 4th finger of the left hand and an ECG triode at V2 precordial lead connected to a *bioPLUX research* data acquisition system (PLUX 2010). The acquisition of ECG and BVP signals was performed synchronously, with the subjects seated and with their left forearm resting on an horizontal platform. The data collected along with the correspondent ECG QRS annotations is available on the Open Signals database (http://www.opensignals.net).

2.3 *Algorithm evaluation procedure*

The method used to assess the accuracy of the algorithm is based on the comparison of the number of maxima detected in the BVP signal with the number of ECG pulse annotations. The comparison was performed by visual inspection when a critical point was detected. To find a critical point we used two different approaches. In both approaches we verified if the number of maxima detected in the BVP signal was the same as the annotated in the correspondent ECG.

In the first approach, if the number of maxima in the BVP was equal to the number of ECG pulse annotations, we checked if there were some discrepancies in the time intervals between consecutive maxima in both BVP and ECG. The discrepancies were identified as critical points and visually inspected in order to decide if they corresponded or not to lost maxima in the BVP signal.

In the second approach, if the number of maxima in the BVP was different from the number of ECG pulse annotations, we had to visually inspect the signal and look for critical points because we could not compare the time intervals directly.

We have applied this method to determine the number of true and false positives as well as true and false negatives, which will be used to evaluate the sensitivity and specificity of two versions of the algorithm: (a) with backsearch routine and (b) without backsearch routine.

3 RESULTS AND DISCUSSION

Sensitivity and specifity results of the two versions of the algorithms are listed in Table 1 and 2.

The version with backsearch routine presents a sensitivity of 99.94% for the 20 210 peaks annotated in the ECG while the second version showed a sensitivity of only 99.60% for the same dataset. On the other hand, specificity was 100% for both versions.

Analyzing these results it is valid to induce that our strategy revealed high levels of performance

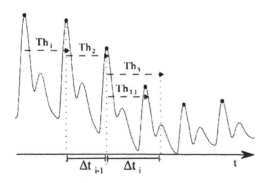

Figure 1. BVP signal with a regular pulse detection and with a backsearch pulse detection.

Tabel 1. Sensitivity and specificity of the algorithm with the backsearch routine.

	Sen (%)	Spe (%)
Gross	99.94	100
Average	99.93	100

Tabel 2. Sensitivity and specificity of the without the backsearch routine.

	Sen (%)	Spe (%)
Gross	99.60	100
Average	99.58	100

and that the backsearch routine increased the sensitivity of the algorithm.

Our study also revealed that the algorithm's sensitivity is highly affected by physiological phenomena like Premature Ventricular Contraction (Keany and Desai 2010) which can lead to attenuation and suppression of some BVP pulses. This situation has been the cause of most of non-detected BVP pulses.

Excluding those events we can conclude that the present algorithm showed an excellent performance.

REFERENCES

Haahr, R. 2006. Reflectance Pulse Oximetry Sensor for the Electronic Patch. Technical University of Denmark.

Keany, J.E. & Desai, A.D. Premature Ventricular Contraction: eMedicine Emergency Medicine. Available at: http://emedicine.medscape.com/article/761148-overview [Accessed May 13, 2010].

Peper, E. et al. 2007. Is There More to Blood Volume Pulse Than Heart Rate Variability, Respiratory Sinus Arrhythmia, and Cardiorespiratory Synchrony? Biofeedback, 35(2), 54–61.

PLUX, bioPLUX Research. PLUX Wireless Biosignals. Available at: www.plux.info [Accessed April 5, 2010].

Reisner, A. et al. 2008. Utility of the Photoplethysmogram in Circulatory Monitoring. Anesthesiology, 108(5), 950–958.

Webster, J.G. 1997. Design of pulse oximeters, IOP Publishing Ltd.

Zong, W. et al. 2003. An Open-source Algorithm to Detect Onset of Arterial Blood Pressure Pulses. *Computers in Cardiology*, 30, 259–262.

Technology and Medical Sciences – Natal Jorge et al. (eds)
© *2011 Taylor & Francis Group, London, ISBN 978-0-415-66822-4*

Bilateral study on arterial stiffness assessment by a non-invasive optical technique of Photoplethysmography

V. Vassilenko
Center of Physics and Technological Research—CEFITEC, Physics Department, Faculty of Sciences and Technology, Universidade Nova de Lisboa, Caparica, Portugal

A.C. Silva
NMT, Lda., Madan Parque—Parque de Ciência e Tecnologia de Almada, Caparica, Portugal

A.M. Martin
Faculty of Mathematics, University of Sevilha, Sevilha, Spain

J.G. O'Neill
Faculdade de Ciências Médicas, Universidade Nova de Lisboa, Lisboa, Portugal

ABSTRACT: The great potential of Photoplethysmography (PPG) for vascular assessment, such as arterial disease, arterial compliance and ageing, was recently recognized. In this paper we describe a prototype apparatus based on the low cost, simple and portable PPG technology. Also, we are present a new protocol for the experimental measurements of arterial stiffness as a potential tool for early diagnostic of the atherosclerosis.

A bilateral pulse measurements system simultaneously acquired PPG pulses from left and right arms, electrocardiographic (ECG) and pressure electrical signals. The PPG reflectance mode sensors utilize low cost semiconductor technology with LED and photodetector devices working at the near infrared wavelength of 940 nm. The principal parameters of LED sensor and its importance for signal sensitivity optimization are also discussed.

Keywords: Arterial blood vessels, Stiffness, Photoplethysmography (PPG), Pulse Wave Velocity (PWV), Stiffness Index (SI) and Reflection Index (RI)

1 INTRODUCTION

Cardiovascular diseases are the leading cause of death worldwide. That condition has a close relationship with changes in the elastic properties of blood vessels. Increased arterial stiffness is a characteristic of the elderly population. However, recently is noted an increasing number of young people with manifestations of vascular disorders such as atherosclerosis, diabetes mellitus, and others. Thus, the main motivation of this study was the development of methods and devices for screening and early diagnosis of these diseases.

Currently, the most common parameter for assessing in vivo mechanical properties of arteries is the Pulse Wave Velocity (PWV). However, the value of this index varies not only depending on the location of sensors for detection of this wave along the different arteries, but even in anatomically symmetric points of the ends he has certain differences, which makes it impossible to compare the limited existing data in literature. Accordingly, a bilateral study of the wave pulse signal was conducted, measured in the radial arteries on the right and left, in order to determine the quantitative relationship between them.

2 EXPERIMENTAL RESULTS

The experimental data were acquired using a prototype apparatus, method and protocol, previously developed in our group, based on a cheap, fast, portable and non-invasive measurements technique Photoplethysmography (PPG). This optical technique can be used to detect blood volume changes in the microvascular bed of tissue. PPG has been applied in many different clinical settings, including clinical physiological monitoring, such as blood oxygen saturation, heart rate, blood pressure, cardiac output and respiration. The great potential of PPG for vascular assessment, such as arterial disease, arterial compliance and ageing, was also recently recognized (Allen, 2007).

Optical PPG reflectance mode sensors (Stojanovic & Karadaglic, 2007), which utilize low cost semiconductor technology with LED and photodetector devices, operating at a near infrared wavelength of 920 nm, were adapted for acquiring the pulse wave in the peripheral zone of the carpus and then tested for quality and repeatability of the signal (Vale, et al., 2008).

Special attention in protocol elaboration were given to the minimization of factors which affect reproducibility of PPG measurements, including the method of probe attachment to the tissue, probe-tissue interface pressure, minimization of movement artifact, subject posture and room temperature (Vassilenko, et al., 2008). The main parameters analyzed were the Pulse Wave Velocity (PWV), the Stiffness Index (SI) and the Reflection Index (RI) and the measurements were made on a sample of 23 healthy adult volunteers and without an associated diagnosis of both sexes, aged between 22 and 65.

The obtained experimental results for PWV, SI and RI were analyzed statistically according to age and sex to determine a quantitative relationship between the values of those parameters for symmetrical ends points of the Right Hand Side (RHS) and Left Hand Side (LHS) was used the Pearson Correlation test and the Paired Samples test (T-Student test).

From our results there is a significant linear Correlation (the variables are significantly dependent on each other) between parameters SI RHS & SI LHS ($r = 0.722$, $p < 0.001$) and RI RHS & RI LHS ($r = 0.668$, $p < 0.001$), and a little lower for the PWV RHS & PWV LHS ($r = 0.582$, $p = 0.004$).

3 CONCLUSIONS

Obtained experimental results for the PWV are in good agreement with the similar ones from the literature. However there are no data in the literature for comparison for other parameters.

Statistical analysis all tested parameters show that there is no variability, so experimentally measures valuesfor Pulse Wave Velocity (PWV), the Stiffness Index (SI) and the Reflection Index (RI) are uniform.

In general, results shows that PWV and SI, both given in m/s, are strongly correlated with aging, as a principal factor. From other hand, the Reflection Index shows to be more sensitive to the individual arterial characteristics. This suggests that they are promising parameters for the assessment and early diagnostics of atherosclerosis and other arterial diseases

Furthermore, the investigation on more statistically significant population could be done in order to define the normative ranges for these parameters for the healthy people, and also estimate the accuracy of arterial disease detection.

BIBLIOGRAPHY

Allen, J. 2007. Photoplethysmography and its application in clinical physiological measurement, *Physiological Measurement*, Vol. 28: R1–R39.

Stojanovic, R. & Karadaglic, D. 2007. A LED-LED based photopletysmography sensor.—*Physiol. Meas.* Vol. 28: N19–N27.

Vale, A.C., Silva, A.C., Ferreira, J.L. & Vassilenko, V. 2008. Parametrização de sensores de sinal fotopletismográfico para o estudo de vasos sanguíneos. *Proc. 16th National Conference of Physics, 6–8, September, Caparica, Portugal*: 168.

Vassilenko, V., Vale, A.C., Silva, A.C. & Pavlov, S. 2008. Improvement of PPG methodology for arterial stiffness assessment, *Proc. IV Intern. Conf. on Optoelectronic Information Technologies—'Photonics ODS, 29, September-2, October, Vinnytsia, Ukraine*: 65.

Technology and Medical Sciences – Natal Jorge et al. (eds)
© 2011 Taylor & Francis Group, London, ISBN 978-0-415-66822-4

A biomimetic strategy to prepare silica- and silica/biopolymer-based composites for biomedical applications

R.B. Chim, M.E.M. Braga, M.M. Figueiredo & H.C. de Sousa
CIEPQPF, Chemical Engineering Department, FCTUC, University of Coimbra, Coimbra, Portugal

C.R. Ziegler & J.J. Watkins
Department of Polymer Science and Engineering, University of Massachusetts, Amherst, USA

ABSTRACT: Green and biomimetic strategies were developed for the formation and processing of silica and silica/biopolymer-based composites and for the immobilization of bioactive species such as drugs and proteins on those materials. This may lead to the future development of valuable composite materials for several biomedical, drug delivery and hard tissue engineering applications. These strategies involved the use of recently discovered bioinspired catalysts for tetraethylorthosilicate (TEOS) hydrolysis and condensation, the use of biopolymers from natural, biological and renewable sources and, finally, and the use of Supercritical Fluids (SCFs) to process the biomimetically generated composites.

Green and non-harsh sol-gel methods such as one-pot aqueous procedures at near room temperature/pressure and at near-neutral/neutral pH conditions were employed. Biomimetic catalysts are non-toxic and widely available biomolecules and, due to their different pH character in water solutions, they were employed alone or titrated against one another for the formation of silica and of silica-based composites over broad and tunable ranges of pH, including neutral pH. This methodology was also used to attain a desired final pH taking in consideration the most advantageous value in terms of the stability of the employed bioactive species as well as to make possible the dissolution of those biopolymers which dissolve at different pH values, thus allowing the simultaneous silica and bioactive composite formation. These procedures presented evident advantages when compared to the current conventional methods (using HCl, p-TSA, ammonia, high temperatures/pressures) in terms of avoiding the use and the residual presence of organic/inorganic potentially toxic substances and when the immobilization of pH- and thermo-labile biopolymers and bioactive species is intended. Furthermore, the incorporation of other inorganic osteoconductive materials (such as calcium hydroxyapatite) was also easily performed concurrently. An innovative sequential and continuous SCF extraction procedure was tested to remove residuals and to dry some of the generated materials, thus avoiding the use of high drying temperatures which may degrade the involved thermo-labile substances as well as to prevent the shrinkage of formed composites.

Silica and silica/biopolymer-based composites were prepared at room temperature and at 37°C, and at pH values between 2.9 and 9.8. Several biopolymers and proteins were evaluated as composite organic materials such as chitin, chitosan, *N*-carboxymethyl chitosan, dextran and oxidized dextran, starch and amylopectin, pectin, sodium alginate, gelatin, soy protein and bovine albumin. Calcium hydroxyapatite and several polyphenolic compounds from different natural origins were also tested. TEOS was the preferred silica precursor despite the fact that several other vinylic orthosilicates were also used. Water-soluble vinylic monomers and initiators were also added and polymerized during or after silica formation. Finally, dexamethasone (widely used as an anti-inflammatory and as an osteogenic differentiation substance for bone marrow stem cells) was incorporated in silica and in some silica/biopolymer composites and its release profile was studied.

Some selected composite materials were characterized using several chemical, physical and thermal analytical techniques. The effects of pH, stirring and of employed drying conditions/methods (including supercritical fluid drying) on synthesis yields and on some of the obtained materials properties were evaluated.

Preliminary results indicated that some of these green and biomimetic methodologies may have a great potential for the development and preparation of silica-based composite materials that can be used for several biomedical and hard tissue engineering applications. Presently, more work is being carried out on these most promising materials in terms of their obtained and intended functional properties for biomedical applications.

Keywords: Green and biomimetic methods, silica, silica-based composites, biomedical applications

Technology and Medical Sciences – Natal Jorge et al. (eds)
© 2011 Taylor & Francis Group, London, ISBN 978-0-415-66822-4

Non-invasive biomonitoring of human health: Technical developments in breath analysis

Valentina Vassilenko
Center of Physics and Technological Research (CEFITEC), Physics Department, Faculdade de Ciências e Tecnologia, Universidade Nova de Lisboa, Caparica, Portugal
NMT, Lda, Madan Parque daFCT-UNL, Caparica, Portugal

The detection and monitoring of biomarkers for oxidative stress by measurement of endogenous compounds in exhaled breath has received increasing attention in the past decade. Numerous studies have been performed in order to establish the physiological and pathophysiological meaning of Volatile Organic Compounds (VOCs) emission in human breath. Results obtained in these studies indicate that the analysis of VOCs in breath gas may become a promising non-invasive tool for medical diagnosis and for monitoring the success of therapy.

Breath gas analysis is difficult to perform because of low VOC concentrations in breath air (at the level of parts per billion by volume (ppbv) and even lower), high humidity of breath gas, lack of suitable sampling techniques, and absence of sensitive and capable measuring techniques. These difficulties have partly been overcome by improvements in sampling and combiningsophisticated equipment with new, improved analytical methods. However, in order to introduce breath analysis into clinical practice, analytical devices have to be brought to the bedside. So, large-scale clinical use of breath analysis requires portable, on-site instruments that provide information on well-understood biomarkers, and preferably in real time.

In this talk will be present state-of-arte of the recent technical developments and outlines potential clinical applications of breath analysis. Special attention will be done to the new generation of instruments such as Ion Mobility Spectrometer (IMS), which due to its high sensitivity (low ppb range), portability and low cost maintenance could be useful as a screening test for many different diseases. IMS evolved into an inexpensive and powerful analytical technique for sensitive detection of many trace compounds that has recently started being applied in the medical field. This technique is based on the drift of ions given their mobility in the gas phase, at ambient pressure, under the influence of an electric field. The fact that is does not require vacuum or further sample preparation and the analysis is performed in a few minutes makes this technique suit\e to be used in hospitals and healthcare centers.

Although the application of IMS in the medical field is recent, its efficiency in the diagnosis and detection of several pathologies has been proved in a number of studies. Diseases like lung cancer, sarcoidosis, pneumonie and Chronic Obstructive Pulmonary Disease (COPD) were successfully detected/diagnosed using ion mobility spectrometry.

Presented devices carry also an in-system computer unit and can be operated as stand alone devices. They show outstanding user friendliness through a self explaining menu. Operational steps as well as settings of measurements are visualized on the 6.4″ TFT display and can be executed or changed by a rotary pulse encoder.

This stand-alone unit can be also integrated with computer. Software controlled switching allow access to all relevant parameters for method development. Manual or fully-automatic operation include data acquisition, analysis, visualization and data storage on internal memory or itstransfer to external devices or network shares.

Considering the potential of the technique, further clinical trials will be implemented in the near future in order to generate a data base with partners from hospitals for the early non-invasive detection and its cure monitoring for different pathologies like a cancer, pneumonie, diabetes, cholesterol, tuberculosis, liver diseases, among others.

Author index

Abrantes, J.M.C.S. 177, 197
Almeida, H.A. 327, 337, 339
Almeida, J.B. 79
Altoé, M.L. 107
Alvarez-Lorenzo, C. 313
Alves, Jr. S. 325
Amorim, P. 169
António, C.C. 57, 191
Atalaia, T.J.V. 177
Aya, J.C. 143

Barros, R. 239
Bártolo, P.J. 327, 337, 339
Będziński, R. 63, 321
Belo, O. 135
Bernardes, R. 215, 221
Bertemes-Filho, P. 119
Botelho, M.F. 329
Braga, M.E.M. 313, 315, 319, 351
Bragança, A.M. 317
Brás, L. 129
Brito, P. 329

Cabrita, A.S. 233
Caldeira, L. 151
Camargo, E.D.L.B. 143
Caramelo, F.J. 329, 333
Cardoso, A. 23
Carvalho, A. 329
Carvalho, P. 43
Castro, C.F. 57, 191
Castro, M.P. 285
Cavalheiro, J. 123
Chim, R.B. 351
Clemente, M. 267
Coelho, J.F.J. 319
Completo, A. 147
Concheiro, A. 313
Convales, D. 289
Cordeiro, C.R. 209
Corrêa, Jr. F.L. 95, 205
Costa, H. 23
Cunha, L.T. 341

Cunha-Vaz, J. 215, 221
Curado, M. 111

da Roza, T.H. 39
da Silva, T.G. 325
de Araújo, R.C. 205
de Sousa, H.C. 313, 315, 319, 351
Dias, A.G. 341
Dias, A.M.A. 315, 319
dos Santos, L.R. 205
Dostálek, M. 15
Duarte, A.C. 257
Duarte, C.M.M. 313, 319
Duarte, R. 129
Duarte, S. 39
Dušek, J. 15

Esperança, J.M.S.S. 319

Fantoni, D.T. 143
Fernandes, J. 173
Ferreira, A.G.M. 319
Ferreira, A.J.M. 101, 227
Ferreira, J. 111
Ferreira, N.C. 333
Ferreira, S. 43
Figueiredo, M.M. 351
Fiorina, E. 301
Flores, P. 83
Franco, S. 79
Freitas, A.C. 257
Freitas, D.M. 339
Freitas, D.R. 251

Gabriel, J. 169, 267
Gambôa, F. 209
Gamboa, H. 345
Garbe, C. 101, 271
García-Aznar, J.M. 307
Gentil, F. 101, 271
Gil, M.H. 313, 315
Gomes, A.M. 257
Gomes, E.F. 129

Gómez-Benito, M.J. 307
Gonçalves, A.M.D. 293
Gonçalves, P.J.S. 245, 293
Gonsalves, A.M.d'A.R. 209
Gramacho, S. 209

Hellmuth, R.A.P. 69
Hoffmann, I.O. 143

Isaías, P. 29

Janela, F. 151, 239
Jindra, T. 15
Jorge, A.M. 129

Krowicki, P. 63, 321
Krysztoforski, K. 63, 321

Lavrador, R. 151
Leal, G. 297
Lecca, P. 3
Lencart, J. 341
Lima, M. 83
Lima, R.G. 69, 143
Lori, N.F. 151
Loureiro, J. 39

Macedo, M. 29
Macedo, R. 279
Machado, J. 111
Machado, L.S. 157
Maduro, C. 221
Marceneiro, S. 319
Marques, A.T. 285
Marques, M.A. 19
Marrucho, I.M. 319
Martin, A.M. 349
Martins, A.R.C. 143
Martins, P. 101, 173, 271
Martins, P.A.L.S. 227
Martins, R. 345
Mascarenhas, T. 39, 227
Massafra, A. 51
Medeiros, J. 345

Mesnard, M. 147
Moraes, R.M. 157
Morais, M.V.G. 107
Moura, C.S. 327
Moura, D. 257
Moura, F.S. 143

Natal Jorge, R.M. 39, 101, 169,
    173, 227, 271, 285, 309
Neto, V.F. 341
Neves, C. 297
Nunes, B. 233
Nunes, P. 163

Oliveira, C. 79
Oliveira, R. 333
O'Neill, J.G. 349

Pais, A.A.C.C. 209
Palma, S. 345
Parente, M. 271
Parente, M.P.L. 39, 101, 173
Pascoal, A.G. 275
Paterno, A.S. 119
Pereira, M.E. 257
Pérez, M.A. 307
Piñeiro, M. 209
Pinheiro, H. 257
Pinho, J.C. 267
Pinotti, M. 95, 205, 309
Pintado, M.M. 257
Pinto, V.C. 19
Pires, J.N. 329
Pontes, A.J. 89, 261
Portela, A. 123

Quintas, M. 169

Rafael, A. 233
Ramos, A. 147, 341
Ramos, I.M. 251
Ramos, N.V. 19
Rato, L.M. 233
Rebelo, L.P.N. 319

Reina-Romo, E. 307
Reis, M. 345
Relvas, B. 57
Relvas, C. 147, 341
Ribeiro, A.M. 275
Rocha, D.N. 95, 205, 309
Rocha, L.A. 35, 89, 261
Rocha-Santos, T.A.P. 257
Rodriguez, S. 143
Roncon-Albuquerque, R. 35
Rosa, S.S.R.F. 107
Ruzsanyi, V. 317

Sá, V. 23
Sales, B.R.A. 157
Sampaio, S.M. 35
Santos, A. 173, 215, 227
Santos, I.B.V. 325
Santos, I.C.T. 35, 89, 261
Santos, J. 329
Santos, J.A.M. 341
Santos, L. 173, 227
Santos, L.F.F. 197
Santos, L.S. 107
Santos, R. 43, 115, 279
Santos, S. 173
Santos, T. 215, 221
Sanz-Herrera, J.A. 307
Seabra, E. 83
Seabra, I.J. 315
Sepulveda, A. 261
Sepúlveda, A.T. 89
Serranho, P. 221
Sielemann, S. 317
Silva, A. 43, 169, 267
Silva, A.C. 349
Silva, C. 43
Silva, C.P. 107
Silva, F.C. 233
Silva, L.F. 83
Silva, L.I.B. 257
Silva, O.L. 143
Silva-Filho, A.L. 227
Simões, J.A. 147

Simões, P.N. 319
Simoes, R. 183
Slade, A.P. 289
Smirnov, G. 23
Soares, D.P. 285
Soares, F. 111
Soldati, Jr. J.B. 95
Sono, T.S.P. 95, 205
Sousa, A. 267
Sousa, A.S.P. 279
Sousa, L.C. 57, 191
Sousa, T.H.S. 143
Świątek-Najwer, E. 63, 321
Szmuchrowski, L.A. 95

Tavares, A.A.S. 311
Tavares, J.M.R.S. 35, 89, 251,
    261, 279, 311
Teixeira, J. 169
Thomson, G. 289
Torres, P.M.B. 245
Trindade, V.L.A. 173

Van Petten, A.M.V.N. 205
Vasconcelos, B. 329
Vasconcelos, M. 123
Vassilenko, V. 317, 349, 353
Vaz, M.A.P. 19
Veiga, G. 329
Ventura, S.R. 251
Viana, J.C. 89, 261
Vieira, P. 163, 297
Vimieiro, C.B.S. 95
Vincence, V.C. 119
Voinescu, M. 285
Vorstius, J. 289

Watkins, J.J. 351

Yañez, F. 313

Ziegler, C.R. 351

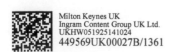

9 781138 112896